D1758610

Jorge L. Alió · Dimitri T. Azar (Eds.)

Management of Complications in Refractive Surgery

Jorge L. Alió · Dimitri T. Azar (Eds.)

Management
of Complications
in Refractive Surgery

With 250 Figures and 44 Tables

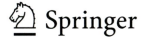 Springer

Jorge L. Alió, M.D., Ph.D.
Professor and Chairman of Ophthalmology
Medical Director
Vissum Corporation
Avda de Denia s/n
Edificio Vissum
03016 Alicante, Spain
E-mail: jlalio@vissum.com

Dimitri T. Azar, M.D.
Professor and Head
Department of Ophthalmology and Visual Sciences
Illinois Eye and Ear Infirmary
University of Illinois at Chicago
3.138 EEI MC 648
1855 W. Taylor Street
Chicago, IL 60612, USA
E-mail: dazar@uic.edu

ISBN 978-3-540-37584-5 (eBook)
DOI 10.1007/978-3-540-37584-5

Library of Congress Control Number: 2007939906

Cover design: Frido Steinen-Broo, eStudio Calamar, Spain

Printed on acid-free paper

9 8 7 6 5 4 3 2 1

springer.com

Foreword

My interest in corneal lamellar surgery began in 1985 when I observed Lee Nordan perform a freeze keratomileusis in Houston with Josè Ignacio Barraquer's freeze technique. At that time, however, I realized that this type of surgery was subject to too many variables, and that for the most part these were independent of the ability and the competence of the surgeon. A more controllable technique was necessary.

Luck would have it that just a few months later I was invited by Philippe Sourdille to Nantes to perform live cataract surgery. In the adjoining room, Jorg Krumeich performed a no-freeze keratomileusis. My interest for corneal lamellar surgery was stimulated further, where a few weeks later in Germany, I observed this new technique, and started to use it myself just a few months after.

But times were hard, particularly when I look back on them now.

The microkeratomes were precise instruments, but they were rudimentary, they were difficult to use and were also potentially risky. The lamellar cut had to have a thickness of at least 300 µm, the lamella had to be fixed to a workbench, and the refractive cut had to be performed on the stromal face with the microkeratome. The optic zones were extremely small particularly in consideration that the target corrections were in excess of 10 D.

Thinking about all that today makes me cringe…

However, Barraquer's idea was brilliant, and what followed on later proved that it was a winner.

The technique with the surgical correction of refraction, with the variant by Antonio Ruiz and others, stayed alive until the excimer laser appeared on the scene. At that point, everything changed–luckily for surgeons over the world and to the enormous satisfaction of the patients!

When Theo Seiler in Berlin demonstrated the use of this machine and despite the fact that everyone had their attention fixed on its use on the surface tissue, I had an idea…finally, I would be able to perform the refractive step of keratomileusis with a repetitive instrument of micrometric precision. Then in 1989, I performed the first operation (the first case anywhere in the world) of intrastromal ablation, using the excimer laser.

At that time, we were all still tied to the concept of performing the refractive step on the stroma of the cut lamella and that is what I did. However, this was not the road to the future, and it was Joannis Pallikaris who had the brilliant idea of performing the step on the in situ stroma. The idea was to cut a thinner lamella and ingeniously preserve a hinge to avoid losing continuity with the cornea.

However, the hinge was in a nasal position because the cut progressed from the temporal side to the internal canthus. Unquestionably, it would have been preferable to have the uncut zone at the top to avoid dislocation of the flap during blinking. I decided to perform the operation with a "traditional" microkeratome–again the first ever worldwide in 1989–proceeding with the microkeratome, in an extremely well-exposed eye, from downward up.

Immediately afterwards, we saw the appearance of the first microkeratome with a fixed plate. What a relief! Finally, the anxiety and worry of creating a perforating lamellar cut had disappeared; we had the option of creating a superior hinge. The laser-assisted in situ keratomileusis (LASIK) down-up technique was born.

We then reached the modern era where improvements to the excimer laser appeared every couple of months; there was the transition from the mono-zone to the multi-zone, from a flying-spot treatment to a wave front, with the subsequent addition of the eye tracker and the recognition of the iris, as well as a whole series of minor innovative changes all geared to improving the end result.

We have reached the state of surgical fiction. However, unfortunately, patients do not participate correspondingly. In fact, laser refractive surgery went extremely well for a number of years and then unexpectedly hit a period of calm or stagnation.

Had we possibly created excessively high expectations?

Had we possibly operated on patients who were not suitable?

Had we possibly induced too many complications?

There is no doubt that on reading this book we can find the solution to many of the mistakes that all of us, to a greater or lesser degree, had made in the past, and we can find many useful and positive suggestions. However, more importantly, we find the necessary information for preventing or reducing the complications, both intraoperative and postoperative, even through the more attentive selection of the patients to be subjected to surgery.

In today's world, refractive surgery commands an extremely important place in eye-surgery practice.

Some techniques are still in their infancy, others have been used for more than 10 years, some have almost disappeared totally from the operating rooms, and more will be developed in the future.

The results of any surgical procedure, even those not related to ophthalmology, were evaluated exclusively from a quantitative point of view; in our specific case, the measurement was how many decimals were recovered by the eye after surgery.

Then surgeons realized that the quality of vision is also extremely important and only an evaluation of this could explain some of the often-incomprehensible complaints the patients would make.

Having a clear picture of how a person's quality of life can be changed by the onset of complications becomes of utmost importance, even in consideration of the person's job or leisure activities, as these can be contraindications to certain types of surgery.

The most popular operation is LASIK: The surgical step that, more than any other, causes problems is the cut with the microkeratome.

Are there still problems with the flap?

Yes! Thin flap, non-uniform flap, perforated flap, incomplete flap, etc. This is due to the fact that this step is mechanical, and by definition not precise, and also because it depends on the surgeon skills.

So who makes more mistakes, the surgeon or the machine?

One essential ingredient of refractive surgery is that the treatment is efficacious and achieves the preset objectives. However, even more important is that it is associated with very few complications, and that these will be acceptable to both the patient and the surgeon. This is particularly true if we consider that these operations are not essential but a question of choice; they are not strictly necessary from a medical point of view.

It is therefore important to publish a book that deals specifically with the complications of refractive surgery, their treatment, and how to prevent them.

The first chapter is essential; it presents the refractive results and the complications from surgery. It describes the risk–benefit ratio that allowed refractive surgery to be accepted and listed among the most popular surgical techniques being used at present.

The second of the introductory chapters is original and specific; it takes a separate look at the effect the complications may have on the quality of life.

A number of chapters on the complications of LASIK follow. It makes sense that these form the main bulk of the book, given that this is the most widespread technique on the international scenario.

First, we have an encyclopedic review of the intraoperative problems of the flap, and then the precocious and late-onset postoperative problems.

All the well-known complications are described.

The problems of complications associated with the flap have been greatly reduced since the currently available microkeratomes have been used. These are more reliable and safer; however, possibly a cut that was independent of mechanical instruments would be a better solution. This led to the development and launch of the femtosecond laser that could perform the work of the microkeratome but with greater precision and fewer risks.

In addition to the anatomical complications, specific chapters examine the calculation errors in refractive correction; again, in the past these topics were not dealt with in sufficient detail.

Finally, there are chapters on the complications of the eye, which actually create the subjective problems for the patients and leave them dissatisfied with the results of the operation.

The femtosecond laser can contribute to reducing these and other problems.

What are the advantages associated with this laser? First of all, the lack of blades! In addition, the possibility of no complications in the event of technical problems, and the option of repeating the operation just a short time later.

Potentially, it can also prevent ectasia; subject to the precise preoperative measurement of the corneal thickness, the cut can be performed uniformly over the entire area and that is not all…

Further improvements to the equipment and the software permit greater improvements to the ablation techniques; aberrometers that are more suitable allow the elimination of the optical aberrations; more advanced pupillometers will reduce the patients' functional problems and improve the end result.

However, additional problems persist: scarring, melting, etc., the etiopathogenesis of which must be examined in depth to enable surgeons to identify the key factors for resolving them.

The book also contains descriptions of topics that were previously not treated specifically: nummular keratitis, fluid in the interface, and ptosis. The latter complication is rightly considered, given the complaints it elicits from patients.

Then, ample space is given to the problem of dry eye, which was underestimated when this surgical technique was initially developed.

Rare complications are also examined such as optic neuropathy and the problems of eye motility.

Can any problems related to infection be resolved with the use of disposable instruments, on the understanding that these must have the same validity and competitive costs as their repeated-use/sterilizable counterparts? Will that be enough? I do not think so. However, if we improve the preoperative diagnosis and the medical preparation of the patient, there is no doubt that we will be able to reduce the frequency of the problems.

The photorefractive keratectomy (PRK) technique, which is still popular, is examined with its main complications, namely haze and regression.

Improvements in laser-assisted sub-epithelial keratectomy (LASEK) are unquestionably linked to finding a way, probably chemical, to attain, precise detachment of the corneal epithelium while respecting the cell vitality.

Will EpiLASIK be able to distance the doctor and patient from the postoperative difficulties similar to those associated with PRK and bring them closer to LASIK?

What will the future hold for the techniques with phakic intraocular lenses (IOLs)?

Surgery that began more than 20 years ago, and then abandoned because of too many complications, has come back into fashion not merely because elevated defects could not be suitably treated with the laser, but mainly due to the improvements in the materials and the design of the phakic IOLs in addition to the better knowledge in the anatomy and physiology of the eye.

Further improvements in the shape, thickness, and dimensions of the IOL and their foldability can avoid complications such as glaucoma, cataract, and corneal decompensation. However, the reduction in problems is also associated by better pre- and postoperative instrumental analysis of the eye; instruments such as Visante and the like must be constantly used and applied in this type of surgery, taking into consideration that, generally speaking, a phakic IOL is not designed to remain in the eye for the rest of the patient's life.

The manufacturers must also aim to develop an IOL that is easy to remove if necessary.

Possibly the most important step will be to produce a precise definition for contraindications for the phakic IOLs and whether the existence of three types of IOLs is justified. The future will tell whether only one of these should be used. By analyzing the complications associated with each one of them, we should be able to provide answers to these questions.

In addition, the more recent surgical techniques for the correction of severe visual defects and presbyopia will be increasingly oriented to the replacement of a human crystalline with a multifocal artificial lens.

However, is this ethically and deontologically correct? And will it be possible to further reduce the residual problems associated with this surgery, namely, capsular opacity and problems with the retina?

The definition of the etiopathogenesis of macular edema and neovascularization present in the eye will allow us to reduce some of these problems.

Dedicated software will avoid the refractive surprises associated with previous corneal refractive surgery.

Four chapters on lesser-used techniques follow: radial keratotomy, conductive keratoplasty, intracorneal segments, and intracorneal inserts.

Specifically for radial keratotomy, a technique that is no longer being used, the chapter describes the problems the surgeon has to face in the event of a repeat refractive operation and/or cataract surgery.

Last but not of least importance in today's scenario, the final three chapters.

Understanding whether the patient will be happy with the result or not is essential for surgery of this type, and associated with this problem is the informed consent.

The final chapter compares the complications presented in the literature over the past 10 years, permitting a comparison of the various techniques and a visualization of how experience and technological progress has led to a reduction in the complications that resulted from the initial inexperience of the surgeons and the learning curve associated with this new technique.

In other words, this book summarizes in a clear, complete, and updated manner all the information associated with this subject. It provides a practical and not an empirical approach to the various problems examined. It is more comprehensive with respect to previous publications, covering every aspect of refractive surgery.

The high quality of the images only serves to augment the validity of the book.

The various chapters were written impartially by experts on the specific subject.

The updated, complete information contained in this book makes it an important publication for all our colleagues who are specialized in this field of ocular surgery.

Another important stimulus from this book is that we must fuel the desire to continue along this road of improvement for these refractive techniques.

However, this subject is constantly evolving and therefore the various chapters will act as a stimulus for additional research and improvements to the techniques: The book contains all we know to date and highlights the areas that still need to be explored.

On behalf of all refractive surgeons, I would like to thank the Aliò Foundation and its staff for its enormous contribution to the improvements and the developments seen in refractive surgery. I would also like to thank them for the effort and commitment to improving the expertise of our colleagues, which in the final analysis is translated into an advantage for the patients.

Lucio Buratto

Preface

The reader will find in this book a modern perspective on complications in refractive surgery. The environment and the perspective of the topic have been changing continuously in the last 10 years, most notably in the last 5 years. Many traditional complications such as flap complications are now in decline, whereas other new complications are appearing. The overall frequency and epidemiology of the different complications of refractive surgery have dramatically changed with the different technological innovations that have been introduced into the practice of corneal refractive surgery. However, not all complications followed this decrease, but rather have increased in their frequency; traditional problems such as endothelial cell loss and cataract induction in some phakic IOL models remain concerns of refractive surgeons, and new forms of inflammatory complications of refractive surgery have emerged. Refractive complications such as aberrations induced by previous procedures, decentrations, and others are now properly treated due to significant technological improvement and knowledge of the performance of eye physiology and optics. This book is aimed at providing current and future refractive surgeons with up-to-date information on the pathogenesis of potential refractive surgical complications and at offering an approach to their prevention and treatment.

In addition to our own experience in refractive surgery, we have relied on the invaluable experience of many friends and colleagues who have authored several chapters within this book. Our author list represents the best of the best in refractive surgery. This unique panel of unparalleled international experts has clearly contributed to the science and the practice of refractive surgery. We would like to thank them for the service and contributions to refractive surgery, to patients, and through their respective chapters, to advancing the knowledge of refractive surgery.

It is our hope that the reader will find in this book the requisite links between the science and practice of refractive surgery. The acceptance of refractive surgery as a separate subspecialty in ophthalmology is higher than ever, thanks to the attention being paid to surgical complications and their management. The surgical outcomes and quality of life of patients undergoing refractive surgery has steadily improved.

The promise of refractive surgery rests in our singular focus on our patients' quality of life and quality of vision. Continued improvements in our field are dependent on enhanced technologies and superior training. To this end, we offer this book as a complement in order to assist our field in becoming better educated about the complications that we face, by providing better tools to solve them, and by increasing knowledge of how to prevent them, all to benefit our patients.

We would like to thank Springer for its support to this edition and ongoing support for refractive surgery. We also offer our heartfelt thanks to our families for their support, which has allowed us to devote our attention to the edition of this book.

Jorge L. Alió
Alicante, Spain

Dimitri Azar
Chicago, Illinois

January 2008

Contents

Chapter 13

Chapter 13.1

Chapter 13.2

Chapter 13.3

List of Contributors

Natalie A. Afshari, M.D.
Assistant Professor of Ophthalmology
Duke University Medical Center
Box 3802
Durham, NC 27710, USA
Email: Natalie.afshari@duke.edu

César Albarrán, O.D.
Vissum Corporation
Avda de Denia s/n
Edificio Vissum
03016 Alicante, Spain
and
Refractive Surgery Department
Instituto Oftalmológico de Alicante
Miguel Hernández University
Alicante, Spain

Jorge L. Alió, M.D., Ph.D.
Professor and Chairman of Ophthalmology
Miguel Hernández University, Medical School
Vissum Corporation
Avda de Denia s/n
Edificio Vissum
03016 Alicante, Spain
E-mail: jlalio@vissum.com

Waleed A. Allam, M.D.
Research Fellow, Ophthalmology
Refractive Surgery Department
New England Eye Center,
Tufts University School of Medicine
750 Washington St., Box 450
Boston, MA 02111, USA
E-mail address: WAllam@tufts-nemc.org

Norma Allemann, M.D.
Professor, Department of Ophthalmology
Federal University of São Paulo
Paulista School of Medicine
São Paulo, Brazil

Noel Alpins, M.D., F.R.A.C.S., F.R.C.Ophth., F.A.C.S.
Centre for Eye Research Australia
The University of Melbourne
Departmentof Ophthalmology
c/- Royal Victorian Eye & Ear Hospital
Locked Bag 8
East Melbourne, VIC 8002, Australia
E-mail: nalpins@unimelb.edu.au

Renato Ambrosio, Jr., M.D., Ph.D.
Department of Ophthalmology
Fluminense Federal University
Niterói, Brazil
and
Medical Director
Instituto de Olhos Renato Ambrósio
Visare Personal Laser & Refracta-RIO
Rua Conde de Bonfim 211/712
Rio de Janeiro, Brazil 20520-050
E-mail: renatoambrosiojr@terra.com.br

J. Fernando Arevalo, M.D., F.A.C.S.
Edif. Centro Caracas PH-1
Av. Panteon, San Bernardino
Caracas 1010, Venezuela
E-mail address: arevalojf@movistar.net.ve

Jean Louis Arne, M.D.
Professor of Ophthalmology and Head of Department
Service d'Ophtalmologie
Hôpital Purpan
Toulouse, France
University of Toulouse
Toulouse, France
E-mail: Jean-louis.arne@wanadoo.fr

Dimitri Azar, M.D.
Professor and Head
Department of Ophthalmology and Visual Sciences
Illinois Eye and Ear Infirmary
University of Illinois at Chicago
3.138 EEI MC 648
1855 W. Taylor Street
Chicago, IL 60612, USA
E-mail: dazar@uic.edu

Julio Baviera, M.D.
Paseo de la Castellana 20
28046 Madrid, Spain
E-mail: jbaviera@clinicabaviera.com

Michael W. Belin, M.D.
Professor
Director of Refractive Surgery
Albany Medical College
Cornea Consultants of Albany
1220 New Scotland Rd., Suite 101
Slingerlands, NY 12159, USA

Laurie Brown, C.O.M.T., C.O.E.
1550 Oak St., Suite 5
Eugene, OR 97401, USA
E-mail: finemd@finemd.com

Marlane J. Brown, O.D., F.A.A.O.
Minnesota Eye Consultants
710 E. 24th Street, Suite 106
Minneapolis, MN 55404, USA

Lucio Buratto, M.D.
Piazza Repubblica 21
20124 Milano, Italy
E-mail: lucio@buratto.com

Wallace Chamon, M.D.
Professor, Department of Ophthalmology
Federal University of São Paulo
Paulista School of Medicine
São Paulo, Brazil
E-mail: visus@pobox.com

Arturo S. Chayet, M.D.
CODET Vision Institute
Padre Kino 10159
Tijuana, Mexico 22320
E-mail: arturo.chayet@codetvision.com

Beatrice Cochener, M.D.
Centre Hospitalier Universitaire de Brest
Brest Cedex, France
E-mail: Beatrice.Cochener-lamard@chu-brest.fr

Antonio Calossi, D.O.
via 2 Giugno 52
50053 Certaldo (FI), Italy
E-mail: calossi@tin.it

José de la Cruz, M.D.
Assistant Professor
Department of Ophthalmology
and Visual Sciences
Illinois Eye and Ear Infirmary
University of Illinois at Chicago
3.164 EEI MC 648
1855 W. Taylor Street
Chicago, IL 60612, USA
E-mail: josedlc@uic.edu

Elizabeth A. Davis, M.D.
Assistant Clinical Professor of Ophthalmology
Minnesota Eye Consultants
710 E. 24th Street, Suite 106
Minneapolis, MN 55404, USA
and
University of Minnesota
Minneapolis, MN USA

David Fahd, M.D.
Research Fellow
Department of Ophthalmology and Visual Sciences
Illinois Eye and Ear Infirmary
University of Illinois at Chicago
3.138 EEI MC 648
1855 W. Taylor Street
Chicago, IL 60612, USA

I. Howard Fine, M.D.
Clinical Professor of Ophthalmology
Casey Eye Institute
1550 Oak St., Suite 5
Eugene, OR 97401, USA
E-mail: finemd@finemd.com

Eric E. Gabison, M.D.
Fondation Ophtalmologique A.
de Rothschild and Bichat Hospital, APHP
25–29 rue Manin
75940 Paris Cedex 19, France
and
CNRS UMR 7149
University Paris XII
Paris, France

Reinaldo A. Garcia, M.D.
Clinica Oftalmologica Centro Caracas
Edif. Centro Caracas PH-1
Av. Panteon, San Bernardino
Caracas 1010, Venezuela

Bruno M. Fontes, M.D.
Instituto de Olhos Renato Ambrósio
Visare Personal Laser & Refracta-RIO
Rua Conde de Bonfim 211/712
Rio de Janeiro, Brazil 20520-050
and
Department of Ophthalmology
Federal University of São Paulo
"Escola Paulista de Medicina"
São Paulo, Brazil

Rafael A. Garcia-Amaris, M.D.
Clinica Oftalmologica Centro Caracas
Edif. Centro Caracas PH-1
Av. Panteon, San Bernardino
Caracas 1010, Venezuela

Javier Gaytan, M.D.
Instituto de Microcirugía Ocular
Departamento de Cornea
c/Munner 10, 10 CP 08022,
Barcelona Spain

Oscar Gris, M.D.
Instituto de Microcirugía Ocular
Departamento de Cornea
c/Munner 10, 10 CP 08022,
Barcelona Spain

José L. Güell, M.D., Ph.D.
Instituto de Microcirugía Ocular
Departamento de Cornea
c/Munner 10, 10 CP 08022,
Barcelona Spain
E-mail: guell@imo.es

Joelle Hallak, B.Sc.
Research Specialist
Department of Ophthalmology and Visual Sciences
Illinois Eye and Ear Infirmary
University of Illinois at Chicago
3.138 EEI MC 648
1855 W. Taylor Street
Chicago, IL 60612, USA
E-mail: joelle@uic.edu

David R. Hardten, M.D.
Adjunct Associate Professor of Ophthalmology
Minnesota Eye Institute
710 E. 24th Street, Suite 106
Minneapolis, MN 55404, USA
Email: drhardten@mneye.com,
with copy to srrust@mneye.com

Sadeer Hannush, M.D.
Attending Surgeon
Wills Eye Hospital
Department of Ophthalmology
Philadelphia, PA
and
Cornea Consultants of Albany
1220 New Scotland Rd., Suite 101
Slingerlands, NY 12159, USA
E-mail: SBHannush@comcast.net

Thanh Hoang-Xuan, M.D.
Professor of Ophthalmology
University of Paris 7
Director, Cornea, External Diseases
and Refractive Surgery Services
Fondation Ophtalmologique A.
de Rothschild and Bichat Hospital, APHP
25–29 rue Manin
75940 Paris Cedex 19, France
E-mail: hoangxuant@aol.com

Richard S. Hoffman, M.D.
1550 Oak St., Suite 5
Eugene, OR 97401, USA
E-mail: finemd@finemd.com

Teresa S. Ignacio, M.D.
IntraLase Corp.
9701 Jeronimo Rd.
Irvine, CA 92618, USA
E-mail: tignacio@intralase.com

Sandeep Jain, M.D.
Assistant Professor in Ophthalmology
Department of Ophthalmology and Visual Sciences
Illinois Eye and Ear Infirmary
University of Illinois at Chicago
3.164 EEI MC 648
1855 W. Taylor Street
Chicago, IL 60612, USA
E-mail: jains@uic.edu

Daniela Jardim, M.D.
Instituto de Olhos Renato Ambrósio
Visare Personal Laser & Refracta-RIO
Rua Conde de Bonfim 211/712
Rio de Janeiro, Brazil 20520-050

Vikentia J. Katsanevaki, M.D., Ph.D.
Head of Refractive Department
Vardinoyannion Eye Institute
University of Crete Medical School
Voutes P.O. Box 1352
Heraklion, Crete, Greece
E-mail: vikatsan@med.uoc.gr

Bharavi Kharod, M.D.
Duke University Medical Center
Box 3802
Durham, NC 27710, USA

Michael Knorz, M.D.
Professor of Ophthalmology
FreeVis LASIK Center
Medical Faculty Mannheim
of the University of Heidelberg
Femto LASIK Professional
Theodor Kutzer Ufer 1–3
68167 Mannheim, Germany
E-mail: knorz@eyes.de

Takashi Kojima, M.D.
Research Fellow, Ophthalmology
Department of Ophthalmology and Visual Sciences
Illinois Eye and Ear Infirmary
University of Illinois at Chicago
3.138 EEI MC 648
1855 W. Taylor Street
Chicago, IL 60612, USA

Richard Lindstrom, M.D.
Professor of Ophthalmology
Minnesota Eye Consultants
710 E. 24th Street, Suite 106
Minneapolis, MN 55404, USA
and
Medical Director
University of Minnesota
Minneapolis, MN USA
E-mail: rllindstrom@mneye.com

Carlo F. Lovisolo, M.D.
San Raffaele University Hospital
Quattroelle Eye Centres
Milan, Italy
E-mail: loviseye@fastwebnet.it

Antonio A.P. Marinho, M.D., Ph.D.
R. Crasto 708
4150-243 Porto, Portugal
E-mail: marin@mail.telepac.pt

Marguerite McDonald, M.D., F.A.C.S.
Clinical Professor of Ophthalmology Tulane University
School of Medicine
New Orleans, LA, USA
and
Rockville Centre
Ryan Medical Arts Building
2000 North Village Avenue, Suite 402
Rockville Centre,
NY 11570, USA
Margueritemcdmd@aol.com

Merce Morral, M.D.
Instituto de Microcirugía Ocular
Departamento de Cornea
c/Munner 10, 10 CP 08022,
Barcelona Spain

Felicidad Manero, M.D.
Instituto de Microcirugía Ocular
Departamento de Cornea
c/Munner 10, 10 CP 08022,
Barcelona Spain

Fabio Mazzolani, M.D.
Quattroelle Eye Centers
Via Cusani 7
20121 Milano, Italy
E-mail: carlo.lovisolo@quattroelle.org

Orkun Muftuoglu, M.D.
Vissum Corporation
Avda de Denia s/n
Edificio Vissum
03016 Alicante, Spain

Alessandro Mularoni, M.D.
Ospedale Maggiore
Largo Negrisoli 2
40133 Bologna, Italy
E-mail: alessandro.mularoni@ausl.bologna.it

M. Emilia Mulet, M.D., Ph.D.
Department of Ophthalmology
Miguel Hernández University, Medical School
Vissum Corporation
Avda de Denia s/n
Edificio Vissum
03016 Alicante, Spain

Rudy M.M.A. Nuijts, M.D., Ph.D.
Department of Ophthalmology
Academic Hospital Maastricht
P. Debyelaan 25
6202 AZ, Maastricht, The Netherlands
E-mail: rnu@compaqnet.nl

David P.S. O'Brart, M.D., F.R.C.S., F.R.C.Ophth.
Department of Ophthalmology
St. Thomas' Hospital
London, UK
DavidOBrart@aol.com

Tatsuya Ongucci, M.D.
Research Fellow, Ophthalmology
Department of Ophthalmology and Visual Sciences
Illinois Eye and Ear Infirmary
University of Illinois at Chicago
3.138 EEI MC 648
1855 W. Taylor Street
Chicago, IL 60612, USA

Mark Packer, M.D., F.A.C.S.
Clinical Associate Professor
Oregon Eye Institute
1550 Oak St., Suite 5
Eugene, OR 97401, USA
E-mail: finemd@finemd.com

David Piñero, O.D.
Department of Ophthalmology
Miguel Hernández University, Medical School
Vissum Corporation
Avda de Denia s/n
Edificio Vissum
03016 Alicante, Spain

Konrad Pseudovs, Ph.D.
NH&MRC Centre for Clinical Eye Research,
Department of Ophthalmology,
Flinders Medical Centre and Flinders University
Bedford Park, South Australia 5045, Australia
E-mail: Konrad.Pesudovs@flinders.edu.au

Jerome C. Ramos-Esteban, M.D.
Eye Institute
Cleveland Clinic
9500 Euclid Avenue
Cleveland, OH 44195, USA

J. Bradley Randleman, M.D.
Assistant Professor of Ophthalmology
Emory University Department of Ophthalmology
1365 B Clifton Road NE, Suite 4500
Atlanta, GA 30322, USA
E-mail: Jrandle@emory.edu

Emanuel Rosen, M.D., F.R.C.S.Ed.
10 St. John Street
Manchester M3 4DY, UK
E-mail: ERosen9850@aol.com

José Mª Ruiz-Moreno, M.D., Ph.D.
Miguel Hernández University, Medical School
Vissum Corporation
Avda de Denia s/n
Edificio Vissum
03016 Alicante, Spain

James J. Salz, M.D.
Medical Director
Laser Vision Medical Associates
240 South La Cienega Blvd., Suite 250
Beverly Hills, CA 90211, USA
E-mail: drsalz@drsalz.com

Juan G. Sanchez, M.D.
Clinica Oftalmologica Centro Caracas
Edif. Centro Caracas PH-1
Av. Panteon, San Bernardino
Caracas 1010, Venezuela

Mohamed H. Shabayek, M.D, M.Sc.
Department of Ophthalmology
Miguel Hernández University, Medical School
Vissum Corporation
Avda de Denia s/n
Edificio Vissum
03016 Alicante, Spain
and
Research Institute of Ophthalmology
Giza, Egypt

Bryan S. Sires, M.D., Ph.D.
Allure Facial Laser and Medispa
University of Washington
Clinical Associate Professor
Kirkland, WA 98033, USA
E-mail: bsires@u.washington.edu

Stephen Slade, M.D.
3900 Essex Lane, Suite 101
Houston, TX 77027, USA
E-mail: sgs@visiontexas.com

Roger F. Steinert, M.D.
Professor of Ophthalmology
Professor of Biomedical Engineering
Department of Ophthalmology
118 Med Surge I
University of California, Irvine
Irvine, CA 92697-4375, USA
E-mail: steinert@uci.edu

Charles Wm. Stewart, D.O.
LIGI Tecnologie Medicali S.p.A.
via Luigi Corsi, 50
74100 Taranto, Italy

Karl G. Stonecipher, M.D.
Medical Director
TLC Greensboro
3312 Battleground Ave.
Greensboro, NC 27410, USA
E-mail: StoneNC@aol.com

Kody G. Stonecipher
1009 Country Club Drive
Greensboro, NC 27408, USA
E-mail: stonenc@gmail.com

R. Doyle Stulting, M.D., Ph.D.
Professor of Ophthalmology
Emory University Department of Ophthalmology
1365 B Clifton Road NE, Suite 4500
Atlanta, GA 30322, USA
E-mail: ophtrds@emory.edu

Jonathan H. Talamo, M.D.
Associate Clinical Professor of Ophthalmology
Harvard Medical School
Talamo Laser Eye Consultants
Reservoir Place, Suite 184
1601 Trapelo Rd.
Waltham, MA 02451, USA
E-mail: jht1@comcast.net; jtalamo@lecb.com

Gustavo E. Tamayo, M.D.
Bogota Laser Refractive Surgery
Calle 114 #9-45 Torre B, Suite 906
Bogota, Colombia
E-mail: gtvotmy@telecorp.net

Nayyirih G. Tahzib, M.D.
Department of Ophthalmology
Academic Hospital Maastricht
P. Debyelaan 25
6202 AZ, Maastricht, The Netherlands

Luis F Torres, M.D., Ph.D.
INOVA Vision Institute
Department of Surgery,
Biomedical Center, Autonomous
University of Aguascalientes
Sierra Morena 238, Bosques del Prado
Aguascalientes, Ags, Mexico 20127
E-mail: ftorresb@yahoo.com

Vance Thompson, M.D., F.A.C.S.
Director
Sioux Valley
Clinic, Talley Building
Sioux Falls, SD, USA
and
Sanford Clinic Vance Thompson Vision
1310 West 22nd Street, 2nd Floor
Sioux Falls, SD 57105, USA
E-mail: thompsov@siouxvalley.org

Gemma Walsh, B.Optom.
Centre for Eye Research Australia
The University of Melbourne
Department of Ophthalmology
c/- Royal Victorian Eye & Ear Hospital
Locked Bag 8
East Melbourne, VIC 8002, Australia

Steve Wilson, M.D.
Eye Institute
Cleveland Clinic
9500 Euclid Avenue
Cleveland, OH 44195, USA
E-mail: WILSONS4@ccf.org

Helen K. Wu, M.D.
Assistant Professor of Ophthalmology
New England Eye Center,
Tufts University School of Medicine
750 Washington St., Box 450
Boston, MA 02111, USA
E-mail: HWu@tufts-nemc.org

George O. Waring III, M.D., F.A.C.S., F.R.C.Ophth.
Clinical Professor of Ophthalmology
Emory University, School of Medicine
Atlanta, Georgia, USA

Refractive Surgery Outcomes and Frequency of Complications

Wallace Chamon and Norma Alleman

Contents

Core Messages

■ There is no risk-free surgical procedure.

■ There are enough data in literature to determine the risk for the majority of the refractive surgery procedures.

■ Refractive surgery risks and benefits should be evaluated individually in order to choose the surgical approach properly.

■ Not only incidence, but also morbidity of each possible complication should be considered in this choice.

■ Decision making in refractive procedure is an individualized process that should be based on scientific knowledge, patient's characteristics, and surgeon experience.

1.1 Common Complications Associated with Refractive Surgery

Some complications are implicit to any surgical procedure, varying only in their incidence and morbidity. Such complications will be evaluated here according to their characteristics in each group of refractive surgical procedures.

1.1.1 Refractive Imprecision and Loss of Spectacle-Corrected Visual Acuity

The most frequent complication observed in any refractive procedure is the lack in achieving accurate refraction outcome. As a rule, accuracy decreases with the amount of refractive error. Photoablative procedures tend to be the most accurate ones for low ametropias. Photorefractive keratectomy (PRK) and laser-assisted in situ keratomileusis (LASIK) deal with different variables that may affect predictability: corneal wound healing and stromal bed elasticity, respectively [1].

Although results minimally favor LASIK, we may expect that in any photoablative procedure, approximately 60–70% of eyes will achieve 20/20 uncorrected visual acuity and will be within +/−0.50 D after surgery. If we analyze only low myopias (under 6.00 D), approximately 70–80% will achieve 20/20 uncorrected visual acuity (Table 1.1) [1–9].

A general evaluation of surgical safety should consider spectacle-corrected visual acuity (SCVA). One to 5% of eyes will lose at least two lines of SCVA 6 months after surgery, but 1% or less of all eyes will achieve less than 20/40 of SCVA. One to 2% of eyes that achieved, preoperatively, 20/20 of SCVA will achieve less than 20/25 SCVA after surgery (Table 1.2) [1–9].

Phakic intraocular lenses (IOLs) tend to present less accurate refractive correction; although, since they are nor-

Table 1.1. LASIK versus PRK for correction of myopia

	UCVA 20/20				+/- 0.50 D				UCVA 20/20 (low myopia)			
	LASIK		PRK		LASIK		PRK		LASIK		PRK	
	n	%	n	%	n	%	n	%	n	%	n	%
Literature: 6 months postoperative												
Wang et al. [4]	109	81.7	335	71.6					109	81.7	335	71.6
Hersh et al. [5]	61	26.2	68	19.1								
El-Magrabi et al. [7]	28	67.9	28	42.9	59	27.1	68	29.4				
Forseto et al. [6]	8	100	9	88.9	8	87.5	9	88.9	8	100	9	88.9
Hjordtal et al. [1]	25	4	20	15	25	20	20	25				
Literature: 12 months postoperative												
Wang et al. [4]	103	82.5	307	72	103	70.9	307	61.2	103	82.5	307	72
El-Magrabi et al. [7]	30	66.7	30	53.3	30	73.3	30	66.7				
el Danasuri et al. [8]	24	79.2	24	62.5	24	87.5	24	83.3	24	79.2	24	62.5
Forseto et al. [6]	15	73.3	15	53.3	15	93.3	15	86.7	15	73.3	15	53.3
Hjordtal et al. [1]	25	4	20	15	25	16	20	30				
FDA: 6 months postoperative	6,615	59.4	3,173	59.9	7,207	69.9	3,296	62.7				
FDA: 12 months postoperative	2,774	58.1	2,094	54.5	2,985	61	2,065	56.3				
6 months total	6,846	59.4	3,633	59.9	7,299	69.4	3,393	61.9	117	82.9	344	72.1
6 months literature total	231	57.6	460	60	92	30.4	97	34	117	82.9	344	72.1
6 months FDA total	6,615	59.4	3,173	59.9	7,207	69.9	3,296	62.7	0	NA	0	NA
12 months total	2,971	58.8	2,490	56.4	3,182	61.4	2,461	57.3	142	81	346	70.5
12 months literature total	197	69	396	66.4	197	68	396	62.4	142	81	346	70.5
12 months FDA total	2,774	58.1	2,094	54.5	2,985	61	2,065	56.3	0	NA	0	NA

Data set modified from Shortt et al. [3]

PRK photorefractive keratectomy, UCVA 20/20 eyes that achieved post treatment uncorrected visual acuity (UCVA) of 20/20, +/- 0.50 D eyes within 0.50 D of target refraction, UCVA 20/20 (low myopia) eyes that achieved post treatment UCVA of 20/20 in a subgroup of myopia $\leq$6 D, FDA US Food and Drug Administration, NA not applicable

Table 1.2 LASIK versus PRK for spectacle-corrected visual acuity (SCVA)

	Loss of ≥2 lines				SCVA < 20/40				SCVA < 20/25			
	LASIK		PRK		LASIK		PRK		LASIK		PRK	
	n	%	n	%	n	%	n	%	n	%	n	%
Literature: 6 months postoperative												
Wang et al. [4]	307	3.9	103	1								
Hersh et al. [5]	68	11.8	59	3.4	68	1.5	61	0	68	1.5	59	1.7
El-Magrabi et al. [7]	27	7.4	27	7.4	27	3.7	27	0	27	3.7	27	3.7
Forseto et al. [6]	24	0	24	0	24	0	24	0	24	0	24	0
Hjordtal et al. [1]	20	10	25	4	20	0	25	0	20	0	25	0
FDA: 6 months postoperative	4,412	3.2	7,554	1.1	4,414	0.3	7,810	0.3	4,299	2.4	7,612	1.4
6 months total	4,858	3.4	7,792	1.2	4,553	0.4	7,947	0.3	4,438	2.3	7,747	1.4
6 months literature total	446	5.4	238	2.5	139	1.4	137	0	139	1.4	135	1.5
6 months FDA total	4,412	3.2	7,554	1.1	4,414	0.3	7,810	0.3	4,299	2.4	7,612	1.4

Data set modified from Shortt et al. [3]

PRK photorefractive keratectomy, loss of ≥2 lines eyes that lost of ≥2 lines of SCVA, SCVA < 20/40 final SCVA worse than 20/40, SCVA < 20/25 final SCVA worse than 20/25 when preoperative best SCVA ≥ 20/20, FDA US Food and Drug Administration, NA not applicable

mally used to correct higher ametropias, an expected result with most of the patients within +/−1.00, should be appreciated [10–14]. Image magnification after correcting high-myopic eyes with IOLs generate a confounding factor in evaluating pre- and post-SCVA; therefore, information published on this subject lacks credibility [15].

The only procedure that does not rely on clinical refraction to determine total correction is clear lens extraction. Its predictability depends on how accurately we can determine corneal power, axial length, and the effective position of the implanted IOL. Approximately 95% of normal eyes should present less than 1.00 D of refractive error [16]. Predictability reduces greatly when operating eyes that underwent corneal refractive surgery, but new approaches for calculating IOL power have improved the results [17, 18].

1.1.2 Infection

Determining the risk of infection on photoablative procedures is a difficult task due to misdiagnoses and lack in laboratorial information. We may expect an incidence between 0.1:10,000 and 1:10,000, favoring LASIK over PRK [19–21]. Infection has been reported after LASIK with femtosecond laser [22]. Bilateral simultaneous keratorefractive procedures are considered standard of care [23, 24], but the risk of bilateral infection may add extra damage to this po-

tentially devastating complication. Risk of infection in intraocular surgeries should follow the incidence of infection in cataract surgery that is approximately 1:1,000 [25–27]. Intracorneal implants are theoretically more susceptible to infection due the difficulty of the immune system to act in an intrastromal fashion [28–30].

1.1.3 Infection and Contact Lenses

Risk of infection in contact lenses wearers should be considered when evaluating incidence of infection in refractive surgery. The risk of keratitis in contact lenses wearers depends on the modality of use (daily wear or extended wear) and the lens type. Literature has shown that, per year, the risk of presenting a severe keratitis will vary from 3:10,000 to almost 100:10,000 [31], and the risk of presenting loss of visual acuity is 3.6:10,000 among silicone hydrogel extended wearers [32].

1.1.4 Subjective Complaints

Subjective complaints such as halos, glare, starburst, and low-contrast sensitivity maybe correlated to low- and high-order optical aberrations [33, 34] as well as to optical characteristics of the implanted IOL [35–38] and the diameter of the pupil [39]. All refractive procedures present the risk of subjective complaints, but special attention should be paid in keratorefractive surgeries in eyes with larger pupil diameter, since this procedure is performed further from the pupil plane, when compared with phakic intraocular implants or clear lens extraction.

1.1.5 Retinal Detachment

Retinal detachment has been associated with LASIK [40–44]; but, so far, it is not possible to detect a cause–effect relationship nor to determine a higher incidence of vitreoretinal pathological conditions post-LASIK.

Cataract extraction increases the cumulative risk of retinal detachment an average of fourfold. There is no difference between patients who underwent extracapsular cataract extraction and phacoemulsification. The risk increases in myopic [45], younger men (less than 50 years old) [46, 47]. It has been suggested that phakic IOLs implantation may be related to a higher risk of retinal detachment [48, 49].

1.2 Keratorefractive Procedures

1.2.1 Photorefractive Keratectomy

1.2.1.1 Haze
Incidence of haze and treatment regression is associated to the attempted correction and may be expected to be up to 2% in the first year post-PRK [50]. Although it is commonly suggested that haze may be less incident with newer lasers, there is no scientific evidence that it is true [51].

1.2.1.2 Mitomycin C
The use of intraoperative mitomycin C has raised the expectation for treating higher ametropias with PRK [52–57]. Potential risks associated to its use are the consequences of keratocyte depletion [58] as well as endothelium and anterior chamber toxicity [59, 60].

1.2.1.3 Keratectasia
Although there are reports of keratectasia that occurred in normal eyes after PRK [61], most the few cases reported so far are of forme fruste keratoconus that progressed after PRK [62–64] or phototherapeutic keratectomy (PTK) [65, 66]. It is still to be proven if the procedure influences the progression of the disease.

1.2.2 LASIK

1.2.2.1 Microkeratome-Related Complications
Irregular flaps related to the microkeratome cut maybe presented as incomplete flaps, free caps, buttonholed flaps [67], thin flaps, thick flaps, and partially cut flaps. Irregular flaps

are expected in less than 1% of the procedures performed with new microkeratomes [23, 68–72]. Microkeratome-related complications depend on the learning curve and may be two or three times more frequent in the first 1,000 surgeries [69]. Initial microkeratomes had a complication rate of up to 6%; their evolution, with new safety concerns, decreased the incidence [70, 72]. Outcomes after an irregular flap are improved if photoablation is not carried out at the time of the complication [73, 74].

1.2.2.2 Femtosecond Laser
Most of the literature shows that reliability in flap creation has increased with the use of femtosecond laser [75–77], but some articles do not differentiate the outcomes between microkeratome and femtosecond laser [78, 79]. A new entity, transient light-sensitivity syndrome (TLSS), was reported in approximately 1% of the eyes with femtosecond laser-created flaps [80, 81].

1.2.2.3 Dislocated Flap
Flap dislocation is a complication encountered in approximately 2% of the procedures [71, 82] and has been reported up to 30 months after the surgery [83–85].

1.2.2.4 Diffuse Lamellar Keratitis
Diffuse lamellar keratitis (DLK) is a disease of unknown pathophysiology [86–88] that was first described in 1998 [89]. It occurs in an average of 0.7% of the procedures, and it is most frequently present in outbreaks [90]. A hyperopic shift and increased optical aberrations are expected in patients that presented DLK [91, 92].

1.2.2.5 Keratectasia
Although there are reports of ectasia that occurred in eyes without known risk factors [93], approximately 90% of the eyes that develop ectasia have preoperative signs of forme fruste keratoconus [94]. Besides the diagnosis of forme fruste keratoconus and residual stromal bed of less than 250 μm [94], known topographical risk factors for corneal ectasia post-LASIK are corneal curvature, pachymetry, oblique astigmatism, posterior corneal surface elevation, difference between inferior and superior corneal dioptric power, and correlation between anterior and posterior best-fit sphere [95]. Treatments for corneal ectasia include rigid contact lenses, intrastromal corneal rings [96], keratoplasty, and collagen cross-linking [97, 98].

1.3 Phakic Intraocular Lenses

1.3.1 Endothelial Cell Loss

Anterior chamber angle-supported phakic IOLs present an initial decrease in endothelium cell density of 5–10% in 2 years, with a slightly higher than normal decrease after that [99–102]. Iris-supported lenses appear to present continuous decrease in cell density at longer follow-up, achieving between 10 and 15% at 2 years [99, 103, 104]. Although posterior-chamber IOLs have a lower risk of endothelial cell loss, a decrease of 5 to 10% may be expected 2 years after surgery [105]. Careful follow-up of patients who have undergone phakic implants should allow lenses to be removed before any clinical symptoms present, if damage of the endothelium persists.

1.3.2 Pupillary Block Glaucoma

Pupillary block glaucoma has been reported in anterior chamber iris-supported [106], angle-supported [107, 108], and posterior chamber phakic IOLs [109–111]. Preoperative iridectomy is mandatory, but pupillary block has been reported even in the presence of effective iridectomy [111].

1.3.3 Iris Atrophy and Pupil Ovalization

Eyes with anterior chamber angle-supported phakic IOLs have a tendency to present sectorial iris atrophy and consequent pupil ovalization [100–102, 107]. Its frequency depends on the limits accepted, but up to 40% ovalization (difference of 0.5 mm in orthogonal diameters) may be expected [101].

1.3.4 Chronic Inflammation

Chronic inflammation is present in all phakic IOL models. It has been reported to be higher than are controls in anterior chamber iris-supported and anterior chamber angle-supported at 12, 18, and 24 months after surgery [101, 112]. Aqueous flare was slightly better for the angle-supported group.

In posterior chamber IOLs, aqueous flare increased by 49.19% in the first postoperative month in relation to preoperative values, decreasing afterward, but remaining above preoperative values up to 2 years postoperatively [105].

1.3.5 Intraocular Lens Dislocation

Traumatic and spontaneous IOL dislocations have been described in anterior chamber iris-supported phakic IOLs [113, 114].

1.3.6 Cataract

Anterior subcapsular cataracts are related to posterior chamber phakic IOLs implants and are present in 8.2% of the eyes [115–118]. Most of the eyes that presented cataract were operated on in the beginning of the surgeon's learning curve [117]. Nuclear cataract has been reported in ante-

rior chamber angle-supported IOLs [118, 119], but it has not possible to determine a cause–effect relationship.

1.3.7 Pigment Dispersion

Pigment dispersion has been observed in approximately 3% of eyes that underwent posterior chamber phakic IOL implants [110, 120, 121]. There are no reports of glaucoma in eyes that presented pigment dispersion.

1.3.8 Posterior Luxation (in Phakic Refractive Lens™)

Spontaneous luxation to the vitreous of one specific model of silicone posterior chamber phakic IOL (Phakic Refractive Lens, PRL™) is a severe complication related to the weakening of the zonule [122, 123].

Take-Home Pearls

■ Refractive surgery provides a variety of elective procedures to be performed in otherwise healthy eyes. The knowledge of their possible complications is mandatory to inform our patients of their options.

References

1. Hjortdal JO, Moller-Pedersen T, Ivarsen A, Ehlers N (2005) Corneal power, thickness, and stiffness: results of a prospective randomized controlled trial of PRK and LASIK for myopia. J Cataract Refract Surg 31:21–29
2. Shortt AJ, Allan BD (2006) Photorefractive keratectomy (PRK) versus laser-assisted in-situ keratomileusis (LASIK) for myopia. Cochrane Database Syst Rev CD005135
3. Shortt AJ, Bunce C, Allan BD (2006) Evidence for superior efficacy and safety of LASIK over photorefractive keratectomy for correction of myopia. Ophthalmology 113:1897–1908
4. Wang Z, Chen J, Yang B (1997) Comparison of laser in situ keratomileusis and photorefractive keratectomy to correct myopia from –1.25 to –6.00 diopters. J Refract Surg 13:528–534
5. Hersh PS, Brint SF, Maloney RK, Durrie DS, Gordon M, Michelson MA (1998) Photorefractive keratectomy versus laser in situ keratomileusis for moderate to high myopia. A randomized prospective study. Ophthalmology 105:1512–1522, discussion 1522–1523
6. Forseto AS, Nosé RA, Nosé W (2000) PRK versus LASIK for correction of low and moderate myopia [in Portuguese]. Arq Bras Oftalmol 63:257–262
7. El-Maghraby A, Salah T, Waring GO III, Klyce S, Ibrahim O (1999) Randomized bilateral comparison of excimer laser in situ keratomileusis and photorefractive keratectomy for 2.50 to 8.00 diopters of myopia. Ophthalmology 106:447–457
8. el Danasoury MA, el Maghraby A, Klyce SD, Mehrez K (1999) Comparison of photorefractive keratectomy with excimer laser in situ keratomileusis in correcting low myopia (from –2.00 to –5.50 diopters): a randomized study. Ophthalmology 106:411–420; discussion 420–421

1

9. US Food and Drug Administration (2006) Lasik eye surgery. Available via http://www.fda gov/cdrh/LASIK/. Cited 22 March 2007

10. Roy S, Tritten JJ (2002) [Myopic implant of the posterior chamber using a flexible Collamer lens]. Klin Monatsbl Augenheilkd 219:196–200

11. Liekfeld A, Friederici L, Klotz O (2005) [Monocentric two-year results after phakic posterior chamber lens (PRL) implantation in myopic patients]. Klin Monatsbl Augenheilkd 222:888–893

12. Leroux-Les-Jardins S, Ullern M, Werthel AL (1999) [Myopic anterior chamber intraocular lens implantation: evaluation at 8 years]. J Fr Ophtalmol 22:323–327

13. Lackner B, Pieh S, Schmidinger G, Hanselmayer G, Dejaco-Ruhswurm I, Funovics MA, (2003) Outcome after treatment of ametropia with implantable contact lenses. Ophthalmology 110:2153–2161

14. Benedetti S, Casamenti V, Marcaccio L, Brogioni C, Assetto V (2005) Correction of myopia of 7 to 24 diopters with the Artisan phakic intraocular lens: two-year follow-up. J Refract Surg 21:116–126

15. Garcia M, Gonzalez C, Pascual I, Fimia A (1996) Magnification and visual acuity in highly myopic phakic eyes corrected with an anterior chamber intraocular lens versus by other methods. J Cataract Refract Surg 22:1416–1422

16. Holladay JT, Prager TC, Chandler TY, Musgrove KH, Lewis JW, Ruiz RS (1988) A three-part system for refining intraocular lens power calculations. J Cataract Refract Surg 14:17–24

17. Aramberri J (2003) Intraocular lens power calculation after corneal refractive surgery: double-K method. J Cataract Refract Surg 29:2063–2068

18. Chamon W (2004) A new approach to correct an inherent error in IOL calculation formulas for eyes submitted to keratorefractive procedures. Invest Ophthalmol Vis Sci 45(Abstr):341

19. de Oliveira GC, Solari HP, Ciola FB, Lima AL, Campos MS (2006) Corneal infiltrates after excimer laser photorefractive keratectomy and LASIK. J Refract Surg 22:159–165

20. Wroblewski KJ, Pasternak JF, Bower KS, Schallhorn SC, Hubickey WJ, Harrison CE (2006) Infectious keratitis after photorefractive keratectomy in the United States army and navy. Ophthalmology 113:520–525

21. Moshirfar M, Welling JD, Feiz V, Holz H, Clinch TE (2007) Infectious and noninfectious keratitis after laser in situ keratomileusis Occurrence, management, and visual outcomes. J Cataract Refract Surg 33:474–483

22. Lifshitz T, Levy J, Mahler O, Levinger S (2005) Peripheral sterile corneal infiltrates after refractive surgery. J Cataract Refract Surg 31:1392–1395

23. Gimbel HV, van Westenbrugge JA, Penno EE, Ferensowicz M, Feinerman GA, Chen R (1999) Simultaneous bilateral laser in situ keratomileusis: safety and efficacy. Ophthalmology 106:1461–1467, discussion 1467–1468

24. Huang D, Krueger R, Stulting RD (2000) Correlation between eyes in bilateral LASIK. Ophthalmology 107:1962–1963

25. Kattan HM, Flynn HW, Jr., Pflugfelder SC, Robertson C, Forster RK (1991) Nosocomial endophthalmitis survey. Current incidence of infection after intraocular surgery. Ophthalmology 98:227–238

26. Marty N, Malavaud S (2002) [Epidemiology of nosocomial infections after cataract surgery and role of the Infection Control Committee in prevention]. Bull Acad Natl Med 186:635–645, discussion 645–648

27. Haapala TT, Nelimarkka L, Saari JM, Ahola V, Saari KM (2005) Endophthalmitis following cataract surgery in southwest Finland from 1987 to 2000. Graefes Arch Clin Exp Ophthalmol 243:1010–1017

28. McAlister JC, Ardjomand N, Ilari L, Mengher LS, Gartry DS (2006) Keratitis after intracorneal ring segment insertion for keratoconus. J Cataract Refract Surg 32:676–678

29. Mondino BJ, Rabin BS, Kessler E, Gallo J, Brown SI (1977) Corneal rings with gram-negative bacteria. Arch Ophthalmol 95:2222–2225

30. Hofling-Lima AL, Branco BC, Romano AC, Campos MQ, Moreira H, Miranda D (2004) Corneal infections after implantation of intracorneal ring segments. Cornea 23:547–549

31. Morgan PB, Efron N, Hill EA, Raynor MK, Whiting MA, Tullo AB (2005) Incidence of keratitis of varying severity among contact lens wearers. Br J Ophthalmol 89:430–436

32. Schein OD, McNally JJ, Katz J, Chalmers RL, Tielsch JM, Alfonso E (2005) The incidence of microbial keratitis among wearers of a 30-day silicone hydrogel extended-wear contact lens. Ophthalmology 112:2172–2179

33. Chalita MR, Chavala S, Xu M, Krueger RR (2004) Wavefront analysis in post-LASIK eyes and its correlation with visual symptoms, refraction, and topography. Ophthalmology 111:447–453

34. Chalita MR, Krueger RR (2004) Correlation of aberrations with visual acuity and symptoms. Ophthalmol Clin North Am 17:135–42, v–vi

35. Chiam PJ, Chan JH, Aggarwal RK, Kasaby S (2006) ReSTOR intraocular lens implantation in cataract surgery: quality of vision. J Cataract Refract Surg 32:1459–1463

36. Casprini F, Balestrazzi A, Tosi GM, Miracco F, Martone G, Cevenini G (2005) Glare disability and spherical aberration with five foldable intraocular lenses: a prospective randomized study. Acta Ophthalmol Scand 83:20–25

37. Bellucci R, Morselli S, Pucci V (2007) Spherical aberration and coma with an aspherical and a spherical intraocular lens in normal age-matched eyes. J Cataract Refract Surg 33:203–209

38. Tester R, Pace NL, Samore M, Olson RJ (2000) Dysphotopsia in phakic and pseudophakic patients: incidence and relation to intraocular lens type(2). J Cataract Refract Surg 26:810–816

39. Oshika T, Tokunaga T, Samejima T, Miyata K, Kawana K, Kaji Y (2006) Influence of pupil diameter on the relation between ocular higher-order aberration and contrast sensitivity after laser in situ keratomileusis. Invest Ophthalmol Vis Sci 47:1334–1338

40. Ruiz-Moreno JM, Perez-Santonja JJ, Alio JL (1999) Retinal detachment in myopic eyes after laser in situ keratomileusis. Am J Ophthalmol 128:588–594

41. Arevalo JF, Freeman WR, Gomez L (2001) Retina and vitreous pathology after laser-assisted in situ keratomileusis: is there a cause-effect relationship? Ophthalmology 108:839–840

42. Lin J, Xie X, Du X, Yang Y, Yao K (2002) [Incidence of vitreoretinal pathologic conditions in myopic eyes after laser in situ keratomileusis]. Zhonghua Yan Ke Za Zhi 38:546–549

43. Suzuki CR, Farah ME (2004) Retinal peripheral changes after laser in situ keratomileusis in patients with high myopia. Can J Ophthalmol 39:69–73

44. Faghihi H, Jalali KH, Amini A, Hashemi H, Fotouhi A, Esfahani MR (2006) Rhegmatogenous retinal detachment after LASIK for myopia. J Refract Surg 22:448–452

45. Sheu SJ, Ger LP, Chen JF (2006) Axial myopia is an extremely significant risk factor for young-aged pseudophakic retinal detachment in taiwan. Retina 26:322–327

46. Erie JC, Raecker MA, Baratz KH, Schleck CD, Burke JP, Robertson DM (2006) Risk of retinal detachment after cataract extraction, 1980–2004: a population-based study. Ophthalmology 113:2026–2032

47. Olsen G, Olson RJ (2000) Update on a long-term, prospective study of capsulotomy and retinal detachment rates after cataract surgery. J Cataract Refract Surg 26:1017–1021

48. Martinez-Castillo V, Boixadera A, Verdugo A, Elies D, Coret A, Garcia-Arumi J (2005) Rhegmatogenous retinal detachment in

phakic eyes after posterior chamber phakic intraocular lens implantation for severe myopia. Ophthalmology 112:580–585

49. Navarro R, Gris O, Broc L, Corcostegui B (2005) Bilateral giant retinal tear following posterior chamber phakic intraocular lens implantation. J Refract Surg 21:298–300

50. Kuo IC, Lee SM, Hwang DG (2004) Late-onset corneal haze and myopic regression after photorefractive keratectomy (PRK). Cornea 23:350–355

51. Fiore T, Carones F, Brancato R (2001) Broad beam vs. flying spot excimer laser: refractive and videokeratographic outcomes of two different ablation profiles after photorefractive keratectomy. J Refract Surg 17:534–541

52. Bedei A, Marabotti A, Giannecchini I, Ferretti C, Montagnani M, Martinucci C (2006) Photorefractive keratectomy in high myopic defects with or without intraoperative mitomycin C: 1-year results. Eur J Ophthalmol 16:229–234

53. Netto MV, Chalita MR, Krueger RR (2007) Corneal haze following PRK with mitomycin C as a retreatment versus prophylactic use in the contralateral eye. J Refract Surg 23:96–98

54. Netto MV, Mohan RR, Sinha S, Sharma A, Gupta PC, Wilson SE (2006) Effect of prophylactic and therapeutic mitomycin C on corneal apoptosis, cellular proliferation, haze, and long-term keratocyte density in rabbits. J Refract Surg 22:562–574

55. Carones F, Vigo L, Scandola E (2006) Wavefront-guided treatment of symptomatic eyes using the LADAR6000 excimer laser. J Refract Surg 22:S983–S989

56. Chalita MR, Roth AS, Krueger RR (2004) Wavefront-guided surface ablation with prophylactic use of mitomycin C after a buttonhole laser in situ keratomileusis flap. J Refract Surg 20:176–181

57. Carones F, Vigo L, Scandola E, Vacchini L (2002) Evaluation of the prophylactic use of mitomycin-C to inhibit haze formation after photorefractive keratectomy. J Cataract Refract Surg 28:2088–2095

58. Netto MV, Mohan RR, Ambrosio R, Jr., Hutcheon AE, Zieske JD, Wilson SE (2005) Wound healing in the cornea: a review of refractive surgery complications and new prospects for therapy. Cornea 24:509–522

59. Torres RM, Merayo-Lloves J, Daya SM, Blanco-Mezquita JT, Espinosa M, Nozal MJ (2006) Presence of mitomycin-C in the anterior chamber after photorefractive keratectomy. J Cataract Refract Surg 32:67–71

60. Morales AJ, Zadok D, Mora-Retana R, Martinez-Gama E, Robledo NE, Chayet AS (2006) Intraoperative mitomycin and corneal endothelium after photorefractive keratectomy. Am J Ophthalmol 142:400–404

61. Malecaze F, Coullet J, Calvas P, Fournie P, Arne JL, Brodaty C (2006) Corneal ectasia after photorefractive keratectomy for low myopia. Ophthalmology 113:742–746

62. Lovisolo CF, Fleming JF (2002) Intracorneal ring segments for iatrogenic keratectasia after laser in situ keratomileusis or photorefractive keratectomy. J Refract Surg 18:535–441

63. Javadi MA, Mohammadpour M, Rabei HM (2006) Keratectasia after LASIK but not after PRK in one patient. J Refract Surg 22:817–820

64. Seiler T, Koufala K, Richter G (1998) Iatrogenic keratectasia after laser in situ keratomileusis. J Refract Surg 14:312–317

65. Miyata K, Takahashi T, Tomidokoro A, Ono K, Oshika T (2001) Iatrogenic keratectasia after phototherapeutic keratectomy. Br J Ophthalmol 85:247–248

66. Dean SJ, McGhee CN (2002) Keratectasia after PTK. Br J Ophthalmol 86:486

67. Leung AT, Rao SK, Cheng AC, Yu EW, Fan DS, Lam DS (2000) Pathogenesis and management of laser in situ keratomileusis flap buttonhole. J Cataract Refract Surg 26:358–362

68. Nakano K, Nakano E, Oliveira M, Portellinha W, Alvarenga L (2004) Intraoperative microkeratome complications in 47,094 laser in situ keratomileusis surgeries. J Refract Surg 20(Suppl): S723–S726

69. Tham VM, Maloney RK (2000) Microkeratome complications of laser in situ keratomileusis. Ophthalmology 107:920–924

70. Walker MB, Wilson SE (2000) Lower intraoperative flap complication rate with the Hansatome microkeratome compared to the Automated Corneal Shaper. J Refract Surg 16:79–82

71. Yildirim R, Devranoglu K, Ozdamar A, Aras C, Ozkiris A, Ozkan S (2001) Flap complications in our learning curve of laser in situ keratomileusis using the Hansatome microkeratome. Eur J Ophthalmol 11:328–332

72. Jacobs JM, Taravella MJ (2002) Incidence of intraoperative flap complications in laser in situ keratomileusis. J Cataract Refract Surg 28:23–28

73. Pallikaris IG, Katsanevaki VJ, Panagopoulou SI (2002) Laser in situ keratomileusis intraoperative complications using one type of microkeratome. Ophthalmology 109:57–63

74. Sharma N, Ghate D, Agarwal T, Vajpayee RB (2005) Refractive outcomes of laser in situ keratomileusis after flap complications. J Cataract Refract Surg 31:1334–1337

75. Talamo JH, Meltzer J, Gardner J (2006) Reproducibility of flap thickness with IntraLase FS and Moria LSK-1 and M2 microkeratomes. J Refract Surg 22:556–561

76. Montes-Mico R, Rodriguez-Galietero A, Alio JL (2007) Femtosecond laser versus mechanical keratome LASIK for myopia. Ophthalmology 114:62–68

77. Binder PS (2006) One thousand consecutive IntraLase laser in situ keratomileusis flaps. J Cataract Refract Surg 32:962–969

78. Lim T, Yang S, Kim M, Tchah H (2006) Comparison of the IntraLase femtosecond laser and mechanical microkeratome for laser in situ keratomileusis. Am J Ophthalmol 141:833–839

79. Patel SV, Maguire LJ, McLaren JW, Hodge DO, Bourne WM (2007) Femtosecond laser versus mechanical microkeratome for LASIK: a randomized controlled study. Ophthalmology 114:1482–1490

80. Munoz G, Albarran-Diego C, Sakla HF, Javaloy J, Alio JL (2006) Transient light-sensitivity syndrome after laser in situ keratomileusis with the femtosecond laser Incidence and prevention. J Cataract Refract Surg 32:2075–2079

81. Stonecipher KG, Dishler JG, Ignacio TS, Binder PS (2006) Transient light sensitivity after femtosecond laser flap creation: clinical findings and management. J Cataract Refract Surg 32:91–94

82. Recep OF, Cagil N, Hasiripi H (2000) Outcome of flap subluxation after laser in situ keratomileusis: results of 6-month follow-up. J Cataract Refract Surg 26:1158–1162

83. Aldave AJ, Hollander DA, Abbott RL (2002) Late-onset traumatic flap dislocation and diffuse lamellar inflammation after laser in situ keratomileusis. Cornea 21:604–607

84. Booth MA, Koch DD (2003) Late laser in situ keratomileusis flap dislocation caused by a thrown football. J Cataract Refract Surg 29:2032–2033

85. Tumbocon JA, Paul R, Slomovic A, Rootman DS (2003) Late traumatic displacement of laser in situ keratomileusis flaps. Cornea 22:66–69

86. Kocak I, Karabela Y, Karaman M, Kaya F (2006) Late onset diffuse lamellar keratitis as a result of the toxic effect of Ecballium elaterium herb. J Refract Surg 22:826–827

87. Lazaro C, Perea J, Arias A (2006) Surgical-glove-related diffuse lamellar keratitis after laser in situ keratomileusis: long-term outcomes. J Cataract Refract Surg 32:1702–1709

88. Shen YC, Wang CY, Fong SC, Tsai HY, Lee YF (2006) Diffuse lamellar keratitis induced by toxic chemicals after laser in situ keratomileusis. J Cataract Refract Surg 32:1146–1150

89. Smith RJ, Maloney RK. Diffuse lamellar keratitis (1998) A new syndrome in lamellar refractive surgery. Ophthalmology 105:1721–1726

90. Bigham M, Enns CL, Holland SP, Buxton J, Patrick D, Marion S (2005) Diffuse lamellar keratitis complicating laser in situ keratomileusis: post-marketing surveillance of an emerging disease in British Columbia, Canada, 2000–2002. J Cataract Refract Surg 31:2340–2344

91. Dada T, Pangtey MS, Sharma N, Vajpayee RB, Jhanji V, Sethi HS (2006) Hyeropic shift after LASIK induced diffuse lamellar keratitis. BMC Ophthalmol 6:19

92. Beer SM, Campos M, Lopes PT, Andre JA, Jr., Schor P (2007) Ocular wavefront aberrations in patients after diffuse lamellar keratitis. Cornea 26:6–8

93. Klein SR, Epstein RJ, Randleman JB, Stulting RD (2006) Corneal ectasia after laser in situ keratomileusis in patients without apparent preoperative risk factors. Cornea 25:388–403

94. Randleman JB, Russell B, Ward MA, Thompson KP, Stulting RD (2003) Risk factors and prognosis for corneal ectasia after LASIK. Ophthalmology 110:267–275

95. Tabbara KF, Kotb AA (2006) Risk factors for corneal ectasia after LASIK. Ophthalmology 113:1618–1622

96. Kymionis GD, Siganos CS, Kounis G, Astyrakakis N, Kalyvianaki MI, Pallikaris IG (2003) Management of post-LASIK corneal ectasia with Intacs inserts: one-year results. Arch Ophthalmol 121:322–326

97. Wollensak G, Sporl E, Seiler T (2003) [Treatment of keratoconus by collagen cross-linking]. Ophthalmologe 100:44–49

98. Kohlhaas M, Spoerl E, Speck A, Schilde T, Sandner D, Pillunat LE (2005) [A new treatment of keratectasia after LASIK by using collagen with riboflavin/UVA light cross-linking]. Klin Monatsbl Augenheilkd 222:430–436

99. Perez-Santonja JJ, Iradier MT, Sanz-Iglesias L, Serrano JM, Zato MA (1996) Endothelial changes in phakic eyes with anterior chamber intraocular lenses to correct high myopia. J Cataract Refract Surg 22:1017–1022

100 Baikoff G, Arne JL, Bokobza Y, Colin J, George JL, Lagoutte F (1998) Angle-fixated anterior chamber phakic intraocular lens for myopia of –7 to –19 diopters. J Refract Surg 14:282–293

101. Allemann N, Chamon W, Tanaka HM, Mori ES, Campos M, Schor P (2000) Myopic angle-supported intraocular lenses: two-year follow-up. Ophthalmology 107:1549–1554

102. Alio JL, de la Hoz F, Perez-Santonja JJ, Ruiz-Moreno JM, Quesada JA (1999) Phakic anterior chamber lenses for the correction of myopia: a 7-year cumulative analysis of complications in 263 cases. Ophthalmology 106:458–466

103. Menezo JL, Cisneros AL, Rodriguez-Salvador V (1998) Endothelial study of iris-claw phakic lens: four year follow-up. J Cataract Refract Surg 24:1039–1049

104. Saxena R, Landesz M, Noordzij B, Luyten GP (2003) Three-year follow-up of the Artisan phakic intraocular lens for hypermetropia. Ophthalmology 110:1391–1395

105. Jimenez-Alfaro I, Benitez del Castillo JM, Garcia-Feijoo J, Gil de Bernabe JG, Serrano de La Iglesia JM (2001) Safety of posterior chamber phakic intraocular lenses for the correction of high myopia: anterior segment changes after posterior chamber phakic intraocular lens implantation. Ophthalmology 108:90–99

106. Budo C, Hessloehl JC, Izak M, Luyten GP, Menezo JL, Sener BA (2000) Multicenter study of the Artisan phakic intraocular lens. J Cataract Refract Surg 26:1163–1171

107. Leccisotti A (2005) Angle-supported phakic intraocular lenses in hyperopia. J Cataract Refract Surg 31:1598–1602

108. Ardjomand N, Kolli H, Vidic B, El-Shabrawi Y, Faulborn J (2002) Pupillary block after phakic anterior chamber intraocular lens implantation. J Cataract Refract Surg 28:1080–1081

109. Smallman DS, Probst L, Rafuse PE (2004) Pupillary block glaucoma secondary to posterior chamber phakic intraocular lens implantation for high myopia. J Cataract Refract Surg 30:905–907

110. Hoyos JE, Dementiev DD, Cigales M, Hoyos-Chacon J, Hoffer KJ (2002) Phakic refractive lens experience in Spain. J Cataract Refract Surg 28:1939–1946

111. Bylsma SS, Zalta AH, Foley E, Osher RH (2002) Phakic posterior chamber intraocular lens pupillary block. J Cataract Refract Surg 28:2222–2228

112. Perez-Santonja JJ, Iradier MT, Benitez del Castillo JM, Serrano JM, Zato MA (1996) Chronic subclinical inflammation in phakic eyes with intraocular lenses to correct myopia. J Cataract Refract Surg 22:183–187

113. Menezo JL, Avino JA, Cisneros A, Rodriguez-Salvador V, Martinez-Costa R (1997) Iris claw phakic intraocular lens for high myopia. J Refract Surg 13:545–555

114. Perez-Santonja JJ, Alio JL, Jimenez-Alfaro I, Zato MA (2000) Surgical correction of severe myopia with an angle-supported phakic intraocular lens. J Cataract Refract Surg 26:1288–1302

115. Trindade F, Pereira F (1998) Cataract formation after posterior chamber phakic intraocular lens implantation. J Cataract Refract Surg 24:1661–1663

116. Fink AM, Gore C, Rosen E (1999) Cataract development after implantation of the Staar Collamer posterior chamber phakic lens. J Cataract Refract Surg 25:278–282

117. Sanchez-Galeana CA, Smith RJ, Sanders DR, Rodriguez FX, Litwak S, Montes M (2003) Lens opacities after posterior chamber phakic intraocular lens implantation. Ophthalmology 110:781–785

118. Menezo JL, Peris-Martinez C, Cisneros AL, Martinez-Costa R (2004) Phakic intraocular lenses to correct high myopia: Adatomed, Staar, and Artisan. J Cataract Refract Surg 30:33–44

119. Alio JL, de la Hoz F, Ruiz-Moreno JM, Salem TF (2000) Cataract surgery in highly myopic eyes corrected by phakic anterior chamber angle-supported lenses. J Cataract Refract Surg 26:1303–1311

120. Baikoff G, Bourgeon G, Jodai HJ, Fontaine A, Lellis FV, Trinquet L (2005) Pigment dispersion and Artisan phakic intraocular lenses: crystalline lens rise as a safety criterion. J Cataract Refract Surg 31:674–680

121. Trindade F, Pereira F, Cronemberger S (1998) Ultrasound biomicroscopic imaging of posterior chamber phakic intraocular lens. J Refract Surg 14:497–503

122. Eleftheriadis H, Amoros S, Bilbao R, Teijeiro MA (2004) Spontaneous dislocation of a phakic refractive lens into the vitreous cavity. J Cataract Refract Surg 30:2013–2016

123. Hoyos JE, Cigales M, Hoyos-Chacon J (2005) Zonular dehiscence two years after phakic refractive lens (PRL) implantation. J Refract Surg 21:13–17

Chapter 2

Influence of Refractive Surgery Complications on Quality of Life

Konrad Pesudovs

2

Contents

Core Messages

- A number of questionnaires exist for the measurement of quality of life (QOL) in the refractive surgery patient, but not all questionnaires are equal in validity.

- Rasch analysis is important in the development of questionnaires to optimize question inclusion, unidimensionality, and to provide valid linear scoring.

- A quality of life instrument should include a breadth of content areas, e.g., well-being, convenience, and concerns, not just functioning or satisfaction.

- QOL instruments readily demonstrate the benefits of refractive surgery.

- A sound QOL instrument is also sensitive to the negative impacts of surgical complications, providing an insight into the real impact of the intervention on the person.

2.1 Introduction

It has been customary to evaluate the success of refractive surgery using objective clinical measures such as postoperative uncorrected visual acuity (UCVA) and residual refractive error [19]. However, these measures do not necessarily correlate well with patients' postoperative subjective impressions [13]. Ultimately, the patient's perspective is an important outcome of refractive surgery and a number of instruments have been developed to assess quality of life (QOL), including the Quality of Life Impact of Refractive Correction (QIRC) questionnaire [15], the Refractive Status Vision Profile (RSVP) [17], and the National Eye Institute Refractive Quality of Life (NEI-RQL) [12]. While these instruments and others have chiefly been used to show the improvement in QOL that occurs with laser refractive surgery [2, 5, 7, 12, 13, 18], a sound QOL instrument should also be sensitive to the effect of complications from refractive surgery.

The purpose of this chapter is to outline the key issues in QOL measurement, discuss the instruments available for use, and to summarize specifically what is known about the impact of the complications of refractive surgery on QOL.

2.2 Measurement Concepts

Perhaps the most important issue in questionnaire selection is the validity of the scoring system. Without this, the information gathered is meaningless. The RSVP and NEI-RQL instruments use traditional summary scoring, in which an overall score is derived through summative scoring of responses [9]. Summary scoring is based on the hypotheses that all questions have equal importance, and response categories are accordingly scaled to have equal value with uniform increments from category to category. For example, in a summary-scaled visual disability questionnaire, the Activities of Daily Vision Scale (ADVS) [10], "a little difficulty" scores 4, while "extreme difficulty" is twice as bad and scores 2, and "unable to perform the activity due to vision" is similarly two times worse, with a score of 1. The same scale is applied across all questions. This rationale of "one size fits all" is flawed, and Rasch analysis has been used to confirm that differently weighted response categories are necessary to provide a valid and contextual scale that truly represents QOL. For instance, the ADVS questionnaire ascribes the same value to "a little difficulty" regarding visual ability "driving at night" as "a little difficulty" with "driving during the day," though the former is by far the more difficult and complex task, and it defies logic to equate the two.

Rasch analysis is a new approach to questionnaire development that utilizes modern statistical methods to measure health outcomes in a meaningful way by incorporating an appropriate weighting factor for each QOL measure to provide true linear scoring, and through improved validity in terms of question inclusion and demonstration of unidimensionality [11, 20].

2.3 Instruments

2.3.1 Quality of Life Impact of Refractive Correction Questionnaire

Pesudovs et al. developed and validated the QIRC questionnaire [15] to measure the impact of refractive correction on QOL. Visual function, symptoms, convenience, cost, health concerns, and well-being are included in the content of this instrument, which was rigorously developed using literature review, expert opinion, and focus groups. Content was determined using a pilot questionnaire with Rasch analysis for item reduction [20]; this resulted in the final 20-item questionnaire (Table 2.1, available in full at http://konrad. pesudovs.com/konrad/questionnaire.html). QIRC is ratified as a valid and reliable measure of refractive correction-related QOL by both Rasch analysis and standard psychometric techniques [15]. QIRC scores are reported on a 0–100 scale, which is free of floor and ceiling effects, with a higher score representing better QOL, and the average score being close to 50 units. QIRC has been used for measuring outcomes of refractive surgery [5] and for comparing the QOL of patients wearing spectacles, contact lenses, or post–refractive surgery [16].

The QIRC questionnaire effectively differentiates between spectacle wearers, contact lens wearers, and post–refractive surgery patients, with the refractive surgery group having a better QIRC score (50.23±6.31) than did contact lens wearers (46.70±5.49, $p < 0.01$) and spectacle wearers (44.13±5.86, $p < 0.001$) [16]. There were significant differences between scores on 16 of the 20 questions; of the remaining 4 questions, 2 health concerns and 2 well-being questions did not detect differences between groups. QIRC scores have also been shown to improve after laser assisted in situ keratomileusis (LASIK) refractive surgery from a mean ±SD of 40.07±4.3 to 53.09±5.25 [5.]

Individual item analysis showed 15 of the 20 items demonstrated statistically significant improvement. Patients reported improved QOL on all 5 convenience items, both economic items, all 4 health concern items, and on 4 of the 7 items in the well-being domain (Fig. 2.1).

Table 2.1. The 20 items included in the QIRC questionnaire

Item description
1. How much difficulty do you have driving in glare conditions?
2. During the past month, how often have you experienced your eyes feeling tired or strained?
3. How much trouble is not being able to use off-the-shelf (non-prescription) sunglasses?
4. How much trouble is having to think about your spectacles or contact lenses or your eyes after refractive surgery before doing things, e.g., traveling, sport, going swimming?
5. How much trouble is not being able to see when you wake up, e.g., to go to the bathroom, look after a baby, see alarm clock?
6. How much trouble is not being able to see when you are on the beach or swimming in the sea or pool, because you do these activities without spectacles or contact lenses?
7. How much trouble are your spectacles or contact lenses when you wear them when using a gym/doing keep-fit classes/circuit training etc?
8. How concerned are you about the initial and ongoing cost to buy your current spectacles/contact lenses/refractive surgery?
9. How concerned are you about the cost of unscheduled maintenance of your spectacles/contact lenses/refractive surgery, e.g., breakage, loss, new eye problems?
10. How concerned are you about having to increasingly rely on your spectacles or contact lenses since you started to wear them?
11. How concerned are you about your vision not being as good as it could be?
12. How concerned are you about medical complications from your choice of optical correction (spectacles, contact lenses, and/or refractive surgery)?
13. How concerned are you about eye protection from ultraviolet (UV) radiation?
14. During the past month, how much of the time have you felt that you have looked your best?
15. During the past month, how much of the time have you felt that you think others see you the way you would like them to (e.g., intelligent, sophisticated, successful, cool, etc.)?
16. During the past month, how much of the time have you felt complimented/flattered?
17. During the past month, how much of the time have you felt confident?
18. During the past month, how much of the time have you felt happy?
19. During the past month, how much of the time have you felt able to do the things you want to do?
20. During the past month, how much of the time have you felt eager to try new things?

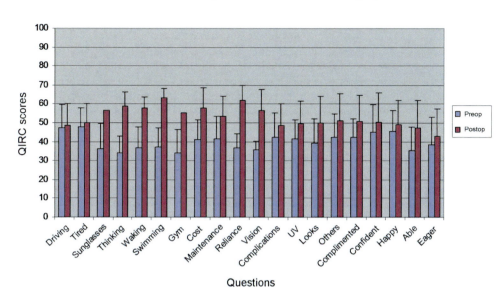

Pre- and Postoperative LASIK Refractive Surgery

Fig. 2.1. Pre- and post-LASIK mean (error bars ±1 SD) responses on each QIRC question

2.3.2 Refractive Status Vision Profile

The RSVP was developed almost exclusively on a refractive surgery population (92% of subjects), so it is really only valid for refractive surgery [17]. Its 42 items fall into the domains of concern (6 items), expectations (2), physical/social functioning (11), driving (3), symptoms (5), glare (3), optical problems (5), and problems with corrective lenses (7 items) [18]. The RSVP has been shown to be sensitive to QOL changes related to visual functioning and refractive error, and is responsive to refractive surgery [18]. Improvements after refractive surgery occurred in the subscales: expectations, physical and social functioning and problems with corrective lenses.

The RSVP was developed using traditional techniques, but its psychometric properties were re-evaluated by Garamendi et al., using Rasch analysis. The original 42-item questionnaire showed poor targeting of item impact to patient QOL, items with a ceiling effect, underutilized response categories, and a high level of redundancy. Rasch analysis guided response-scale restructuring and item reduction to a 20-item instrument, with improved internal consistency and precision for discriminating between groups. Fourteen items relating to functioning and driving were reduced to five items and eight related to symptoms and glare were reduced to three. This is consistent with the content of the QIRC questionnaire, in which Rasch analysis identified that patients with corrected refractive error experienced few problems with visual function, and issues of convenience, cost, health concerns, and well-being were more influential on QOL [15]. Perhaps the reason why the original RSVP was so heavily weighted with functioning and symptoms questions was because the items were principally determined by clinicians [17], who tend to deal with patients' presenting complaints of symptoms or functional difficulties instead of using more objective methodology to discover the less acute but still important QOL issues.

2.3.3 National Eye Institute Refractive Quality of Life Instrument

The NEI-RQL instrument is a conventionally developed 42-item questionnaire that includes subscales related to clarity of vision, expectations, near and far vision, diurnal fluctuations, activity limitations, glare, symptoms, dependence on correction, worry, suboptimal correction, appearance, and satisfaction. The development and validation of the NEI-RQL was spread across three papers and despite rigorous work with focus groups, there is no report on how the final 42 items were selected [3, 6, 12]. However, the NEI-RQL can discriminate between modes of refractive correction and is sensitive to QOL changes related to visual functioning and refractive error. Two studies have used the NEI-RQL to demonstrate improved QOL after refractive surgery [12, 14]. The NEI-RQL has not been tested or scaled using Rasch analysis.

2.3.4 Others

The Myopia Specific Quality of Life and the Canadian Refractive Surgery Research Group Questionnaires have been conventionally validated and shown to be responsive to refractive surgery [4, 8]. Other studies that report QOL issues before and after refractive surgery have used informal, non-validated questionnaires,[1, 2, 7, 13] so really only provide limited evidence.

2

2.4 Complications and QOL

2.4.1 QIRC

Two studies using the QIRC questionnaire have highlighted QOL problems after LASIK. In a cross-sectional comparison of spectacle, contact lens, and refractive surgery patients, the post–refractive surgery group was also asked to report any visual disturbances that arose after surgery, and a small number optionally reported postoperative complications. Nine (8.6%) LASIK patients volunteered written comments regarding their postoperative status (including poor vision in low light, dry eyes, regression, and haloes at night); five of these nine were very negative about their refractive surgery. Seven patients (6.7%) had a very low QIRC score (37.86±2.13), which included the five who volunteered negative comments and two who did not comment. Three of these patients were still wearing spectacles all day every day, and two suffered from significant dry eye [16]. In another study, looking at the outcome of LASIK, large improvements in QOL were found in the majority of subjects [5]. Three (4.5%) subjects had decreased QIRC scores, and these were associated with complications. All reported decreased quality of vision including driving at night, and one reported light sensitivity. Low scores were manifested in visual function, symptoms, concerns, and well-being items. None of the patients with improved QIRC scores experienced any serious complications after LASIK.

2.4.2 RSVP

Schein et al. investigated laser refractive surgery outcomes using the RSVP and found a worsening of overall score in 4.5% of patients [18]. With regard to individual subscales, poorer postoperative scores occurred for 29.5% of subjects on the driving subscale, 19.9% for optical problems, 16.3% for glare, 12.7% for symptoms, 7.4% for concern, 5.9% for functioning, and 2.3% had trouble with corrective lenses. A worsening of at least one subscale score was found in 26% of patients, and 15% reported dissatisfaction with vision postoperatively. Increased age at surgery was the strongest predictor of poorer RSVP scores or dissatisfaction with vision.

2.4.3 NEI-RQL

McDonnell et al. found QOL, as measured with the NEI-RQL, improved overall after LASIK, but symptoms of glare were significantly worse, and clarity of vision showed no significant change [12]. Nichols et al. also looked at the NEI-RQL and did not report any adverse outcomes [14]. These results raise the possibility that the NEI-RQL is not very sensitive to the negative QOL impacts of complications of refractive surgery.

2.4.4 Outcomes Reported with Other Instruments

In early PRK outcomes research, 77.5% of 173 patients reported improvement in their general QOL, but 16.8% were debilitated by subjective visual symptoms [2]. The only significant preoperative predictor was refractive error—higher preoperative refraction leads to lower satisfaction rates. In another large PRK study, 31.7% of 690 patients reported worsening night vision after surgery, and 30% reported dissatisfaction with night vision [4]. The frequency of each of the reported symptoms was 34.3% for starbursts, 52.4% for halos, and 61.5% for glare from oncoming headlights. For the patients who experienced glare, 55.6% reported that it was more debilitating post-PRK. These findings are in contrast to those reported after LASIK.

McGhee et al. reported only 3 of 50 LASIK patients experienced night vision symptoms, and only 1 reported dissatisfaction or that their QOL was not improved [13]. They also reported that patients who aimed for a residual myopic refraction expressed disappointment with UCVA, and that presbyopia experienced suboptimal near vision. However, limitations of this study are that the only content area tested was functioning, and no patients had any serious complications. Hill found that only 3 in 200 subjects would not have LASIK again despite 24% reporting worsening night vision and 27% reporting light sensitivity [7]. The 3 individuals cited worsening night vision, presbyopia, and psychological distress as reasons for opting against the intervention. Bailey et al., in a patient satisfaction survey, found 16 of 604 patients were dissatisfied after LASIK, and a high percentage of these reported symptoms of glare, halos, or starbursts (81.3%) [1]. Those who had surgical enhancement were found to be more likely to experience these symptoms, and along with those with increased age, greater corneal toricity, or smaller pupil size were less likely to be satisfied with the intervention.

Lee et al. developed the Myopia Specific Quality of Life Questionnaire, which contains four domains: visual function, symptoms, social role function, and psychological well-being [8]. They identified eight adverse symptoms that were most frequently reported after LASIK: eye dryness, blurred vision, lowered indoor or night vision, halos, regression, glare, temporary reduction in near vision, and infection. Multivariate analysis showed that patients having symptoms that are more adverse experienced significantly less improvement in QOL, so they concluded that freedom from adverse effects is one of the most important requirements for achieving excellent outcomes.

2.5 Implications

The caveat with the usually high QOL afforded by refractive surgery is the associated risk. Common complications of laser refractive surgery such as loss of contrast vision, loss of best-corrected vision, regression, and dry eye problems are effectively identified by QOL instruments, with patients requiring spectacle or contact lens correction or experiencing severe dry eye faring the worst. Night vision symptoms are common, but these do not necessarily negatively affect QOL. While QOL research has identified some risk factors for poorer outcome, e.g., older age and multiple treatments, this information does not translate into an altered patient selection strategy. While these results suggest that night vision symptoms are less prevalent with LASIK than PRK, there is no evidence that newer laser treatment paradigms provide any QOL benefit compared to older systems. Ongoing evaluation of refractive surgery outcomes using QOL measurement is required to demonstrate the benefits of technological increments.

Take-Home Pearls

- ■ Questionnaires can effectively demonstrate improved QOL from laser refractive surgery.

- ■ Serious complications of refractive surgery lead to markedly reduced QOL, but minor complications, like night vision disturbances, may not negatively affect QOL.

- ■ Routine evaluation of refractive surgery outcomes should include QOL measurement.

- ■ The ideal QOL outcome measure for refractive surgery would contain broad content, be developed and validated with Rasch analysis and have valid linear scoring, e.g., QIRC.

Acknowledgment

Konrad Pesudovs is supported by National Health and Medical Research Council (Canberra, Australia) Career Development Award 426765.

References

1. Bailey MD, Mitchell GL, Dhaliwal DK et al (2003) Patient satisfaction and visual symptoms after laser in situ keratomileusis. Ophthalmology 110:1371–1378
2. Ben-Sira A, Loewenstein A, Lipshitz I et al (1997) Patient satisfaction after 5.0-mm photorefractive keratectomy for myopia. J Refract Surg 13:129–134
3. Berry S, Mangione CM, Lindblad AS et al (2003) Development of the National Eye Institute refractive error correction quality of life questionnaire: focus groups. Ophthalmology 110:2285–2291
4. Brunette I, Gresset J, Boivin JF et al (2000) Functional outcome and satisfaction after photorefractive keratectomy. Part 2: survey of 690 patients. Ophthalmology 107:1790–1796
5. Garamendi E, Pesudovs K, Elliott DB (2005) Changes in quality of life after laser in situ keratomileusis for myopia. J Cataract Refract Surg 31:1537–1543
6. Hays RD, Mangione CM, Ellwein L et al (2003) Psychometric properties of the National Eye Institute-Refractive Error Quality of Life instrument. Ophthalmology 110:2292–2301
7. Hill JC (2002) An informal satisfaction survey of 200 patients after laser in situ keratomileusis. J Refract Surg 18:454–459
8. Lee J, Park K, Cho W et al (2005) Assessing the value of laser in situ keratomileusis by patient-reported outcomes using quality of life assessment. J Refract Surg 21:59–71
9. Likert RA (1932) A technique for the measurement of attitudes. Arch Psychol 140:1–55
10. Mangione CM, Phillips RS, Seddon JM et al (1992) Development of the "Activities of Daily Vision Scale." A measure of visual functional status. Med Care 30:1111–1126
11. Massof RW (2002) The measurement of vision disability. Optom Vis Sci 79:516–552
12. McDonnell PJ, Mangione C, Lee P et al (2003) Responsiveness of the National Eye Institute Refractive Error Quality of Life instrument to surgical correction of refractive error. Ophthalmology 110:2302–2309
13. McGhee CN, Craig JP, Sachdev N et al (2000) Functional, psychological, and satisfaction outcomes of laser in situ keratomileusis for high myopia. J Cataract Refract Surg 26:497–509
14. Nichols JJ, Twa MD, Mitchell GL (2005) Sensitivity of the National Eye Institute Refractive Error Quality of Life instrument to refractive surgery outcomes. J Cataract Refract Surg 31:2313–2318
15. Pesudovs K, Garamendi E, Elliott DB (2004) The Quality of Life Impact of Refractive Correction (QIRC) questionnaire: development and validation. Optom Vis Sci 81:769–777
16. Pesudovs K, Garamendi E, Elliott DB (2006) A quality of life comparison of people wearing spectacles or contact lenses or having undergone refractive surgery. J Refract Surg 22:19–27
17. Schein OD (2000) The measurement of patient-reported outcomes of refractive surgery: the refractive status and vision profile. Trans Am Ophthalmol Soc 98:439–469
18. Schein OD, Vitale S, Cassard SD et al (2001) Patient outcomes of refractive surgery. The refractive status and vision profile. J Cataract Refract Surg 27:665–673
19. Waring GO, 3rd (2000) Standard graphs for reporting refractive surgery. J Refract Surg 16:459–466
20. Wright BD, Masters GN (1982) Rating Scale Analysis. MESA Press, Chicago

Chapter 3

LASIK: Intraoperative (Flap) Complications

3

Contents

Core Messages

- A thin, irregular, or buttonhole flap is a significant complication of lamellar surgery that typically calls for aborting the case.

- Thin, irregular or buttonhole flaps can occur with all keratomes, including the new femtosecond devices.

- The cause of a thin, irregular, or buttonhole flap is often unclear and can be multifactorial.

- Causes of a thin, irregular, or buttonhole flap may include low pressure, poor corneal lubrication, poor blade quality, preexisting corneal pathology, or a keratome malfunction.

- Most thin, irregular, or buttonhole flap cases can be redone with either LASIK or PRK and do have a good prognosis.

- Remember, the key when faced with a poor flap typically is not to ablate.

3.1 Thin, Irregular, Buttonhole Flaps
Stephen G. Slade

Many of the serious complications of laser assisted in situ keratomileusis (LASIK) are related to the use of the keratome. In this chapter, we will at the causes, prevention, diagnosis, and treatment of thin, irregular, or buttonhole flaps of poor quality or "poor-quality flaps." These poor-quality flaps are a significant concern with lamellar surgery, for example, the incidence of buttonhole flaps using a mechanical microkeratome ranges between 0.3 and 2.6% of general LASIK procedures [1]. The incidence with the femtosecond laser seems lower. No buttonhole flaps were reported during the clinical evaluation of the IntraLase® FS laser. To date, IntraLase has received one confirmed buttonhole flap report out of 873,777 procedures performed. This represents an incidence of 0.0001%. This is still serious, as various sources state that of all of the flap complications, the occurrence of a buttonhole flap is the most likely to result in a poor refractive outcome, if not managed properly (Fig. 3.1.1).

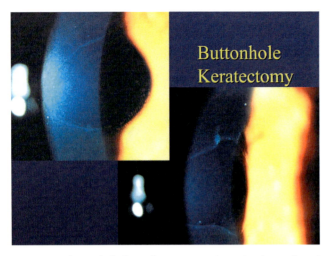

Fig. 3.1.1 A buttonhole flap is shown in two views, this donut-shaped flap has an "island" of uncut cornea directly over the pupil

3.1.2 Causes

Complications due to poor keratectomy can cause major visual problems. Keratectomies can be incomplete, decentered, or uneven. An incomplete keratectomy is usually caused by a suction break. It is critical to have good suction for the duration of the keratome pass. If the keratome stops before the pass is complete, then there might not be room to place the ablation. The keratectomy can be extended by hand but will not be of the same quality of the microkeratome section. A bad or damaged blade can cause a grossly irregular keratectomy.

Poor-quality flaps are mainly related to metal microkeratomes but, as reported above, may also occur with femtosecond laser keratomes. During creation of the corneal flap using the IntraLASIK procedure, the flap may be cut, leaving a hole in the center or mid-periphery of the flap. This irregular cut is similar to a "buttonhole" or donut-shaped flap that can occur with a mechanical keratectomy. The buttonhole flap is created when the focus of the laser beam begins the cut at the desired depth in the stroma but breaks through the surface of the epithelium at some position in the flap, and then returns to the stroma. This occurrence creates a flap with a "donut hole" or "buttonhole" in the flap. Buttonhole flaps can be caused by one or more of the following factors in IntraLase procedures:

- Attempted creation of very thin corneal flap (<100 μm)
- Poor applanation with contact glass
- Patient movement during the procedure

In summary, poor-quality flaps can be caused by one or more of the following factors in mechanical keratectomies:

- Loss of suction during the transverse cut
- Patient cornea steeper than 46 D prior to surgery [2]

- Low or reduction in patient intraocular pressure [2]
- Poor lubrication of the corneal surface or keratome malfunction
- Excess tissue being compressed beyond applanation by the keratome foot plate, causing buckling of the cornea [3]

3.1.3 Diagnosis

A poor-quality flap should be suspected whenever the keratome cut does not proceed as expected. A buttonhole or thin flap often can be seen without manipulating the flap at all. Sometimes allowing the corneal surface to dry slightly or wiping off the tear film will reveal the edges of a buttonhole, for example. If the diagnosis is uncertain, then carefully inspect the flap. Always use caution in lifting such a flap. Buttonhole flaps can be incomplete with a continuous layer of epithelium overlying the hole in Bowman's.

One advantage of diagnosing a poor-quality flap with the femtosecond laser is that a poor-quality flap can often be seen during its creation as discussed below (Fig. 3.1.2).

3.1.4 Prevention

The inspection, set-up, and preoperative testing of these instruments are critical. Careful attention to minute detail is essential to minimize and avoid potential complications, as well as to obtaining an excellent flap. Exposure is also vital to the keratectomy. This is largely dependent on orbital anatomy. The deep-set eye with an overhanging brow is best avoided in early cases. Proper anesthesia and sedation will aid in achieving good exposure. The main goal is to

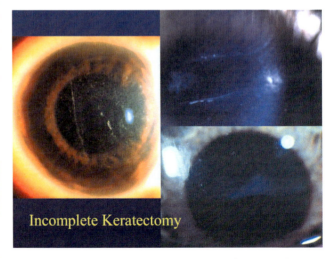

Fig. 3.1.2 Three incomplete flaps are shown. Left a partial flap with the hinge in the pupil space, right top a strip of uncut cornea directly over the visual axis caused by debris on the blade, and right bottom a hemi-flap with the entire bottom half of the cornea uncut due to a damaged blade

provide a clear path and gear track. Fluid management is important to avoid a false meniscus in the measurement of the cap diameter and intraocular pressure (IOP). The cornea should be wet for the pass, but a little dry for the applanation. Always take a moment to inspect the eye before the placement of the suction ring. There should be no chemosis, and the pupil should be centered between the speculum. If chemosis is present, then the fluid should be milk out with curved tiers down beneath the lid speculum. A speculum that provides maximum exposure with reasonable patient comfort is desirable. The pupil should be constricted only with the light from the microscope. Again, the case should be set up for maximum exposure; good suction must be present, good centration, a slow, controlled pass of the keratome, and a sharp, accurate blade. The keratome must be checked for smooth operation, a perfect blade, and a good suction sterile field and overall clean technique must be used.

The femtosecond laser offers a unique advantage to the prevention of complications from poor-quality flaps. Quite often, a poor-quality flap can be actually detected during the creation of the flap with a femtosecond laser. This is because the flap takes longer to create (20 s vs. 6 s), and the flap is visible at all times during the procedure. With experience, a thin flap or buttonhole flap can be seen in its creation and the procedure stopped.

Of course, avoidance and awareness of patients at risk is the best way to prevent flap complications. Patients with the following conditions may be more prone to experiencing flap quality complications:

- History of collagen vascular disease
- Patient cornea steeper than 46 D prior to surgery
- Conjunctival scarring after prior ocular surgery
- Previous incisional keratotomy

- Prior ocular, specifically cornea injury
- History of keratoconus
- Previous scleral buckling surgery
- Patient with unusually thick epithelial layer (>90 μm)

3.1.5 Treatment

Clinical concerns when dealing with poor-quality flaps include the potential for epithelial cells to infiltrate the stroma, causing epithelial ingrowth in the central axis. This may result in corneal scarring in the visual field, affecting visual acuity. In addition, invasive epithelial ingrowth can lead to more severe complications, such as stromal melt.

If a keratectomy has an irregular surface, then there is an important safety feature of lamellar surgery that should be well known by now. No matter how irregular the surface of the bed might be, there is a perfect match in the underside of the flap. Therefore, if the flap is simply replaced the patient will return to the preoperative refraction and best-corrected vision by the next morning. The femtosecond laser is even friendlier in this regard, in that the flap is held

in place by the microtissue bridges of uncut stroma. These "tags" hold the flap in place so that once the diagnosis is made, the flap is securely attached and can be allowed to wait until a retreatment is advisable. The advantage is that the epithelium and Bowman's is cut last with a femtosecond laser so the procedure may be aborted, leaving epithelium and Bowman's intact. Problems are created when the bed is altered with an attempted ablation such that the flap no longer matches. This is important to remember with incomplete resections also. When in doubt, put the flap back and do not ablate. One of the more pleasant features of lamellar surgery is that the eye can be back to the exact preoperative state the next day, and then reoperated on in the next few weeks or months depending on the situation. If an incomplete resection is present and there is room for the ablation, then one can proceed.

With resections that stop short of the needed diameter, surgeons have extended the flap by hand; but this is dangerous and will not give as smooth as a surface as the microkeratome (Fig. 3.1.3). Remember that incomplete resections can also be caused by a blade that has been damaged, dulling the cutting edge so that a lunette, vertically incomplete resection is produced. With severe suction breaks and very small eccentric resections never attempt to ablate, just try to replace the cap as best as possible.

To avoid loss of best-corrected visual acuity (BCVA), it is recommended that the ablation portion of the procedure be cancelled and the corneal flap replaced to its original position. If it is apparent during the IntraLase cut itself that a buttonhole is forming, then the procedure should be terminated at once. The advantage of the IntraLase in this situation is that the epithelium will remain uncut and the potential flap undisturbed. In this case, the flap should not be lifted or explored. In order to minimize epithelial ingrowth, some surgeons prefer to remove the epithelium from the central button or island of Bowman's membrane [4]. Again, *ablation should not be performed.* Usually, a bandage lens is placed over the buttonhole flap. A deeper flap may be cut again (20–60 μm deeper) approximately 3–6 months later, once BCVA returns, and the refraction is stable. Some surgeons advocate scraping the epithelium and performing photorefractive keratectomy (PRK) laser ablation. However, this procedure "may not be feasible in higher myopes due to the appearance of subepithelial haze" [5]. Many surgeons feel that any ablation over a flap does carry a higher risk of haze, and should be covered with mitomycin.

Take-Home Pearls
- Identify patients at risk for flap complications.
- Carefully set up and review your microkeratome, laser, and surgical protocol.
- Be aware of these complications and suspect them in any uncertain situation.
- Do not ablate a poor quality bed.

Poor-quality flaps can be caused by one or more of multiple conditions that are patient-related, surgeon related, and/or

3

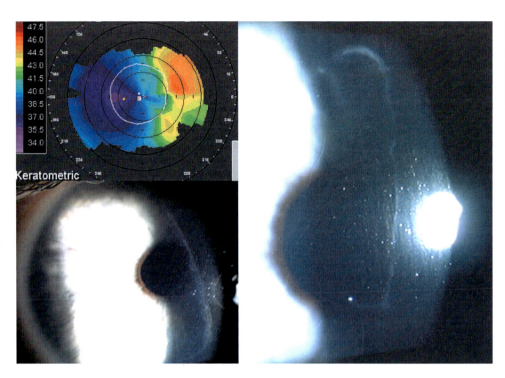

equipment related. Regardless of the cause, a thin, irregular, or buttonhole flap has a higher potential to cause or contribute to a sight-threatening outcome than do many other flap complications. These complications would be corneal scarring in the central visual axis, and/or severe epithelial ingrowth, with possible corneal melting of tissue.

It would be expected that the surgeon might need to perform additional medical and or surgical interventions, such as the removal of epithelial tissue from the central island or Bowman's membrane in order to prevent severe epithelial ingrowth. In some cases, the surgeon may choose to perform a PRK procedure to smooth any corneal irregularities that have developed postoperatively. Other interventions may include scraping of tissue from the central island or Bowman's membrane or suturing of the flap to secure its position. Luckily, these flap complications are largely manageable with careful attention to patients at risk, cautious flap inspection, and willingness to abort the planned ablation.

References

1. Leung ATS, Rao SK, Cheng ACK et al (2000) Pathogenesis and management of laser in situ keratomileusis flap buttonhole. J Cataract Refract Surg 26:358–362
2. Ambrosio R Jr, Wilson SE (2001) Complications of laser in situ keratomileusis: etiology, prevention, and treatment. J Refract Surg 17:350–379
3. Gimbel HV, Anderson Penno EE, van Westenbrugge JA et al (1998) Incidence and management of intraoperative and early postoperative complications in 1000 consecutive laser in situ keratomileusis cases. Ophthalmology 105:1839–1847
4. Updegraff SA, Kritzinger MS (2000) Laser in situ keratomileusis technique. Curr Opin Ophthalmol 11:267–272
5. Melki SA, Azar DT (2001) LASIK complications: etiology, management, and prevention. Surv Ophthalmol 46:95–116

Core Messages

■ An incomplete LASIK flap results from premature stopping of the microkeratome head before reaching the intended hinge position. This is commonly due to mechanical obstacles such as drapes, lashes, or loose epithelium. Microkeratome malfunction or facial features of the patient, such as deep-seated eyes or tight lids, may also play a role.

■ Skilled surgeons have had a much lower incidence of incomplete flaps.

■ Incomplete flaps are best managed by repositioning the flap, postponing the procedure, and considering another intervention later on.

■ Delayed management consists of one of two options, repeating the microkeratome pass or doing surface ablation (PRK or LASEK). The best option depends on the etiology of the original problem.

3.2 Incomplete LASIK Flap

Helen K. Wu and Waleed A. Allam

3.2.1 Introduction

Laser in situ keratomileusis (LASIK) is currently the refractive surgery procedure of choice for most patients with low-to-moderate refractive errors [13]. Thanks to the lamellar corneal flap, LASIK offers rapid visual recovery and minimal postoperative discomfort to the patient, as well as refractive stability and good long-term results. However, creation of the corneal flap is the single most important step in LASIK [8], and flap-related complications occur in as many as 5% of cases [16].

Complications such as free flaps, incomplete flaps, buttonholes, decentered flaps, irregular flap edges, irregular stromal surface, and epithelial abrasions have been reported to affect the visual and refractive outcomes of the procedure and may cause loss of best-corrected visual acuity (BCVA) [16]. Such complications could be serious, especially given the elective nature of LASIK.

Incomplete flaps occur due to premature stopping of the microkeratome head before reaching the intended hinge location. Visual aberrations are more likely to occur when the created hinge results in scarring in proximity to the visual axis [11].

3.2.2 Incidence

Several studies have investigated the incidence of incomplete flap formation with overall incidence ranging between 0.3% [9] and 1.2% [4].

The variation in incomplete flap incidence from one center to another and from one surgeon to another depends on many factors, such as the surgeon's experience and the type of microkeratome used. Unlike other flap-related complications such as buttonholes, thin flaps, and free caps, which result mainly from a combination of anatomical and mechanical factors, incomplete flap occurrence is highly related to the surgeon's own experience (i.e., experienced LASIK surgeons have had a much lower incidence of incomplete flaps than have novice surgeons) [4].

In addition to surgeon experience, another factor affecting the incidence of incomplete flaps is the type of microkeratome used for flap creation. Even with the marked improvements in the newer microkeratome designs, there is still a small but real risk for such types of complications. The use of the femtosecond laser (IntraLase) in the creation of LASIK flaps may reduce the occurrence of incomplete flaps and other flap-related complications [1, 3, 7, 15]; however, even with this technology, incomplete flaps can occur due to suction loss or inappropriate energy and flap settings.

3.2.3 Etiology

Many factors are responsible for the occurrence of incomplete flaps during LASIK. The most common cause of incomplete flaps is jamming of the microkeratome due to either electrical failure or mechanical obstacles. Lashes, drapes, loose epithelium, and precipitated salt from the irrigating solution have been recognized as possible impediments to smooth microkeratome head progress [11].

Less common causes may include suction loss during the microkeratome pass and gear-advancement mechanism jams [11].

3.2.4 Management

3.2.4.1 Immediate Measures

In cases of incomplete flap where there is sufficient surface area in the stromal bed for laser ablation, using a reasonable ablation zone, the procedure can be completed as usual.

In other cases with a small stromal bed with inadequate room for ablation, management is best accomplished by immediate careful repositioning of the partial flap and postponing the procedure. Topical antibiotic and steroid drops should be started immediately. Patients must be followed up regularly until the refractive error is stabilized, and then a second intervention may be performed.

Applying excimer laser treatment to an inadequate stromal bed with a short or incomplete flap is contraindicated. Serious visual and refractive complications may take place, such as irregular astigmatism leading to loss of BCVA, monocular diplopia, and distorted vision, especially at night [5].

If the hinge is beyond the visual axis and the stromal bed is still smaller than intended, then some surgeons consider

3

manual dissection of the flap using a blade to advance it to the intended position. However, this technique is risky and many complications may occur, such as an irregular stromal bed and flap edge, and buttonholing of the flap.

Other surgeons prefer an immediate second microkeratome pass to advance the flap to the intended position [6]. Careful inspection of the microkeratome should be performed to exclude any mechanical dysfunction, inadequate suction, or any obstacles before considering this procedure. However, this technique carries the risk of flap maceration and bileveled stromal bed.

3.2.4.2 Delayed Management

There are two main options for the second intervention in cases of incomplete flaps. First, the microkeratome pass may be repeated after a period. Second, surface ablation may be performed over the abnormal flap by utilizing either photorefractive keratectomy (PRK) or laser subepithelial keratomileusis (LASEK).

There is no widespread agreement among surgeons regarding the appropriate time interval between the primary procedure and the second intervention. Waiting for long periods may be intolerable for the patient, especially in the presence of anisometropia and/or contact lens intolerance. On the other hand, applying excimer laser treatment immediately to the surface of the flap was reported to induce marked subepithelial fibrosis manifesting clinically as haze [10]. Some surgeons [18] recommend an interval of at least 2 weeks prior to performing PRK as a second procedure, so that the epithelial surface will be adequately healed with less irregularity. A minimum of 3 months should be allowed after the initial procedure before considering a second microkeratome pass [14].

Generally, a second intervention is recommended as soon as a consistent refraction and stable flap are obtained. This may range from 2 weeks up to 6 months [17].

Repeating the microkeratome pass carries significant risks and disadvantages. The main risk resides in the possibility of the new microkeratome cut intersecting with the initial one, leading to formation of stromal fragments, with the potential loss of corneal tissue and subsequent irregular astigmatism. When contemplating this maneuver as a second intervention, larger and deeper flaps should be considered. Also, the initial cause that led to the incomplete flap must be ascertained and corrected before attempting the new procedure; otherwise the problem may be repeated [12].

Phototherapeutic keratectomy (PTK) combined with PRK, as described by Wilson [18], is strongly recommended as a second intervention in cases of incomplete flaps. The advantages of such a procedure are a shorter time interval before the second procedure, avoidance of a second microkeratome pass with its potential risks, and the ability to concomitantly treat corneal surface irregularities. This procedure can be carried out 2–4 weeks after the primary procedure. Longer intervals may be associated with a higher incidence of subepithelial fibrosis and haze formation.

However, adjunctive application of mitomycin C (MMC), an antimetabolite agent, has been described to be successful in minimizing corneal haze associated with refractive surgery [2].

Transepithelial PTK aims at treating corneal irregularities as well as removing the corneal epithelium, without the need for vigorous manual scraping that may dislodge the abnormal and unstable corneal flap. The PRK treatment nomogram should include a reduction in the spherical element of the intended correction by approximately 10% to account for the weak healing response induced by the no-touch PTK technique used to remove the epithelium [18]. However, this nomogram should be modified to offset 20–50% of the intended treatment if further stromal PTK is to be performed in cases with corneal irregularities. The aim of this offset is to compensate for the additional corneal flattening and consequent hyperopic shift from PTK [12].

After performing laser treatment, MMC 0.02% (0.2 mg/ml) is applied to the central 6 mm of the cornea with a 6-mm circular sponge for 2 min, after which it is thoroughly irrigated. Care should be taken to avoid limbal and scleral exposure to MMC [12].

Another method to remove the corneal epithelium that can be used in cases without marked corneal irregularity is to use a 20% ethyl alcohol solution for 20–25 s. This helps facilitate removal of the epithelium with less likelihood of flap dislodgement [17]. LASEK may also be used as long as the LASEK flap hinge is opposite the original LASIK flap hinge position, so that the original LASIK flap is not disturbed.

3.2.5 Prevention

As with all refractive surgery complications, the prevention of the problem is preferable to the treatment. Securing a safe path for the microkeratome head is the most important measure to prevent an incomplete flap. This can be achieved by proper draping in a way that prevents the lashes or lids from obstructing the path and using an adjustable eyelid speculum (such as the Lieberman speculum) instead of a wire one, such as the Barraquer wire speculum. Gentle lifting of the globe after suction activation helps in clearing the keratome head path away from the bony orbital margins, especially in persons with deep-seated eyes.

Another critical step that should be done before starting the procedure is careful cleaning and inspection of the microkeratome head and gear system. The whole system should be tested before application to the patient's eye.

The possibility of suction loss must be ruled out by verifying adequate IOP before starting corneal flap creation. This should be done with a tonometer, such as the Barraquer tonometer. Also, subtle clinical signs, such as dilation of the pupil, and symptoms of dimming of vision, confirm the presence of sufficiently elevated IOP to create an adequate flap.

Recently, the use of the femtosecond laser in flap creation has been proven safer and more predictable than the mechanical microkeratomes, with reduction in the incidence of intraoperative flap complications [1, 3, 7, 15].

Take Home Pearls

■ As with other LASIK complications, prevention is preferable to treatment. Preventive measures include securing a wide and safe path for the microkeratome head until it reaches the intended hinge position by careful draping, using adjustable specula in patients with tight eyelids, and gently lifting the globe after suction activation.

■ Always test your microkeratome prior to application to the patient's eye. Confirm that suction is sufficient by use of a tonometer, as well as confirming the concomitant symptoms and signs of dimming of vision and pupil dilation.

■ Never proceed to laser ablation unless you have adequate stromal exposure to result in an ablation with a sufficient optical zone.

■ Wait for a stable refraction before the second intervention.

■ If a second microkeratome pass is chosen, then it should be at a deeper level and with larger flap diameter than the first attempt.

■ If surface ablation is chosen, MMC 0.02% (0.2 mg/ml) should be applied after the ablation for up to 2 min to reduce haze and scarring. A reduction in the amount of treatment also must be considered to compensate for the diminished healing response due to MMC and the hyperopic shift associated with PTK.

References

1. Binder PS (2006) One thousand consecutive IntraLase laser in situ keratomileusis flaps. J Cataract Refract Surg 32:962–969
2. Carones F, Vigo L, Scandola E et al (2002) Evaluation of the prophylactic use of mitomycin-C to inhibit haze formation after photorefractive keratectomy. J Cataract Refract Surg 28:2088–2095
3. Durrie DS, Kezirian GM (2005) Femtosecond laser versus mechanical keratome flaps in wavefront-guided laser in situ ker-
atomileusis: prospective contralateral eye study. J Cataract Refract Surg 31:120–126
4. Gimbel HV, Penno EE, van Westenbrugge JA et al (1998) Incidence and management of intraoperative and early postoperative complications in 1000 consecutive laser in situ keratomileusis cases. Ophthalmology 105:1839–1847
5. Holland SP, Srivannaboon S, Reinstein DZ (2000) Avoiding serious corneal complications of laser assisted in situ keratomileusis and photorefractive keratectomy 107:640–652
6. Katsanevaki VJ, Tsiklis NS, Astyrakakis NI et al (2005) Intraoperative management of partial flap during LASIK. Ophthalmology 112:1710–1713
7. Kezirian GM, Stonecipher KG (2004) Comparison of the IntraLase femtosecond laser and mechanical keratomes for laser in situ keratomileusis. J Cataract Refract Surg 30:804–811
8. Lim T, Yang S, Kim M et al (2006) Comparison of the IntraLase femtosecond laser and mechanical microkeratome for laser in situ keratomileusis. Am J Ophthalmol 141:833–839
9. Lin RT, Maloney RK (1999) Flap complications associated with lamellar refractive surgery. Am J Ophthalmol 127:129–136
10. Majmudar PA, Forstot SL, Dennis RF et al (2000) Topical mitomycin-C for subepithelial fibrosis after corneal refractive surgery. Ophthalmology 107:89–94
11. Melki SA, Azar DT (2001) LASIK complications: etiology, management, and prevention. Surv Ophthalmol 46:95–116
12. Muller LT, Candal EM, Epstein RJ et al (2005) Transepithelial phototherapeutic keratectomy/ photorefractive keratectomy with adjunctive mitomycin-C for complicated LASIK flaps. J Cataract Refract Surg 31:291–296
13. Schwartz GS, Park DH, Lane SS (2005) CustomCornea wavefront retreatment after conventional laser in situ keratomileusis. J Cataract Refract Surg 31:1502–1505
14. Slade SG (1996) LASIK complications. In: Machatt JJ (ed) Excimer laser refractive surgery. Practice and principles. Slack, Thorofare, N.J., pp 360–368
15. Stonecipher K, Ignacio TS, Stonecipher M (2006) Advances in refractive surgery: microkeratome and femtosecond flap creation in relation to safety, efficacy, predictability, and biomechanical stability. Curr Opin Ophthalmol 17:368–372
16. Stulting RD, Carr JD, Thompson KP et al (1999) Complications of laser in situ keratomileusis for the correction of myopia. Ophthalmology 106:13–20
17. Weisenthal RW, Salz J, Sugar A et al (2003) Photorefractive keratectomy for treatment of flap complications in laser in situ keratomileusis. Cornea 22(5):399–404
18. Wilson SA (2001) Transepithelial PRK/PTK for treatment of donut-shaped flaps in LASIK. Refract Surg Outlook Summer 2001.

Core Messages

■ Is free flap really a complication, or just an inconvenience?

■ Try to avoid or prevent free flap. Be careful with flat corneas.

3.3 Dislocated Flaps: How to Solve Free Flaps with No Marks or Flap Malposition
Julio Baviera

3.3.1 Introduction

Although most refractive surgeons consider the appearance of a free flap during laser in situ keratomileusis (LASIK) surgery a complication, this should not be the case. Free

3

flap is part of the history [1–3] of the LASIK procedure as we know it today.

In a retrospective study of 70 patients with free flap in one eye and a nasally hinged flap in the fellow eye, we did not find statistically significant differences in efficacy, safety, predictability, or percentage of enhancements between one eye and the other (Eleftheriadis et al., unpublished).

More than a complication, free flap should be considered an inconvenience that slows the procedure and forces the surgeon to manage the flap more delicately and meticulously. However, a simple inconvenience can become a serious complication when the surgeon loses the flap reference marks, or if they have not been made correctly. This can happen for several reasons.

Situation 1: The marks, which are made using ink on the corneal epithelium, are erased. This happens when the ink marks are too superficial, when surgery has gone on too long, or when there has been a total dislocation of the flap after the procedure during the postoperative rest.

Situation 2: The marks are outside the flap (Fig. 3.3.1). This happens when the marks are made on the sclerocorneal limbus, but are too peripheral, with minimal entry into the center of the cornea. The free flap, which now has a smaller diameter than expected, lies within the marks and is not crossed by them.

Situation 3: The marks lie totally within the free flap. This is very uncommon. It occurs in eyes with a reduced corneal diameter in which the ink marks fall completely within the free flap and do not cross the sclerocorneal limbus (Fig. 3.3.2).

Situation 4: The marks are symmetrical with respect to the radius of the cornea in such a way that when the flap is lifted, they do not form a distinct mirror image, and we are not capable of distinguishing by the marks whether the flap is correctly repositioned or not (stroma vs. stroma)

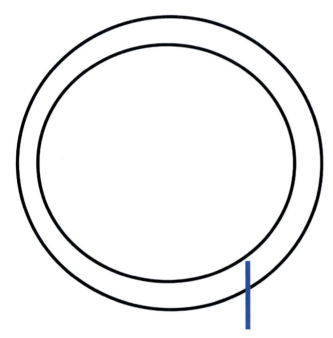

Fig. 3.3.1 The mark does not reach the edge of the flap, and remains completely outside

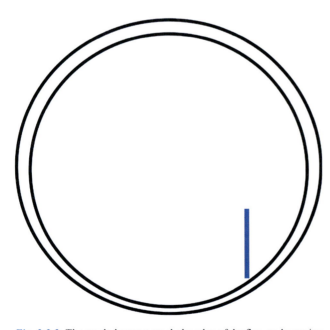

Fig. 3.3.2 The mark does not reach the edge of the flap, and remains completely inside

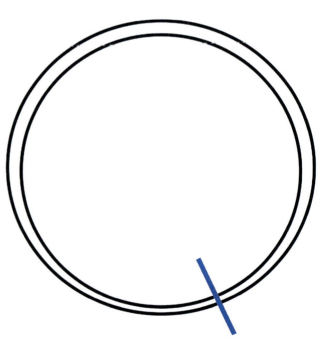

Fig. 3.3.3 When the free flap is repositioned, the mark continues to be observed thanks to the transparency of the flap. As it is radial, the flap fits regardless of whether it is repositioned correctly (stroma vs. stroma) or whether it is repositioned inversely (epithelium vs. stroma)

(Fig. 3.3.3). It may seem strange that it is difficult to distinguish the epithelial side, but it can happen, especially if the stroma has been hydrated. If this situation coincides with marks such as those in Fig. 3.3.3, then we could reposition the flap inversely with the subsequent lack of adherence and the risk of loss of the flap.

3.3.2 Prevention

Situation 1 (the marks are erased): Once the free flap has been obtained, our first systematic maneuver should be to reposition the flap correctly and accurately on the stromal bed by making the visible parts of the original marks coincide. Next, we should always make new marks with ink,

or better still, inerasable marks. These can be made at 12 o'clock using a 300-μm precalibrated knife, as is the case in radial keratotomy. It would be necessary to carry out a peripheral mini-keratotomy, ideally slanting, within the area of the flap, crossing its thickness and penetrating the stromal bed without perforating it. This inerasable mark, which is our standard practice in the case of a free flap, allows us to reposition the flap if all the ink marks are subsequently erased (Fig. 3.3.4).

Situations 2 and 3 (the marks are inside or outside the flap): The best approach is to prevent this situation by making marks that clearly cross the sclerocorneal limbus centrifugally and also approach the center of the cornea enough to allow the situation to be avoided (Fig. 3.3.5). If we do not

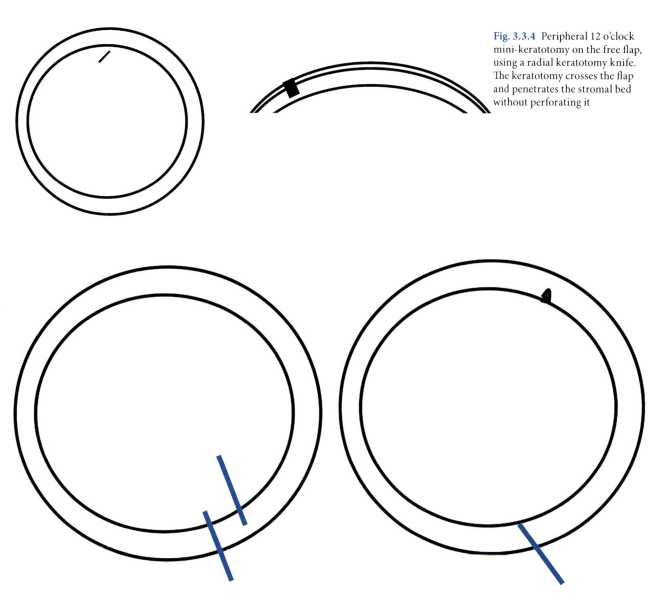

Fig. 3.3.4 Peripheral 12 o'clock mini-keratotomy on the free flap, using a radial keratotomy knife. The keratotomy crosses the flap and penetrates the stromal bed without perforating it

Fig. 3.3.5 Making two marks, one more central and the other more peripheral, guarantees us that, in any case, the edge of the flap will be crossed by one of them

Fig. 3.3.6 Repositioning of a free flap from which the mark has been excluded using a small epithelial notch on the edge of the flap, at 1 o'clock, which coincides with its negative image on the cut receptor edge

3

take this precaution, and the marks are inside or outside the flap, we must try to reposition it correctly, using even the smallest physical details on the edge of the flap, which must coincide with the negative image of the peripheral edge of the cut bed (Fig. 3.3.6). This is often very difficult, as the primary flaps are very regular with perfect edges (this is completely different from LASIK enhancement, with irregularly edged flaps, which are very easy to fit). Once the flap is perfectly repositioned, we should make the new marks (as in situation 1) before performing the laser ablation.

Situation 4 (symmetrical marks): The best prevention is to make the marks in such a way that, when the flap is repositioned inversely, non-coinciding marks are observed between the flap and the peripheral cornea (Fig. 3.3.7). If we do not take this precaution and this situation arises, then we must take the time necessary to reposition the flap safely and correctly (stroma vs. stroma). The patient must be kept under observation until we are completely sure that the flap has been correctly repositioned.

3.3.3 Experience

In our multicenter experience (the Baviera Clinic has 19 surgical centers in Spain), and out of a total of 132,980 LASIK procedures performed from January 2003 until July 2006, the number of free flaps was 1,738 (1.31%). Of these, we found six cases of free flap with loss of marks. The Moria-One microkeratome and Technolas 217 excimer laser from Bausch & Lomb were used in all cases.

Case 1 (situation 4, symmetrical marks): For a 45-year-old woman with refraction in OD (right eye) –2.5 sph(erical) + 3.75 cyl(indrical) × 110°, visual acuity (VA) = 20/20, LASIK was programmed in this eye for –1 D (monovision). A free

flap was obtained using a single circular ink mark. When the free flap was withdrawn from the head of the microkeratome, the surgeon lost the orientation on the epithelial/stromal side of the flap and, during repositioning, the only circular mark made did not allow the flap to be repositioned on the correct side. Finally, and without the help of the mark, the correct orientation was found.

Result: *–1 sph + 0.5 cyl × 20°, VA = 20/20*

Case 2 (situation 2, marks outside the flap): For a 47-year-old woman with –7.5 sph in OS (left eye), VA = 20/20, LASIK was programmed in this eye for –1.25 D (monovision). The free flap obtained did not include marks. The surgeon, with some difficulty, repositioned the flap using the small details of the epithelial edge.

Result: *–1.75 sph + 0.25cyl × 170, VA = 20/20*

Cases 3, 4, 5, and 6 (situation 1, erased marks): The marks were erased, and the flap was not repositioned correctly, leading to mixed astigmatism caused by the rotation of the flap.

3.3.4 Free-Flap Rotation Study

Theoretically, a free flap has parallel faces that are the result of a perfect cut, leaving a flap with a uniform thickness. If this were 100% true, then there would be no optical effects. The rotation of the flap would be similar to the rotation on the eye of a therapeutic contact lens with neutral dioptric power. However, it is virtually impossible to obtain a flap with these characteristics. The flap is usually thinner at the beginning and gradually becomes thicker at the center as the microkeratome advances, in the same way as a radial keratotomy knife that makes shallower cuts at the beginning (beach effect).

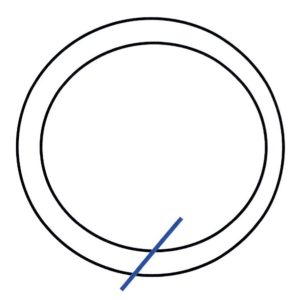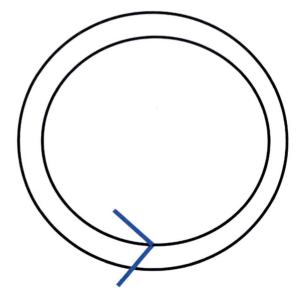

Fig. 3.3.7 As it is not radial, the mark forms a distinguishable non coincident mirror image when the flap is repositioned inversely (epithelium vs. stroma)

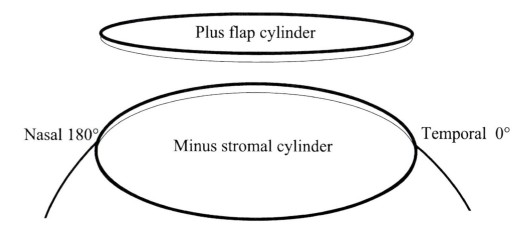

Fig. 3.3.8 Consequence of an irregular microkeratome cut. This leads to a thicker flap in the center and a thinner one at the periphery (*plus cylinder*). The stromal bed contains the negative image of the flap (*minus cylinder*)

0°	**−0.25 +0.5 × 45°**	100°	−3 +6 × 96°
10°	−0.75 +1.5 × 50°	110°	−3 +5.75 × 100°
20°	−1.25 +2.5 × 57°	120°	−2.75 +5.25 × 104°
30°	−1.5 +3 × 62°	130°	−2.5 +4.75 × 111°
40°	−2 +3.75 × 67°	140°	−2 +4 × 116°
50°	−2.25 +4.5 × 70°	150°	−1.75 +3.25 × 118°
60°	−2.5 +5.25 × 75°	160°	−1.25 +2.25 × 126°
70°	−2.75 +5.5 × 80°	170°	−0.75 +1.5 × 132°
80°	−3 +6 × 87°	**180°**	**−0.25 +0.5 × 135°**
90°	**−3 +6 × 90°**		

Fig. 3.3.9 Readings obtained from an auto lens meter after turning in 10° steps a plus-power glass cylinder with +3 D, on a minus-power glass cylinder with −3 D fixed on an axis of 180°. Maximum induced astigmatism when they cross at 90°, and minimum when they cross at 0 or 180°

So as not to complicate the reasoning, if we suppose that the flap once again becomes thinner at the end of the cut, when the blade leaves the eye, we will obtain a flap that behaves optically like a plus-power cylindrical lens, with its axis at 90° and power at 0° (microkeratome pass along the 0–180° axis). Logically, the resulting corneal bed would be the negative image of the flap, and would behave like a minus-power cylinder of the same power and axis (Fig. 3.3.8). If the flap was reset in its original position, then both cylinders would balance and the optic result would be neutral.

Now, if, due to loss of the marks, the cylinders do not fit back into their original position, then we have crossed cylinders in which the plus-power cylinder (flap) has rotated on the minus-power cylinder (corneal bed), resulting in mixed astigmatism with a neutral spherical equivalent, and whose axis and power depend on the angle of rotation, and the power of the cylinders provided by the cut of the microkeratome. Figure 3.3.9 shows the mixed astigmatisms resulting from rotating a plus-power lens cylinder of +3 D on

a minus-power lens cylinder of −3 D fixed at 180°. In the figure, we can see how the induced astigmatism is minimum or non-existent when the axis of both cylinders coincides and maximum when they cross at 90°.

If we assume that the laser ablation has not induced astigmatism, and that it has eliminated any preexisting astigmatism, then the astigmatism that appears after an undesired rotation of the flap would be a consequence of this bicylindrical effect between the flap and the corneal bed.

According to Rubin [4], the bisector of the cylinders that have rotated on one another coincides with the bisector formed between the steep and flat axes of the refractive mixed astigmatism resulting from the rotation. Therefore, the steep axis of the resulting refractive astigmatism would be at 45° counterclockwise of the bisector formed by the two cylinders that have rotated on one another (Fig. 3.3.10).

We could derive the following formula: postoperative axis (in plus cyl) = initial axis (MQ pass) + 45 + angle of flap rotation / 2. Thus: flap angle rotation = 2 × postoperative axis − 90.

- If the resulting value of the angle of flap rotation is positive, then we would consider the turn clockwise, and if it is negative, counterclockwise.
- If a microkeratome with an up–down cut was used, then the initial axis (MQ pass) would not be 0, but 90°, therefore the formula would be: flap angle rotation = 2 × postoperative axis −270.

Returning to our cases:

Case 3 (situation 1, loss of marks): For a 33-year-old woman with OD −2.25 sph, VA = 20/25, LASIK was programmed for emmetropia. A free flap was obtained on which the marks were erased.

Result at 6 weeks: *−2.25 sph + 4.25 cyl × 15°*

The following formula was applied: flap angle rotation = 2 × postoperative axis − 90° = 2 × 15 − 90 = −60.

As the sign was negative, the rotation was considered counterclockwise. The patient was taken into the operating room, and after the relevant ink marks were made on the

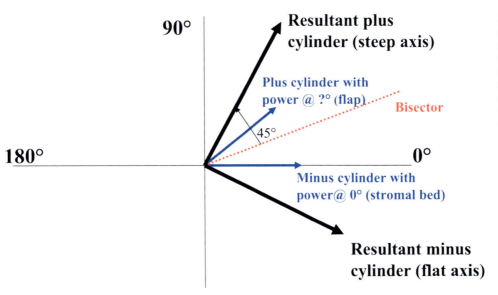

Fig. 3.3.10 Cross cylinders share the bisector with the flat and steep axes of the mixed astigmatism resulting from the turn of the first two. The resultant plus cylinder (*steep axis*) is at 45° counterclockwise from the bisector of the two cross cylinders

flap, it was lifted and turned 60° counterclockwise with the help of a 360° graduated ring.

> **Result after 4 weeks:** *neutral VA = 20/20*

Case 4 (situation 1, loss of marks): For a 30-year-old woman, OS −1 sph + 4 cyl × 75°, VA = 20/20, LASIK was programmed for emmetropia. A free flap was obtained on which the marks were erased.

> **Result at 5 weeks:** *−2 sph + 6 cyl × 4, VA = 20/30⁺*

The following formula was applied: flap angle rotation = 2 × postoperative axis − 90 = 2 × 4 − 90 = −82. As the sign was negative, rotation was considered counterclockwise. The patient was taken to the operating room, and after the relevant ink marks were made on the flap, it was lifted and turned 82° counterclockwise in the same way as the previous case (Figs. 3.3.11, 3.3.12).

> **Result:** *−0.75 sph + 1 cyl × 96,*
> *with improvement in VA to 20/20⁻*

Case 5 (situation 1, loss of marks): For a 40-year-old man, OS with −3.75 sph + 4.5 cyl × 75°, VA = 20/30⁻, LASIK was programmed for emmetropia. A free flap in which the marks were erased was obtained.

> **Result at 4 weeks:** *−1 sph + 2.75 cyl × 55°, VA = 20/30⁻*

If the following formula had been applied: flap angle rotation = 2 × postoperative axis − 90 = 2 × 55 − 90 = 20, then the flap would have had to be turned 20° clockwise. However, the surgeon chose to carry out an astigmatic keratotomy (AK) on the axis of 55°, with a 6-mm optic zone and 3 mm of cordal length.

> **Result after 2 months:**
> *+0.5 sph −0.5 cyl × 60°, VA = 20/25*

Case 6 (situation 1, loss of marks): For a 44-year-old woman, OD with −1.5 sph + 0.25 cyl × 137°, VA = 20/20,

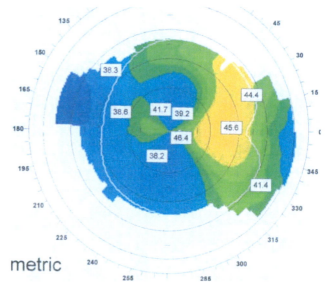

Fig. 3.3.11 Corneal topography shows the inverse astigmatism resulting from incorrect repositioning of the free flap

LASIK was programmed for emmetropia. The results was a free flap with loss of marks.

> **Result at 6 weeks:** *−1 sph +2.5 cyl × 57°, VA = 20/25⁻*

If the following formula had been applied: flap angle rotation = 2 × postoperative axis − 90 = 2 × 57 − 90 = 24, then the flap would have had to be turned 24° clockwise. Nevertheless, the surgeon chose to carry out LASIK enhancement.

> **Result:** *+ 0.5 cyl × 165°, VA = 20/20⁻*

A review of the literature revealed three similar cases reported by Hovanesian [5]. All three finished with induced

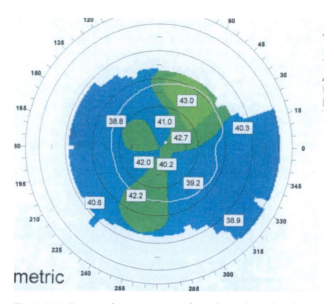

Fig. 3.3.12 Topographic appearance after solving the induced astigmatism by lifting and rotating the flap 82° counterclockwise

mixed astigmatism accompanied by a reduction in best-corrected visual acuity (BCVA). The cases were solved using rotation of the free flap and applying the formula described, although the third case needed a second rotation, which the authors attribute to the fact that the microkeratome did not pass exactly on the usual 0–180° axis.

In our experience, and taking into account cases 5 and 6, the astigmatism resulting from rotation of the flap due to loss of marks can be solved by conventional techniques such as AK or LASIK enhancement. Nevertheless, the best procedure for avoiding a new stromal ablation, and especially for correcting the problem where it occurs, is lifting of the flap and rotation based on the optical principle of astigmatism induced by the cross between two cylinders of the same power and opposite sign.

Core Messages

- Prevention of a distorted flap is mainly focused on prevention of patient eye rubbing early after surgery, but also includes reducing dry eye, especially in the first 3–4 h after the surgery.

- If a distorted flap occurs with significant striae early after the surgery, then lifting the flap and stretching striae works well in most cases.

- Late distortion of the flap may require other techniques including flap suturing or surface phototherapeutic keratectomy.

Take Home Pearls

- Make sufficiently long-lasting ink marks.

- Make marks sufficiently long, to allow the edge of the flap to be crossed by the marks.

- Make non-radial marks that are distinguishable in the event that the flap is repositioned inversely (epithelium vs. stroma).

- In the case of a free flap, reinforce the marks or even make stromal incisions.

- If the marks are lost completely, then try to reposition the free flap using the epithelial details from the edge of the flap.

- Inadequate repositioning (rotation) leads to mixed astigmatism, generally accompanied by reduced BCVA.

- Solve this astigmatism induced by rotation of the flap, using the optical genesis of the astigmatism induced by rotation of equal cylinders with opposite signs.

- Always pass the microkeratome on the same axis (0–180° or 90–270°), so that if there is rotation when repositioning the flap, then this can be corrected as described.

References

1. Barraquer JI, Generalidades sobre las técnicas quirúrgicas actuales. (1980) In: BarraquerJI, Queratomileusis y Queratofaquia. Litografía ARCO, Bogota, pp 97–100
2. Krumeich JH (1983) Indications, techniques and complications of myopic keratomileusis. Int Ophthalmol Clin 23:75–92
3. Buratto L, Ferrari M, Genisi C (1993) Keratomileusis for myopia with the excimer laser (Buratto technique): short-term results. Refract Corneal Surg 9(Suppl):S130–S133
4. Rubin ML (1971) Optics for Clinicians. Triad Scientific, Gainesville, Fla., pp 179–181
5. Hovanesian JA, Maloney RK (2005) Treating astigmatism after a free laser in situ keratomileusis cap by rotating the cap. J Cataract Refract Surg 31:1870–1876

3.4 Management of the Distorted Flap
David R. Hardten

3.4.1 Introduction

The low rate of complications with LASIK has driven patient acceptance of, as well as expectations with, this procedure. Most of the severe complications associated with the procedure are associated with the initial creation of the flap, although some are due to later manipulation of the corneal lamellar flap by the patient. Distortion, striae, or folds in the corneal flap are one of the most commonly encountered flap complications with LASIK. (Figs. 3.4.1, 3.4.2) The pres-

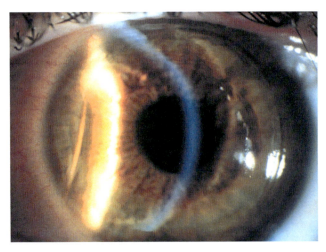

Fig. 3.4.1 Large striae in the flap with distortion of the flap. This patient inadvertently rubbed his eye on the first day after LASIK

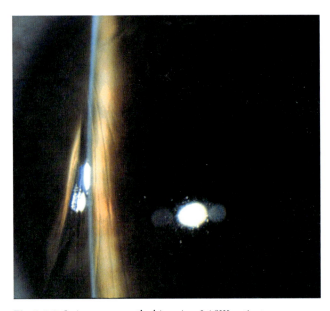

Fig. 3.4.2 Striae seen near the hinge in a LASIK patient

ence of this distortion can result in patient dissatisfaction due to quality of vision complaints, or even loss of BCVA.

3.4.2 Frequency

Distortion of the corneal flap has occurred in 1–4% of cases in reported studies [1–4]. Because striae can often be very mild or peripheral and may be subclinical and not noted by the patient or physician, these studies probably underreport the frequency of any visible striae. More severe striae can be associated with discomfort and very distorted vision and so are more easily detected. They may be more common in eyes with thicker or thinner flaps than average. They have even been reported after femtosecond laser flap

creation, and may be more common after keratoplasty, as the endothelial cell function is poor in the periphery [5, 6]. They become more difficult to manage in the presence of a free corneal cap, or when an epithelial defect is present.

3.4.3 Etiology and Prevention

Factors that increase the potential for flap striae can be present intraoperatively. If the flap becomes desiccated during the portion of the case when the flap is retracted back, then when the flap is replaced, it is contracted compared with its original state and can be difficult to reposition properly. Trying to maintain neutral hydration of the flap is important, as this may lessen the tendency toward flap distortion. If the flap is dehydrated prior to repositioning, taking extra care to rehydrate the flap with balanced saline solution, and then carefully stretching the flap so that the edge of the flap is in line with the gutter created by the microkeratome entry site should reduce the striae. (Figs. 3.3.3, 3.3.4, 3.3.5, 3.3.6) It may take time for the flap to stick well in the proper position, and the flap should be stretched until it no longer retracts out of position. This will occur when the interface tension between the flap and underlying stromal bed is greater than the retraction tension caused by the striae from dehydration. Similarly, if the flap is wrinkled due to intraoperative manipulation or initial misalignment intraoperatively during the initial case, this may result in flap irregularities. Immediate repositioning once this is identified intraoperatively makes permanent striae less likely to be an issue, and allows the flap to be repositioned with alignment of the gutter to flap interface.

Flap distortion may also occur after the procedure, such as during removal of the lid speculum or drapes, or if the patient rubs the eye or touches the eye with an eyedropper tip after surgery [4, 7, 8]. If the patient is looking straight ahead and tries not to squeeze the eyelids during speculum or drape removal, then this may reduce the incidence of flap dislocation during this stage of the surgery.

If the patient takes a long nap or goes a long time without lubrication postoperatively, then the lid may stick to the flap and cause distortion of the flap when the patient opens his/her eye. We usually have the patient try to nap no longer than 2 h postoperatively, without lubrication to reduce the frequency of this cause of a distorted flap. Patients that are very photophobic, or squeeze or tear excessively may also dislocate their flaps postoperatively.

Postoperative examination of the flap after removal of the speculum at the operating microscope or at the slit lamp prior to discharge and on the first postoperative day is useful in the detection of flap striae. To detect fine striae, retroillumination through the dilated pupil may be necessary to identify these more subtle flap irregularities, which are typically not clinically significant. Fluorescein stain may be useful to detect the negative staining pattern seen in striae due to elevation alternating with depression of the flap [9]. Striae are most often perpendicular to the orientation of the hinge. For example, horizontal striae are more frequent

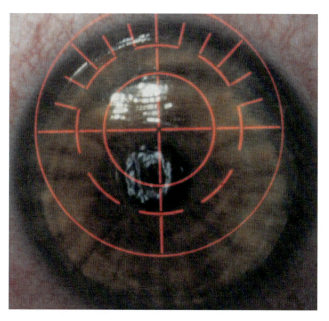

Fig. 3.4.3 Intraoperative striae indicating that the gutter is too large inferiorly, with distortion of the flap and bunching of the flap centrally

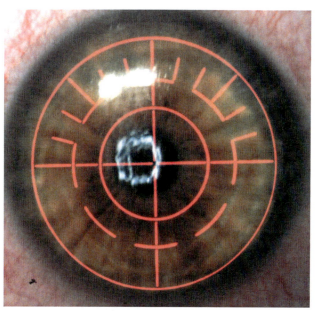

Fig. 3.4.5 Striae are improved after stretching, yet are still present as seen in the ring light reflection

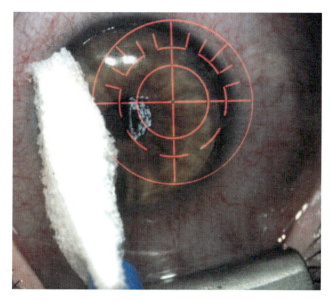

Fig. 3.4.4 A Merocel sponge is used to stretch the flap to close the gutter

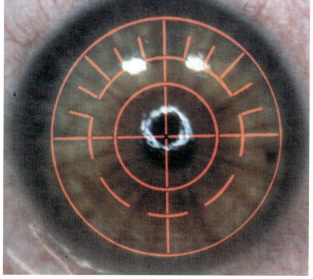

Fig. 3.4.6 Striae resolved after stretching

with nasal hinges are and vertical striae are more typical in flaps made with a vertical hinge.

Prior to creating the corneal flap, ink marks may be placed on the cornea to provide visual marks that may aid in flap repositioning. Care must be taken to make the marks long enough to allow for a range of flap diameters that may end up being created. If the epithelium, however, shifts at the periphery of the flap, then these marks may no longer be useful. The marks may also prove toxic to the epithelium; so, many surgeons have abandoned marking the

flap surface. Asymmetric hydration of the flap, with excessive hydration in one region, and excessive dehydration in another region can result in asymmetry in the size of the flap with resultant striae. In the area of excessive hydration, the flap may be swollen and therefore thicker, which causes the flap to be shorter. If it were to dry in this position, then the gutter would be larger than normal, causing striae. Poor interface adherence due to excessive hydration may also cause retraction of the flap with distortion and misalignment. Instruments such as the Johnston flap applanator (RheinMedical, Tampa, Fla.) or the Lindstrom LASIK flap roller (BD Visitec, Franklin Lakes, N.J.) can be used to roll or massage or depress the flap center at the end of the procedure to remove excess fluid from the flap interface, which some feel may reduce the incidence of striae. At the end of the case, the cornea outside of the flap can be depressed with a forceps to assure that the flap moves with the underlying bed and is identified by the presence of striae radiating from the peripheral cornea into the flap. We prefer to use dry Merocel sponges to stretch the flap from center to periphery to assure that the flap does not move when stretched gently, and that the gutter is visible and well opposed for the entire length of the gutter. Thick lubricating drops are placed over the cornea, and the lid speculum is left in place for a few minutes before removing. The thick drops such as Celluvisc (Allergan, Irvine, Calif.) protect the flap from lid movement when the lid speculum is removed. After removal of the surgical drapes and lid speculum, we have the patient blink to make sure that no movement or displacement of the flap is observed during blinking.

3.4.4 Management

If striae exist after LASIK, then the first step is to identify whether the visual acuity or the quality of vision is affected. If striae are peripheral or minimal enough that they do not affect vision, then they do not require intervention. Visual symptoms can include induced astigmatism (the cornea is thicker in peripheral striae, and this can cause flattening in the meridian of the striae). Visual symptoms can also include ghosting or shadowing due to irregular astigmatism when central. Striae that are going to affect the vision over the long term are best dealt with soon, as the longer they are present, the more difficult they become to remove [4, 7, 8]. Mild striae that only minimally affect the vision may become less symptomatic with time, as the epithelium thickens and reduces their visual significance by smoothing the anterior corneal surface. Contact lens fitting can be considered to improve vision in those patients where surgical intervention is not desired [10]. Fine flap distortion may be from mismatch of the flap and stromal bed, especially in high myopes, and may not influence the vision significantly, nor respond to flap repositioning [11]. Significant striae identified intraoperatively or immediately postoperatively are best dealt with at that time. This reduces the incidence of long-term striae, or epithelial ingrowth, which can be caused by the epithelium growing into the gutter where the edge of the flap should have been. Most striae are identified on the first postoperative day, as patient rubbing, inadvertent touch of the eye with the eye dropper bottles, or drying during sleep with the lid distorting the flap are the most common reasons for striae. Some have advocated addressing the striae at the slit lamp by either stretching with a cotton-tip applicator, or lifting the flap fully at the slit lamp [12, 13]. Care should be taken in these settings to prevent pulling the flap over epithelium that may have grown onto the stromal bed. If striae are found to be visually significant in the early period, we prefer lifting of the flap, removing the epithelium from the gutter and stromal bed where the flap should have been, and stretching the flap back into position with Merocel sponges at the operating microscope. Because the flap now has wrinkles that have been present for some time, and the compressed areas are relatively dehydrated compared with the expanded areas, the striae are more difficult to remove, and the flap is more difficult to position so that there are no gaps in the gutter. The endpoint of repositioning should be a tight gutter with no gap for 360°. It may appear that there are still some striae at the end of the repositioning, as the flap may be more dehydrated in the compressed areas when it was distorted before lifting the flap. Some report good success with hydration of the flap with a hypotonic solution. They advocate lifting the flap, refloating it, and then compressing the flap [4]. We have not found this technique as useful, as the flap is not as adherent when very swollen, and the striae appear to return after 2–3 days if the flap position is not resolved through stretching the flap to maintain a small tight gutter.

For striae present a long time, we still initially manage these striae in the same manner as described above, with lifting of the flap, removing epithelium from the gutter, and then careful stretching of the flap to reestablish a tight gutter. Some recommend epithelial debridement to break epithelial attachments that may be holding the flap in a distorted position [14]. We have successfully reduced striae up to 18 months after surgery, with lifting and stretching without epithelial debridement. In some cases, they can be recalcitrant to several methods, and some have recommended suturing of the flap to hold the flap in a taught position to reduce recalcitrant striae [15, 16]. Suture tension symmetry is important if this is performed. Warming the flap may be useful in manipulating flaps that have striae [17]. Transepithelial PTK can be used to Bowman's layer to remove the striae [18]. The endpoint for the PTK should not be total removal of the striae, as the epithelium can still smooth a significant degree of striae, and hyperopia can result from removal of central corneal tissue. We prefer to use mitomycin C in this situation to reduce the incidence of flap haze.

Flap distortion with reduction in visual quality or best-corrected visual acuity is infrequent but important intraoperative and early postoperative complications with lamellar surgery such as LASIK. Early recognition and treatment are beneficial to aid in resolution of this complication. There are varieties of methods to improve flap striae, and there is no consensus as to which one works the best, so familiarity with all techniques is useful.

Take-Home Pearls

- Manage significant striae early by lifting and stretching the flap.
- Mild striae or flap distortion may improve with time through epithelial remodeling, but may require lifting the flap to realign the flap, or phototherapeutic keratectomy.

References

1. Gimbel HV, Basti S, Kaye GB, Ferensowicz M (1996) Experience during the learning curve of laser in situ keratomileusis. J Cataract Refract Surg 22:542–550

2. Gimbel HV, Penno EE, van Westernbrugge JA, Ferensowicz M, Furlong MT (1998) Incidence and management of intraoperative and early postoperative complications in 1000 consecutive laser in situ keratomileusis cases. Ophthalmology 105:1839–1848

3. Lin RT, Maloney RK (1999) Flap complications associated with lamellar refractive surgery. Am J Ophthalmol 127:129–136

4. Pannu JS (1997) Incidence and treatment of wrinkled corneal flap following LASIK. J Cataract Refract Surg 23:695–696

5. Biser SA, Bloom AH, Donnenfeld ED, Perry HD, Solomon R, Doshi S (2003) Flap folds after femtosecond LASIK. Eye Contact Lens 29:252–254

6. Chan CC, Rootman DS (2004) Corneal lamellar flap retraction after LASIK following penetrating keratoplasty. Cornea 23:643–646

7. Hernandez-Matamoros J, Iradier MT, Moreno E (2001) Treating folds and striae after laser in situ keratomileusis. J Cataract Refract Surg 27:350–352

8. Probst LE, Machat JJ (1998) Removal of flap striae following laser in situ keratomileusis. J Cataract Refract Surg 24:153–155

9. Rabinowitz YS, Rasheed K (1999) Fluorescein test for the detection of striae in the corneal flap after laser in situ keratomileusis. Am J Ophthalmol 127:717–718

10. Lin JC, Rapuano CJ, Cohen EJ (2003) RK4 lens fitting for a flap striae in a LASIK patient. Eye Contact Lens 29:76–78

11. Carpel EF, Carlson KH, Shannon S (2000) Fine lattice lines on the corneal surface after laser in situ keratomileusis (LASIK). Am J Ophthalmol 129:379–380

12. Lichter H, Russell GE, Waring GO III (2004) Repositioning the laser in situ keratomileusis flap at the slit lamp. J Refract Surg 20:166–169

13. Solomon R, Donnenfeld ED, Perry HD, Doshi S, Biser S (2003) Slitlamp stretching of the corneal flap after laser in situ keratomileusis to reduce corneal striae. J Cataract Refract Surg 29:1292–1296

14. Kuo IC, Ou R, Hwang DG (2001) Flap haze after epithelial debridement and flap hydration for treatment of post-laser in situ keratomileusis striae. Cornea 20:339–341

15. Mackool RJ, Monsanto VR (2003) Sequential lift and suture technique for post-LASIK corneal striae. J Cataract Refract Surg 29:785–787

16. Jackson DW, Hamill MB, Koch DD (2003) Laser in situ keratomileusis flap suturing to treat recalcitrant flap striae. J Cataract Refract Surg 29:264–269

17. Donnenfeld ED, Perry HD, Doshi SJ, Biser SA, Solomon R (2004) Hyperthermic treatment of post-LASIK corneal striae. J Cataract Refract Surg 30:620–625

18. Steinert RF, Ashrafzadeh A, Hersh PS (2004) Results of phototherapeutic keratectomy in the management of flap striae after LASIK. Ophthalmology 111:740–746

Contents

4

■ Infection after LASIK surgery, although rare, may cause significant visual loss.

■ Infections presenting early after LASIK (within 1 week) are commonly caused by gram-positive organisms, whereas delayed onset infections (presenting 2–3 weeks after LASIK) are commonly caused by atypical mycobacteria.

■ Persistence of interface inflammation or appearance of corneal infiltrate after LASIK should be presumed infectious unless proven otherwise.

■ Fungal infections should be considered in those cases lacking improvement after early broad-spectrum therapy, as they are associated with severe visual loss.

■ A high index of suspicion and aggressive management, which includes early lifting of the flap, scrapings for microbiological investigation, and irrigation, and aggressive antibiotic therapy, may lead to better outcomes.

4.1 Infections after Refractive Surgery

José de la Cruz, Joelle Hallak,
Dimitri Azar, and Sandeep Jain

4.1.1 Introduction

Nearly 1.3 million laser in situ keratomileusis (LASIK) procedures were performed in the United States during the year 2000. Although LASIK is a relatively safe procedure [1, 2], infection can be a rare but sight-threatening complication. Case reports of infection after LASIK have appeared periodically in the literature. A few descriptive reviews that have been published as part of articles reporting new cases recognize the importance of effective management of this potentially serious complication after LASIK [3–7]. In this chapter, we first present a general discussion on infection after LASIK, followed by relevant excerpts from our systematic review of published literature.

Infections after LASIK are rare. Although prophylactic postoperative broad-spectrum antibiotics like fluoroquinolones and tobramycin are routinely prescribed after almost every LASIK case, infections still occur. The frequency of LASIK infection reported in case series varies from 0.02 to 1.5%. Several large LASIK case series have reported no infectious complications. Early onset infections (within 1 week of surgery) are mainly caused by gram-positive bacteria (*Staphylococcus aureus*). Later onset infections (2–3 weeks after surgery) are mainly caused by atypical mycobacteria (*Mycobacterium chelonae*). Fungal infections (*Candida, Fusarium*) are rare and are usually late onset. In few cases, the infections may be polymicrobial.

Patients with infection after LASIK usually complain of pain, decreased or blurry vision, photophobia, irritation, or redness; however as many as 10% may be asymptomatic. Symptoms and signs such as pain, discharge, flap separation, epithelial defects, and anterior chamber reaction are strongly associated with gram-positive infections, and redness and tearing are more common with fungal infections. However, symptoms such as pain, photophobia, decreased vision, and irritation are nonspecific indicators of ocular surface disease, therefore may not have specific association with particular infections (bacterial, mycobacterial, or fungal). Infections after LASIK often present with inflammation in the corneal interface, which can mimic diffuse lamellar keratitis (DLK). Because of the DLK misdiagnosis, many cases may be initially treated with frequent topical corticosteroid therapy, and there may even be a transient improvement in the inflammation. However, unlike DLK, the inflammation associated with infections usually persists despite topical corticosteroids, and worsen with corticosteroid tapering. The appearance of an interface inflammation more than 1 week after LASIK should be presumed to be of an infectious etiology until proven otherwise. Although the DLK infiltrates may also coalesce, any focal infiltrate surrounded by inflammation should be presumed infectious until proven otherwise. Infections presenting early after LASIK are associated with more severe reductions in visual acuity. However, severe visual acuity reductions are more associated with fungal infections than with gram-positive or mycobacterial infections. Therefore, in cases of suspected infection, if no response or worsening is observed despite 7 days of broad-spectrum antibiotics, the possibility of a fungal infection should be considered.

Corneal infiltrates are present in almost all cases of infections after LASIK. The infiltrates are most commonly in the flap interface followed by infiltrates within the lamellar flap. Infiltrates in the stromal bed and flap margins are less common. An overlying epithelial defect may be present in a third of the cases. In most cases, corneal infiltrates are not accompanied by an epithelial defect. This is contrary to the dogma that an epithelial defect is necessary for the diagnosis of an infectious infiltrate. In other types of refractive surgery, epithelial defects usually serve as a portal for organisms to establish infections in the stroma. However, in LASIK patients, creating the lamellar flap may introduce organisms into the stroma, and an epithelial defect may not be necessary for infection to occur. Infection should be suspected if infiltrates are seen in LASIK patients, and antibiotic therapy should be commenced before an epithelial defect occurs. In severe infections anterior chamber reaction or flap melting may occur. Clinical features that should raise the suspicion of infection with mycobacteria after LASIK include a delayed onset of keratitis (>2 weeks after LASIK) and an indolent course. Presenting symptoms can include any of the following: pain, redness, photophobia, decreased vision, a "white spot" in the cornea, a foreign body sensation, and/or mild irritation. Presenting clinical signs include infiltrates in the corneal interface that can be either multiple white granular opacities <0.5 mm in diameter or single white round lesion (0.1–2 mm in diameter).

Some factors to consider in the differential diagnosis of infectious keratitis:

- DLK
- Interface debris
  - Meibomian/lipid secretions
- Edema
  - Due to bandage contact lens
  - Due to trauma
  - Due to epithelial defect
- Sterile peripheral infiltrate
  - *Staphylococcus* marginal
- Epithelial ingrowth
- Post-viral reactivation
- Post–photorefractive keratectomy haze

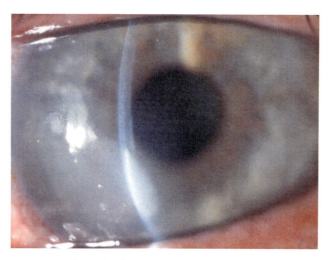

Fig. 4.1.1 Infiltrate development near LASIK flap

Sources for infection after LASIK are multiple, and may include the patient's eyelids, the microkeratome blade or other surgical instruments, and postoperative inoculation by the patient. Possible predisposing factors to infection such as HIV status, break in aseptic technique, previous refractive surgery including RK, and change in microkeratome blade are evident. It is unclear whether lack of microkeratome blade change between eyes in simultaneous bilateral LASIK is a risk factor for infection. Some surgeons operate without changing the blade between eyes; more LASIK performed under these conditions would explain the higher number of infections, independent of whether blade change is a factor. Three clusters of *Mycobacterium* infection were reported from three separate LASIK centers, with contaminated tap water as a likely source. There may also be some association between bilateral infection and HIV positivity and lack of microkeratome blade change. It is possible that epithelial retention patients with previous RK are predisposed to infection after LASIK. Other potential risk factors for infection include epithelial defects during surgery, interface debris, and bandage contact lens usage.

Due to the sequestered nature of infections following LASIK, it may be difficult to rely solely on topical treatment. Antibiotic penetration, especially antifungal agents, may not be sufficient to reach infections that lie at the interface. There may be an association between early flap lift and identification of the organism with a better outcome. Any focal infiltrate after LASIK should be considered infectious, and the practice of empirical antibiotic treatment without culturing should be discouraged. We recommend lifting and repositioning of the flap early after symptom onset for culture, scraping, and irrigation of the stromal bed, especially when the infiltrate involves the interface (Fig. 4.4.1). This allows greater antibiotic penetration and removes the sequestered nidus of infection. Culture media should include blood agar, chocolate agar, Sabouraud's agar, and thioglycolate broth. Cultures for fungus and mycobacteria should not be neglected. Corneal scrapings should be cultured on Lowenstein-Jensen media or Middlebrook 7H-9 agar. Smear stains should include Ziehl-Neelsen or fluorochrome stains for acid-fast bacilli (Fig. 4.4.2). Gram stains,

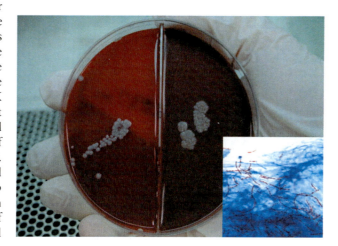

Fig. 4.1.2 The culture plate shows mycobacterial colonies and acid-fast bacilli

Giemsa stains, and KOH preparations at the time of scraping may provide valuable insight into the proper antibiotic therapy before culture results become available (Fig. 4.4.3). Infiltrates confined to the flap, or those associated with full-thickness ulcers, may not benefit greatly from early flap lift, although scrapings for culture should still be taken. Biopsy may be considered in those circumstances, especially if there is no improvement with medical treatment. Flap amputation for therapeutic reasons may limit the amount of vision regained after resolution of infection. However, it is also possible that the extent of injury to the cornea due to the infectious process may be limited by flap amputation, and that there may be greater penetration of antimicrobials. In addition, the lamellar flap may be sent for culture, which may help clarify the cause of infection.

The first step in the treatment of rapid-onset (usually due to gram-positive bacteria) as well as delayed-onset (usually due to atypical mycobacteria) infections after LASIK is to lift the corneal flap and culture as described above. Treatment recommendations that are described herein are based

4

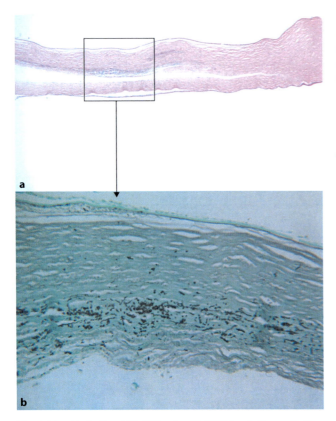

Fig. 4.1.3 a Periodic acid Schiff stain of LASIK flap. **b** Grocott's silver stain with evidence of intrastromal hyphae. (Courtesy of Dr. Douglas Buxton, New York Eye and Ear Infirmary, New York, N.Y.)

on the recommendations in the ASCRS white paper on infections after LASIK [8]. Initial treatment in all cases (described below) should be modified based on culture and scraping results, and clinical response to therapy. Irrigation of the flap interface with an appropriate antibiotic solution (fortified vancomycin 50 mg/ml for rapid-onset keratitis and fortified amikacin 35 mg/ml for delayed-onset keratitis) may be helpful. For rapid-onset keratitis, the recommendation is to use a fourth-generation topical fluoroquinolone such as 0.3% gatifloxacin or 0.5% moxifloxacin given in a loading dose every 5 min for 3 doses, and then every 30 min, alternating with an antimicrobial that is rapidly bactericidal and has increased activity against gram-positive organisms, such as fortified cefazolin 50 mg/ml every 30 min [8]. In patients who work in a hospital environment, there is an added risk for methicillin-resistant *S. aureus* (MRSA). In these patients, the recommendation is to substitute fortified vancomycin 50 mg/ml for cefazolin every 30 min to provide therapy more effective against MRSA. In addition, the use of oral doxycycline 100 mg twice a day to inhibit collagenase production, and discontinuation of corticosteroids is advocated. For delayed-onset keratitis, the recommendation is to begin therapy with amikacin 35 mg/ml every 30 min, alternating with a fourth-generation fluoroquinolone (0.3% gatifloxacin or 0.5% moxifloxacin) every 30 min, starting oral doxycycline 100 mg twice a day, and discontinuing corticosteroids [8].

It should be noted that the recommended initial treatment is ineffective against fungal infections. The treatment for fungal infections is initiated after positive smears or cultures. Also, note that medical treatment of atypical mycobacterial keratitis is often difficult. Treatment for atypical mycobacteria may include topical or oral antibiotic clarithromycin.

4.1 Suspected infection

Several steps may help prevent infectious keratitis following LASIK. Meibomian gland disease should be treated before LASIK. Proper sterilization of instruments and intraoperative sterile techniques should be used, including sterile gloves and drapes, and disinfection of the skin and eyelids with povidone iodine. During the procedure, instruments should be sterile. Efforts should be made to avoid irrigating meibomian secretions into the flap interface (use of a Chayet LASIK drainage ring is helpful). Suction lid specula may be helpful in removing excessive fluids and debris. Postoperatively, patients should be instructed to wear plastic protective shields and not to rub the eye. Prophylactic antibiotics are likely helpful and should be used for a few days postoperatively. Patients should be instructed to avoid sleeping with pets, do gardening, or swimming in the perioperative and early postoperative period. Patients with dry eyes should be instructed to use frequent artificial tears, or, if indicated, punctal plugs may be placed.

4.1.2 Review of Published Literature

We have systematically reviewed published case reports of infection occurring after LASIK, and examined the associations between the microbiologic profile of the infection, risk factors for infection, presentation symptoms and signs, treatment strategies, and the severity of reduction in visual acuity. The original article was published by Chang et al. in *Survey of Ophthalmology* [9]. The authors reproduce relevant details below. A total of 106 infections involving 90 patients were described in 45 articles analyzed. Of all 90 patients, 67 were referrals. Sixteen patients had bilateral infection, and unilateral infection occurred in 74 patients. Eighty-five percent of infections occurred after primary LASIK.

4.1.2.1 Onset and Frequency of Infection

Out of the reported cases, identified by the literature, on infectious keratitis after refractive surgery [3–71], 49% had symptom onset within 7 days of the last refractive procedure. The mean time of presentation in this early onset group was 2.7±4.2 days (range: 0–7 days). Gram-positive bacteria were cultured in 53.7% of the infections, of which during this time period, the predominant reason for infection was of bacterial origin, gram positive being the one of highest percentage (53.7%), *S. aureus*, *Streptococcus pneumoniae*, *Streptococcus viridans*, *Staphylococcus epidermidis*,

Table 4.1.1 Frequency of infection after LASIK

Authors	Frequency of infection (no. of cases/total)
Miller et al. (ARVO abstract) [11]	1.50% (1/1679)
Pirzada et al. [12]	1.20% (1/83)
Dada et al. [13]	0.20% (1/500)
Stulting et al. [14]	0.19% (2/1062)
Perez-Santonja et al. [15]	0.12% (1/801)
Lin and Maloney 16]	0.10% (1/1019)
Seedor et al. (ARVO Abstract) [17]	0.02% (1/6312)
Gimbel et al. [18]	0 (0/2142)
Kawesch and Kezirian [19]	0 (0/290)
Price et al. [20]	0 (0/1747)

Rhodococcus, and *Nocardia*. Other infections identified at similar times, but with lower incidence rates, were *Candida* and atypical mycobacteria (12.2 and 7.3%, respectively).

As time from the onset of symptoms extends, slower organisms find an encouraging environment for growth, changing the infectious etiology. For cases that lasted for more than 10 days, atypical mycobacteria appeared in more than half of them. The majority of ocular infections caused by mycobacteria are from the atypical mycobacteria group. Of this group, only six species have been reported to cause LASIK-related infectious keratitis. Four of the six mycobacteria that have been involved in LASIK infections are rapid growers, *M. chelonae*, and *Mycobacterium fortuitum* (both Runyon type IV) being the two most common. The other two, *Mycobacterium terrae* and *Mycobacterium szulgai* are slow growers. The variation of clinical symptoms is significant when comparing slow growing versus fast growing mycobacterium. Hence, this underscores the importance of late onset symptoms after LASIK with atypical mycobacteria, and its wide range period of presentation from 2 to 14 weeks after surgery. This is in contrast to the shorter period to clinical onset of symptoms for bacteria and even fungus. In the case of fungal keratitis, even though it presents with an indolent course, it most often manifests itself clinically within 24–36 h after trauma as with bacterial etiologies.

The frequency of LASIK infection reported in several case series varied from 0.02 to 1.5% [11– 16]. Several large LASIK case series have reported no infectious complications (Table 4.1.1) [17–20].

4.1.2.2 Characteristics of Infection

The presenting signs and symptoms of infectious keratitis in the setting of refractive surgery are pain, blurred vision, photophobia, redness, foreign-body sensation, and discharge. Information about specific presenting symptoms was available for 81 of the eyes infected after LASIK. Thirty-

nine (48.1%) of the 81 eyes presented with pain, 33 (40.7%) had decreased or blurry vision, 25 (30.9%) had photophobia, 21 (25.9%) presented with irritation, 21 (25.9%) had redness, 7 (9%) complained of discharge, and 10 (12.8%) were asymptomatic.

Corneal infiltrate was present in 102 (96.2%) of 106 eyes. Of the eyes without infiltrate, pain, photophobia, and discharge were presenting symptoms. Eleven (11.5%) infiltrates were entirely within the lamellar flap, 70 (68.6%) were found in the interface, 3 (3.2%) were located in the stroma, 8 (7.8%) involved the flap, interface, and stroma, and 6 (6.3%) involved the flap margin and adjacent cornea (data missing for four eyes). Twelve (11.3%) of 106 eyes were noted to have ulcers, and 4 (3.8%) had abscesses. Anterior chamber (AC) reactions were documented in 24 (22.6%) eyes, and 38 (35.8%) new-onset epithelial defects were found on initial presentation. Infiltrates were present in all eyes without epithelial defects. Flap separation was noted in 11 (10.4%) eyes, and 6 (5.7%) had epithelial ingrowth on presentation. One case of endophthalmitis was reported. In 12 (11.3%) cases, the lamellar flap melted due to the infection.

Gram-positive infections are more likely to be present with pain and discharge than other microorganisms. They are also more strongly associated with epithelial defects, flap separation, and anterior chamber reactions. Fungal infections are significantly more likely than others to present with redness and tearing. Mycobacterial infections were not significantly associated with a particular symptom or sign, but some reports have described the crack windshield appearance of these infiltrates (Fig. 4.4.4). Decreased vision, photophobia, and irritation were nonspecific symptoms of infection that were not associated with any particular microorganism.

4.1.2.3 Microbiological Profile

Infections caused by a single gram-positive organism were found in 27 (26.2%) of the 103 eyes that were cultured, and included *S. aureus*, *S. pneumoniae*, *S. viridans*, *S. epider-*

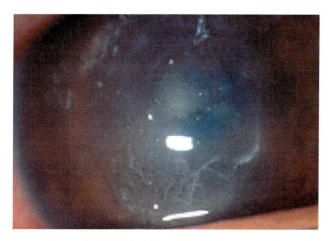

Fig. 4.1.4 Cracked-windshield appearance of corneal infiltrate in atypical mycobacterial infection

Table 4.1.2 Microbiological profile

Organism type	No. of eyes
Gram-positive bacteria	27
Staphylococcus aureus	17
Streptococcus pneumoniae	3
Streptococcus viridans	2
Staphylococcus epidermidis	2
Nocardia	2
Rhodococcus	1
Fungi	9
Fusarium	3
Aspergillus	2
Curvularia	2
Scedosporium	1
Candida	5
Mycobacterium spp.	49
M. chelonae	33
M. abscessus	7
M. szulgai	5
M. fortuitum	2
M. mucogenicum	2
Other	2
Pseudomonas aeruginosa	1
Acanthamoeba	1
Polymicrobial	4
Staphylococcus epidermidis and Fusarium solani	1
S. epidermidis and Aspergillus	1
S. epidermidis/Curvularia spp./acid-fast bacilli	1
Staphylococcus and M. chelonae	1

midis, *Rhodococcus*, and *Nocardia* (Table 4.2.2). Fungus, such as *Fusarium*, *Aspergillus*, *Curvularia*, and *Scedosporium*, was the sole cause of infection in nine eyes (one was not further classified). Forty-nine mycobacterial infections were due to *M. chelonae*, *Mycobacterium abscessus*, *M. szulgai*, *M. fortuitum*, and *Mycobacterium mucogenicum* were found. There were four polymicrobial infections. Seven cultures were sterile.

4.1.2.4 Outcomes and Sequelae

Final visual acuity was available in 99 of the 106 eyes. Clinically nonsignificant reductions in visual acuity occurred in 50 (55.6%) eyes, 25 (25.3%) had moderate reductions, and 24 (24.7%) suffered severe reductions in visual acuity. Thirty-four percent of infections resulting in nonsignificant reductions in acuity were caused by gram-positive bacte-

ria, 42% by mycobacterium, 4% were caused by fungus, 4% were polymicrobial, and 6.1% were culture-negative

Of the eyes with moderate visual acuity reduction, 32% infections were due to gram positives, mycobacterium was found in 52% eyes, 8% were culture negative, 4% were fungal, 4% were not cultured. Gram positives caused three (12.5%) infections in the severe reduction group, six (25 %) were due to fungus, eight (33.3%) were mycobacterial, two (8.3%) were polymicrobial, one (4.2%) eye was culture-negative, and two (8.3%) eyes were not cultured.

Of the 32 gram-positive infections for which information was available, including polymicrobial infections involving gram-positive organisms, the mean final Snellen VA was 20/45. The mean VA of eyes after fungal infections was 20/297, and after mycobacterial infections, the mean acuity was 20/55. Fungus was significantly associated with severe reductions in visual acuity ($p = 0.002$).

Sixteen total keratoplasties, including 2 lamellar keratoplasties and 14 penetrating keratoplasties, were performed. Thirteen were performed for therapeutic reasons, and three were performed for optical reasons (scarring and irregular astigmatism). Eight of the 13 therapeutic keratoplasties were performed for persistent, worsening infiltrate despite 2–12 weeks of intensive medical therapy; 3 keratoplasties were performed after perforation after 3–4 weeks of medical therapy, 1 was performed for corneal thinning and progression of infection after 7 months, and there was no indication available for 1 keratoplasty.

Four percent of eyes were noted to develop epithelial ingrowth after resolution of infection. Information about scarring and irregular astigmatism was available for 75 eyes, after excluding those with therapeutic penetrating keratoplasty.

4.1.3 Conclusion

Although infection after LASIK is a rare complication, serious consequences such as moderate or severe reductions in visual acuity are common after infection. It may be difficult in some cases to distinguish between infection and diffuse lamellar keratitis. However, we emphasize that a high index of suspicion must be maintained whenever inflammation persists after LASIK surgery or a corneal infiltrate develops. Treatment should not be empirical. Cultures and smears should be performed after flap lifting and aggressive topical antibiotic therapy initiated. The initial treatment should be modified based on culture and scraping results and clinical response to therapy.

Take-Home Pearls

- ■ A high index of suspicion for infection must be maintained whenever interface inflammation persists or acorneal infiltrate develops after LASIK.
- ■ Early-onset (less than 1 week after LASIK) infections are usually due to gram-positive bacteria. Late-onset infections are usually due to atypical mycobacteria.

- Early lifting of corneal flap for microbiological tests (smear and cultures) precedes aggressive topical antibiotic therapy.
- Cultures for fungus and atypical mycobacteria should not be neglected.
- Initial therapy may be modified based on culture results and clinical response.
- The most important factor within our control is prevention of infection.

References

1. Choi RY, Wilson SE (2001) Hyperopic laser in situ keratomileusis: primary and secondary treatments are safe and effective. Cornea20:388–393
2. Farah SG, Azar DT, Gurdal C et al (1998) Laser in situ keratomileusis: literature review of a developing technique. J Cataract Refract Surg 24:989–1006
3. Alió JL, Perez-Santonja JJ, Tervo T(2000) Postoperative inflammation, microbial complications, and wound healing following laser in situ keratomileusis. J Refract Surg 16:523–538
4. Ambrosio R Jr., Wilson SE (2001) Complications of laser in situ keratomileusis: etiology, prevention, and treatment. J Refract Surg 17:350–379
5. Garg P, Bansal AK, Sharma S et al (2001) Bilateral infectious keratitis after laser in situ keratomileusis: a case report and review of the literature. Ophthalmology 108:121–125
6. Quiros PA, Chuck RS, Smith RE (1999) Infectious ulcerative keratitis after laser in situ keratomileusis. Arch Ophthalmol 117:1423–1427
7. Wilson SE (1998) LASIK: management of common complications laser in situ keratomileusis Cornea 17:459–467
8. Donnenfeld ED, Kim T, Holland EJ, Azar DT, Palmon FR, Rubenstein JB, Daya S, Yoo SH; American Society of Cataract and Refractive Surgery Cornea Clinical Committee. ASCRS white paper: management of infectious keratitis following laser in situ keratomileusis. J Cataract Refract Surg 10:2008–2011
9. Chang MA, Jain S, Azar DT (2004) Infections following laser in situ keratomileusis: an integration of the published literature. Surv Ophthalmol 49:269-80
10. MacRae SM, Rich LF, Macaluso DC (2002) Treatment of interface keratitis with oral corticosteroids. J Cataract Refract Surg 28:454–461
11. Miller D, Newton J, Alfonso E (2000) Surveillance and infection control standards for refractive surgery centers? ARVO abstract no. 1679
12. Pirzada WA, Kalaawry H (1997) Laser in situ keratomileusis for myopia of −1 to −3.50 diopters. J Refract Surg 13:S425–S426
13. Dada T, Sharma N, Dada VK et al (2000) Pneumococcal keratitis after laser in situ keratomileusis. J Cataract Refract Surg 26:460–461
14. Stulting RD, Carr JD, Thompson KP (1999) Complications of laser in situ keratomileusis for the correction of myopia. Ophthalmology 106:13–20
15. Perez-Santonja JJ, Sakla HF, Abad JL (1997) Nocardial keratitis after laser in situ keratomileusis. J Refract Surg 13:314–317
16. Lin RT, Maloney RK (1999) Flap complications associated with lamellar refractive surgery. Am J Ophthalmol 127:129–136
17. Seedor JA, Shapiro DE, Ritterband DC, et al (2001) LASIK complication rates. ARVO abstract no. 2668
18. Gimbel HV, van Westengrugge JA, Penno EE (1999) Simultaneous bilateral laser in situ keratomileusis: safety and efficacy. Ophthalmology 106:1461–1467
19. Kawesch GM, Kezirian GM (2000) Laser in situ keratomileusis for high myopia with the VISX star laser. Ophthalmology 107:653–661
20. Price FW, Willes L, Price M (2001) A prospective, randomized comparison of the use versus non-use of topical corticosteroids after laser in situ keratomileusis. Ophthalmology 108:1236–1244
21. al-Reefy M (1999) Bacterial keratitis following laser in situ keratomileusis for hyperopia. J Refract Surg 15:216–217
22. Alvarenga L, Freitas D, Holfing-Lima AL (2002) Infectious post-LASIK crystalline keratopathy caused by nontuberculous mycobacteria. Cornea 21:426–429
23. Aras C, Ozdamar A, Bahcecioglu H et al (1998) Corneal interface abscess after excimer laser in situ keratomileusis. J Refract Surg 14:156–157
24. Chung MS, Goldstein MH, Driebe WT Jr et al (2000) Fungal keratitis after laser in situ keratomileusis: a case report. Cornea 19:236–237
25. Chung MS, Goldstein MH, Driebe WT Jr et al (2000) Mycobacterium chelonae keratitis after laser in situ keratomileusis successfully treated with medical therapy and flap removal. Am J Ophthalmol 129:382–384
26. Cuello OH, Carolin MJ, Reviglio VE (2002) Rhodococcus globerulus keratitis after laser in situ keratomileusis. J Cataract Refract Surg 28:2235–2237
27. Dada T, Sharma N, Dada VK et al (2000) Pneumococcal keratitis after laser in situ keratomileusis. J Cataract Refract Surg 26:460–461
28. Gelender H, Carter HL, Bowman B (2000) Mycobacterium keratitis after laser in situ keratomileusis. J Refract Surg 16:191–195
29. Giaconi J, Pham R, Ta CN (2002) Bilateral Mycobaterium abscessus keratitis after laser in situ keratomileusis. J Cataract Refract Surg 28:887–890
30. Gupta V, Dada T, Vajpayee RB (2001) Polymicrobial keratitis after laser in situ keratomileusis. J Refract Surg 17:147–148
31. Hovanesian JA, Faktorovich EG, Hoffbauer JD (1999) Bilateral bacterial keratitis after laser in situ keratomileusis in a patient with human immunodeficiency virus infection. Arch Ophthalmol 117:968–970
32. Karp KO, Hersh PS, Epstein RJ (2000) Delayed keratitis after laser in situ keratomileusis. J Cataract Refract Surg 26:925–928
33. Kim EK, Lee DH, Lee K. et al (2000) Nocardia keratitis after traumatic detachment of a laser in situ keratomileusis flap. J Refract Surg 16:467–469
34. Kim HM, Song JS, Han HS et al (1998) Streptococcal keratitis after myopic laser in situ keratomileusis. Korean J Ophthalmol 12:108–111
35. Kouyoumdjian GA, Forstot SL, Durairaj VD et al (2001) Infectious keratitis after laser refractive surgery. Ophthalmology 108:1266–1268
36. Kuo IC, Margolis TP, Cevallos V (2001) *Aspergillus fumigatus* keratitis after laser in situ keratomileusis. Cornea 20:342–344
37. Lam DS, Leung AT, Wu JT (1999) Culture-negative ulcerative keratitis after laser in situ keratomileusis. J Cataract Refract Surg 25:1004–1008
38. Levartovsky S, Rosenwasser G, Goodman D (2001) Bacterial keratitis following laser in situ keratomileusis. Ophthalmology 108:321–325
39. Maldonado MJ, Juberias JR, Moreno-Montanes J (2002) Extensive corneal epithelial defect associated with internal hordeolum after uneventful laser in situ keratomileusis. J Cataract Refract Surg 28:1700–1702
40. Moon SJ, Mann PM, Matoba AY (2003) Microsporidial keratoconjunctivitis in a healthy patient with a history of LASIK surgery. Cornea 22:271–272
41. Mulhern MG, Condon PI, O'Keefe M (1997) Endophthalmitis after astigmatic myopic laser in situ keratomileusis. J Cataract Refract Surg 23:948–950

4

42. Parolini B, Marcon G, Panozzo GA (2001) Central necrotic lamellar inflammation after laser in situ keratomileusis. J Refract Surg 17:110–112

43. Ramirez M, Hernandez-Quintela E, Betran F et al (2002) Pneumococcal keratitis at the flap interface after laser in situ keratomileusis. J Cataract Refract Surg 28:550–552

44. Read RW, Chuck RS, Rao NS (2000) Traumatic *Acremonium atrogriseum* keratitis following laser-assisted in situ keratomileusis. Arch Ophthalmol 118:418–421

45. Reviglio V, Rodriguez ML, Picotti GS (1998) *Mycobacterium chelonae* keratitis following laser in situ keratomileusis. J Refract Surg 14:357–360

46. Ritterband D, Kelly J, McNamara T (2002) Delayed-onset multifocal polymicrobial keratitis after laser in situ keratomileusis. J Cataract Refract Surg 28:898–899

47. Rubinfeld RS, Negvesky GJ (2001) Methicillin-resistant *Staphylococcus aureus* ulcerative keratitis after laser in situ keratomileusis. J Cataract Refract Surg 27:1523–1525

48. Rudd JC, Moshirfar M (2001) Methicillin-resistant *Staphylococcus aureus* keratitis after laser in situ keratomileusis. J Cataract Refract Surg 27:471–473

49. Sridhar MS, Garg P, Bansal AK (2000) *Aspergillus flavus* keratitis after laser in situ keratomileusis. Am J Ophthalmol 129:802–804

50. Sridhar MS, Garg P, Bansal AK, et al (2000) Fungal keratitis after laser in situ keratomileusis. J Cataract Refract Surg 26:613–615

51. Suresh PS, Rootman DS (2002) Bilateral infectious keratitis after a laser in situ keratomileusis enhancement procedure. J Cataract Refract Surg 28:720–721

52. Verma S, Tuft SJ (2002) *Fusarium solani* keratitis following LASIK for myopia. Br J Ophthalmol 86:1190–1191

53. Watanabe H, Sato S, Maeda N (1997) Bilateral corneal infection as a complication of laser in situ keratomileusis. Arch Ophthalmol 115:1593–159

54. Webber SK, Lawless MA, Sutton GL et al (1999) Staphylococcal infection under a LASIK flap. Cornea 18:361–365

55. Winthrop KL, Steinberg EB, Holmes G (2003) Epidemic and sporadic cases of nontuberculous mycobacterial keratitis associated with laser in situ keratomileusis. Am J Ophthalmol 135:223–224

56. Chandra NS, Torres MF, Winthrop KL (2001) Cluster of *Mycobacterium chelonae* keratitis cases following laser in situ keratomileusis. Am J Ophthalmol 132:819–830

57. Chang SW, Ashraf FM, Azar DT (2000) Wound healing patterns following perforation sustained during laser in situ keratomileusis. J Formos Med Assoc 99:635–641

58. Freitas D, Alvarenga L, Sampaio J (2003) An outbreak of *Mycobacterium chelonae* infection after LASIK. Ophthalmology 110:276–285

59. Fulcher SFA, Fader RC, Rosa RH et al (2002) Delayed-onset mycobacterial keratitis after LASIK. Cornea 21:546–554

60. Karp CL, Tuli SS, Yoo SH (2003) Infectious keratitis after LASIK. Ophthalmology 110:503–510

61. Pache M, Schipper I, Flammer J et al (2003) Unilateral fungal and mycobacterial keratitis after simultaneous laser in situ keratomileusis. Cornea 22:72–75

62. Peng Q, Holzer MP, Kaufer PH (2002) Interface fungal infection after laser in situ keratomileusis presenting as diffuse lamellar keratitis. J Cataract Refract Surg 28:1400–1408

63. Pushker N, Dada T, Sony P (2002) Microbial keratitis after lasik in situ keratomileusis. J Refract Surg 18:280–286

64. Solomon A, Karp CL, Miller D (2001) *Mycobacterium interface* keratitis after laser in situ keratomileusis. Ophthalmology 108:2201–2208

65. Sharma N, Dada T, Dada VK et al (2001) Acute hemorrhagic keratoconjunctivitis after LASIK. J Cataract Refract Surg 27:344–345

66. Tripathi A (2000) Fungal keratitis after LASIK. J Cataract Refract Surg 26:1433

67. Patel NR, Reidy JJ, Gonzalez-Fernandez F (2005) Nocardia keratitis after laser in situ keratomileusis: clinicopathologic correlation. J Cataract Refract Surg 31:2012–2015

68. Chung SH, Roh MI, Park MS, Kong YT, Lee HK, Kim EK (2006) *Mycobacterium abscessus* keratitis after LASIK with IntraLase femtosecond laser. Ophthalmologica 220:277–280

69. Hamam RN, Noureddin B, Salti HI, Haddad R, Khoury JM (2006) Recalcitrant post-LASIK Mycobacterium chelonae keratitis eradicated after the use of fourth-generation fluoroquinolone. Ophthalmology 113:950–954

70. John T, Velotta E (2005) Nontuberculous (atypical) mycobacterial keratitis after LASIK: current status and clinical implications. Cornea 24:245–255

71. Solomon R, Donnenfeld ED, Azar DT, Holland EJ, Palmon FR, Pflugfelder SC, Rubenstein JB (2003) Infectious keratitis after laser in situ keratomileusis: results of an ASCRS survey. J Cataract Refract Surg 29:2001–2006

Core Messages

- DLK is an early postoperative complication appearing as an inflammatory response of the corneal lamellae.

- Occurrence is rare.

- Postoperative examination at 24 h after the LASIK procedure is critical.

- Careful cleaning techniques and avoidance of contaminants may reduce outbreaks.

- Treatment of stages 1 and 2 includes aggressive topical steroids and careful daily monitoring.

- Treatment of stage 3 includes lifting the flap, gentle rinsing, and careful daily monitoring thereafter.

4.2 Diffuse Lamellar Keratitis

Marlane J. Brown, David R. Hardten,
Elizabeth A. Davis, and Richard L. Lindstrom

4.2.1 Diffuse Lamellar Keratitis

LASIK surgery continues to be a popular and effective refractive surgery option for patients. LASIK is a safe and effective alternative to spectacle and contact lens correction of refractive error, but eye care providers must be familiar with potential complications. DLK is an uncommon complication that can occur in the early postoperative period. This complication can cause scarring and an adverse visual outcome. Once considered a mystery, much more is now understood regarding the etiology and treatment of this disease. Understanding the time course of the disease, along with proper identification, staging, and intervention can help eliminate visual loss associated with this condition.

This early post-LASIK inflammatory syndrome was first reported at the October 1997 American Academy of Ophthalmology (AAO) meeting by Smith and Maloney. Their findings were later published in the March 1998 issue of *Ophthalmology* [1]. This condition was characterized by a whitish, granular, diffuse, culture negative lamellar keratitis occurring in the first days after surgery. In some patients' eyes, the inflammation would disappear spontaneously, in some the condition worsened, followed by flap melt, scarring, and adverse visual outcome. This initial report documented 13 eyes with this condition, which the authors termed "diffuse lamellar keratitis."

Other early reports at the 1998 ASCRS meeting also described cases of this peculiar inflammatory reaction occurring in the lamellar interface shortly after LASIK. Names such as "shifting sands," "sands of the Sahara," "PLIK (post-LASIK interface keratitis)," "NSDIK (nonspecific diffuse intra lamellar keratitis)", and "DIK (diffuse intralamellar keratitis)" were applied to the condition [2, 3]. Some of these names like the shifting sands, and sands of the Sahara tried to describe the appearance of the condition, which was whitish, granular, with the appearance of waves of increased density.

DLK can still be a troublesome complication after LASIK. It can occur after uneventful surgery, and progress quickly. Patients with this rare complication can develop the typical cascade of problems despite treatment.

4.2.2 Etiology and Prevalence

DLK is an inflammatory response in the corneal lamella. Its typical pathologic characteristic is inflammatory cell infiltration in the lamella. There has been considerable focus on the etiology of DLK. Contaminants in the lamellar interface introduced at the time of surgery may stimulate the condition in some patients. Oil, wax, metallic, and other foreign particles in the LASIK interface have been documented by investigators using scanning and confocal and electron microscopy, and liquid chromatography [3]. Other cases seemed to be associated with epithelial defects at the time of surgery [4]. It has also been proposed that DLK represents a hypersensitivity reaction to bacterial cell proteins that have accumulated on the autoclaved instruments. The bacteria multiply on the wet instruments or the autoclave overnight [5]. While the sterilization kills the bacteria, the cell walls persist on the instruments, and this material is transferred to the corneal interface. Avoiding the use of stagnant fluids in instrument cleaning and sterilizing protocols has been shown to minimize the occurrence of DLK [6]. Wiping the microkeratome blades with alcohol before mounting may also prevent DLK. One study showed that wiping 100% alcohol on the blade with a Merocel spear and then rinsing with balanced salt solution (BSS) before mounting may remove unwanted substances from the manufacturing or sterilization process [7].

When the LASIK flap is created with the femtosecond laser versus a microkeratome, there may be greater inflammation. A study comparing corneal flaps made with a femto-second laser with those made with a mechanical microkeratome in rabbits measured early postoperative inflammation [8]. Inflammatory cell infiltration in the central cornea and at the peripheral interface was significantly greater in the femtosecond group than the microkeratome group at 4 and 24 h postoperatively. This DLK-like inflammation may require stronger anti-inflammatory drugs to be used postoperatively. However, recent biomechanical studies show improved healing and improved outcomes in vision in general with the femtosecond laser flap creation compared with blade-assisted flap created [9].

It is also known that epithelial defects, either intraoperatively or postoperatively can cause acute or late onset DLK. One study evaluated six DLK cases after an epithelial defect and showed alterations in the keratocyte phenotype. Not all cases showed inflammatory cells in the flap interface, and may have originated from sterile epithelial stromal or inflammatory cell–stromal cell interactions [10].

Other proposed sources that may cause DLK include betadine, BSS, environmental agents, lubricant, topical medications, benzene, contaminants from eyelids such as meibomian gland secretions, laser thermal effect, or talc. What is clear only is that no one source is responsible for the condition.

Confocal microscopy has been used to try to identify the pathogenesis of DLK [11]. In this evaluation, in stages 1 and 2 DLK the epithelium, posterior stroma, and endothelium were found to be normal. In the lamella in front of the incision, many round or oval shaped cells with diameter approximately 12–20 μm were detected. The number of cells varied between the eyes with stage 1. Corneas with stage 2 DLK had dense infiltrates. The cells had eccentric, highly reflective nuclei and less reflective intracellular structures, were mostly mononuclear, and were distributed diffusely or arranged in lines. In the lamella, clusters and lines of small, highly reflective, irregular shaped cells 8–10 μm in diameter were reportedly seen. They were similar to granulocytes of lymphocytes. Seven days postoperatively, these cells almost disappeared. If stage 3 DLK developed, it appeared 3–5 days postoperatively, and more dense infiltration and more highly reflective shape materials showed in the lamella. One microscopist stated this appeared as an aggregation of decayed cells, most likely granulocytes, and was noticed clinically and by confocal microscopy [12].

In those rare corneas that went on to stage 4 DLK, it developed 5–7 days postoperatively. Anterior stromal structure was unclear at this level of inflammation, with highly reflective and folded corneal flaps seen, and highly reflective scarring in some.

The prevalence of DLK has been minimally studied. One study out of Canada over a 2-year period reported DLK incidence of 0.67 cases per 100 procedures ($n = 72,000$ procedures), with 64% occurring in outbreaks. The outbreaks decreased dramatically from the first year to the end of the second year (72–40%), indicating perhaps that reporting and then following prevention and control measures that were recommended may have helped reduce the outbreaks [13].

4.2.3 Identification and Appearance

Examining the patient at day one is critical in identifying DLK. The cellular reaction will usually be apparent in the first 24 h. It will appear as a fine, white, granular reaction in the lamellar interface, and on the first day is most often in the periphery. It is important to differentiate DLK from punctate epithelial keratopathy (PEK), which can appear on day one as well. Swelling of the LASIK flap (flap edema) or epithelial edema may look similar. Using a small amount of fluorescein and paying close attention to where the slit lamp is focusing should help eliminate confusion. It also may be confused with meibomian gland debris and or tear film debris, which occasionally may get trapped under the patients' flaps. Meibomian gland debris looks more grayish in color and may shine more than the flat-white, granular appearance of DLK.

It is uncommon to see DLK after the first 24 h without a causative agent. Causes of late onset DLK have been reported. One case described onset of DLK 3 years after uneventful bilateral LASIK in one eye of a 56-year-old woman. There was no epithelial defect, no trauma, and no other apparent cause, suggesting that DLK can occur several years after LASIK without obvious cause. This particular case was identified as stage 3, and responded well to topical steroids [14]. Another case reported a 58-year-old male Caucasian who developed delayed onset diffuse lamellar keratitis, seemingly in the absence of an epithelial defect, 25 days after an enhancement LASIK procedure to his right eye. In this case, treatment was complicated by the fact that the patient was a steroid responder and experienced an intraocular pressure rise that had to be managed with pressure-lowering drops [15]. It has also been shown that DLK can be associated with viral pseudomembranous keratoconjunctivitis. One case of a 47-year-old woman developing DLK 2 years after uneventful LASIK indicates that perhaps the plane created by the microkeratome may remain unhealed for at least this many months. Aggressive treatment with topical steroids resolved the inflammation; corneal clarity and visual acuity was completely restored in this case [16].

4.2.4 Staging

Four stages have been used to categorize diffuse lamellar keratitis. Once DLK is identified, a staging of severity and location can then be made. The following staging system has proven helpful [17].

Stage 1: Stage 1 is defined by the presence of white, granular cells in the periphery of the lamellar flap, with sparing of the visual axis. This is the most common presentation of DLK at day 1, and with careful inspection, may be present in as many as 1 in 25–50 cases (Figs. 4.2.1, 4.2.2).

Stage 2: Stage 2 is defined by the presence of white, granular cells in the center of the flap, involving the visual axis.

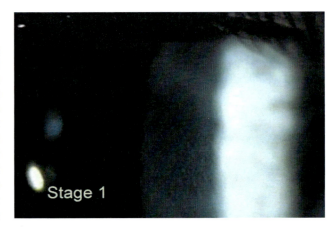

Fig. 4.2.1 Stage 1 DLK is characterized by fine, white cells in the stroma, usually in the inferior periphery. No clumping of cells in the interface or cells in the central portion of the cornea is present

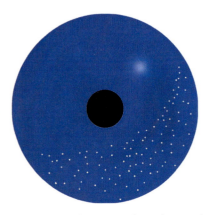

Fig. 4.2.2 Cells are mainly in the periphery and in the stroma in stage 1 DLK

This appearance, occasionally present at day 1, is more frequently seen on day 2 or 3; the result of central migration of cells along the path of least resistance, giving it the so-called shifting-sands appearance. This occurs in approximately 1 in 200 cases (Figs. 4.2.3, 4.2.4).

Stage 3: Stage 3 DLK appears as the aggregation of more dense, white, clumped cells in the central visual axis, with relative clearing in the periphery. This is often, but not always, associated with a subtle decline in visual acuity by one or two lines. Often, but not always, this is accompanied by a subjective description of haze by the patient. The cellular reaction collects in the center of the ablation, and may settle slightly inferior to the visual axis with gravity. The frequency of Stage 3 DLK may be as high as 1 in 500 cases (Figs. 4.2.5, 4.2.6).

Identification of this stage 3, a more intense, central reaction of cells, is paramount to preventing an unwanted outcome. If left untreated, a significant portion of these eyes will go on to develop permanent scarring. Our sur-

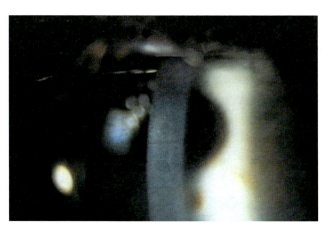

Fig. 4.2.3 Stage 2 DLK is characterized by fine, white cells in the stroma, which now extend to the center of the cornea. No clumping of cells in the interface of the cornea is present

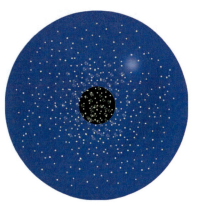

Fig. 4.2.6 Cells are clumping paracentrally and are now in the LASIK flap interface in stage 3 DLK

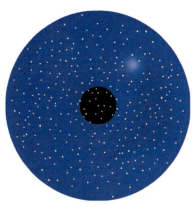

Fig. 4.2.4 Cells are distributed throughout the cornea, even centrally and yet are still in the stroma in stage 2 DLK

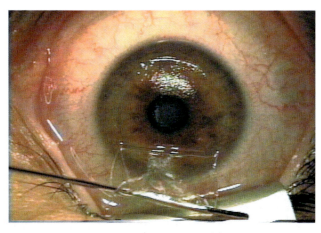

Fig. 4.2.7 Lifting of the LASIK flap and gentle irrigation is helpful in stage 3 DLK

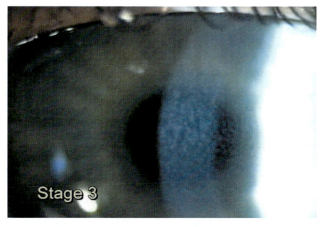

Fig. 4.2.5 Stage 3 DLK is characterized by fine, white cells that have now clumped slightly centrally or just inferior to the center of the cornea. They are no longer only in the stroma, but have now layered slightly in the LASIK interface. At this stage, they may actually start to clear in the periphery. This is the most important stage of DLK to recognize

geons found that lifting the LASIK flap promptly after the appearance of stage 3, or when threshold DLK is present, can effectively blunt the inflammatory response, and prevent permanent scarring from occurring (Fig. 4.2.7). No eyes in the series of this group of surgeons' 10,000 patients had any loss of best-corrected visual acuity (BCVA) attributable to DLK when the interface was irrigated promptly at the identification of stage 3 [17].

Stage 4: Stage 4 DLK is the rare result of a severe lamellar keratitis with stromal melting, permanent scarring, and associated visual morbidity. The aggregation of inflammatory cells and release of collagenases results in fluid collection in the central lamellae, with overlying bullae formation and stromal volume loss. A hyperopic shift due to central tissue loss, along with the appearance of corrugated "mud cracks" are an ominous sign. Lifting and irrigation at this point is of little benefit, and may actually be harmful. Lifting and irrigation at stage 4 may result in additional stromal volume loss if aggressive tissue manipulation is performed. Prop-

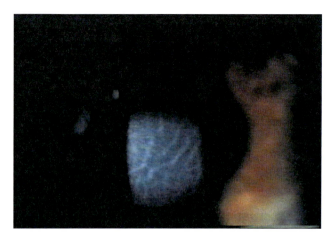

Fig. 4.2.8 Stage 4 DLK is characterized by scarring and loss of stromal volume

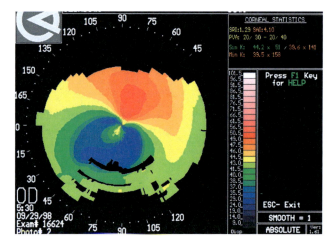

Fig. 4.2.9 Topography from stage 4 DLK can often show irregular astigmatism from extra flattening in the area of stromal volume loss. Often this will improve over the year after the DLK episode

er identification, grading, and appropriate intervention can prevent this from occurring. The incidence of a severe stage 4 DLK is approximately 1 in 5,000 (Figs. 4.2.8, 4.2.9).

4.2.5 Intervention and Treatment

Although each case may show a different level of severity or inflammation, the time course of diffuse lamellar keratitis is consistent. The experience of these authors has shown that the cellular reaction is nearly always present at postoperative day 1, and peaks at approximately day 5. DLK can best be thought of as a threshold disease; after a certain level of inflammation is reached, it is likely that there will be permanent scarring.

Stages 1 and 2 DLK will follow a self-limited course, resolving in 7–10 days. These authors manage both stage 1

and stage 2 by using an aggressive course of topical steroid drops, usually Pred Forte 1% (Allergan, Irvine, Calif.), one drop administered every hour while awake, and by using a steroid ointment applied to the eye at bedtime. Of note is that no randomized study has concluded that this is of benefit. Prompt follow up of the patient in 24 and 48 h will identify the small number of cases that will progress to stage 3.

If stage 3 is identified, management becomes more imperative and aggressive. It either involves either more aggressive topical and oral steroids [18], or, as these authors prefer, lifting the flap and debulking the inflammatory reaction by careful irrigation of the bed and undersurface of the cap. This should be done as soon as stage 3 is identified, which is usually at postoperative day 2 or 3 (48–72 h postoperatively). This should blunt the inflammatory response and it is hoped prevent permanent scarring. If the flap is lifted too soon, then the cells are still in the stroma, and lifting will not debulk the cells.

Lifting the flap is performed by the following method. First, delineate the edges of the flap with a blunt spatula. Lift and retract the flap peripherally to its hinge. This usually is relatively easy in the first 72 h. Once the flap is retracted, gently but thoroughly rinse the bed and undersurface of the cap with BSS on a blunt tipped cannula (see Fig. 4.2.7). Gently cleanse the bed and cap with a lightly moistened Merocel sponge. Aggressive scraping of the flap or stromal bed and using bladed instruments should be avoided. After gentle rinsing and cleansing, carefully reflect and float the flap back into position, and allow the flap to dry in place. Maintain the patient on the aggressive topical steroid use (the authors recommend one drop of Pred Forte 1% every hour while awake) while closely monitoring over the next several days. Often the clinical picture at 24 h after this flap lift shows significant flap edema and not much change in the level of inflammation. As the cellular reaction resolves, this may be tapered.

Lifting the flaps of those eyes showing any stage of DLK at day 1 may be tempting but should be avoided. This would miss the peak inflammatory reaction and would most likely be overtreatment of the majority of stages 1 and 2 cases that would have been self-limited or responsive to topical treatment. However, waiting until day 5 or 6 will risk the development of stage 4 DLK, which does result in permanent scarring. Thus, lifting stage 3 DLK at 48–72 h after the procedure is most effective.

If the most rare and more severe stage 4 DLK has occurred, then lifting the LASIK flap is of little benefit. It may actually add to stromal volume loss as the collagenolytic enzymes have begun to digest the collagen, and lifting the flap may remove more of the soggy, boggy collagen.

Some cases of DLK may be atypical such as the aforementioned late onset DLK or those cases associated with pain, decreased vision, or more dense infiltrates. Be aware that these cases may not be true DLK, or may be infectious in etiology. When in doubt, appropriate culture of the LASIK flap, undersurface, and bed, as well as prompt institution of antibiotic therapy is important.

4.2.6 GAPP Syndrome

GAPP syndrome (good acuity plus photophobia), is a characteristic and transient complication of femtosecond LASIK. William Maloney described it as a toxic non-inflammatory corneal reaction after femtosecond LASIK. (American Academy of Ophthalmology Refractive Surgery Subspecialty Day Meeting, November 2006). This is not DLK, but should be mentioned here as an early complication to LASIK performed with the femtosecond laser. This has also been referred to as transient light sensitivity. As of the writing of this chapter, the precise cause of GAPP is unknown. It is bilateral and appears 6–8 weeks after femtosecond LASIK. Its only symptom is an extreme sensitivity to light without loss of visual acuity. Some patients report pain on upgaze. Patients report no dryness or redness, and examination reveals no DLK, iritis, or scleritis. Reports of GAPP show an incidence of between 1 and 20%, and the syndrome appears more common in women and patients with blue eyes. The prevailing opinion is that GAPP syndrome has an inflammatory base and can be treated with corticosteroids. Administering corticosteroids for 3 days prior to surgery might help prevent this complication. It has been suggested that minimizing femtosecond laser energy may avoid inflammation [19].

One study reported an incidence of 1.1% ($n = 5,667$) of this transient light sensitivity after LASIK performed with femtosecond flap creation. The average age of patient in this study was 41, and about half were women. Onset of symptoms was from 2 to 6 weeks after uneventful LASIK. Most patients' symptoms resolved within 1 week of beginning topical steroid treatment. Patients' symptoms were prolonged if there was a delay in treatment. This study also indicated that reducing raster and side-cut energy settings by an average of 24– 33% significantly reduced the incidence of this syndrome [20].

4.2.7 Steroid-Induced Glaucoma after LASIK

Another complication associated with DLK and its treatment is steroid-induced glaucoma after LASIK. Since treatment of DLK involves aggressive and frequent use of steroid, the possibility of steroid response including elevated intraocular pressure (IOP) should be considered. While treating the DLK must be primary, steroid-induced glaucoma must be considered a possible secondary unwanted effect. In a study reported in 2002, six eyes of four patients who had DLK develop after uneventful LASIK were treated with aggressive corticosteroids. All six eyes had a pocket of fluid develop in the lamellar interface between the flap and the stromal bed associated with a steroid induced rise in IOP. The increase in pressure caused transudation of aqueous fluid across the stroma that accumulated in the flap interface. However, because of the interface fluid, IOP was normal or low measured by central corneal Goldmann applanation tonometry. Only by measuring the pressure peripherally several months later was a high IOP not-

ed. All six of these eyes developed visual field defects, and three eyes had severe glaucomatous optic neuropathy and decreased visual acuity [21].

4.2.8 Infectious Keratitis versus Noninfectious Keratitis

It is important to differentiate microbial keratitis from DLK. Microbial keratitis is a serious complication after LASIK. DLK is also a serious complication after LASIK, but is noninfectious and not treated with antimicrobial drugs. Most common signs of microbial keratitis after LASIK include ciliary and conjunctival hyperemia and whitish stromal infiltrates in the interface. These infiltrates are usually dense and grayish white, with indistinct edges that may extend into the surrounding stroma. Corneal flap and epithelium are commonly involved, causing an epithelial defect that stains with fluorescein. This is not common in diffuse lamellar keratitis, as there is no epithelial defect with DLK. In DLK, the infiltrates are confined to the interface. They are diffuse and scattered through a large area of the interface, not extending anteriorly into the flap or posteriorly into the stroma. Symptoms of microbial keratitis after LASIK include foreign body sensation, decreased vision, pain, photophobia, redness, and tearing. It is uncommon for the patient with DLK to have any of these symptoms, especially in the early stages of the condition. When a lesion is suspected of being microbial keratitis, the corneal flap must be lifted and the stromal bed scraped for culture and laboratory diagnosis. Prompt management with appropriate antibiotics is critical with microbial keratitis, as this is one of the most vision threatening complications after LASIK. DLK can be distinguished from infectious infiltrates by clinical presentation and close follow-up [22].

4.2.9 Conclusion

In conclusion, eye care providers must be familiar with potential complications of LASIK surgery. DLK is an uncommon complication that can occur in the early postoperative period. Undetected or untreated, it can cause scarring and an adverse visual outcome. Once considered a mystery, much now is understood regarding the etiology and treatment of this disease. Increased awareness of potential contaminants as well as proper maintenance and cleaning of sterilizer water reservoirs has decreased but not eliminated the frequency of occurrence of DLK. Educating patients to the importance of early follow up despite lack of symptoms, educating technical staff, and educating those who follow LASIK patients postoperatively is critical to identifying and treating DLK appropriately. However, occasional cases still occur, and understanding the time course of the disease, along with proper identification, staging, and intervention can help eliminate visual loss associated with this condition.

4

Take-Home Pearls

Staging of DLK:

Stage 1
- Usually identified at 1 day postoperatively
- White, granular cells in the periphery of the lamellar flap

Stage 2
- May be present at 1 day postoperatively; more commonly seen 48–72 h postoperative
- White, granular cells in the center of the flap
- Shifting-sands appearance

Stage 3
- If present, usually seen at 48–72 h postoperatively
- Dense, white, clumped cells in the central visual axis
- Requires flap lifting to prevent permanent scarring

Stage 4
- Rare result of a severe lamellar keratitis
- Stromal melting, permanent scarring, and visual morbidity
- Hyperopic shift, mud cracks
- Treatment may be of little help.

References

1. Smith RJ, Maloney RK (1998) Diffuse lamellar keratitis: a new syndrome in lamellar refractive surgery. Ophthalmology 105:1721–1726
2. Kaufman SC (1999) Post LASIK interface keratitis, Sands of the Sahara syndrome, and microkeratome blades (letter). J Cataract Refract Surg 25:1004–1008
3. Kaufman SC, Maitchouk DY, Chiou AG, Beuerman, RW (1998) Interface inflammation after laser in-situ keratomileusis—Sands of the Sahara Syndrome. J Cataract Refract Surg 24:1589–1593
4. Shah MN, Misra M, Wihelmus KR, Koch DD (2000) Diffuse lamellar keratitis associated with epithelial defects after laser in situ keratomileusis. J Cataract Refract Surg 26:1312–1318
5. Peters NT, Iskander NG, Anderson PEE, Woods DE, Mo RA, Gimbel HV (2001) Diffuse lamellar keratitis: isolation of endotoxin and demonstration of the inflammatory potential in a rabbit model. J Cataract Refract Surg 27:917–923
6. Yuhan KR, Nguyen L, Wachler BS (2002) Role of instrument cleaning and maintenance in the development of diffuse lamellar keratitis. Ophthalmology 1090:400–403; discussion 403–404
7. Levinger S, Landau D, Kremer I, Merin S, Aizenman I, Hirsch A, Douieb J, Bos T (2003) Wiping microkeratome blades with sterile 100% alcohol to prevent diffuse lamellar keratitis after laser in situ keratomileusis. J Cataract Refract Surg 29:1947–1949
8. Kim JY, Kim MJ, Kim TI, Choi HJ, Pak JH, Tchah H (2006) A femtosecond laser creates a stronger flap than a mechanical microkeratome. Invest Ophthalmol Vis Sci 47:599–604
9. Stonecipher K, Ignacio TS, Stonecipher M (2006) Advances in refractive surgery: microkeratome and femtosecond laser flap creation in relation to safety, efficacy, predictability, and biomechanical stability. Curr Opinion Ophthalmol 17:368–372
10. Moilanen JA, Holopainen JM, Helinto M, Vesaluoma MH, Tervo TM (2004) Keratocyte activation and inflammation in diffuse lamellar keratitis after formation of an epithelial defect. J Cataract Refract Surg 30:341–349
11. Guo N, Zhou YH, Qu J, Pan ZQ, Wang L (2006) [Evaluation of diffuse lamellar keratitis after LASIK with confocal microscopy.] Zhonghua Yan Ke Za Zhi 42:330–333
12. Buhren J, Cichocki M, Baumeister M, Kohnen T (2002) Diffuse lamellar keratitis after laser in situ keratomileusis. Clinical and confocal microscopy findings. Ophthalmology 99:176–180
13. Bigham M, Enns CL, Holland SP et al (2005) Diffuse lamellar keratitis complicating laser in situ keratomileusis: post-marketing surveillance of an emerging disease in British Columbia, Canada, 2000–2002. J Cataract Refract Surg 31:2340–2344
14. Jin GJ, Lyle WA, Merkley KH (2005) Late-onset idiopathic diffuse lamellar keratitis after laser in situ keratomileusis. J Cataract Refract Surg 31:435–437
15. Buxey K (2004) Delayed onset diffuse lamellar keratitis following enhancement LASIK surgery. Clin Exp Optom 87102–106
16. Gris O, Guell JL, Wolley-Dod C, Adan A (2004) Diffuse lamellar keratitis and corneal edema associate with viral keratoconjunctivitis 2 years after laser in situ keratomileusis. J Cataract Refract Surg 30:1366–1370
17. Linebarger EJ, Hardten DR, Lindstrom RL (2003) Diffuse lamellar keratitis: recognition and management. In: Buratto L, Brint SF (eds) Custom LASIK surgical techniques and complications. Slack, Thorofare, N.J., pp 745–750
18. Hoffman RS, Fine IH, Packer M (2003) Incidence and outcomes of LASIK with diffuse lamellar keratitis treated with topical and oral corticosteroids. J Cataract Refract Surg 29:451–456
19. Cimberle Michael (2006) (Munoz, Gonzalo) (Report on Alicante International Refractive Meeting) Retinal detachment rates for lens exchange, phakic IOLs comparable. Ocular Surgery News, 15 June 2006, pp 3–6
20. Stonecipher KG, Dishler JG, Ignacio TS, Binder PS (2006) Transient light sensitivity after femtosecond laser flap creation: clinical findings and management. J Cataract Refract Surg 32:91–94
21. Hamilton DR, Manche EE, Rich LF, Maloney RK (2002) Steroid induced glaucoma after laser in situ keratomileusis associated with interface fluid. Ophthalmology 109:659–665
22. Alió JL, Perez-Santonja JJ, Tervo T (2000) Postoperative inflammation, microbial complications, and wound healing following Laser in situ keratomileusis. J Refractive Surg 16:523–538

- The reader must recognize that not all flap interface haze appearing after LASIK represents DLK or infection.

- Interface fluid is usually the result of elevated IOP, frequently steroid-induced. The fluid may be space occupying, resulting in falsely low IOP measurements on applanation tonometry, or non–space occupying, allowing accurate pressure measurement.

- If presumed DLK does not respond to a regimen of frequent topical steroids, then consider elevated IOP as the etiology (pressure-induced interlamellar stromal keratitis).

- Management consists of discontinuation of the topical steroid and lowering of the IOP.

4.3 Pressure-Induced Interlamellar Stromal Keratitis

Sadeer B. Hannush and Michael W. Belin

4.3.1 Introduction

DLK, or sands of the Sahara (SOS), is post–LASIK corneal flap interface infiltration or inflammation that was first described in 1998 by Smith and Maloney [1] in a series of 12 patients. The infiltrates typically present on postoperative days 1 to 3 and may be diffuse, focal, or multifocal. They are confined to the lamellar interface and are not associated with an anterior chamber reaction. Four clinical stages have been described, ranging from non–visually significant interface haze to severe dense infiltration associated with stromal necrosis [2]. Most cases are mild, asymptomatic, and self-limited or responsive to topical steroids. Slit lamp examination typically shows a fine granular infiltrate confined to the flap interface, often in the periphery of the stromal bed. Moderate cases are often accompanied by a decrease in visual acuity and more cellular deposition or haze in the visual axis. Severe cases are associated with significant interface haze, cellular aggregation, and pain. Severe cases not responding to hourly topical steroid drops may require surgical intervention to irrigate the interface, washing off the inflammatory cells, and other potential inflammatory agents. Untreated, severe DLK can lead to flap melting and necrosis [3]. The incidence of DLK has been reported to range from 1 to 4%, but this almost certainly underestimates the true incidence, because very mild cases are often missed or underreported [4]. The cause of DLK remains obscure and is probably multifactorial.

Suspected causes include metallic debris from the microkeratome or blade, sterilizer reservoir biofilms, meibomian gland secretions, bacterial endotoxins, glove talc, cleaning or disinfecting solutions, debris from surgical sponges, and epithelial debris. Rather than being caused by a single agent, DLK probably represents a common inflammatory response in the lamellar interface to a variety of stimuli.

A late-onset DLK picture has also been reported in LASIK patients, weeks, or months after surgery, in the setting of trauma, recurrent erosions, or epithelial abrasions [5–7].

Another condition that may mimic DLK has been described as resulting from the accumulation of interface fluid. Slit lamp examination of these patients reveals a clear zone between the stromal bed and flap that represents a pocket of interface fluid [8–10]. In this entity, central applanation tonometry is very low as can be expected when applanating over a pocket of fluid, while more reliable methods of measuring intraocular pressure such as peripheral applanation or pneumotonometry reveal markedly elevated pressure inside the eye.

In 2002, we reported a series of four patients in whom a clinical picture almost identical to classic DLK developed [11]. All patients described onset of decreased visual acuity after the first post-operative week, all failed to improve with frequent topical steroid drops, and all had clinically significant elevated IOP. No patient exhibited any frank interface fluid or clear zone. Each patient responded with both improvement in visual acuity and decrease in interface haze, with the lowering of intraocular pressure and discontinuation of topical steroids. To describe this condition we coined the term elevated intraocular pressure-induced interlamellar stromal keratitis (PISK) (Figs. 4.3.1, 4.3.2, 4.3.3, 4.3.4).

Since our initial report, several reports have appeared in the ophthalmic literature describing the same phenomenon. In 2003, Davidson et al. [12] described the case of a 53-year-old patient with a history of treated ocular hypertension who underwent uncomplicated LASIK surgery. The postoperative course was complicated by markedly elevated IOP induced by topical corticosteroid drops used to treat what appeared to be diffuse lamellar keratitis. Once the topical steroids were discontinued, the intraocular pressure returned to normal range with complete resolution of the corneal findings. In 2004, Cheng et al. [13] described the in vivo confocal microscopic findings in two patients with ste-

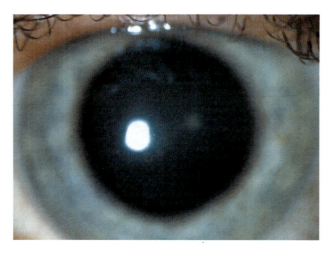

Fig. 4.3.1 Patient with PISK, showing mild diffuse haze

4

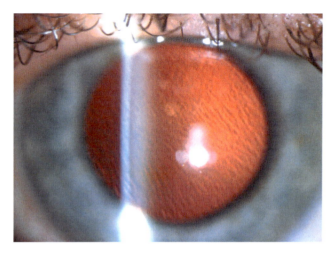

Fig. 4.3.2 Same patient seen with retroillumination: wavy, granular pattern mimics sands of the Sahara (SOS) in diffuse lamellar keratitis (DLK)

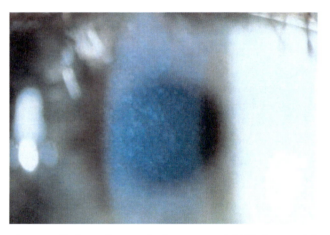

Fig. 4.3.3 Slit lamp photograph of a patient with PISK, showing diffuse interface haze similar to mild-to-moderate DLK

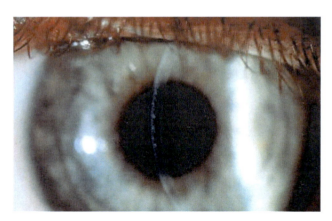

Fig. 4.3.4 Slit lamp photograph of same patient: narrow slit shows haze limited to the interface

roid-induced glaucoma after LASIK. Confocal microscopic examination did not show mononuclear cells and granulocytes typically seen in patients with classic DLK. This was confirmed by a similar report in 2006 by Kurian et al. [14]. They observed swollen and enlarged cellular structures, as well as the presence of microlacunae separating the stromal collagen lamellae. Again, inflammatory mononuclear cells and granulocytes, seen in patients with DLK, were absent. In 2004, Nordlund et al. [15] described 10 eyes of six patients with late-onset interface inflammation and increased IOP. The lamellar inflammation was refractive to topical steroids and did not resolve until the pressure was controlled. In 2006, Galal et al. [16] described the same phenomenon in 13 eyes. They concluded that what they described as interface corneal edema was secondary to elevation of IOP, which developed in steroid responders after LASIK, creating a misleading clinical picture simulating DLK or infectious keratitis. Most recently (March 2007), in a report describing the same phenomenon, Frucht-Pery et al. [17] attributed early transient visual acuity loss after LASIK to steroid-induced elevation of IOP.

The exact cause of DLK remains obscure and is probably multifactorial. DLK represents a clinical presentation rather than a specific disease entity. Previously, associated factors (e.g., bacterial exotoxins, debris, and chemical contamination) were known agents capable of inducing an inflammatory reaction. Even late DLK induced by epithelial defects has a known inflammatory component. The possible cause-and-effect relationship in PISK is less clear. Steroid-induced pressure elevation in non-operated eyes is typically clinically silent and not associated with an inflammatory component. It may be that lamellar keratitis after LASIK represents a common clinical presentation for both inflammatory and non-inflammatory insults to the post-LASIK eye. Alternatively, the DLK-like picture in PISK may represent a mild form of non–space-occupying interface fluid collection (microlacunae) with measurable elevated pressure. This, in contrast to space occupying interface fluid with falsely low or normal intraocular pressure previously described in the literature.

4.3.2 Conclusion

It is important to recognize that PISK occurs beyond the typical immediate postoperative period and is associated with a significantly elevated IOP. All cases respond not to topical steroid therapy, but to lowering of the IOP and a reduction or discontinuation of the topical steroids. Patients may or may not have a history of ocular hypertension. The IOP elevations may occur in some patients earlier than is traditionally associated with steroid-induced IOP elevation.

It is customary for refractive surgeons not to measure IOP on the first postoperative day for fear of causing a flap displacement. It has become too commonplace, however, not to measure IOP on later routine postoperative visits because the refractive population tends to be a younger, healthier group that is at lower risk for ocular disease. The importance of IOP measurement and of maintaining a high level of suspicion when a DLK-like picture occurs after the first postoperative week is not associated with other causative events (e.g., epithelial defect), and does not readily respond to an increase in topical steroids, cannot be overemphasized. IOP measurement in cases of suspected DLK appearing after the first week after LASIK is strongly recommended. If elevated, lowering the pressure and discontinuing the topical steroids frequently results in resolution of the interface changes, paralleled by improvement in vision.

Take-Home Pearls

■ DLK usually appears 1 to 3 days after LASIK, and weeks or months later in the setting of trauma, corneal abrasions, or erosions.

■ A DLK-like picture appearing a week or more after LASIK may not be inflammatory in nature. It may represent interface fluid that may or may not be space occupying.

■ It is important to measure IOP and to maintain a high level of suspicion when a DLK-like picture occurs after the first postoperative week, is not associated with other causative events (e.g., epithelial defect), and does not readily respond to an increase in topical steroids.

■ If IOP is indeed elevated, consider PISK as the etiology.

■ Management consists of lowering the pressure and discontinuation of the topical steroids.

References

1. Smith RJ, Maloney RK (1998) Diffuse lamellar keratitis: a new syndrome in lamellar refractive surgery. Ophthalmology 105:1721–1726
2. Kaufman SC, Maitchouk DY, Chiou AGY, Beuerman RW (1998) Interface inflammation after laser in situ keratomileusis. Sands of the Sahara syndrome. J Cataract Refract Surg 24:1589–1593
3. Linebarger EJ, Hardten DR, Lindstrom RL (2000) Diffuse lamellar keratitis: diagnosis and management. J Cataract Refract Surg 26:1072–107
4. Holland SP, Mathias RG, Morck DW et al (2000) Diffuse lamellar keratitis related to endotoxins released from sterilizer reservoir biofilms. Ophthalmology 107:1227–1233; discussion 1233–1234
5. Chang-Godinich A, Steinert RF, Wu HK (2001) Late occurrence of diffuse lamellar keratitis after laser in situ keratomileusis. Arch Ophthalmol 119:1074–1076
6. Keszei VA (2001) Diffuse lamellar keratitis associated with iritis 10 months after laser in situ keratomileusis. J Cataract Refract Surg 27:1126 –1127
7. Harrison DA, Periman LM (2001) Diffuse lamellar keratitis associated with recurrent corneal erosions after laser in situ keratomileusis. J Refract Surg 17:463–465
8. Rehany U, Bersudsky V, Rumelt S (2000) Paradoxical hypotony after laser in situ keratomileusis. J Cataract Refract Surg 26:1823–1826
9. Najman-Vainer J, Smith RJ, Maloney RK (2000) Interface fluid after LASIK: misleading tonometry can lead to end-stage glaucoma [letter]. J Cataract Refract Surg 26:471–472
10. Parekh JG, Raviv T, Speaker MG (2001) Grossly false applanation tonometry associated with interface fluid in susceptible LASIK patients [letter]. J Cataract Refract Surg 27: 1143–1144
11. Belin MW, Hannush SB, Yau CW, Schultze RL (2002) Elevated intraocular pressure-induced interlamellar stromal keratitis. Ophthalmology 109:1929–1933
12. Davidson RS, Brandt ID, Mannis MJ (2003) Intraocular pressure-induced interlamellar keratitis after LASIK surgery. Glaucoma 12:23–26
13. Cheng AC, Law RW, Young AL, Lam DS (2004) In vivo confocal microscopic findings in patients with steroid-induced glaucoma after LASIK. Ophthalmology 111:768–774
14. KurianM, Shetty R, Shetty BK, Devi SA (2006) In vivo confocal microscopic findings of interlamellar stromal keratopathy induced by elevated intraocular pressure. Cataract Refract Surg 32:1563–1566
15. Nordlund MI, Grimm S, Lane S, Holland EJ (2004) Pressure-induced interface keratitis: a late complication following LASIK. Cornea 23:225-234
16. Galal A, Artola A, Belda I, Rodriguez-Prats I, Claramonte P, Sanchez A, Ruiz-Morenao O, Meravo I, Alió J (2006) Interface corneal edema secondary to steroid-induced elevation of intraocular pressure simulating diffuse lamellar keratitis. J Refract Surg 22:441–447
17. Frucht-Pery J, Landau D, Raiskup F, Orucov F, Strassman E, Blumenthal EZ, Solomon A (2007) Early transient visual acuity loss after LASIK due to streroid-induced elevation of intraocular pressure. J Refractive Surgery 23:244–251

Core Messages

■ Sources of flap surface problems

■ Prevention of flap striae

■ Differentiation of macrostriae and microstriae

■ Medical and office interventions for flap striae

■ Phototherapeutic keratectomy

4.4 Prevention and Management of Flap Striae after LASIK

Roger F. Steinert

4.4.1 Introduction

An optically smooth and clear flap is critical for recovery of vision after LASIK. The anterior flap is the principal optical interface of the eye, dominating the factors influencing the recovery of vision. A smooth surface also leads to patient comfort and overall patient satisfaction with the procedure.

The preoperative assessment must include accurate assessment of the status of meibomian gland and tear production. The presence of external ocular or systemic diseases that influence the stability of the LASIK flap surface must be determined. If the tear film is not optimal, then aggressive preoperative measures must be taken, including lid hygiene, tear supplementation, anti-inflammatory agents, and possibly placement of punctal plugs prior to the LASIK procedure. Prophylaxis is more effective than remedial therapy is once the LASIK flap is in difficulty postoperatively.

Operative factors can also influence the difficulties in a smooth LASIK flap postoperatively. Anesthetic drop administration should be minimized, and when anesthetic is applied, following with an artificial tear and instructing the patient with the eyelids closed in order to prevent drying due to lack of blinking is advisable. Administration of vasoconstrictive agents such as phenylephrine and brimondine (Alphagan, Allergan, Irvine Calif.) has been associated with flap irregularities, possibly due to effects on dryness and mucin in the tear film. If alignment marks are made with ink, then they should be irrigated immediately, as most inks have an alcohol base, which also disrupts the epithelium. If it is compatible with the manufacture's recommendations, use of a non-preserved medium viscosity artificial tear immediately prior to the passage of a microkeratome can reduce some of the frictional damage to the epithelium. In addition, minimizing the duration of elevation of the flap will reduce the potential for induced damage to the surface. Likewise, it is advisable to avoid prolonged irrigation under the flap once it is replaced, as the duration of irrigation is related to the amount of induced flap edema with subsequent striae. Likewise, excessive stroking of the flap may contribute to the development of both surface defects and striae. It is important not to let the flap surface dry at any time. Once the flap is reposition, immediate administration of a high viscosity artificial agent such as Celluvisc (Allergan) is helpful.

The flap should also be protected against physical injury with a shield or goggles. It is important to educate the patient about the proper administration of eye drops in order to avoid disrupting the flap by pressure on the eyelids or direct trauma from an eye drop bottle tip. For the first day, in addition to the pharmacologic medications, frequent administration of an artificial tear maintains lubricity. In the hours immediately following LASIK surgery, naps longer than 1 hour should be interrupted with the administration of artificial tears in order to avoid drying and adhesion of the flap to the underside of the eyelid during sleep. Most patients will have a reduction in tear film quality and/or volume for several months postoperatively, and frequent administration of artificial tears is usually advisable, as well as more aggressive surface treatment if deterioration of the surface is detected.

4.4.2 Flap Striae

Flap striae, or wrinkles, have two general types of configuration. Macrostriae consist of broad undulations of parallel or semi-parallel lines. This appearance is similar to a washboard or wind-swept sand (Fig. 4.4.1). Macrostriae are usually caused by dislocation of the flap. Careful inspection of the slit lamp will typically show a widened gutter. Because the epithelium may have rapidly filled in this area, application of fluorescein will help show the presence of a widened gutter as the fluorescein pools. Microstriae have a more random pattern of fine irregularities easier seen on retroillumination. The appearance is similar to dried, cracked mud or the dry cracks on a salt lake bed (Fig. 4.4.2). Microstriae have an appearance somewhat similar to prominent corneal nerves.

In many cases, flap slippage that results in macrostriae has no identifiable cause. However, some patients will note acute onset of unusual pain if the flap slippage occurs due to drying with subsequent traction on the flap.

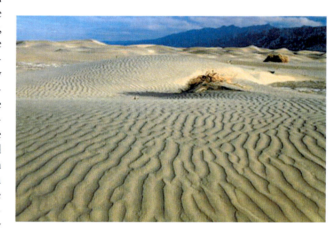

Fig. 4.4.1 Macrostriae have broad undulations similar to wind-swept sand

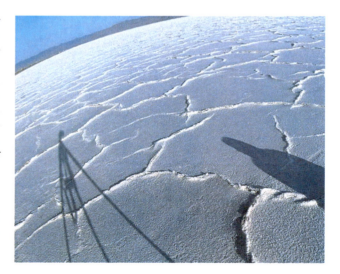

Fig. 4.4.2 Microstriae resemble random fine cracks as seen in a dried salt lake bed

4.4.2.1 Treatment of Macrostriae

If macrostriae are detected soon after occurrence, ideally within the first 24 h, then the surgeon has the opportunity to resolve the problem with immediate treatment. The flap should be lifted, epithelium cleaned from the gutter in order to avoid subsequent epithelial ingrowth into the interface, and then the flap floated with balance salt solution, gently stroked, and smoothed back into position (Fig. 4.4.3). Application of bandage soft contact lens for 1 day helps stabilize the flap and may reduce the potential for epithelial ingrowth.

When macrostriae are undetected and untreated for 1 or more days, the folds tend to become fixed. This occurs due to a filling in effect of the epithelium, followed by contracture of the collagen. Based on the severity and duration of the folds, a sequence of increasingly aggressive interventions may be needed to eliminate the folds. These include de-epithelialization, followed by swelling of the flap with hypotonic solution, stretching with forceps, and suturing with interrupted or running sutures.

De-epithelialization is important in releasing fixed macrostriae because the epithelium has remodeled around the macrostriae and will prevent the folds from relaxing (Fig. 4.4.4). Epithelium can be debrided directly with a spatu-

la or similar instrument, but a gentle and effective way of both debriding epithelium and beginning a swelling of the flap is to drip sterile distilled water over the central cornea for several minutes. This will cause the epithelium to swell and the cell membranes rupture, following which, gentle debridement with a surgical spear sponge will be possible. Further drops of sterile distilled water on the surface will lead to more flap edema anteriorly, which will help relax the fixed macrostriae. The flap itself is refloated with balanced salt solution, not the hypotonic distilled water, because the swelling is desired anteriorly in the flap, but not in the region of the interface. If excessive hydration of the flap occurs, then there is the possibility that swelling in the anteroposterior direction will result in a mechanical contracture of the flap diameter. Initially the flap striae will appear to have been resolved. However, when the flap is repositioned and then subsequently dehydrates due to endothelial pump function, the reduced flap diameter will be fixed in place and then new striae may occur as a result.

After hydration as described above, the macrostriae may not be fully resolved, but should appear improved. By the next day, when the bandage soft contact lens is slipped aside, the macrostriae should be resolved. If the macrostriae appears severe despite the initial hydration, or they have not resolved the next day, then the patient can be instructed to apply drops of sterile distilled water with the bandage contact lens in place on an hourly basis for 1 day. Because these drops are not preserved, it is important that they are discarded after no more than 1 day's use. In addition, prophylactic antibiotic drops and steroid drops are important. These corneas have increased vulnerability to an inflammatory reaction (diffuse lamellar keratitis).

If macrostriae persist despite the hydration treatment, then traction may be necessary. In some cases traction with one or more forceps will be successful. If simple traction with forceps is unsuccessful, then the flap may be sutured with multiple interrupted 10-0 nylon sutures or a tight running circumferential suture. Sutures can be removed within several days or weeks; there is no firm guideline on the timing of suture removal [1, 2]. The surgeon should make the patient aware that the suturing of the flap may create new striae or induce regular or irregular astigmatism. In

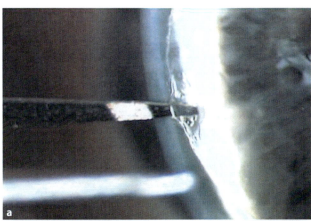

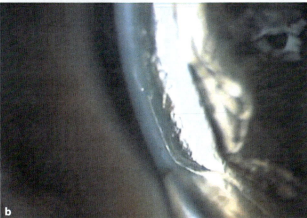

Fig. 4.4.3 Macrostriae. a Lifting the edge of a flap with the tip of a jeweller's forceps. b The flap gutter has been cleaned of an ingrowth of epithelium; the edge is visible near the limbus

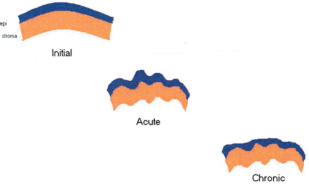

Fig. 4.4.4 Schematic illustration of establishment of macrostriae with epithelial remodelling and collagen contracture

severe cases of recalcitrant striae, amputating and discarding the flap has been advocated [3].

4.4.2.2 Treatment of Microstriae

Before instituting treatment of microstriae, the surgeon must determine whether microstriae are optically significant and responsible for a patient's visual symptoms. Because microstriae are smaller in both elevation and width, compared with macrostriae, the epithelium may be able to mask the presence and reduce the optical impact of microstriae. Most LASIK flaps, in fact, have microstriae that are invisible.

Optically significant microstriae are usually not detected on color corneal topography maps but can be seen disrupting the mires on a Placido image. In addition, optically significant microstriae will typically exhibit "negative staining" of the fluorescein pattern, as well as being visible on retroillumination (Fig. 4.4.5) [4].

Microstriae pathologically represent fine wrinkles in Bowman's layer. This in turn causes disruption of the tear film and the anterior optical surface. Risk factors for optically significant microstriae include thin flaps and high myopia, in which the flattening of the surface of the cornea by the myopic correction causes anterior compression of the flap [5]. However, troublesome microstriae have occurred with no known risk factors.

The initial treatment should be medical, encouraging surface epithelial healing. This includes treatment of any external eyelid disease, frequent administration of nonpreserved artificial tears, and, where needed, puntal plugs or treatment for several weeks with an extended wear bandage soft contact lens.

Numerous treatments have been advocated for persistent optically significant microstriae, including the treatments listed above for macrostriae (hydration, stretching, and suturing) [15]. In addition, heating of the flap and pressure with a cotton-tip applicator have been advocated [6–12].

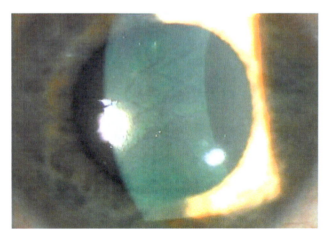

Fig. 4.4.5 Microstriae seen by "negative staining" of fluorescein in the tear film, caused by the disruption of the tear film by the elevated surface over the microstriae, disrupting the tear film

4.4.3 Phototherapeutic Keratectomy

In my experience, the most reliable and predictable results in treating microstriae and persistent macrostriae, occur with use of the technique of excimer laser PTK [13, 14].

The protocol for PTK with a broad beam laser (Visx S4, Advanced Medical Optics, Santa Clara, Calif.) is as follows. Three hundred pulses are programmed at a diameter of 6 mm. In the first phase of the treatment, 200 pulses are applied to perform transepithelial ablation utilizing the pupil tracker. The epithelium acts as a masking agent, as it is thinner over the striae and thicker in areas between the striae. After the initial 200 pulses, the surgeon then turns off the pupil tracker and applies a maximum of 100 further pulses utilizing masking fluid. A medium viscosity preservative free artificial tear (e.g., Refresh Plus, Allergan) is applied with a debris-free microsurgical spear sponge. Ideally, a moderate amount of moisture is applied, such that the cornea appears to glisten, but where the fluid layer is not so thick as to fully obscure the microstriae. If the fluid layer is too thick, the laser pulses will emit a dull, thudding sound rather than a sharper, snapping sound, and bubbling may be seen in the fluid. Five to eight pulses are delivered, followed by rewiping and repeating the process, with the surgeon controlling the pulse delivery with the foot pedal of the laser. Setting the laser repetition rate as low as possible (6 Hz) facilitates the repeat wiping and brief firing of the laser. The PTK is judged to be completed when the appearance of the striae is markedly reduced but not necessarily eliminated, or when the maximum number of 300 pulses is reached, whichever comes first.

Postoperatively, a bandage soft contact lens is applied and antibiotic and steroid drops at a rate of at least four times daily are used until re-epithelialization occurs, typically around the fourth postoperative day.

We have now analyzed and published the results from 44 patients with the mean follow-up after PTK of 297 days (ranging from 70 to 931 days). Mean uncorrected visual acuity improved from 20/43 to 20/33, and mean best spectacle improved from 20/29 to 20/23 at the last follow-up visit. Figure 4.4.6 shows the change in acuity in PTK. Overall there was an average shift in refractive error of +0.80 D after PTK (Fig. 4.4.7).

Refractive stability after PTK could be assessed in 24 eyes that were available at both 1 month and 1 year later (Fig. 4.4.8). The shift in mean refraction from the 1 month to the 12-month later was less than 0.50 D.

The PTK treatment did not result in optically significant haze in the LASIK flaps. Only five (1.6%) eyes reached a haze level of 1.00+; 14 (7.8%) eyes had trace haze at any interval, and 28 (59.6%) eyes had no detectable haze at any interval. No instances of late-onset haze occurred.

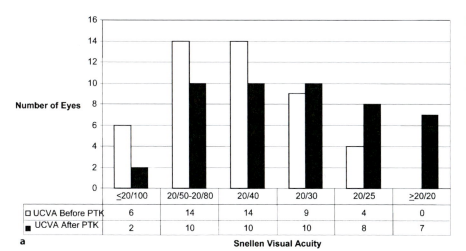

□ UCVA Before PTK	≤20/100	20/50-20/80	20/40	20/30	20/25	>20/20
□ UCVA Before PTK	6	14	14	9	4	0
■ UCVA After PTK	2	10	10	10	8	7

a   Snellen Visual Acuity

Fig. 4.4.6 **a** Distribution of uncorrected vision uncorrected visual acuity before and after phototherapeutic keratectomy. **b** Distribution of BSCVA before and after phototherapeutic keratectomy. **c** Change in best spectacle corrected visual acuity. (From [14], reproduced with permission)

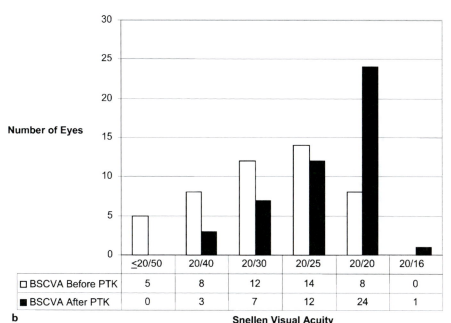

	≤20/50	20/40	20/30	20/25	20/20	20/16
□ BSCVA Before PTK	5	8	12	14	8	0
■ BSCVA After PTK	0	3	7	12	24	1

b   Snellen Visual Acuity

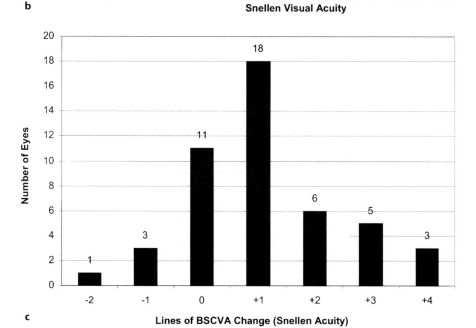

c   Lines of BSCVA Change (Snellen Acuity)

4

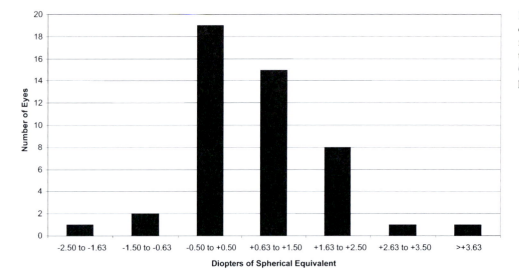

Fig. 4.4.7 Distribution of net change in spherical equivalent refractive error after phototherapeutic keratectomy. (From [14], reproduced with permission)

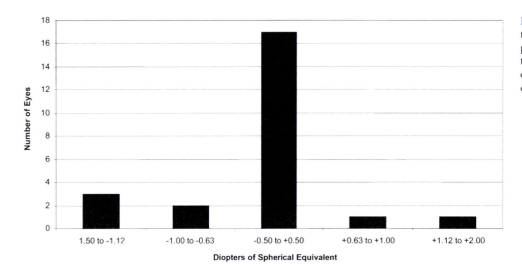

Fig. 4.4.8 Change in refraction from one month post phototherapeutic keratectomy to the last visit at 12 months or later. (From [14], reproduced with permission)

Take-Home Pearls

■ Careful attention to preoperative risk factors, external disease, and proper patient education and training postoperatively can reduce the frequency of macrostriae and microstriae in the LASIK flap.

■ If flap slippage occurs with optically significant macrostriae, treatment should be prompt and definitive, utilizing increasingly aggressive measures as needed. If macrostriae are detected and treated within 24 h, refloating the flap, accompanied by debridement of the epithelium and hydration, is usually successful.

■ In more severe or prolonged cases aggressive stretching or suturing of the flap may be necessary. In contrast, visually significant microstriae may improve by support of the epithelium medically.

■ PTK after a standardized protocol has been proven to be safe and effective in improving acuity in cases of established flap striae.

References

1. Mackool RJ, Monsanto VR (2003) Sequential lift and suture technique for post-LASIK corneal striae. J Cataract Refract Surg 29:785–787
2. Jackson DW, Hamill MB, Koch DD (2003) Laser in situ keratomileusis flap suturing to treat recalcitrant flap striae. J Cataract Refract Surg 29:264–269
3. Lam DSC, Leung ATS, Wu JT et al (1999) Management of severe flap wrinkling or dislodgement after laser in situ keratomileusis. J Cataract Refract Surg 25:1441–1447
4. Rabinowitz YS, Rasheed K (1999) Fluorescein test for the detection of striae in the corneal flap after laser in situ keratomileusis. Am J Ophthalmol 127:717–718
5. Charman WN (2002) Mismatch between flap and stromal areas after laser in situ keratomileusis as source of flap striae J Cataract Refract Surg 28:2146–2152
6. Lin JC, Rapuano CJ, Cohen EJ (2003) RK4 lens fitting for a flap striae in a LASIK patient. Eye Contact Lens 29:76–78
7. Araki-Sasaki K, Tsumura T, Kinoshita T et al (2002) Corneal remodeling by hard contact lenses to manage microstriae after laser in situ keratomileusis. J Cataract Refract Surg 28:2050–2053

8. Solomon R, Donnenfeld ED, Perry HD et al (2003) Slitlamp stretching of the corneal flap after laser in situ keratomileusis to reduce corneal striae. J Cataract Refract Surg 29:1292–1296

9. Lyle WA, Lin GJC (2000) Results of flap repositioning after laser in situ keratomileusis. J Cataract Refract Surg 26:1451–1457

10. Fox ML, Harmer E. Therapeutic flap massage for microstriae after laser in situ keratomileusis (2004) Treatment technique and implications. J Cataract Refract Surg 30:369–373

11. Hernandez-Matamoros J, Iradier MT, Moreno E (2001) Treating folds and striae after laser in situ kertomileusis. J Cataract Refract Surg 27:350–352

12. Donnenfeld ED, Perry HD, Doshi SJ et al (2004) Hyperthermic treatment of post-LASIK corneal striae. J Cataract Refract Surg 30:620–625

13. Steinert RF, Ashrafzadeh A, Hersh PS (2004) Results of phototherapeutic keratectomy in management of flap striae after LASIK. Ophthalmology 111:740–746

14. Ashrafzadeh A, Steinert RF (2007) Results of phototherapeutic keratectomy in the management of flap striae after LASIK before and after developing a standardized protocol: long term follow-up in an expanded patient population. Ophthalmology 114:1118–1123

15 Muñoz G, Alio JL, Perez-Santonja JJ et al (2000) Successful treatment of severe wrinkled corneal flap after laser in situ keratomileusis with deionized water. Am J Ophthalmol 129:91–92

Core Messages

■ Sterile infiltrates represent a rare condition that starts within 1–5 days after LASIK.

4.5 Marginal Sterile Corneal Infiltrates after LASIK

Renato Ambrósio, Jr., Daniela Jardim, and Bruno M. Fontes

4.5.1 Introduction

LASIK remains the first choice for the correction of refractive errors in the majority of patients [10]. Clinical advantages of LASIK over surface ablation techniques are related to the maintenance of an intact healthy epithelium over the central cornea after the lamellar cut is performed to expose the corneal stroma for laser ablation. This technique leads to faster visual rehabilitation, less postoperative discomfort, and less healing response, which tends toward more stability, especially for eyes with higher corrections [5, 24, 32]. LASIK has very high patient satisfaction rates and is associated with significant improvement in the quality of life for the majority of patients [32]. Nevertheless, LASIK technique has limitations and associated complications related to the creation of a hinged flap or to its presence on the cornea after surgery [6, 19]. These complications extend from mere annoyance to catastrophic consequences for the eye that threaten vision. Early recognition and prompt appropriate treatment of such possible complications is critical to maximize the success rates of the procedure (efficiency), as to minimize the chances of visual loss (safety). In addition, it is important to be alert to identify, in the preoperative process, cases at higher risk for complications. This would enable the surgeon to develop strategies to prevent or minimize the impact of such problems on the patients' recovery.

The very high popularity of LASIK over the past decade had motivated basic science and clinical research, which lead to a significant evolution in the technique as in the understanding of its pathophysiology. New complications inherently related to the LASIK flap have been described and better understood. The potential space created by the lamellar dissection creates a corneal environment susceptible of specific inflammatory conditions. The flap interface is a path of least resistance to cell migration, which determines the particular presentation of inflammatory processes as DLK [2, 31]. It is also a determinant of potential lamellar opportunistic infections [1, 2] and other forms of culture-negative keratitis [4, 11, 16, 18, 39]. In addition, the understanding on the mechanisms related to specific LASIK complications had an impact in similar conditions not necessarily related to the procedure. For example, the neurotrophic mechanisms related to LASIK-associated dry eye [35, 38] have provided important insights that have been also relevant to other forms of dry eye [9]. Even though the clinical aspects and pathophysiology of these complications are very different, they all have in common some relation with the lamellar corneal dissection. In this chapter, we review peripheral or marginal sterile infiltrates that follow LASIK, regarding its pathophysiology, clinical aspects, diagnosis, prevention, and treatment.

4.5.2 Defining Sterile Corneal Infiltrates

Marginal or peripheral sterile corneal infiltrates are localized, noninfectious inflammatory processes of the ocular surface that can be associated with a number of etiologies. Classically, this type of peripheral keratitis is also called marginal catarrhal infiltrates or ulcers because of the host's antibody hypersensitivity response to the antigen of bacteria related to chronic blepharoconjunctivitis, usually *Staphylococcus* spp. [18]. However, β-hemolytic *Streptococcus* and other bacteria, and other conditions such as collagen vascular disease may also lead to peripheral sterile corneal ulcers.

There are reports of sterile corneal infiltrates after various refractive procedures (Table 4.5.1) [4, 14–16, 18, 29, 33, 39]. Sterile infiltrates have been described after PRK [14, 15, 29, 33], in association with topical nonsteroidal anti-inflammatory drugs (NSAIDs) without concurrent steroids [29, 33] as well as with patching the eye with bandage contact lenses causing hypoxia [29, 33] and topical anesthetic

4

Table 4.5.1 Reports of sterile corneal infiltrates after various refractive procedures

Case no.	Authors	Eyes	Beginning of symptons	Associated conditions	Visual outcome	Culture	Treatment
1	Haw and Manche [10]	Unilateral OS	Day 1	History of dry eye and chalazion excision	20/20	Obtained	Topical antibiotics and corticosteroids
2	Yu et al. [11]	Bilateral	Day 1	Superior corneal pannus	20/25	Not performed	Topical antibiotics and corticosteroids
3	Ambrosio et al. [12]	Bilateral	Day 6	Meibomian gland dysfunction and blepharitis	20/20	Bacterial and fungal cultures were obtained	Topical antibiotics and corticosteroids
4	Ambrosio et al. [12]	Bilateral	Day 1	Meibomian gland dysfunction and blepharitis	20/25	Bacterial and fungal cultures were obtained	Topical antibiotics and corticosteroids
5	Lahners et al. [13]	Bilateral	Day 1	Small exotropia associated with mild amblyopia and an atypical pterygium	20/25	Cultured by scraping the areas of the infiltrates associated with epithelial defects. Flaps not lifted.	Antibiotic and topical corticosteroid. *Blood work-up ruled out systemic autoimmune/inflammatory etiologies
6	Lahners et al. [13]	Bilateral	Day 5	History of rheumatoid arthritis well controlled. Mild meybomian gland disease and superficial stromal scarring, mild pannus, trace stromal thinning	20/20	Not performed	Antibiotic and corticosteroids
7	Lifshitz et al. [14]	Bilateral	Day 3	No identifiable	20/25	Not performed	Topical antibiotics and corticosteroids
8	Lifshitz et al. [14]	Unilateral OD	Day 1	No identifiable	20/20	Not performed	Topical antibiotics and corticosteroids
9	Singhal et al. [28]	Bilateral	Day 1	No identifiable	20/20	Not performed	Topical antibiotics and corticosteroids

abuse [14]. In this situation, the typical clinical presentation is from the first to third postoperative day, with moderate-to-severe pain, decreased visual acuity, ciliary injection of the globe, and subepithelial white infiltrates in the treated area, often in the shape of an immune ring, with or without peripheral infiltrates [29, 33]. There is a high risk of permanent scarring accompanied by irregular astigmatism and reduced one to two lines of best spectacle corrected visual acuity [14, 29, 33]. The incidence has been reported as abut one case for every 300 PRK procedures [33]. The most accepted mechanism for the development of these infiltrates is related to the use of topical NSAIDs without concomitant use of topical steroids. As NSAIDs block only the cyclo-oxygenase pathway of arachidonic acid metabolism, there is a shift of arachidonic acid metabolism through the alternative lipo-oxygenase pathway. The resulting leukotriene accumulation results in neutrophil chemotaxis and sterile corneal infiltrates [15]. In addition, a Wessely-type peripheral immune ring has also been described after PTK for corneal scarring in a patient that was also treated with diclofenac eye drops and a bandage contact lens after the surgery [34]. In this case, corneal biopsy was performed, which demonstrated infiltration by neutrophils and the presence of an active fibroblastic reaction, without lymphocytes or plasma cells [23]. This case clearly illustrates the role of neutrophil chemotaxis by leukotrienes. The understanding about this causative mechanism and the use of topical steroids, along with NSAIDs, has significantly reduced the occurrence of this entity [7].

However, sterile corneal infiltrates after surface ablation is not exclusively related to topical NSAIDs without concurrent steroids and tight contact lens. Rao and coworkers [26] reported a patient who developed bilateral, marginal-inferior, subepithelial infiltrates of presumed noninfectious etiology after myopic PRK in whom NSAIDs and a soft contact lens were not used postoperatively. In addition, a case of peripheral sterile corneal infiltrates after LASEK has been reported without the use of topical NSAIDs [18]. In this situation, the mechanisms are likely to be different from sterile corneal infiltrates after surface ablations that were caused by the use of topical NSAIDs or tight contact lens wear. There is a high similarity of this condition to marginal catarrhal infiltrates related to staphylococcal lid margin disease. In addition, clinical presentation is also less intense, as usually it does not affect outcome.

Peripheral sterile catarrhal infiltrates have been reported after LASIK (Table 4.5.1) with nasal and superior hinge types of mechanical microkeratome [4, 11, 16, 18, 30, 39] and with the femtosecond laser [18]. The mechanism of this type of sterile corneal infiltrates after refractive procedures is likely related to immune reactions.

4.5.3 Pathophysiology

Local immune reactions, along with mixture effects of the flap creation and laser ablation on the cornea, associated with other ocular surface and/or systemic factors can trigger this complication [4, 11, 16, 18, 30, 39]. Classic marginal catarrhal keratitis resembles sterile peripheral infiltrates very highly. The clinical findings, clinical courses, and response to corticosteroid treatment suggest a similar pathophysiologic mechanism. In the case of classic marginal catarrhal infiltrates, the pathogenesis has been attributed to a localized corneal hypersensitivity reaction to toxins produced by bacteria colonizing the eyelid margins. These lesions represent sterile local deposition of antigen–antibody complexes in the peripheral corneal stroma (Gell & Coombs types II and/or III) [27]. The antigen is most likely an exotoxin elaborated by local bacteria, usually *Staphylococcus aureus*. However, several other organisms have been implicated in marginal keratitis [27].

Mondino et al. [22] created an experimental animal model of catarrhal infiltrates by applying exotoxins from *Staphylococcus* spp. onto the eyes of rabbits previously sensitized to the cell walls antigens. They demonstrated that immunized rabbits expressed humoral immunity against ribitol teichoic acid (RTA), a major antigen of *S. aureus*. Immunoglobulin (Ig)G and IgA antibody levels against RTA were measured in serum, tears, and cornea over a 5-month period, using enzyme-linked immunosorbent assay. Antibody levels were correlated with the development of the lesions [22]. Histologically, polymorphonuclear leukocytes and mononuclear cells were found. Immune complex deposition activates the classic complement pathway, and this was thought to trigger polymorphonuclear leukocyte infiltration, proteolytic enzyme release, and subsequent ulceration.

The clinical findings, clinical courses, and response to corticosteroid treatment suggest a similar pathophysiologic mechanism for peripheral sterile infiltrates after LASIK and marginal catarrhal keratitis from hypersensitivity reaction to toxins produced by bacteria. However, it is not clear how humoral immunity plays a role into this mechanism.

The corneal wound healing response after refractive surgery implicates a complex sequence of events involving cytokine-mediated interactions between epithelial cells, keratocytes, corneal nerves, lacrimal gland, tear film, and cells of the immune system [29–31]. Epithelial injury that is associated with LASIK flap formation and flap lifting triggers cytokine release, including interleukin (IL)-1α and tumor necrosis factor (TNF) α [21, 37] which bind to specific receptors in the keratocyte cells. The subsequent effects include production of pro-inflammatory chemokines, such as monocyte chemotactic and activating factor (MCAF), granulocyte colony-stimulating factor (G-CSF), IL-4, neutrophil-activating peptide (ENA-78), and monocyte-derived neutrophil chemotactic factor (MDNCF). These chemokines attract inflammatory cells into the cornea from the limbal blood vessels and the tear film [13]. It has been hypothesized that in ocular surface inflammatory conditions, such as blepharitis or meibomian gland dysfunction, patients have an inflammatory milieu that predisposes to increased cellular migration into the peripheral cornea following the production of cytokines IL1-α and TNF-α during LASIK procedure [4]. It is also possible that lid manipulation during surgery contribute to an increase of the meibomian secretions containing bacterial toxins into the ocular surface [18].

4.5.4 Clinical Diagnosis and Differential Diagnosis

The patients typically have a sluggish onset of the clinical signs with mild to lack of symptoms because of the gradual evolution of the infiltrates. Usually, the condition presents from the first to the fifth day after the surgery, visual acuity is not severely affected, and the condition affects both eyes if they were operated on the same day. The typical presentation is a localized or circumferential stromal infiltrate peripheral to the flap edge, with intact overlying epithelium and an intervening clear zone between the peripheral corneal infiltrate and the limbus (Fig. 4.5.1a, b) [4, 16, 18, 30]. There is mild-to-moderate redness, and there is no anterior chamber reaction. Blepharitis, meibomian gland dysfunction, or seborrhea is usually found. Usually there are no prominent symptoms, and patients may complain of mild pain, foreign body sensation, and tearing.

4

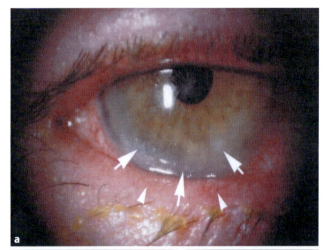

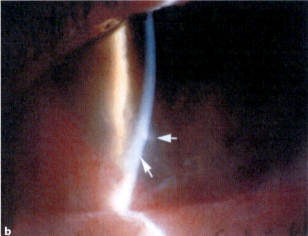

Fig. 4.5.1 **a** Numerous peripheral infiltrates located just outside the flap edge on the first day after LASIK (arrows). **b** Direct slit illumination under high magnification demonstrates the clear zone (also called lucid interval) between the infiltrates and the limbus

Cellular infiltration under the flap as DLK might be also occur in the presence of peripheral infiltrates [4, 18, 30]. These cases are likely to have more aggressive healing and develop refractive regression and undercorrection, which can be observed in corneal topography (Fig. 4.5.2).

Proper differentiation from infectious keratitis is essential for the management of these patients. It is important to maintain a high degree of suspicion for infectious keratitis because the management is very different, and the prognosis could be disastrous if the infection is not properly treated.

Herpes simplex keratitis is also in the differential diagnosis of marginal keratitis [33]. The ultraviolet exposure associated with the excimer laser might trigger for HSV-1 reactivation [17, 25]. Even patients without history of herpetic eye disease can present with this complication. Accordingly, it should always be considered for patients with infiltrates or persistent corneal epithelial defects after excimer laser procedures.

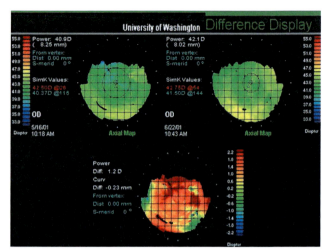

Fig. 4.5.2 Axial corneal topography subtraction maps demonstrating myopic regression between the first and third month after LASIK. Interestingly, the coefficient of irregularity (CIM) decreased from 3.70 to 1.43

4.5.5 Clinical Management and Preventive Measurements

Topical steroids represents as the mainstream for the treatment of peripheral infiltrates after LASIK. We typically use prednisolone acetate 1% every 1–2 h while the patient is awake, and recommend reevaluating the patient every day, until the condition is under control. Short doses of systemic steroids are to be considered (i.e., prednisone 0.5–1 mg/kg/day for 5 days) if the inflammation is not responsive to topical intense treatment.

In situations where the clinical presentation is more severe (as with dense infiltrates, edema, epithelial defect, purulent discharge, considerable pain, and decreased vision), it is advised to get material for microbiological cultures and laboratory workup, as well as to treat these cases empirically as bacterial infections until the cultures come back negative, to increase the use of topical and systemic steroids. We typically use fourth-generation fluoroquinolones. If there is a high suspicious of infective etiology, fortified topical antibiotics can be used (i.e., amikacin 20 mg/ml and vancomycin 50 mg/ml), keeping in mind that local toxicity induced by fortified antibiotics may play a role in corneal inflammation and induce a more severe picture. In the absence of discharge, epithelial ulceration, and anterior chamber reaction, the surgeon might decide not to proceed with invasive investigations such as corneal scraping, increasing topical steroids with a close monitoring of the patients' signs and symptoms.

If DLK is grade III, or if there is aggregation of cells clumped in the visual axis associated with haze and reduced vision the center, flap lift and irrigation is advised [6, 19, 31]. Typically, this maneuver is very effective when combined to intense topical steroids.

During preoperative screening, the surgeon should be alert to identify patients with moderate blepharitis and/or meibomian gland dysfunction to start prophylactic treatment prior to surgery. Acne rosacea and hypercholesterolemia are possible important risk factors [4]. Classically, lid scrubs, hygiene, and tetracycline and its derivatives treatment (i.e., doxycycline 100 mg twice daily) should be considered. Alternatively, ω-3–type essential fatty acid (EFA) nutritional supplementation with flaxseed or fish oil has been shown to be effective in up to 75% of patients with blepharitis and dry eye symptoms (Boerner et al. 2001, unpublished data) [3]. Higher dietary intake of n-3 EFA is associated with a decreased incidence of dry eye in women [20]. However, the use of n-3 EFA oral supplementation to optimize ocular surface prior to LASIK and surface ablation is anecdotal, and controlled trials are needed to confirm efficacy. Preoperative optimization with topical cyclosporine A is an alternative for patients with chronic dry eye and blepharitis. This medication has been demonstrated to be effective in masked, controlled clinical trials for dry eye [28]. We recommend this approach for cases identified as moderate dry eye that are candidates for LASIK as a possible maneuver to turn these candidates into good candidates for LASIK, minimizing the occurrence of LASIK-associated dry eye.

If an enhancement is to be performed for a patient that had sterile infiltrates after the first LASIK procedure, then prophylactic pretreatment with high penetration corticosteroids for 2–3 days prior to LASIK may be helpful in preventing recurrence of the marginal sterile infiltrates. It is also an alternative for eyes with residual signs of blepharitis and meibomian gland dysfunction despite lid hygiene and doxycycline. The surgeon can anticipate the susceptibility for such patients, so that they would be monitored more carefully following surgery.

Oral antiviral prophylaxis and treatment may be appropriate when performing LASIK in patients with a history of ocular or systemic HSV infection. We typically use acyclovir 800 mg a day starting 1 week prior to surgery. HSV cultures may be necessary for definitive diagnosis, and antiviral treatment may be considered for cases that have negative bacterial and fungal cultures with poor response to topical corticosteroid treatment, especially if there are corneal epithelial defects associated [4].

Confocal microscopy is a powerful diagnostic tool as it provides a non-invasive recognition of several pathologic conditions at the cellular level [8]. We believe there is a clinical potential for the confocal microscopy exam to clinically differentiate sterile and infectious keratitis after LASIK, as well as for helping identifying the microorganism. This would be a major improvement for managing such complications after refractive surgery. However, it has not been demonstrated yet.

4.5.6 Conclusion

Surgeons must be aware of sterile infiltrates, which is a distinct complication from corneal infiltrates of infectious etiology after LASIK. Its treatment and outcomes are quite different from those of infectious keratitis, so that we advocate for a high degree of suspicious in cases of peripheral infiltrates, and for a careful evaluation of the patient with daily visits if necessary, to rule out the bacterial or HSV infection.

Although the exact mechanism of this complication remains unclear, recognition of post-LASIK peripheral sterile infiltrates is essential for the management of these patients. Appropriate and early management with intense topical steroids usually results in a rapid disappearance of the infiltrates without affecting the outcome [4, 11, 16, 18, 30, 39]. It is also important to identify cases at higher risk for this complication, so that preoperative treatment would avoid or minimize its development.

> **Take-Home Pearls**
> - Sterile infiltrates after LASIK might occur with mechanical or laser keratomes.
> - Typical presentation is multiple lesions with intact epithelium.
> - Intervening clear zone between peripheral cornea and the limbus (similar to catarrhal infiltrates)
> - Can be complicated by DLK, when flap lift for interface cleaning may be necessary
> - Negative smears and cultures (sterile inflammation)
> - Blepharitis often associated
> - Resolves with intensive high penetration topical corticosteroids
> - Myopic regression often seen after proper treatment
> - Recurrence is likely with LASIK enhancement (consider prophylactic pretreatment with high penetration corticosteroids)
> - Identification of cases at higher risk (blepharitis, ocular rosacea) is important to enable preoperative treatment for prevention of this complication
> - Differential diagnosis
>   Infectious keratitis
>   Herpes simplex keratitis

References

1. Adan CB, Sato EH, Sousa LB, Oliveira RS, Leao SC, Freitas D (2004) An experimental model of mycobacterial infection under corneal flaps. Braz J Med Biol Res 37:1015–1021
2. Alio JL, Perez-Santonja JJ, Tervo T, Tabbara KF, Vesaluoma M, Smith RJ, Maddox B, Maloney RK (2000) Postoperative inflammation, microbial complications, and wound healing following laser in situ keratomileusis. J Refract Surg 16:523–538

3. Ambrósio Jr R, Stelzner S, Boerner C, Honan P, McIntyre DJ (2002) Nutritional treatment of dry eye: lipids. Rev Refract Surg3:29–35

4. Ambrósio R Jr, Periman LM, Netto MV, Wilson SE (2003) Bilateral marginal sterile infiltrates and diffuse lamellar keratitis after laser in situ keratomileusis. J Refract Surg 19:154–158

5. Ambrósio R Jr, Wilson S (2003) LASIK vs LASEK vs PRK: advantages and indications. Semin Ophthalmol 18:2–10

6. Ambrósio R Jr, Wilson SE (2001) Complications of laser in situ keratomileusis: etiology, prevention, and treatment. J Refract Surg 17:350–379

7. Arshinoff SA, Mills MD, Haber S (1996) Pharmacotherapy of photorefractive keratectomy. J Cataract Refract Surg 22:1037–1044

8. Chiou AG, Kaufman SC, Kaufman HE, Beuerman RW (2006) Clinical corneal confocal microscopy. Surv Ophthalmol 51:482–500

9. Dogru M, Stern ME, Smith JA, Foulks GN, Lemp MA, Tsubota K (2005) Changing trends in the definition and diagnosis of dry eyes. Am J Ophthalmol 140:507–508

10. Duffey RJ, Leaming D (2005) US trends in refractive surgery: 2004 ISRS/AAO Survey 21:742–748

11. Haw WW, Manche EE (1999) Sterile peripheral keratitis following laser in situ keratomileusis. J Refract Surg 15:61–63

12. Holland EJ, Schwartz GS (1999) Classification of herpes simplex virus keratitis. Cornea 18:144–154

13. Hong JW, Liu JJ, Lee JS, Mohan RR, Mohan RR, Woods DJ, He YG, Wilson SE (2001) Proinflammatory chemokine induction in keratocytes and inflammatory cell infiltration into the cornea. Invest Ophthalmol Vis Sci 42:2795–2803

14. Kim JY, Choi YS, Lee JH (1997) Keratitis from corneal anesthetic abuse after photorefractive keratectomy. J Cataract Refract Surg 23:447–449

15. Ku EC, Lee W, Kothari HV, Scholer DW (1986) Effect of diclofenac sodium on the arachidonic acid cascade. Am J Med 80:18–23

16. Lahners WJ, Hardten DR, Lindstrom RL (2003) Peripheral keratitis following laser in situ keratomileusis. J Refract Surg 19:671–675

17. Levy J, Lapid-Gortzak R, Klemperer I, Lifshitz T (2005) Herpes simplex virus keratitis after laser in situ keratomileusis. J Refract Surg 21:400–402

18. Lifshitz T, Levy J, Mahler O, Levinger S (2005) Peripheral sterile corneal infiltrates after refractive surgery. J Cataract Refract Surg 31:1392–1395

19. Melki SA, Azar DT (2001) LASIK complications: etiology, management, and prevention. Surv Ophthalmol 46:95–116

20. Miljanovic B, Trivedi KA, Dana MR, Gilbard JP, Buring JE, Schaumberg DA (2005) Relation between dietary n-3 and n-6 fatty acids and clinically diagnosed dry eye syndrome in women. Am J Clin Nutr 82:887–893

21. Mohan RR, Hutcheon AE, Choi R, Hong J, Lee J, Mohan RR, Ambrosio R Jr, Zieske JD, Wilson SE (2003) Apoptosis, necrosis, proliferation, and myofibroblast generation in the stroma following LASIK and PRK. Exp Eye Res 76:71–87

22. Mondino BJ, Adamu SA, Pitchekian-Halabi H (1991) Antibody studies in a rabbit model of corneal phlyctenulosis and catarrhal infiltrates related to Staphylococcus aureus. Invest Ophthalmol Vis Sci 32:1854–1863

23. Mondino BJ (1998) Inflammatory diseases of the peripheral cornea. Ophthalmology 95:463–472

24. Netto MV, Mohan RR, Ambrosio R Jr, Hutcheon AE, Zieske JD, Wilson SE (2005) Wound healing in the cornea: a review of refractive surgery complications and new prospects for therapy. Cornea 24:509–522

25. Pepose JS, Laycock KA, Miller JK, Chansue E, Lenze EJ, Gans LA, Smith ME (1992(Reactivation of latent herpes simplex virus by excimer laser photokeratectomy. Am J Ophthalmol 114:45–50

26. Rao SK, Fogla R, Rajagopal R, Sitalakshmi G, Padmanabhan P (2000) Bilateral corneal infiltrates after excimer laser photorefractive keratectomy. J Cataract Refract Surg 26:456–459

27. Robin JB, Dugel R, Robin SB. Immunologic disorders of the cornea and conjunctiva (1999) In: Kaufman HB, Barron BA, McDonald MB (eds) The cornea, 2nd edn, on CD-Rom. Butterworth-Heinemann, Newton, Mass.

28. Sall K, Stevenson OD, Mundorf TK, Reis BL (2000) Two multicenter, randomized studies of the efficacy and safety of cyclosporine ophthalmic emulsion in moderate to severe dry eye disease. CsA Phase 3 Study Group. Ophthalmology 107:631–639

29. Sher NA, Krueger RR, Teal P, Jans RG, Edmison D (1994) Role of topical corticosteroids and nonsteroidal antiinflammatory drugs in the etiology of stromal infiltrates after excimer photorefractive keratectomy. J Refract Corneal Surg 10:587–588

30. Singhal S, Sridhar MS, Garg P (2005) Bilateral peripheral infiltrative keratitis after LASIK. J Refract Surg 21:402–404

31. Smith RJ, Maloney RK (1998(Diffuse lamellar keratitis. A new syndrome in lamellar refractive surgery. Ophthalmology 105:1721–1726

32. Tahzib NG, Bootsma SJ, Eggink FA, Nabar VA, Nuijts RM (2005) Functional outcomes and patient satisfaction after laser in situ keratomileusis for correction of myopia. J Cataract Refract Surg 31:1943–1951

33. Teal P, Breslin C, Arshinoff S, Edmison D (1995) Corneal subepithelial infiltrates following excimer laser photorefractive keratectomy. J Cataract Refract Surg 21:516–518

34. Teichmann KD, Cameron J, Huaman A, Rahi AH, Badr I (1996) Wessely-type immune ring following phototherapeutic keratectomy. J Cataract Refract Surg 22:142–146

35. Wilson SE, Ambrosio R (2001) Laser in situ keratomileusis-induced neurotrophic epitheliopathy. Am J Ophthalmol 132:405–406

36. Wilson SE, Mohan RR, Mohan RR, Ambrosio R Jr, Hong J, Lee J (2001) The corneal wound healing response: cytokine-mediated interaction of the epithelium, stroma, and inflammatory cells. Prog Retin Eye Res 20:625–637

37. Wilson SE, Netto M, Ambrosio R Jr (2003) Corneal cells: chatty in development, homeostasis, wound healing, and disease. Am J Ophthalmol 136:530–536

38. Wilson SE (2001) Laser in situ keratomileusis-induced (presumed) neurotrophic epitheliopathy. Ophthalmology 108:1082–1087

39. Yu EY, Rao SK, Cheng AC, Law RW, Leung AT, Lam DS (2002) Bilateral peripheral corneal infiltrates after simultaneous myopic laser in situ keratomileusis. J Cataract Refract Surg 28:891–894

Core Messages

■ Ptosis following refractive surgery is increasing in incidence.

■ Refractive and oculofacial plastic surgeons are beginning to recognize this complication.

■ Recognition of refractive surgery induced ptosis is leading to better coordination of care.

■ Multiple etiologic factors cause refractive surgery induced ptosis.

■ Examination elucidates the type of ptosis.

■ Levator dehiscence ptosis is most recognized type of refractive surgery-induced ptosis.

■ Surgical repair is best achieved with levator advancement surgery.

4.6 Ptosis

Bryan S. Sires

4.6.1 Introduction

Postoperative ptosis is becoming a more widely recognized complication, with the increased number of refractive cases being performed worldwide. Understanding the relevance of this relationship will help to provide better-coordinated care between the refractive surgeon and the oculofacial plastic surgeon. The exact frequency of this complication is not known, but is likely underestimated by many surgeons. More awareness of postoperative ptosis will allow the refractive surgeon to develop protocols to hopefully avoid this complication and if still present, know when to refer care to the oculofacial plastic surgeon.

Ptosis after refractive surgery is a complex topic. Factors before, during, and after refractive surgery influence the onset of ptosis. Ptosis type is usually aponeurotic dehiscence after refractive surgery, but can be mechanical or traumatic. Examination of aponeurotic ptosis reveals a low margin reflex distance, good levator function, and an elevated eyelid crease. Small incision external ptosis repair is best suited to achieve desired eyelid height and contour.

4.6.2 Anatomy and Factors Predisposing to Ptosis after Refractive Surgery

The upper eyelid is a structure of great importance with regard to the protection and maintenance of clear vision [2]. The upper eyelid functions to cover the ocular surface from debris and drying caused by air with a blink or eyelid closure. Each blink cycle also evenly spreads tears over the ocular surface and directs the tears toward the lacrimal drain. There are several anatomic layers to the upper eyelid (Fig.

4.6.1). The skin is thin, with minimal subcutaneous tissue compared with other regions of the body. This is helpful in providing well-concealed, fine scars after surgery. Most incisions are made in the lid crease. The eyelid crease is formed by elastic fibers that come from the levator aponeurosis and insert into the dermis of the skin, causing it to indent. Below the skin is the closing muscle of the eye called the orbicularis oculi muscle. This muscle is innervated by the facial nerve. The pretarsal and preseptal components of the orbicularis oculi muscle provide the involuntary blink for ocular surface maintenance, while the orbital component is for the voluntary blink associated with noxious stimuli to the eye. The blink rate can be as high as 24 times per minute [5]. The blink cycle is created by the differential stimulation of the opening/retracting (superior levator muscle and Mueller's muscle) and closing/protracting (orbicularis oculi muscle and inferior tarsal muscle) muscles in coordinated fashion. Mueller's muscle and the inferior tarsal muscle are sympathetically innervated. The superior levator muscle is innervated by the superior division of the oculomotor nerve. The superior levator muscle and Mueller's muscle sit behind the orbital septum. The septum separates the anterior eyelid structures from the orbital space. Behind the septum, the orbital fat and lacrimal gland are encountered above the superior levator muscle and aponeurosis. The nasal fat is white, the preaponeurotic fat is yellow, and the lacrimal gland is gray (Fig. 4.6.2). The preaponeurotic fat usually drapes over the lacrimal gland laterally in the eyelid. These colors are helpful in identifying your location during surgery [9]. Beneath the superior levator aponeurosis sits Mueller's muscle, and beneath Mueller's muscle is the palpebral conjunctiva.

Distinct differences in anatomy exist between the Occidental and Asian eyelids. However, it is not know if this difference influences the frequency of postoperative ptosis following refractive surgery.

The surgical anatomy is divided into the anterior, middle, and posterior eyelid lamellae. The anterior lamella is made up of the skin and orbicularis oculi muscle. The middle lamella is the orbital septum. The posterior lamella is the superior levator muscle, Mueller's muscle, tarsus, and the conjunctiva. When discussing surgical anatomy of the eyelid, it is conceptually easier to think of these three lamellae rather than the several layers independently.

4.6.3 Etiology

Many factors can influence the etiology of aponeurotic ptosis associated with refractive surgery. These factors can be present before, during, and after the refractive surgery.

The most common pre–refractive surgery etiology is related to the use of hard contact lenses [6]. Contact lens–related ptosis is a clinical form of aponeurotic disinsertion usually seen in the elderly population. The relationship between the use of contact lens wear and ptosis was first made in 1981 [3]. Obviously, the refractive surgery population contains a significant number of contact lens users prior to

4

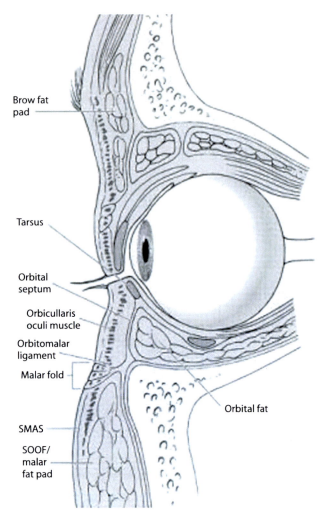

Brow fat pad

Tarsus

Orbital septum

Orbicullaris oculi muscle

Orbitomalar ligament

Malar fold

Orbital fat

SMAS

SOOF/ malar fat pad

Fig. 4.6.1 Illustration of the anatomy of the upper eyelid showing various layers. The anterior surgical lamella is made up of the skin and orbicularis oculi muscle layer. The middle layer is the orbital septum. The posterior lamella is composed of the retractors (Mueller's muscle and levator aponeurosis/muscle), tarsus, and palpebral conjunctiva

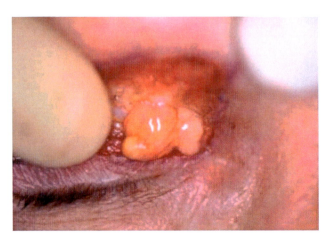

Fig. 4.6.2 External photograph demonstrating the color difference between the nasal fat (*white*) and the preaponeurotic fat (*yellow*). A higher carotenoid content is the cause of the yellow fat

refractive surgery intervention. Ptosis may be manifest prior to or after the refractive surgery. A component of the etiology of this type of ptosis is related to the production of fibrosis in Mueller's muscle plane with contact lens use [10]. However, there has been no study to elucidate whether this phenomenon is related to the actual wearing of the contact lens and/or the placement or removal of the contact lens by creating traction on the eyelids. The use of a plunger for the placement and removal of rigid gas permeable lenses would reduce the traction on the eyelids in hopes of decreasing the incidence of aponeurotic ptosis.

It is also known that people prone to ptosis have decreased amounts of antioxidants in the preaponeurotic fat [1]. This fat pad is characteristically more yellow and is related to a two- to fourfold increase in the amount of carotenoids present [9] (Fig. 4.6.2). The preaponeurotic fat pad sits on the surface of the levator aponeurosis and muscle. Carotenoids may play a protective role for the highly metabolic levator muscle by scavenging free radicals from the 24,000 blink cycles a day [5]. The levator muscle is responsible for the opening of the eye during the blink cycle. Patients who develop ptosis, as the result of contact lens use or refractive surgery, may have been more susceptible to ptosis later in life if neither of these interventions had occurred due to a possible inherent decreased amount of antioxidants in their orbital fat.

During refractive surgery, a lid speculum is used to retract the eyelids. Tension of the eyelids against the speculum has also been suggested as an etiology of ptosis. Another alternative is the stretching of the eyelids with adhesive drape removal after the completion of the refractive procedure. This is avoidable if care is taken when removing the drapes. A minimum of 6 months should be allowed to pass prior to considering eyelid repair since this is the closing stage for recovery in cases in of traumatic ptosis. Refractive surgery uses topical anesthesia and does not require the use of anesthetic injections, avoiding some factors leading to ptosis.

Finally, after the refractive surgery, the patient may have mechanical ptosis from eyelid edema caused by the placement of the lid speculum. This is transient and typically resolves spontaneously.

4.6.4 Examination

The exam of a ptosis patient includes a complete eye exam, with special attention to the upper eyelid, tear lake, and ocular surface. The balance between stimulation of the muscles of retraction and protraction in an open eye determine the resting state of the eyelid margin relative to the eye. The distance from the eyelid margin to a fine light reflection on the central cornea is the called the margin reflex distance (MRD). The maximum height of the upper eyelid is just nasal to the pupil. A normal MRD measurement is 3–5 mm, which places the eyelid margin above the pupil in ambient light. The eyelid crease in the Caucasian eyelid is positioned above the eyelid margin at about 8 mm in men and

10 mm in women. The Asian lid has a lower crease at about 5 mm or none at all in about half of the Asian population. In aponeurotic ptosis seen after refractive surgery, the eyelid crease height is usually higher indicative of attenuation and stretching of the levator aponeurosis. This causes the eyelid crease height to be greater. The complete excursion of the upper eyelid up and down is an indicator of the levator function (LF). A normal measurement is greater than 10 mm. LF is not altered in aponeurotic ptosis. There is usually complete eyelid closure or no lagophthalmos seen in aponeurotic ptosis. Up to 2 mm of lagophthalmos is tolerated in individuals with normal protective mechanisms such as Bell's phenomenon, corneal sensation, and tear lake height.

Tear lake height assessment is important when performing ptosis surgery, especially after refractive surgery. Cutting of the corneal nerves especially with LASIK leads to decreased tear production. After the ptosis surgery, small amount of lagophthalmos can be expected. In a dry eye setting or in keratitis sicca patients' lagophthalmos could be detrimental. If these conditions are known ahead of time, then more conservative surgery (less elevation of the eyelid) should be performed to avoid lagophthalmos. Slit-lamp biomicroscopy and the Schirmer paper strip are useful techniques to determine tear height assessment.

Visual field testing is an important component in the preoperative evaluation. These tests determine the degree to which the superior visual field is obstructed. Insurance companies have specific criteria such as MRD, visual field percentage obstruction, and photographs used to determine coverage. If these are not met, then the ptosis condition is considered cosmetic in nature and not covered by insurance. The current criteria being used by most insurance agencies are greater than 30% of the superior visual field is obstructed. This is determined by performing a visual field in a relaxed state, followed by a repeated field with the lids taped into their normal anatomic position. The difference between these two states determines the percentage of superior visual field obstruction.

Photographs also play a role in determining insurance coverage. Specific fields of view are required to make a photographic assessment of coverage. The first view is a raccoon view or a straight on view of both eyes and periocular regions. Confirmation of the MRD can be made with this view. The second field of view is side views from the right and left. This allows one to determine if the pupil can be seen from the side. If not, then the patient's peripheral vision is blocked as well.

Unilateral ptosis is a special condition requiring further preoperative testing [8]. This is the result of the possibility of Hering's law. The definition states that equal and simultaneous innervation flows to synergistic muscles concerned with the desired direction of movement. If not considered, then there is a possibility that the ptosis pattern can be reversed if only correcting the initially observed ptotic eyelid. The central caudate subnucleus of the third nerve nucleus controls eyelid height. It usually gets its cue from the dominant seeing eye. Thus, it is necessary to determine eye

dominance. Next, it is mandatory to perform a lift test of the droopy eyelid. This is an attempt to manifest the Herring's phenomenon by observing for a reversal of the ptotic eyelid. The test can be done manually or pharmacologically (2.5% phenylephrine). If Hering's phenomenon is present, then both eyelids should be repaired at the same time. If not present during testing, then the patient should be informed that there is a possibility that the opposite eyelid could droop following correction of the unilateral ptotic eyelid.

4.6.5 Treatment

Several surgical techniques exist to repair aponeurotic ptosis. These include open and small incision levator aponeurotic tucks and conjunctiva–Mueller muscle excisions. The surgical treatment of ptosis has evolved considerably with the advent of small incision levator aponeurotic surgery. This section is devoted only to the small-incision approach.

The classic open levator surgery involved an incision across the entire eyelid crease, with opening of the entire septum to expose the horizontal extent of the levator aponeurosis and muscle. Many factors, such as the amount of local anesthesia, the use of epinephrine, overhead lights, patient consciousness, inadvertent injection of the levator muscle, Hering's phenomenon, etc., can influence the outcome of the eyelid height. The small-incision technique uses an incision about a third the size of the classic technique [7]. This means less anesthesia and epinephrine are required, and there is a reduced chance of infiltrating the levator muscle. Also, less of the orbicularis oculi muscle is anesthetized, maintaining a more normal balance between retractors and protractors. The classic open technique and the small-incision technique have been compared side by side on an efficacy basis. The small-incision technique is completed in half the time, with similar results achieved concerning the height of the eyelid [4]. However, the small-incision technique outperformed the classic technique in achieving desirable contour of the upper eyelid.

The small-incision technique involves an eyelid crease incision over the central third of the eyelid crease [7] (Fig. 4.6.3). Dissection is carried through the orbicularis oculi muscle down to the external surface of the central tarsus. Enough tarsus is cleaned so a suture can be passed partial thickness through it. Next, the conjoined tendon (blending of the levator aponeurosis and the septum) is grasped and placed on inferiorly directed traction. The central orbital septum is opened, exposing the preaponeurotic fat. The under surface of the fat is cleaned exposing the musculoaponeurotic junction. At this point, one or two sutures are passed from the tarsus up to the junction. The horizontal position of the sutures is important. The goal is to achieve lift at a point just nasal to the pupil and at the lateral limbus. The tension of the sutures is adjusted with the patient awake and cooperative to determine the set points so the height and contour are symmetric. Once completed, the ends

4

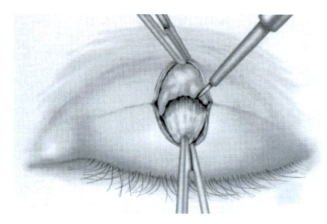

Fig. 4.6.3 Illustration of the small incision surgical approach. The incision is only 8–10 mm in length or a third of the eyelid, and allows exposure of the tarsus and levator aponeurosis after dissection through the orbital septum. The corresponding tarsus is cleaned below for passage of the suture for anchoring

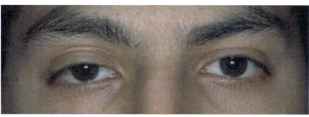

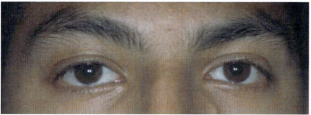

Fig. 4.6.4 Before and after external photographs of a patient who underwent the small-incision approach of the right upper eyelid and achieved a symmetric result

of the suture are tied and cut. A single eyelid-crease reformation suture is then placed from the new inferior edge of the levator aponeurosis to the inferior cut edge of the orbicularis oculi muscle. The skin is then closed (Fig. 4.6.4).

The small-incision ptosis repair technique is easily combined with other upper eyelid procedures such as blepharoplasty and entropion/eyelash ptosis repair.

Take-Home Pearls

■ Ptosis caused by refractive surgery is influenced by many factors including contact lens use, lid speculum and drape use, and patient predisposition.
■ Examination is useful to help determine the ptosis type; aponeurotic ptosis includes a low margin reflex distance, with good levator function and an elevated eyelid crease.
■ Aponeurotic surgical repair is the usual type of ptosis surgery.
■ Repair is best achieved with the small, external-incision levator tuck technique.

References

1. Ahmadi A, Saari J, Mozaffarian D et al (2005) Decreased carotenoid content in preaponeurotic orbital fat of patients with involutional ptosis. Ophthalmol Plast Reconstr Surg 21:46–51
2. Dutton JJ (1994) The eyelids and the anterior orbit. In: Dutton JJ (ed) Atlas of clinical and surgical orbital anatomy. Saunders, Philadelphia
3. Epstein G, Putterman AM (1981) Acquired blepharoptosis secondary to contact lens wear. Am J Ophthalmol 91:634–639
4. Frueh BR, Musch DC, McDonald HM (2004) Efficacy and efficiency of a small-incision, minimal dissection procedure versus a traditional approach for correcting aponeurotic ptosis. Ophthalmology 111:2158–2163
5. Hall A (1945) The origin and purpose of blinking. Br J Ophthalmol 29:455–467
6. Kersten RC, de Conciliis C, Kulwin DR (1995) Acquired ptosis in the young and middle-aged adult population. Ophthalmology 102:924–928
7. Lucarelli MJ, Lemke BN (1999) Small incision external levator repair: technique and early results. Am J Ophthalmol 127:637–644
8. Lyon DB, Gonnering RS, Dortzbach RK et al (1993) Unilateral ptosis and eye dominance. Ophthal Plast Reconstr Surg 9:237–240
9. Sires BS, Saari J, Garwin GG et al (2001) The color difference in orbital fat. Arch Ophthalmol 119:868–871
10. Wantanabe A, Araki B, Noso K et al (2006) Histopathology of blepharoptosis caused by prolonged hard contact lens wear. Am J Ophthalmol 141:1092–1096

Core Messages

■ The cornea, like most tissues, manifests only a limited number of responses to a wide variety of aggressions.

■ One example of such end-stage response is stromal melting, also mentioned in the literature as keratolysis or stromal necrosis.

■ When melting stops, the wounded area is optically dense and hypercellular and seldom returns to normal tensile strength, mainly because of a reduction in thickness.

■ The therapeutic approach must be directed towards the underlying disease or "trigger" phenomenon, and it will depend on the aggressivity of the melt.

■ Stromal melting has been classically associated with LASIK although, occasionally, it has also been seen after other corneal refractive procedures.

■ Both epithelial ingrowth and flap edge melting are more common in LASIK retreatments, when relifting the flap, perhaps more commonly, in hyperopic retreatments.

4.7 Melting

*José L. Güell, Merce Morral, Oscar Gris,
Javier Gaytan, and Felicidad Manero*

4.7.1 Introduction

All the layers of the cornea, like most tissues, manifest only a limited number of responses to the wide variety of diseases and aggressions that assault it [1] and "melting," a relatively new term also named keratolysis or necrosis, is just one of them. In fact, from a descriptive point of view, it may also be named as a defect. Defects can have different durations. A defect is considered acute if it appears suddenly and then heals, as in a corneal laceration; recurrent if it appears repeatedly, as in a recurrent epithelial erosion; and chronic or persistent if healing stops and the defect remains or progresses, as in the case of sterile stromal ulcers associated with herpes simplex keratitis or those associated with epithelial ingrowth, which might be progressive. In order to better understand which the possible mechanisms are involved on its etiopathogenesis, and thus, the appropriate therapeutic strategies, we first review some basic concepts about stromal physiology and healing.

4.7.2 Basic Concepts

The corneal stroma accounts for 90% of the corneal thickness, and it is composed almost entirely of extracellular material. Two zones of tissue are recognized, Bowman's layer, a homogeneous acellular sheet of randomly oriented collagenous fibers, and lamellar stroma, organized in obliquely oriented bundles of collagen containing spindle-shaped cells named keratocytes.

Bowman's layer represents approximately 2% of the corneal thickness. It is composed of an irregular meshwork of filaments made up of collagen types I, III, V, and VI, and possibly type IV collagen.

Stromal fibroblasts, or keratocytes, are neural crest–derived, spindle-shaped cells and produce the majority of the extracellular matrix, both the collagenous and proteoglycan components. Under physiological conditions, keratocytes exhibit minimal mitotic activity and serve mainly to maintain the slow turnover of extracellular components. Normal keratocytes decrease in density from anterior to posterior with a slight increase in the area anterior to Descemet's membrane.

The lamellar stroma is composed to approximately 200 layers of type I collagen, the most abundant in the adult cornea, which are oriented parallel to the corneal surface. The noncollagenous intercellular component of the stroma is composed of glycosaminoglycans. Proteoglycans are acidic macromolecules that are formed of at least one sulfated glycosaminoglycan (GAG) bound to a protein core and associated with collagen fibrils at specific axial locations. As these molecules are extremely hydrophilic, most of the water present in the intercellular stroma is in the form of water associated with GAG molecules. The proteoglycans are located between collagen fibrils and may be regulators of collagen fibril spacing and diameter. Intralamellar adhesive strength of the stroma depends on the relationship between the collagen lamellae and the proteoglycans. Adhesive strength is greater near the periphery, where there is considerably more collagen interweaving.

The stimulus to corneal stromal reaction is cell death. If only a small number of keratocytes are lost, then there may be only a minimal degree of keratocyte response, as may be seen in superficial foreign bodies of the cornea. There may also be no keratocyte response at all. In that case, the defect may be permanently filled with epithelial cells that thicken the epithelial cell layer focally and reestablish the surface contour.

Like the surface epithelial cells, the corneal stromal cells become activated and change their biochemical apparatus from only maintaining surrounding collagen and proteoglycans to actually synthesizing collagen and proteoglycans. The number of keratocytes increase by mitotic division, and other keratocyte-like fibroblasts may also enter the area. After an intact epithelial cover is established, keratocytes migrate from their point of origin to the site of injury and begin to produce collagen. However, although the reparative collagen is of type I, the same as the native collagen, its diameter is generally larger, and the caliber of individual collagen fibers is more variable. The result is that the homogeneity allowing the transmission of light is lost, and the scar is easily identified clinically.

Similarly, the new proteoglycans differ in character and proportion. The newly formed proteoglycans tend to bind water more tightly, resulting in long-term excess hydration of scar tissue. The difference in the nature of the proteoglycans results in irregular spacing of the new collagen fibers, which increases the opacification of the tissue.

Stromal keratocytes undergo a second type of metamorphosis, generally in the latter stages of wound healing. The cells develop intracytoplasmic actinomyosin contractile elements, like those present in muscle cells (myofibroblasts or fibromyoblasts). Fibromyoblasts are responsible of the "contraction" of the corneal wound, which may lead to irregular corneal astigmatism. Maturing the corneal collagen does not create a contractile force, although this change may alter the degree of opacification of the scar.

The initial extracellular matrix of the scar produced is not the same as the final or resting scar. Under the influence of poorly defined stimuli, including mechanically generated forces from surrounding tissues, collagens and proteoglycans are selectively catabolized by specific proteases. New collagen and proteoglycans are then selectively synthesized in a more advantageous orientation, quantity, or proportion. Myofibroblasts revert to cells with maintenance characteristics similar to the native keratocytes. Hypercellularity may be a permanent feature of the scar tissue. The degree of transparency of the scar tissue may be improved, but not to the point of functional rehabilitation.

Although the wounded area is optically dense and hypercellular, corneal scar tissue seldom returns to normal tensile strength. It is estimated that the maximum recovery is 70% of native tensile strength.

Several agents that can inhibit matrix metalloproteinase (MMP) activities in vitro have been tested as topical agents in vivo using the rabbit model of alkali burns. Some MMP inhibitors appear to act by nonspecifically chelating the zinc cation present at the active site of MMPs. These agents include sodium edetic acid (EDTA), tetracycline, cysteine, and acetylcysteine. Thiol-containing synthetic inhibitors of collagenase have been developed that are substantially more potent than the first-generation collagenase inhibitors.

Tissue inhibitor of metalloproteinases type I (TIMP-1) is a protein that is synthesized and secreted by many types of cells and acts endogenously to inhibit the matrix metalloproteinases, collagenase, gelatinase, and stromelysin. Top-

ical application of purified recombinant TIMP-1 significantly reduced the progression of corneal ulceration in rabbits after severe alkali burn. TIMP-1 has not been evaluated in patients affected of corneal burns.

Although much more basic and clinical investigations are needed, treatment of infectious corneal ulcers with a combination of antibiotics and a MMP inhibitor may reduce the risk of extensive necrosis.

Topical anti-inflammatory agents such as corticosteroids or non-steroidal anti-inflammatory agents (NSAIDs) are often associated with delayed stromal healing and acceleration of corneal ulceration. Part of this effect is probably attributable to decreasing DNA synthesis in regenerating stromal fibroblasts. In addition, corticosteroids reduce the synthesis of collagen by fibroblasts in culture. Addition of insulin or epidermal growth factor (EGF), however, may partially preserve the detrimental effect of corticosteroids on wound strength.

4.7.3 Stromal Melting: Classification

From a physiopathological point of view, we can classify stromal melting into several subgroups (Table 4.7.1).

As it is quite common in other clinical situations, some of them may be, obviously, present together.

The therapeutic approach will be directed towards the underlying disease or "triggering" phenomenon, although

Table 4.7.1 Stromal melting

Active	■ Infectious keratitis ■ Culture-negative ulcerative keratitis [2] ■ Caustication (alkali, acid, burn induced) ■ Immunological diseases (rheumatoid arthritis, primary Sjögren's syndrome [3], Vogt-Koyanagi-Harada's syndrome [4], etc.) ■ Vitamin A deficiency [5] ■ DLK ■ Other diseases: paraneoplastic pemphigus [6]
Trophic (dellen phenomenon)	Pterygium or pingeculae After avulsion of a Molteno shunt plate [7]
Neurotrophic keratopathy	After damage to the trigeminal nerve [8]

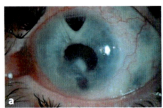
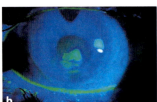
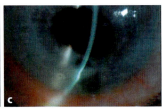

Fig. 4.7.1 a–c Clinically, corneal ulcers are associated with a certain degree of focal or diffuse stromal lysis

some general options might also be considered, especially in those more aggressive and urgent settings: the use of glue and a therapeutic soft or hard contact lens [9, 10], partial keratectomy with amniotic membrane transplantation [11, 12], or a combination of them [13, 14].

For example, as we have previously mentioned, the use of oral tetracyclines (doxycycline) for the control of melting has been a classical approach because of their antimetalloproteinase action and has demonstrated to be useful also in front of infections such as *Pseudomonas* keratitis [15] (Fig. 4.7.1).

Another classical option has been the use of topical medroxyprogesterone (MPG) due to its presumed ability to suppress collagenase enzymes. In some series of keratoprosthesis [16], it has been reported that, although MPG may not influence the underlying incidence of melt-related complications, which are likely to be associated with other risk factors especially HSV (herpes simplex virus) and rheumatic diseases [17], it may also have a protective effect with regard to stromal melt onset and severity.

Platelet-activating factor (PAF) delays corneal epithelial wound healing by inhibiting the adhesion of epithelial cells, increasing apoptosis of stromal cells, and inducing an imbalance in favor of MMP-9 activation. Thus, a novel PAF receptor antagonist, LAUO9O1 (2,4,6-trimethyl,1-4-dibydropyridine-3-5-dicorboxylic acid ester), might be useful in the control of alkali induced stromal melting and in some aggressive cases after LASIK, especially high risk cases.

4.7.4 Stromal Melting after Excimer Laser Refractive Surgery

4.7.4.1 Epidemiology and Etiopathogenesis

Stromal melting has been classically associated with LASIK, although it has also been seen after other corneal refractive procedures occasionally. It is unilateral in most cases and there is an interval between the onset of melting and LASIK of about 2–5 weeks [18]. In 75% of the cases, it has been associated to a surgical error or a problem during the immediate postoperative period, such as epithelial defects, thin and/or irregular flaps including buttonholes, epithelial ingrowth [19], DLK, and so on (Fig. 4.7.2).

In about 50% of the cases, melting may be associated to a systemic disease such as thyroiditis, systemic lupus, Sjögren's disease, rheumatoid arthritis, dry skin, eczema, erythema, and others. Nevertheless, some series have shown that with a proper selection of cases, something difficult to determine, the frequency of melting in rheumatic diseases is extremely low [21–23].

Although topical steroids and cyclosporine A have been frequently used, the classical course of the disease is a self-limited phenomenon of about 21–45 days, ending in variable degrees of opacification (leukoma) and/or regular and irregular astigmatism. In most cases, as we have already explained in this chapter, the melting of the flap is possibly caused by apoptosis initiated by the cells of the implanted layer (epithelial ingrowth) [24] (Fig. 4.7.3).

As it is well known, the use of NSAIDs was rapidly accepted for the treatment of pain, inflammation, and photophobia after PRK some years ago. Due to their possible antiproliferative effect on keratocytes, NSAIDs have also been used for the long-term treatment of post-PRK haze and regression and after LASIK by modulating wound healing [25–28]. There have been numerous published and non-published cases of melting after excimer laser refractive surgery associated with the use of NSAIDs [29–31]. Some investigators think that the mechanism by which epithelial cells secrete MMP-1 and MMP-8 may play a role in the pathogenesis of corneal melting associated with NSAIDs use. In fact, it has been described after cataract surgery, penetrating keratoplasty (PKP), incisional refractive surgery, bullous keratopathy, after pterygium surgery, in the course of bacterial corneal ulcers [32], and after excimer laser surgery. In some severe, extreme cases, melting evolved to acute or late corneal perforation [33].

In the case of LASIK, besides systemic risk factors such as rosacea or rheumatoid arthritis, the associated key point

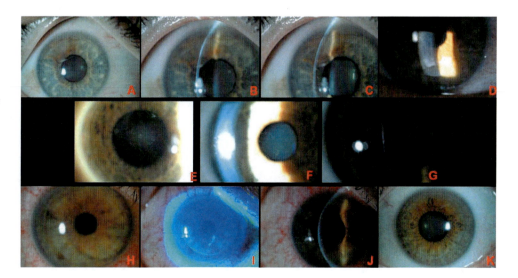

Fig. 4.7.2 A–D Peripheral stromal lysis can occur after epithelial ingrowth. **E–G** Central stromal lysis (end stage) after DLK. **H–J** Another case of DLK (grade IV). If DLK is urgently and intensively treated, then stromal lysis will not occur. **K** Same case 6 months later. No stromal lysis is seen

4

Fig. 4.7.3 High-risk situations of epithelial ingrowth and melting after LASIK.
A Irregular lenticule.
B Epithelial defect, especially over the flap edge. **C** Irregular epithelial edges (reoperation) and DLK

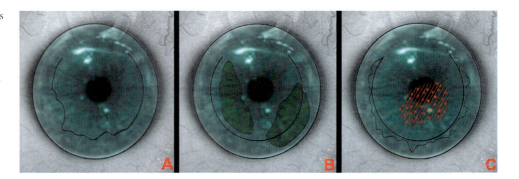

Fig. 4.7.4 Epithelial ingrowth. Clinical photographs pre- and postoperatively (before and after cleaning the epithelium). After cyst resection, the most effective surgical approach is suturing the flap (**A–C**), although it is not always necessary (**D–F**). When epithelial ingrowth is aggressive, stromal flap lysis is very frequent (**G–I**)

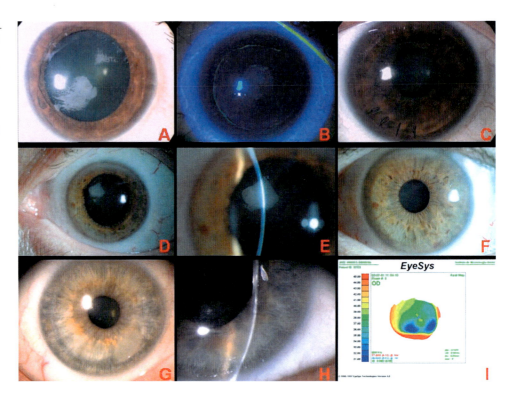

is the exposure of the stroma associated with dislocated flap or severe flap wrinkling or dislodgment [34].

Although multiple factors contribute to corneal melting after LASIK, including dry eye, autoimmune disease, and lack of epithelial and stromal integrity due to neurotrophic, mechanical and biomechanical (MMP, leukotrienes) interactions, the use of diclofenac (and other NSAIDs) after LASIK might potentiate these factors. Whereas MMP expression is a normal component of repair, as we have previously described, excessive or inappropriate MMP activity is associated with corneal keratolysis. Some studies provide evidence that topical application of diclofenac sodium 0.1% and possibly other NSAIDs may be associated with aberrant MMP expression in the cornea [35].

It is widely recognized that both epithelial ingrowth [36] and flap edge melting are more common in LASIK retreatments, when relifting the flap, than in primary cases [37] and, perhaps, this is especially common in hyperopic re-

treatments (30% epithelial ingrowth with 2% melting in some series) (Fig. 4.7.4). This self-limited phenomenon must not be confused with that associated with active infection [38], due to *Nocardia* or *Aspergillus*, for example [39].

The incidence of large intraoperative epithelium sloughing/defects during LASIK might be a diagnostic sign for subclinical epithelial basement membrane dystrophy (EBMD) [40]. These patients, as any other with pre- or postoperative epithelial defects of other etiology, especially at the flap edge level, are predisposed to multiple postoperative complications (Fig. 4.7.5). They include mainly DLK and flap microfolds in the early postoperative period, and/or epithelial ingrowth and flap melting later on. From our point of view, and because of the high risk for epithelial sloughing in the second eye, LASIK should not be performed.

Another relatively common situation associated with stromal melting (both the flap and the bed stroma) is DLK, especially grades III and IV [41].

Fig. 4.7.5 Infections after LASIK: epithelial or interface infections may induce DLK and secondary, focal, or diffuse stromal lysis. Topical treatment must be early and aggressive. **A–C** Herpetic epithelial infection. **D–G** Mycobacteria at the interface. Observe the final focal necrosis of the flap. **H–K** Adenoviral infection. **L–O** Pneumococcal focal

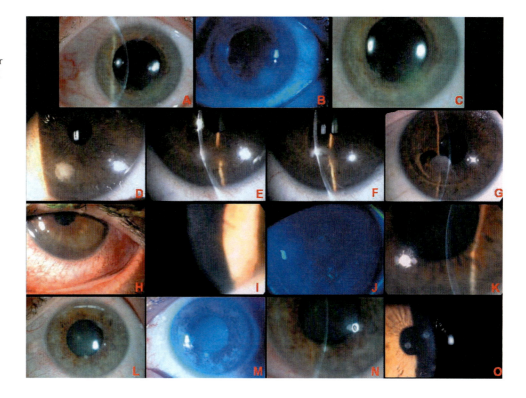

4.7.4.2 Therapeutic Approach

As it has been previously stated, stromal melting after LASIK is usually a self-limited phenomenon, which does not require specific treatment and can only be observed. In fact, for example, most investigators think that, contrary to dense epithelial ingrowth, it does not always require surgical intervention, as it eventually regresses spontaneously. Surgery will only be necessary when it appears to progress, affects directly or indirectly visual function, or causes flap melting [42]. The particular techniques are being covered in another chapter; however, we mention the use of alcohol or antimetabolite drugs such as mitomycin C are contraindicated because the secondary melting might be more common.

We have also previously mentioned the possible role of topical NSAIDs in potentiating other risk factors of melting such as dry eye and certain autoimmune diseases. From our point of view, the use of NSAIDs will only be suggested in some selected cases during the first hours or few days after LASIK or surface techniques, and basically, because of their analgesic capacity. There is no other role for them in this setting.

Both epithelial ingrowth and flap edge melting are more common in LASIK reoperations. That is why an adequate technique maximally preserving the epithelial edges at the time of relifting is very useful in preventing such a complication (Fig. 4.7.6). Circular flap rhexis is a good example of such an approach [43].

A high index of suspicion for epithelial ingrowth, especially when it may masquerade as stromal edema associated with persistent epithelial defect, is essential to avoid a delayed diagnosis, which can result in irreversible visual loss due to stromal melting and/or infectious keratitis (Fig. 4.7.7) [44]. In some advanced cases of melt associated with epithelial ingrowth, the treatment might need to be very aggressive, for example with flap amputation [45].

Finally, in those melting cases associated with DLK, mostly grades III and IV, aggressive treatment will also be mandatory, including relifting the flap, cleaning the interface and intensive topical steroid–antibiotic treatment, in order to control the progression of the melt [40].

Take-Home Pearls

- Corneal melting is the final common response of the stroma to a variety of insults.
- Although multiple factors contribute to corneal melting after LASIK, including dry eye, autoimmune diseases, etc., the use of topical NSAIDs might potentiate these factors.
- The classical course of the disease is a self-limited phenomenon.
- Epithelial ingrowth and flap edge melting are more common in LASIK reoperations, and that is why an adequate and delicate technique is critical in order to avoid them.
- In those very rare and severe cases, associated with advanced epithelial ingrowth or DLK, aggressive treatment will be mandatory.

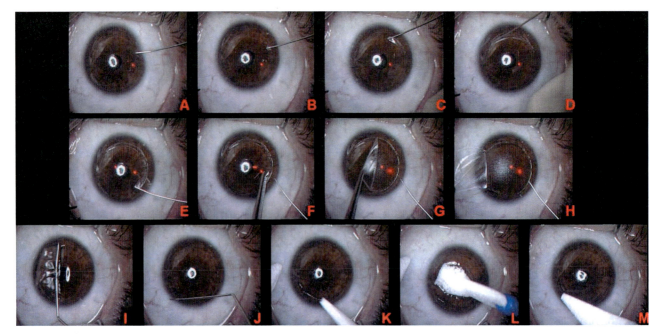

Fig. 4.7.6 A–M A careful surgical technique for reoperation of LASIK is the best way to avoid subsequent complications. Preserving the edges of the flap is especially important

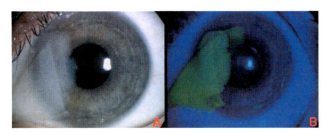

Fig. 4.7.7 A, B For some extensive epithelial defects occurring during LASIK, a good alternative to therapeutic contact lens may be amniotic membrane (patch) in order to avoid postoperative complications

References

1. Waring GO III, Rodrigues MM (1987) Patterns of pathologic response in the cornea. Surv Opthalmol 31:262–266
2. Lam DS, Leung AT, Wu JT, Fan DS, Cheng AC, Wang Z (1999) Culture-negative ulcerative keratitis after laser in situ keratomileusis. J Cataract Refract Surg 25:1004–1008
3. Vivino FB, Minerva P, Huang CH, Orlin SE (2001) Corneal melt as the initial presentation of primary Sjögren's syndrome. J Rheumatol 28:379–382
4. Paroli MP, Pinca M, Speranza S, Marino M, Pivetti-Pezzi P (2003) Paracentral corneal melting in a patient with Vogt-Koyanagi-Harada's syndrome, psoriasis, and Hashimoto's thyroiditis. Ocul Immunol Inflamm 11:309–313
5. Su WY, Chang SW, Huang SF (2003) Amniotic membrane transplantation for corneal perforation related to vitamin A deficiency. Ophthalmic Surg Lasers Imagining 34:140–144
6. Beele H, Claerhout I, Kestelyn P, Dierckxens L, Naeyaert JM, De Laey JJ (2001) Bilateral corneal melting in a patient with paraneoplastic pemphigus. Dermatology 202:147–150
7. Liu SM, Su J, Hemady RK (1997) Corneal melting after ablationn of a Molteno shunt plate. J Glaucoma 6:357–358
8. Nishida T, Nakamura M, Konma T, Ofuji K, Nagano K, Tanaka T, Enoki M, Reid TW, Brown SM, Murphy CJ, Manis MJ (1997) Neurotrophic keratopathy—studies on substance P and the clinical significance of corneal sensation. NipOn Ganka Gakkai Zasshi 101:948–74
9. Spelsberg H, Sundmacher R (2005) Significance of immediate affixation of a hard contact lens in the emergency treatment of severe alkali burns of the cornea (case report) Klin Monatsbl Augenhelilkd 222:905–909
10. Vote BJ, Elder MJ (2000) Cyanoacrylate glue for corneal perforations: a description of a surgical technique and a review of the literature. Clin Experiment Ophthalmol 28:437–442
11. Xi XH,Cao YN, Tang LS, Qin B, Jiang DY (2004) Corneal combined amniotic membrane transplantation for early severe alkali chemical injury of the eye. Zhong Nan Da Xue Xue Bao Yi Xue Ban 29:704–706
12. Ma DH, Wang SF, Su WY, Tsai RJ (2002) Amniotic membrane graft for the management of scleral melting and corneal perforation in recalcitrant infectious scleral and corneoscleral ulcers. Cornea 21:275–283
13. Soong HK, Farjo AA, Katz D, Meyer RF, Sugar A (2000) Lamellar corneal patch grafts in the management of corneal melting. Cornea 19:126–134
14. Su CY, Lin CP (2000) Combined use of an amniotic membrane and tissue adhesive in treating corneal perforation: a case report. Ophthalmic Surg Lasers 31:151–154
15. McElvanney AM (2003) Doxycycline in the management of pseudomonas corneal melting: two case reports and a review of the literature. Eye Contact Lens 29:258–61
16. Celia R Hicks, Geoffrey J Crawford (2003) Melting after keratoprosthesis implantation: the effects of medroxyprogesterone. Cornea 22:497–500
17. Dudenhoefer EJ, Nouri M, Gipson IK, Baratz KH, Tisdale AS, Dryja TP, Abad JC, Dohlman CH (2003) Histopathology of ex-

planted collar button keratoprostheses: a clinicopathologic correlation. Cornea 22:424–428

18. Ly Y, Li HY (2005) Analysis of clinical characteristics and risk factors of corneal melting after laser in situ keratomileusis. Zhonghua Yan Ke Za Zhi 41:330–334

19. Castillo A, Diaz-Valle D, Gutierrez AR, Toledano N, Romero F (1998) Peripheral melt of flap after laser in situ keratomileusis. J Refract Surg 14:61–63

20. Alió JL, Artola A, Belda JI, Perez Santonja JJ, Muñoz G, Javaloy J, Rodríguez-Prats JL, Galal A (2005) LASIK in patients with rheumatic diseases: a pilot study. Ophthalmology 112:1948–1954

21. Smith RJ, Maloney RK (2006) Laser in situ keratomileusis in patients with autoimmune disease. J Cataract Refract Surg 32:1292–1295

22. Kohnen T (2006) Excimer laser refractive surgery in autoimmune disease (Letter to the Editor). J Cataract Refract Surg 32:1241

23. Cobo-Soriano R, Beltran J, Baviera J (2006) LASIK outcomes in patients with underlying systemic contraindications: a preliminary study. Ophthalmology 113:e1–e8

24. Du Z, Guo H, Zheng Q (2001) Immunohistochemical and clinical studies on sub-corneal flap epithelial implantation accompanied by flap melting after excimer laser in situ keratomileusis. Zhonghua Yan Ke Za Zhi 37:84–86

25. Lu KL, Wee WR, Sakamoto T, McDonnell PJ (1996) Comparison of in vitro antiproliferative effects of steroids and nonsteroidal antiinflammatory drugs on human keratocytes. Cornea 15:185–190

26. Nguyen KD, Lee DA (1992) Effects of steroids and nonsteroidal antiinflammatory agents on human ocular fibroblast. Invest Ophthalmol Vis Sci 33:2693–2701

27. Nguyen KD, Lee DA (1993) In vitro evaluation of antiproliferative potential of topical cyclo-oxygenase inhibitors in human Tenon's fibroblast. Exp Eye Res 57:97–105

28. Nassaralla B, Szerenyi K, Wang Xw et al (1995) Effect of diclofenac on corneal haze after photorefractive keratectomy in rabbits. Ophthalmology 102:469–474

29. Joseph KW, Hsu , W Todd Johnston, Russell W Read, Peter J McDonnell, Rey Pangalinan, Narsing Rao, Ronald E Smith (2003) Histopathology of corneal melting associated with diclofenac use after refractive surgery. J Cataract Refract Surg 29:250–256

30. Hsu JK, Johnston WT, Read RW, McDonnel PJ, Pangalinan R, Rao N, Smith RE (2003) Histopathology of corneal melting associated with diclofenac use after refractive surgery. J Cataract Refract Surg 29:250–256

31. Flach AJ (2001) Corneal melts associated with topically applied nonsteroidal anti-inflammatory drugs. Trans Am Ophthalmol Soc 99:205–210; discussion 210–212

32. Tatsuhiko Asai, Tetsushi Nakagami, Mina Mochizuki, Norimasa Hata, Takako Tsuchiya, Yoshihiro Hotta (2006) Three cases of corneal melting after instillation of a new nonsteroidal anti-inflammatory drug. Cornea 25:224–227

33. Gabison EE, Chastang P, Menashi S, Mourah S, Doan S, Oster M, Mauviel A, Hoang-Xuan T (2003) Late corneal perforation after photorefractive keratectomy associated with topical diclofenac: involvement of matrix metalloproteinases. Ophthalmology 110:1626–1631

34. Lam DS, Leung AT, Wu JT, Cheng AC, Fan DS, Rao SK, Talamo JH, Barraquer C (1999) Management of severe flap wrinkling or dislodgment after laser in situ keratomuleusis. J Cataract Refract Surg 25:1441–1447

35. Hargrave SL, Jung JC, Fini ME, Gelender H, Catre C, Guidera A, Udell I, Fisher S, Jester JV, Bowman RW, McCulley JP, Cavanagh HD (2002) Possible role of the vitamin E solubilizer in topical diclofenac on matrix metalloproteinase expression in corneal melting: an analysis of postoperative keratolysis. Ophthalmology 109:343–350

36. Perez-Santonja JJ, Ayala MJ, Sakla HF, Ruiz-Moreno JM, Alió JL (1999) Retreatment after laser in situ keratomileusis. Ophthalmology 106:21–28

37. Alió JL, Galal A, Artola A, Ayala MJ, Merayo J (2006) Hyperopic LASIK retreatments with the Technolas laser. J Refract Surg 22:596–603

38. Patel NR, Reidy JJ, Gonzalez-Fernandez F (2005) Nocardia keratitis after laser in situ keratomileusis: clinicopathologic correlation. J Cataract Refract Surg 31:2012–2015

39. Kuo IC, Margolis TP, Cevallos V, Hwang DG (2001) Aspergillus fumigatus keratitis after laser in situ keratomileusis. Cornea 20:342–344

40. Perez-Santonja JJ, Galal A, Cardona C, Artola A, Ruiz-Moreno JM, Alió JL (2005) Severe corneal epithelial sloughing during laser in situ keratomileusis as a presenting sign for silent epithelial basement membrane dystrophy. J Cataract Refract Surg 31:1932–1937

41. De Rojas Silva MV, Diez Feijo E, Rodríguez Ares MT, Sánchez-Salorio M (2004) Confocal microscopy of stage 4 diffuse lamellar keratitis with spontaneous resolution. J Refract Surg 20:391–6

42. Lin JM, Tsai Y, tseng SH (2005) Spontaneous regression of dense epithelial ingrowth after laser in situ keratomileusis. J Refract Surg 21:300–302

43. Perez-Santonja JJ, Medrano M, Ruiz-Moreno JM, Cardona-Ausina C, Alió L (2001) Circular flap rhexis: a refinement technique for LASIK re-treatment. Arch Soc Esp Oftalmol 76:303–308

44. Azar DT, Scally A, Hannush SB, Soukiasian S, Terry M (2003) Characteristic clinical findings and visual outcomes. J Cataract Refract Surg 29:2358–2365

45. Yang B, Wang Z, Chen J (2001) The management of epithelial ingrowth after laser in situ keratomileusis. Chin Med Sci J 16:241–243

Chapter 5

LASIK: Late Postoperative Complications

Contents

Core Messages

- Dry eye is the most common early and late postoperative complication after LASIK surgery.

- LASIK-induced dry eye is caused by a combination of decreased corneal innervation and chronic ocular surface inflammation.

- LASIK-induced dry eye is manifested clinically by the presence of fluctuation in visual acuity, punctate epithelial erosions, and, in some patients, with decreased tear production.

- LINE is the preferred term to describe this condition when it occurs after LASIK or LASIK enhancement in an eye with no symptoms or signs of dry eye prior to surgery. Some eyes likely have both LINE and underlying inflammatory dry eye disease.

- Optimization of the ocular surface is an important step to improving patient satisfaction and outcomes after LASIK surgery.

5.1 Dry Eye

*Jerome C. Ramos-Esteban
and Steven Wilson*

5.1.1 Introduction

LASIK is the most commonly performed refractive surgery procedure for the correction of myopia, hyperopia, and astigmatism in the United States [1]. Dry eye is the most common early and late postoperative complication after LASIK [2]. The purpose of this chapter is to review the epidemiology, risk factors, clinical manifestations, diagnostic techniques, and management of dry eye in patients undergoing LASIK surgery.

5.1.2 Epidemiology of Dry Eye in LASIK Patients

Estimating the incidence and prevalence of dry eye that occurs after LASIK is difficult since a significant proportion of patients who have this procedure develop a subtle, difficult-to-diagnose form of the disease. There is also a lack of standardized criteria to define this condition. Also, the signs and symptoms of dry eye after LASIK are more prevalent in the early phases of the disease, with a natural tendency for the disorder to resolve over time [3].

5.1.2.1 Primary Procedures

5.1.2.1.1 Myopic LASIK

The incidence of dry eye after LASIK has been estimated to range between 5% [4] and 52% [5] among Caucasian patients, with a higher reported incidence among Asians [4]. This transitory condition, which typically resolves within 6–9 months after surgery [3], is thought to result from a combination of mechanisms.

Direct mechanical microkeratome and laser-induced photoablative damage to the corneal nerve plexuses can lead to sensory denervation of the cornea. Damage to the epithelial, subepithelial, and superficial stromal nerve plexuses occurs at the edge and along the flap interface, sparing the deeper stromal nerves [6]. Decreased corneal sensation can contribute to the development of LASIK-induced dry eye by affecting the functional unit composed by the ocular surface–trigeminal nerve–brain stem–facial nerve–lacrimal gland axis responsible for decreased tear production [3, 7–14] and modulation of the expression of lacrimal gland derived cytokines. These cytokines such as hepatocyte growth factor (HGF) and epidermal growth factor (EGF) have been implicated in the modulation of corneal epithelial wound healing [15]. Actual decreases in tear secretion noted in the first few months after LASIK are, however, relatively modest [7–9].

Dry eye after LASIK may also have a chronic ocular surface inflammatory etiology, manifested by loss of conjunctival goblet cells that may in turn reduce mucin production [16]. Chronic ocular surface inflammation can now be treated with topical cyclosporine 0.05%, which primarily functions to interrupt IL-2 signaling and decrease T-cell activation and the subsequent release of pro-inflammatory cytokines [17]. A small proportion of patients with dry eye attributable to underlying chronic inflammation may be cured of their disease with topical cyclosporine 0.05%. Cyclosporine 0.05% has also been used in the management of LASIK patients with preoperative dry eye and has been

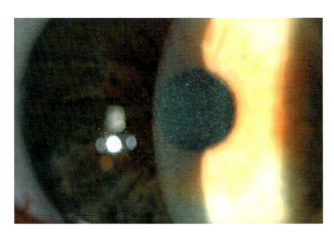

Fig. 5.1.1 Slit lamp photo of punctate epithelial erosions in a cornea at one week after LASIK. The patient had no symptoms or signs of dry eye prior to surgery, suggesting that this represents a relatively pure case of LASIK-induced neurotrophic epitheliopathy

shown to improve refractive predictability (mean postoperative refractive spherical equivalent closer to target refraction) at 3 and 6 months after surgery compared with artificial tears–treated patients [17, 18].

However, LASIK-induced dry eye cannot be solely explained based on decreased tear production. This is further evidenced in patients undergoing LASIK or LASIK enhancement, who frequently do not complain of dry eye symptoms, despite marked punctate epithelial erosions and basic tear production (measured using the Schirmer's test) that is normal and not significantly different compared with preoperative levels [7, 19]. Wilson [7, 9] coined the term LASIK-induced neurotrophic epitheliopathy (LINE) to describe this condition occurring after LASIK or LASIK enhancement that lasts 6–9 months after surgery. We believe this is the most dominant etiology underlying symptoms associated with LASIK dry eye disorder.

Thus, dry eye after LASIK likely represents a multifactorial spectrum of conditions that includes in all cases a neurotrophic epitheliopathy component and, at least in some cases, underlying inflammatory dry eye, in addition to several other potential disorders affecting the ocular surface.

5.1.2.1.2 Hyperopic LASIK

The development of punctate epithelial keratopathy after LASIK for hyperopia is more prevalent after high hyperopic corrections compared with similar myopic corrections [20]. In addition to increased corneal staining, hyperopic corrections can also result in a reduction in tear film stability and reduced tear volume [13]. Hyperopic ablations require larger flaps and more peripheral ablations, which affect the magnitude and duration of corneal sensitivity loss to a greater extent [13]. Furthermore, the central corneal steepening induced by hyperopic ablations can also lead to alterations in blink dynamics and ocular surface tear spreading.

5.1.2.2 LASIK Enhancements

LASIK enhancements are traditionally performed between 3 and 6 months after surgery when patients are thought to have achieved refractive stability. Despite technological advances in excimer laser ablation profiles and microkeratome design, refractive regression still occurs after LASIK surgery, primarily due to wound healing–related factors such as epithelial hyperplasia and stromal remodeling [21]. Patients experiencing refractive regression can be retreated by lifting the LASIK flap and reapplying the excimer laser to further reshape the stromal bed.

The incidence of regression after myopic LASIK can be as high as 27% and, in some studies, has been found to be associated with the presence of chronic dry eye [14]. In this patient population, female sex, higher attempted refractive correction, and greater ablation depth have also been correlated with myopic regression [14]. Preoperative increased ocular surface staining, lower tear volume, tear instability, decreased corneal sensation, and dry eye symptoms have also been correlated with regression in myopic patients [14].

Regression rates for patients undergoing hyperopic LASIK have been calculated to be close to 32%, with similar correlations between dry eye symptoms, greater preoperative ocular surface staining scores, and lower tear volumes [13].

Dry eye symptoms have not been shown to increase after myopic LASIK enhancements despite of documented higher ocular surface fluorescein staining scores. Interestingly, in this patient population, both Schirmer's test and tear break up time (TBUT) have been reported to be within normal limits, despite a documented reduction in corneal sensitivity up to 6 months after surgery compared with pre-enhancement levels [19]. This further supports the theory that LASIK-induced dry eye may be partially caused by a neurotrophic epitheliopathy of the cornea [7, 9]. Interestingly the presence of clinically controlled underlying rheumatic diseases, which predisposes to dry eye, does not seem to increase the rate of refractive regression or enhancements after LASIK surgery [22].

5.1.3 Risk Factors

Several preoperative (female gender, race, preexisting dry eye syndrome) as well as intraoperative (hinge-related, highly attempted corrections, and ablation depth) risk factors have been correlated with the development of dry eye after LASIK. Understanding these risk factors can assist the refractive surgeon in selecting effective strategies to optimize the ocular surface prior to surgery, which in turn can result in improved refractive outcomes.

5.1.3.1 Patient Population

5.1.3.1.1 Gender and Age

The incidence of dry eye in female patients has been shown to be significantly higher than for male patients in large population–based epidemiologic studies [23]. Female gender has been found to correlate with higher rates of myopic [14] and hyperopic [13] regression after LASIK. Female patients over the age of 40 have also been found to be more likely to develop intraoperative epithelial defects during LASIK surgery [24], which in turn has been associated with postoperative complications such as epithelial ingrowth [25, 26] and DLK [27].

Hormonal differences, more specifically a reduction in androgen levels in peri- or postmenopausal females, may also account for the increased overall prevalence of dry eye symptoms after LASIK surgery [13, 28]. Androgen deficiency in females has been associated with inflammation of the lacrimal gland [29] and, possibly, meibomian glands [30] leading to alterations of the ocular surface leading to dry eye. The benefit of hormone replacement therapy for the management of dry eye symptoms and its role in refractive outcomes remains to be clearly defined in LASIK surgery.

5.1.3.1.2 Race

Asian patients have been found to have a higher prevalence of dry eye symptoms after LASIK compared with Caucasians patients [4]. Clinically, Asian eyes may experience a longer recovery time for their preoperative dry eye parameters (TBUT, PRT, Schirmer's test 1, staining score, and corneal sensation) to return to baseline values after LASIK [4] and, thus, experience a more prolonged and severe form of the disease. This notion holds true even when patients are matched for laser surgical ablation depth with Caucasian eyes [4].

Several mechanisms have been postulated to explain the higher incidence of dry eye among Asian patients undergoing LASIK, including reduced blink rate after LASIK from to 3 to 12 months after surgery [3], contact lens–induced surface lid abnormalities [31], narrower palpebral fissures [32], and microkeratome-related conjunctival trauma during flap creation [33].

5.1.3.2 Preexisting Dry Eye Syndrome

Diagnosing the presence of preexisting dry eye syndrome (DES) is one of the most important evaluations for any patient seeking LASIK surgery. As was previously emphasized, the presence of an underlying DES can affect corneal wound healing leading to refractive regression [21] and increased need for enhancements [13, 14].

Preexisting dry eye of different degrees of severity has been documented in 38% [34] to 75% [35] of patients seeking myopic LASIK surgery. Even though visual outcomes in patients with preexisting dry eye and those with probable and no dry eye have not been shown to be significantly different in terms of BCVA and uncorrected visual acuity (UCVA) up to 12 months after surgery [35], these patients tend to have more dry eye symptoms, higher ocular surface staining scores, and lower Schirmer's test results [35]. In addition, patients without preoperative dry eye have been shown to undergo earlier recovery of corneal sensitivity (3

vs. 6 months) compared with patients with preexisting dry eye [35].

Finally, preoperative optimization of the ocular surface can also help to reduce the risk of intraoperative complications and facilitate the performance of LASIK surgery in patients with moderate forms of preoperative dry eye [35, 36].

5.1.3.3 Hinge-Related Factors

Creation of a LASIK flap with a microkeratome blade transects the epithelial/subepithelial and superficial stromal nerve plexuses located at the edge of the flap and along the flap interface, resulting in decreased corneal sensitivity [6]. The loss of corneal sensitivity is not uniform between the different areas of the cornea, and is more deeply depressed in the central cornea [37]. The nerves located in the area adjacent to the hinge are not transected by the microkeratome blade, nor are they ablated by the excimer laser, as demonstrated by the greater corneal sensitivity measured near the hinge compared with the central and peripheral cornea after LASIK surgery [37]. Based on these observations, corneal sensitivity can potentially vary according to the location and width of the LASIK flap hinge. Several studies have been conducted in order to determine whether the location and width of the LASIK flap affects the incidence and severity of dry eye symptoms [5, 38–40]. Several considerations such as the definition of dry eye used in the study, anatomical differences in nerve leash distribution within the cornea, possible different patterns of corneal nerve regeneration in response to mechanical injury, and differences in corneal sensitivity testing methods must be weighed before drawing any conclusions from these studies, which report conflicting results.

5.1.3.3.1 Hinge Location

The location of the hinge determines the orientation of the LASIK flap–which typically is either superior (vertical) or nasal (horizontal). Superior hinge flaps can be created with a Hansatome microkeratome (Bausch & Lomb), whereas the Amadeus microkeratome (Advanced Medical Optics) can be used to create nasal hinge flaps.

Conflicting reports have been published regarding the exact location of the point of entry, distribution, and orientation of sensory (long ciliary) corneal nerves at the limbus [41, 42]. Sensory [41] and anatomical [42] arguments have been postulated to explain differences in corneal sensitivity between different areas of the cornea. Based on the greater corneal sensitivity of the nasal and temporal corneal limbus compared with the inferior limbus, corneal innervation has been thought to be the highest in these two areas [41]. A recent study using in vivo confocal microscopy contradicted this previous concept, where it demonstrated that nerves predominantly extend across the corneal apex preferentially following a 6-to-12 o'clock orientation [42]. Furthermore, this study also demonstrated that nerve trunks are equally distributed around the corneal circumference, with no predilection for the 3 and 9 o'clock positions [42].

Therefore, the lack of consensus in this practical point likely accounts for differences between studies regarding the effect of hinge location on the return of corneal sensitivity and duration of this neurotrophic state which can range anywhere from 3 [35, 43], 6 [3, 38], 9 [44], to 18 months [8] after LASIK surgery.

In one study, myopic LASIK patients with superior hinge flaps were shown to have more severe postoperative corneal staining scores and a significant reduction in corneal sensation for up to 6 months after surgery compared with nasal flaps [40]. Superior hinged flaps were also correlated with higher Schirmer's test results compared with nasal flaps [40, 45]. In a different study, patients with superior hinge flaps were also found to have worse uncorrected visual acuity at 1 week after surgery, along with higher topographical surface regularity index (SRI), greater total corneal fluorescein staining scores, greater symptom severity scores (Ocular Surface Disease Index), and lower TBUT compared with preoperative levels [5].

In contrast, nasal hinge flaps have been shown to have significantly higher mechanical corneal sensitivity thresholds (gas esthesiometry) in the early (1 week and 1 month) postoperative period compared with superior hinge flaps. Nevertheless, this difference did not achieve statistical significance using Kaplan-Meier survival analysis for the development of dry eye between fellow eyes [5]. In a different study, measured corneal sensitivity in nasal hinge flaps was shown significantly reduced compared with superior hinges [46].

In yet a different study, central corneal sensitivity was shown equally decreased between superior or nasal hinge flaps up to 6 months after surgery [38]. Quadratic analysis of corneal sensitivity has further suggested that nasal hinges may preserve corneal sensitivity better over the hinge area compared with superior flaps at 1 month postoperatively [38].

On the balance, studies favoring one hinge position over the other with regard to predisposition to development of LASIK dry eye are inconclusive. This is probably related to the recent appreciation that corneal nerves penetrate the cornea with equivalent frequency around the circumference of the cornea [42].

5.1.3.3.2 Hinge Width

The width of the LASIK flap hinge represents another important consideration that can potentially affect corneal sensitivity and may contribute to the development of dry eye after surgery.

The effect of hinge width has been studied in patients undergoing myopic LASIK with nasal hinged flaps. Wide nasal hinges (average: 6.48 mm) compared with narrow hinges (average: 4.22 mm) have been shown to have significantly higher mean corneal sensation for up to 6 months after surgery compared with narrow hinged flaps [39]. Interestingly, in a paper comparing the effect of superior hinges against nasal hinges on corneal sensitivity and dry eye after LASIK, superior hinged flaps were noted to have statis-

tically significant wider hinges compared with nasal hinges [40]. In this study, patients with superior hinge flaps (wider) had even more important reduction in corneal sensitivity and more corneal staining with fluorescein compared with the nasal hinged group [40]. Thus, hinge width may influence corneal sensitivity, but more importantly, hinge location may play a more important role in the complex flap related mechanisms leading to dry eye after LASIK.

5.1.3.4 High Attempted Corrections and Ablation Depth

High refractive errors by themselves do not correlate with increased risk of dry eye, although prolonged use of contact lenses to correct these errors can lead to alterations in tear secretion [10] and clearance [8], and prolonged recovery of corneal sensitivity up to 16 months after LASIK [8].

Higher refractive errors necessitate deeper ablations and larger treatment zones to minimize postoperative optical aberrations. The deeper the laser ablation, the greater the distance required for the regenerating nerve trunks to travel in order to re-innervate the corneal epithelium following surgery [5]. Deeper ablations may also lead to more pronounced [47] and prolonged [44] reductions in corneal sensitivity.

Regression analysis has estimated that for every diopter of treated spherical equivalent of myopia there is a 20% greater chance of developing dry eye (based on fluorescein staining alone) in low myopic corrections [5]. In addition, laser-calculated ablation depth, combined ablation depth, and flap thickness have also been correlated with dry eye [5]. High attempted myopic correction has also been shown to increase the incidence of myopic regression and further need for LASIK enhancements [14]. The same can be said for patients with high hyperopic corrections in whom punctate epithelial keratopathy after LASIK is more prevalent compared with similar magnitudes of myopic correction [20].

5.1.4 Diagnostic Approach to Patients with Dry Eye after LASIK

5.1.4.1 Clinical Manifestations

Clinical manifestations of dry eye after LASIK are better characterized by exploring the patients' symptoms, performing a comprehensive clinical examination, and understanding the mechanisms leading to dry eye after LASIK surgery.

In general, dry eye has been defined as a disorder of the tear film caused by either tear deficiency or excessive tear evaporation, which in turn causes damage to the ocular surface and is associated with symptoms of ocular discomfort [31]. Dry eye can be further classified into tear-deficiency states (production), increased evaporative loss (lipid dysfunction), or poor blink distribution (mechanical) over the ocular surface. Recently, however, it has become clear that tear composition is also an important factor in the pathophysiology of dry eye disease [15–17, 31]. Following LASIK

5

surgery, the additional factor of the neurotrophic contribution of transient loss of innervation to the flap is also an important factor [7–9].

5.1.4.2 Pathophysiology

The creation of the LASIK flap along with the photoablation of corneal nerve plexuses by the excimer laser during LASIK surgery can lead to the development of a neurotrophic state of the ocular surface [7–9]. Decreased corneal sensitivity can lead to both quantitative [31] and qualitative [15–17, 31] tear film abnormalities. Chronic sensory denervation of the cornea can also lead to increased cytokine and growth factor expression [15, 17], increased tear osmolarity [48], mucin deficiency states [16], as well as alterations in blink frequency [3]– all contributing to abnormalities of the ocular surface. These changes can also contribute to the development of chronic inflammation of the ocular surface, which can be demonstrated histologically by the presence of activated lymphocytes [49] and loss of conjunctival goblet cells in LASIK patients [50]. Therefore, conceptually, the pathogenesis of dry eye after LASIK should be considered multifactorial.

5.1.4.3 Dry Eye Symptoms after LASIK

A high proportion of patients undergoing LASIK surgery develop dry eye symptoms during their early postoperative course. Patients' dry eye symptoms have been shown, however, to correlate poorly with the results of clinical tests for dry eye [51[. Since the cornea becomes neurotrophic after LASIK [7–9], patient complaints can be different from classic dry eye patients. Visual fluctuation which is exacerbated during certain times of the day (e.g., glare at night or night vision problems) is probably the most common presenting symptom of dry eye after LASIK [14]. In addition, patients may also complain of dryness, foreign-body sensation, and tearing. In severe cases, patients can also develop symptoms related to recurrent erosion syndrome after LASIK, which, although rare, are a source of significant patient morbidity when it occurs [52]. Moreover, the presence of chronic dry eye has been correlated with the development of refractive regressions in both myopic [14] and hyperopic [13] patients–which may also be a source of visual fluctuation in these patients.

5.1.4.4 Clinical Signs

Clinical signs of dry eye after LASIK can be divided into three groups: tear film–related abnormalities, ocular surface staining, and corneal sensation abnormalities. In practice, patients with LASIK-induced dry eye usually present with a combination of the above-described signs of dry eye.

5.1.4.4.1 Tear Film–Related Abnormalities

Evaluation of the tear film can be divided into four basic components: tear secretion, tear volume, tear osmolarity, and tear stability.

Tear Secretion

Tear secretion is sometimes divided into basal and reflex components, although many experts believe that all tear production is, to an extent, reflexive. The Schirmer's test is considered by many clinicians to be the gold standard for the measurement of tear secretion [51], although its limitations in individual patients have been well characterized. The Schirmer's test is performed by placing a thin strip of filter paper at the junction of the middle and lateral third of the patient's lower lid for 5 min. The amount of paper wetting is then measured using millimeter ruler. There are three types of Schirmer's tests: basic tear secretion and Schirmer's tests I and II. Basic tear secretion measures tear secretion after the instillation of a topical anesthetic to the conjunctival fornix. In contrast, the Schirmer's tests I and II are performed without anesthetic and they measure both basic and reflex tear secretion. The difference between the Schirmer's tests I and II consists in the stimulation of the nasal mucosa with a cotton tip applicator during Schirmer's test II. Abnormal filter paper wetting after 5 minutes is considered less than 10 mm with either basic tear secretion or the Schirmer's test I, or less than 15 mm with Schirmer's test II.

Tear secretion measured by either basic tear secretion or Schirmer's test I has been shown to decrease after LASIK surgery compared with preoperative levels [3, 8, 10, 12, 53], although the measured decreases have been modest. This decrease in tear secretion has been consistently observed in several studies at 1 month after LASIK surgery [3, 8, 10, 12] with some studies returning to baseline levels by 3 [3] and 6 months [3, 8] respectively. The cutoff established by the investigator (measured filter paper wetting) can significantly alter both the sensitivity and specificity of these tests and, therefore, the results of clinical trials [51]. However, in some patients with signs and symptoms of dry eye after LASIK, no statistically significant differences in tear secretion (Schirmer's test I) have been found compared with asymptomatic eyes from 1 to 6 months after surgery despite of the presence of ocular surface staining with fluorescein and rose bengal [9].

Tear Film Volume

Tear volume can be measured using the phenol red test (PRT). Briefly, this test uses a 0.2-mm-wide and 50-mm-long white cotton thread, which is stained with 0.1% phenol red solution [54, 55]. The thread is placed on the outer third portion of the patient's lower eyelid after asking the patient to look up. The patient is then asked to look straight ahead and the thread is removed 15 s to 2 min later [54–56]. The direct effect of the tear film pH causes discoloration of the thread, which can be easily measured using a millimeter ruler and indicates the volume of tears flowing in the eye. A PRT value of less than 11 mm over 15 s is considered diagnostic of tear deficiency [56]. Although this test has some potential for providing valuable information regarding tear deficiency states (tear volume), it is still unclear whether it really only measures tear volume and not other factors such as tear secretion and turnover [55]. Therefore, this test is probably better suited as a way of assessing the tear meniscus [56].

PRT has not been shown to decrease in eyes after myopic LASIK surgery compared with control eyes [11]. Tear volume, as measured with this technique, has not been shown to correlate with either age or decrease in corneal sensitivity in age-matched control patients with myopia [11]. In contrast, when preoperative PRT values are compared with postoperative PRT values in the same patients with myopia undergoing LASIK, PRT has been shown to decrease compared to baseline at 1 and 2 weeks, 1 month, and 3 months after surgery [34]. Similar results have been observed in hyperopic patients with chronic dry eye who have undergone LASIK surgery. Thus, PRT values at 2 weeks, 1 month, and 3 months have also been shown to decrease after hyperopic LASIK [13]. In addition, hyperopic regression has also been correlated with lower PRT results at 2 weeks and 1 month in patients with preexisting reduced PRT values prior to surgery [13].

Tear Film Osmolarity

Tear film osmolarity measurements are performed by collecting the patient's tear film meniscus at the slit lamp with a polyester rod. The patient is asked to look up and the rod is used to absorb the lower tear meniscus for 3 min [53]. Once the tear meniscus is collected, it undergoes several manipulations that require a laboratory setting that includes a centrifugation machine, micropipettes, and an ohmmeter, among other instruments [53]. The elaborate and technical nature of this test makes it unavailable for the busy clinician and, therefore, its use is not widespread. This is unfortunate since tear osmolarity is thought to be more sensitive and specific than Schirmer's test and lactoferrin test in differentiating between keratoconjunctivitis sicca patients and normal controls [57].

Tear film osmolarity has been shown to significantly increase after LASIK for myopia compared to preoperative levels at 3 and 6 months after surgery [53]. The increase in tear osmolarity seen after LASIK surgery can be explained by two different mechanisms. These include decreased tear production or increased tear evaporation.

Tear Film Stability

Tear stability is assessed clinically by measuring tear breakup time (TBUT). TBUT is performed by applying a premoistened fluorescein strip with balanced salt solution to the inferior conjunctival fornix. The patient is asked to blink several times to evenly spread the fluorescein dye over the corneal surface. The patient is then instructed to stop blinking and to look straight ahead while the ocular surface is illuminated with the cobalt blue light of the slit lamp. TBUT measures the time interval between the last blink and the appearance of the first random dry spot in the patient's precorneal tear film. The reproducibility of this test is low and, therefore, requires multiple sequential assessments [12, 53]. In addition, differences in methodology, such as the use of commercially available fluorescein drops or especially designed fluorescein strips, can alter the results of this test [58].

TBUT values have been consistently shown to decrease after LASIK surgery [3, 12–14, 53, 59]. Decreased TBUT can be measured as early as 1–7 days [12], and 1 [3] and 3 months [3, 12] after LASIK surgery, with variable recovery times to baseline preoperative levels. TBUT recovery can occur as early as 1 [12] or 3 months [53], and as late as 6 months [3, 12, 13, 53] after LASIK surgery. Decreased TBUT has also been correlated with subjective scores of dryness during the first 3 months after LASIK surgery [3]. In addition, lower TBUT values have been associated with regression after myopic LASIK at both 6 and 12 months after surgery, which is possibly due to disruption of the epithelial barrier during surgery [13].

TBUT can be reduced after LASIK due to a reduction in corneal sensitivity, which in turn can lead to decreased tear secretion and increased evaporative tear loss [3]. Moreover, surgical injury (intraoperative trauma to the corneal epithelium and postoperative toxicity from eye drops) can also lead to an irregular ocular surface and affect TBUT values [12]. An irregular tear film interface can also lead to patient dissatisfaction after LASIK surgery by inducing higher order aberrations such as coma and trefoil [60].

The use of the TMS (Topographic Modeling System) software, which measures both TMS–TBUT and TMS–tear breakup area (TMS-BUA) [61, 62], can also be used to assess tear film stability with the use of videokeratography. In a pilot study, both TMS-BUT and TMS-BUA were found to have higher sensitivity and specificity for the detection of tear film stability abnormalities compared with traditional slit lamp TBUT. Furthermore, preoperative TMS-BUT and TMS-BUA values have been shown to correlate with the development of dry eye signs and symptoms after LASIK surgery [61]. Nevertheless, the results obtained with this technology remain to be validated in larger independent clinical trials.

5.1.4.4.2 Ocular Surface Staining

Ocular surface staining after the instillation of dyes is considered as an important element in the evaluation of patients with dry eye. Staining patterns of the cornea and conjunctiva can be graded using different methods such as the Oxford grading scheme [51]. The Oxford grading scheme, or a modified version of this test, has been used in several clinical trials to assess the presence of dry eye before and after LASIK surgery [3, 4, 8, 13, 39, 40, 63] fluorescein sodium [3, 4, 8, 13, 14, 28], rose bengal [3, 7, 9], and lissamine green [39, 40, 63] have all been used as staining agents to evaluate the severity and distribution of ocular surface abnormalities related to dry eye in LASIK patients. The order in which these tests are performed is important, since both rose bengal and lissamine green can affect the results of the Schirmer's and tear breakup time (TBUT) tests due to the induction of reflex tearing [64].

Surface Dyes

Fluorescein Sodium

Fluorescein sodium is a xanthine-derived dye (yellow colored), which is routinely used to stain the pre-corneal tear

5

meniscus and ocular surface. Fluorescein has the advantage of being well tolerated and relatively nontoxic to corneal epithelial cells. Fluorescein is applied as a solution or after moistening the tip of a fluorescein-impregnated paper strip, which is applied to the inferior conjunctival fornix. The patient is then asked to blink several times, and the presence and pattern of staining is assessed with the use of a cobalt blue exciter filter. Fluorescein stains were basement membrane or underlying stroma is exposed by epithelial injury. A disadvantage of this technique is the rapid penetration of fluorescein into the corneal stroma in the presence of epithelial defects, which can blur the margins of the staining defect.

Rose Bengal

Rose bengal is a fluorinated dye (pink in color), which causes dose-dependent staining of the cornea and conjunctiva. Instillation of a drop of rose bengal should be performed while the patient is looking down and after topical anesthetic administration in order to minimize patient discomfort. Rose bengal staining of the ocular surface can be enhanced using a red-free (green) light source. Since rose bengal does not diffuse beyond the conjunctival epithelium, the staining pattern can be visualized for a longer period of time compared to fluorescein. Rose bengal stains areas where there is disruption of the mucinous protective layer covering of conjunctival or corneal epithelial cells [65]. A major disadvantage of rose bengal use is related to its intrinsic toxicity to corneal epithelial cells.

Lissamine Green

Lissamine green is a synthetic dye that causes dose-dependent staining of the ocular surface but induces less toxicity to the ocular surface compared with rose bengal [64]. Lissamine green should be applied after administration of a topical anesthetic drop and while the patient is looking down. Lissamine green staining lasts as long as rose bengal since it does not diffuse into the substantia propria of the conjunctiva [64]. The staining, however, takes longer to develop, and the clinician should wait 45 s to 1 min after application before assessing the staining pattern. The staining pattern in an individual eye is very similar with rose bengal and lissamine green. Therefore, although it has not been systematically studied, lissamine green likely also stains areas on the conjunctivae and cornea where there is disruption of the mucinous protective layer covering these cells.

Oxford Grading Scheme

The Oxford grading scheme was developed to quantify the amount of corneal and conjunctival epithelial surface damage in patients with dry eye [64]. This grading scheme uses a standardized chart with a series of panels depicting the distribution of ocular surface staining in increasing order of severity. The examiner compares the overall pattern of staining seen during the clinical examination with the appearance of each panel and grades the severity of ocular staining accordingly.

Significance of Ocular Surface Staining in LASIK Patients

Ocular surface staining related to LASIK surgery is usually confined to the area of the flap, often sparing the flap edges. Punctate epithelial erosions (PEE) can develop as early as 1 week [8] and usually peak by 1 to 3 months after LASIK surgery [8, 13, 34]. Ocular staining scores have a tendency to return to preoperative baseline levels by 6 [8, 34] to 12 [13] months after surgery.

5.1.4.4.3 Ocular Sensation Abnormalities

The integrity of the ocular surface–trigeminal nerve–brain stem–facial nerve–lacrimal gland axis [3, 7–14] is essential for the maintenance of the basic refractive properties of the cornea. This complex neuronal network regulates among other functions tear production (basal and stimulated) and blink rate, which are essential for optimal refraction of light at the air–tear interface.

Corneal sensitivity measured by esthesiometric techniques has been shown greatly reduced before and after LASIK surgery [3–5, 8, 11, 14, 19, 35, 38–40, 63]. This reduction in corneal sensation has been associated with contact lens use, decreased tear production, higher ocular staining scores, tears instability, and reduced blink rate in some patients after LASIK surgery.

Esthesiometry Methods

Cochet-Bonnet Esthesiometer

The Cochet-Bonnet esthesiometer is considered the gold standard for the assessment of corneal sensitivity for touch sensation. Briefly, this technique uses a 60-mm-long and 0.12-mm-wide adjustable nylon monofilament. The monofilament is soft when fully extended and becomes rigid as the length is shortened with a hand piece in 5-mm decrements. The monofilament is then applied to the surface of the cornea in a perpendicular plane while the patient looks straight ahead. The length of the monofilament is shortened until the patient feels it for the first time, and then the monofilament length is subsequently recorded. In principle, the higher the number recorded (longer filament length), the more sensitive the cornea. It is important to remember to perform this test at the beginning of the exam and prior to anesthetic drop use.

Role of Corneal Sensitivity in the Pathogenesis of Dry Eye Loss of corneal sensitivity after LASIK is not uniform between the different areas of the cornea, and is more deeply depressed in the central cornea [37]. Factors responsible for decreased corneal sensation after LASIK include direct microkeratome or femtosecond laser transection and excimer laser photoablation of epithelial/subepithelial and superficial stromal nerve plexuses located at the edge of the flap and along the flap interface [6]. Loss of corneal sensitivity produces to a neurotrophic state that lasts anywhere from 3 [35, 43], 6 [3, 38], 9 [44] to 18 months [8] after LASIK surgery.

Predictably, corneal sensitivity after LASIK enhancements is reduced compared to pre-enhancement values. This significant difference is detectable from 1 to 6 months after surgery [19]. LASIK-induced corneal denervation may take years to return to preoperative levels in some patients, in parallel with the low number of re-innervated fibers observed after LASIK surgery observed in the flap in some eyes using confocal microscopy at 1 year or more after surgery [66].

5.1.4.5 Conjunctival Goblet Cell Density

Conjunctival goblet cell density can be determined by obtaining superficial conjunctival epithelial cell samples collected by impression cytology. Goblet cell density has been shown to decrease after both myopic [16] and hyperopic LASIK [13]. Depletion of conjunctival goblet cells can lead to a reduction in mucin production. Goblet cells loss has been shown to inversely correlate with dry eye symptoms in LASIK patients who have not had management of their ocular surface prior to surgery [16].

Loss of goblet cells is probably multifactorial and results from a combination of several factors. These may include a neurotrophic conjunctiva and resulting loss of nerve influences on goblet cell differentiation, tear film and epithelial cytokine-mediated deficiency states, in addition to suction-induced, microkeratome-related mechanical trauma.

5.1.4.6 Subjective Evaluation of the Ocular Surface Disease

The Ocular Surface Disease Index (OSDI) was developed by the outcomes research group at Allergan (Irvine, Calif.). This index has been validated in a prospective clinical trial and has been shown to effectively discriminate and grade the severity of dry eye symptoms [67].

Briefly, the OSDI consists of 12 questions that have been designed to gather information regarding the severity of dry eye symptoms. The completed questionnaire is graded using a severity scale ranging from 0 to 4. Items 1–5 consist of symptom related questions, items 6–9 assess how much dry eye symptoms interfere with daily tasks, and items 10–12 assess environmental conditions that can potentially exacerbate dry eye symptoms. The frequency of symptoms is recorded using the severity scale previously mentioned. A score of 0 indicates that symptoms are present none of the time, a score 1 some of the time, a score of 2 half of the time, a score of 3 most of the time, and a score of 4 all of the time [68]. The OSDI is then scored using the following formula: OSDI = sum of severity scores for all of the questions answered / total number of questions answered × 4 [68].

In our experience, the OSDI provides a valuable tool for detecting patients with occult dry eye during the screening process for refractive surgery. We have included it as a routine component in our first encounter with the patient.

5.1.5 Management

Optimization of the ocular surface is an important step to improving patient satisfaction and outcomes after LASIK surgery. The management of dry eye begins during the preoperative screening examination, when patients' signs and symptoms are assessed, and an individualized treatment regimen devised to prepare ascertain whether the patient is a candidate for LASIK and, if so, the ocular surface optimized prior to surgery.

Assessment begins with the diagnosis and treatment of rosacea–blepharitis. Either of these conditions may exacerbate the dry eye condition and increase the overall inflammatory milieu of the ocular surface. Treatment of these conditions includes lid hygiene regimens and in some cases the use oral doxycycline and topical antibiotics.

In patients who present symptoms and signs or signs alone of dry eye disease, including onset of contact lens intolerance and conjunctival and/or corneal staining with rose bengal or lissamine green, it is imperative to treat the underlying condition, these patients are predisposed to the development of severe LASIK-induced neurotropic epitheliopathy after LASIK surgery [7, 9]. In addition, any punctate epithelial erosions of the corneal surface may induce artifact in wavefront measurements used for custom corneal ablations. Although artificial tears and several other treatment modalities may be helpful in these patients, topical cyclosporine A 0.05% (Restasis, Allergan) has become the mainstay of treatment for many refractive surgeons, since pretreatment prior to LASIK surgery and continued treatment in the months after surgery has been found to markedly reduce LASIK-induced dry eye and improve the visual outcomes of LASIK surgery [17].

5.1.5.1 Topical Preparations

5.1.5.1.1 Artificial Tears

Lubrication of the ocular surface is a mainstay of treatment of LASIK-induced dry eye prior to and after surgery. Lubrication of the ocular surface with non-preserved artificial tears may be beneficial the corneal microenvironment and lead to a reduction of dry eye symptoms before and after LASIK. Several commercially available artificial tear preparations such as 0.5% carboxymethylcellulose in lactate buffer (Refresh Plus, Allergan), 0.3% hydroxypropyl methylcellulose and 1% dextran bicarbonate buffer (Bion Tears, Alcon) and hydroxypropyl-guar and polyethylene glycol preparations (Systane, Alcon) have been used for the optimization of the ocular surface before and after LASIK surgery. Recently, Allergan has introduced a new artificial tear (Optive) that contains components that lubricate the ocular surface and provide osmo-protection for corneal and conjunctival epithelial cells. This new concept may offer significant advantages over other artificial tear formulations.

5.1.5.1.2 Lid Scrubs

Management of rosacea–blepharitis and meibomian gland dysfunction (MGD) also represents a very important step for the optimization of the ocular surface. As a first step, blepharitis should be managed with the use of commercially available lid scrubs and warm compresses, along with lid hygiene with neutral detergents such as baby shampoo. As a second step, oral tetracyclines (doxycycline) 100 mg twice a day can also be used due to its matrix metalloproteinase inhibition properties, which have been shown to be increased in patients with rosacea-associated corneal complications [69].

5.1.5.1.3 Topical Cyclosporine A

Cyclosporine A 0.05% ophthalmic solution (Restasis) has been successfully used for the management of dry eye and has found increasing acceptance among refractive surgeons for optimizing the ocular surface prior to surgery and treatment of LASIK-induced dry eye [17]. Our approach is to institute treatment with topical cyclosporine in any patient who has preoperative signs and/or symptoms of dry eye, especially if there is conjunctival or corneal staining with rose bengal or lissamine green. These patients are reevaluated at 1-month intervals for resolution of their dry eye symptoms and signs prior to completion of the preoperative evaluation (obtaining wavefront measurements, etc.). In our experience, over 50% of patients with preoperative symptoms and signs will have complete resolution within 1 month of instituting treatment and can complete their preoperative evaluation and proceed to LASIK surgery with continued administration of cyclosporine for 6 months after surgery. Some patients take several months of treatment with cyclosporine before there is complete resolution of symptoms and signs and surgery can be performed. Approximately 10–15% of patients will continue to have symptoms and/or signs of dry eye despite topical cyclosporine treatment for 6 months or more. In our opinion, these individuals are not candidates for refractive surgery.

Topical cyclosporine A treatment has proven to be very safe. Some patients (approximately 10–15%) have stinging upon initial instillation of cyclosporine. This typically occurs in more severe patients with moderate to severe conjunctival and/or corneal staining. Stinging can be minimized by concurrently applying a topical corticosteroid such as prednisolone acetate 1% or loteprednol etabonate 0.5% for 10–14 days [70]. The corticosteroid drop is then discontinued, and the cyclosporine maintained through surgery, stopping only on the day of surgery and for 2 days, out of concern the vehicle could somehow diffuse beneath the flap.

Patients who are pretreated with topical cyclosporine A rarely develop LASIK-induced neurotrophic epitheliopathy (LINE). If LINE develops despite cyclosporine treatment, then cyclosporine A should be continued and augmented with other modalities including non-preserved artificial tears and ointments, oral α–ω omega fatty acids, and punctual plugs.

Some patients with no symptoms or signs of dry eye disease prior to LASIK will develop LINE after LASIK surgery. Surprisingly, topical cyclosporine A twice a day has proven to be highly effective in treating the condition in these patients. Presumably, these eyes had underlying inflammatory dry eye prior to surgery that did not produced symptoms or signs, but transecting the corneal nerves add-

ed another stressor that tipped the eye over the threshold to clinical disease. Once the treatment is instituted, the cyclosporine is typically continued for 6–8 months and, in our experience, is highly effective in treating the disorder. Subsequent LASIK enhancements should include cyclosporine pretreatment because the LINE recurs in virtually one hundred percent of cases without treatment.

5.1.5.2 Punctal Plugs

Our use of punctal plugs has declined markedly since topical cyclosporine treatment became available. Punctal plug occlusion is not recommended in patients with an underlying inflammatory etiology responsible for the development of their dry eye until the inflammation has been controlled with anti-inflammatory treatment. Tears containing inflammatory cytokines can become stagnant in the conjunctival cul-de-sac through the action of punctal plugs can further exacerbate damage to the ocular surface.

In LASIK patients who continue to demonstrate signs of dry eye such as punctate epithelial erosions and visual fluctuation, punctal plugs are a reasonable alternative, especially if topical cyclosporine A treatment is not available. If despite cyclosporine A treatment a patient continues to have LINE, then punctal plugs may be a helpful addition to augment treatment. Thus, punctal plug occlusion has been shown to reduce wavefront aberrations in myopic patients with post-LASIK dry eye [71].

5.1.5.3 Oral Dietary Supplements

Nutrition supplementation with ω-3 fatty acids (flaxseed oil) has been associated with a reduction in chronic dry eye symptoms [72]. Although the role of nutritional supplementation has not yet been evaluated in the context of LASIK surgery, dietary supplementation represents a logical addition, especially in moderate-to-severe patients who do not respond adequately to topical cyclosporine or if topical cyclosporine is not available.

5.1.5.4 Autologous Serum

The use of autologous serum should be exceedingly rare after LASIK because most patients who might need this form of treatment should have been effectively screened in the preoperative evaluation. Thus, if a patient fails cyclosporine A treatment or this treatment is not available and they continue to have punctate ocular surface staining with rose bengal despite intensive non-preserved artificial tears and punctal plugs, then they should not undergo LASIK surgery. Occasionally, however, there may be patients who have symptoms and signs develop after LASIK that are unresponsive to other treatments, and treatment with autologous serum becomes an option. Autologous serum tear preparation diluted to 20% concentration with sterile saline solution has been used for the management of persistent epithelial defects [73], Sjögren's syndrome [74] and dry eye after graft-versus-host disease [75]. Autologous serum uses the patient's own blood products, and presumably the cytokines such as epidermal growth factor, transforming growth factor, and vitamin A contained in them to heal the ocular surface [74]. When necessary, treatment with 20% autologous serum solution may increase tear stability (increase tear break up time) at 6 months after surgery and reduce rose bengal staining of the ocular surface after LASIK surgery [76].

5.1.6 Conclusion

Dry eye is the most common complication associated with LASIK surgery. LASIK-induced dry eye represents a multifactorial condition that is manifested clinically by the presence of fluctuation in visual acuity, punctate epithelial erosions and, in some patients, decreased tear production. Patients with LINE can develop punctate epithelial erosions and rose bengal staining of the ocular surface in the presence of normal Schirmer's test. Damage to corneal nerves, induced by the creation of the LASIK flap and excimer laser tissue ablation, induces a transient dry eye state via a combination of denervation leading to decreased tear production; altered cytokine expression, which modulates wound healing; loss of conjunctival goblet cells, which reduces mucin production; and decreased blink rate, causing mechanical problems with tear distribution over the ocular surface.

Management of dry eye after LASIK begins during the screening visit, with optimization of the ocular surface using artificial tears, warm compresses, and lid hygiene and treating the underlying ocular surface inflammation with immunomodulatory agents such as cyclosporine A 0.05%.

> **Take-Home Pearls**
> - The ocular surface should be optimized prior to LASIK surgery.
> - Recognition and treatment of rosacea–blepharitis should include lid hygiene regimens, and in some cases oral doxycycline and topical antibiotics.
> - Lubrication of the ocular surface with non-preserved artificial tears is a mainstay of treatment of LASIK-induced dry eye prior to and after surgery.
> - Topical cyclosporine A 0.05% (Restasis) is helpful in the prophylaxis and treatment of LASIK-induced dry eye. Patients who are pretreated with topical cyclosporine A rarely develop LINE.
> - Although helpful, punctal plug occlusion is not recommended as first-line treatment in patients with an underlying inflammatory-based dry eye, since inflammatory cytokines may be maintained at high levels within the tears.

References

1. Duffey RJ, Leaming D (2005) US trends in refractive surgery: 2004 ISRS/AAO Survey. J Refract Surg 21:742–748
2. Solomon KD, Holzer MP, Sandoval HP et al (2002) Refractive Surgery Survey 2001. J Cataract Refract Surg Feb 28:346–355
3. Toda I, Asano-Kato N, Komai-Hori Y, Tsubota K (2001) Dry eye after laser in situ keratomileusis. Am J Ophthalmol Jul 132:1–7
4. Albietz JM, Lenton LM, McLennan SG (2005) Dry eye after LASIK: comparison of outcomes for Asian and Caucasian eyes. Clin Exp Optom Mar 88:89–96
5. De Paiva CS, Chen Z, Koch DD et al (2006) The incidence and risk factors for developing dry eye after myopic LASIK (Exp Eye Res) Am J Ophthalmol 141:438–445
6. Linna TU, Perez-Santonja JJ, Tervo KM, Sakla HF, Alio y Sanz JL, Tervo TM (1998) Recovery of corneal nerve morphology following laser in situ keratomileusis. Exp Eye Res 66:755–763
7. Wilson SE, Ambrosio R (2001) Laser in situ keratomileusis-induced neurotrophic epitheliopathy. Am J Ophthalmol 132:405–406
8. Battat L, Macri A, Dursun D, Pflugfelder SC (2001) Effects of laser in situ keratomileusis on tear production, clearance, and the ocular surface. Ophthalmology 108:1230–1235
9. Wilson SE (2001) Laser in situ keratomileusis-induced (presumed) neurotrophic epitheliopathy. Ophthalmology 108:1082–1087
10. Benitez-del-Castillo JM, del Rio T, Iradier T, Hernandez JL, Castillo A, Garcia-Sanchez J (2001) Decrease in tear secretion and corneal sensitivity after laser in situ keratomileusis. Cornea 20:30–32
11. Patel S, Perez-Santonja JJ, Alio JL, Murphy PJ (2001) Corneal sensitivity and some properties of the tear film after laser in situ keratomileusis. J Refract Surg 17:17–24
12. Yu EY, Leung A, Rao S, Lam DS (2000) Effect of laser in situ keratomileusis on tear stability. Ophthalmology 107:2131–2135
13. Albietz JM, Lenton LM, McLennan SG (2002) Effect of laser in situ keratomileusis for hyperopia on tear film and ocular surface. J Refract Surg 18:113–123
14. Albietz JM, Lenton LM, McLennan SG (2004) Chronic dry eye and regression after laser in situ keratomileusis for myopia. J Cataract Refract Surg 30:675–684
15. Wilson SE, Liang Q, Kim WJ (1999) Lacrimal gland HGF, KGF, and EGF mRNA levels increase after corneal epithelial wounding. Invest Ophthalmol Vis Sci 40:2185–2190
16. Albietz JM, McLennan SG, Lenton LM (2003) Ocular surface management of photorefractive keratectomy and laser in situ keratomileusis. J Refract Surg 19:636–644
17. Salib GM, McDonald MB, Smolek M (2006) Safety and efficacy of cyclosporine 0.05% drops versus unpreserved artificial tears in dry-eye patients having laser in situ keratomileusis. J Cataract Refract Surg 32:772–778
18. Wilson S, Perry HD (2007) Long-term resolution of chronic dry eye symptoms and signs after topical cyclosporine A treatment. Ophthalmology 114:76–79
19. Toda I, Kato-Asano N, Hori-Komai Y, Tsubota K (2006) Dry eye after LASIK enhancement by flap lifting. J Refract Surg 22:358–362
20. Davidorf JM, Zaldivar R, Oscherow S (1998) Results and complications of laser in situ keratomileusis by experienced surgeons. J Refract Surg 14:114–122
21. Wilson SE, Mohan RR, Hong JW, Lee JS, Choi R, Mohan RR (2001) The wound healing response after laser in situ keratomileusis and photorefractive keratectomy: elusive control of biological variability and effect on custom laser vision correction. Arch Ophthalmol 119:889–896
22. Alio JL, Artola A, Belda JI et al (2005) LASIK in patients with rheumatic diseases: a pilot study. Ophthalmology 112:1948–1954
23. Moss SE, Klein R, Klein BE (2000) Prevalence of and risk factors for dry eye syndrome. Arch Ophthalmol 118:1264–1268

24. Tekwani NH, Huang D (2002) Risk factors for intraoperative epithelial defect in laser in-situ keratomileusis. Am J Ophthalmol 134:311–316

25. Asano-Kato N, Toda I, Hori-Komai Y, Takano Y, Tsubota K (2002) Epithelial ingrowth after laser in situ keratomileusis: clinical features and possible mechanisms. Am J Ophthalmol 134:801–807

26. Wang MY, Maloney RK (2000) Epithelial ingrowth after laser in situ keratomileusis. Am J Ophthalmol 129:746–751

27. Mulhern MG, Naor J, Rootman DS (2002) The role of epithelial defects in intralamellar inflammation after laser in situ keratomileusis. Can J Ophthalmol 37:409–415

28. Albietz JM, Lenton LM (2004) Management of the ocular surface and tear film before, during, and after laser in situ keratomileusis. J Refract Surg 20:62–71

29. Sullivan DA, Krenzer KL, Sullivan BD, Tolls DB, Toda I, Dana MR (1999) Does androgen insufficiency cause lacrimal gland inflammation and aqueous tear deficiency? Invest Ophthalmol Vis Sci 40:1261–1265

30. Krenzer KL, Dana MR, Ullman MD et al (2000) Effect of androgen deficiency on the human meibomian gland and ocular surface. J Clin Endocrinol Metab 85:4874–4882

31. Lemp MA (1995) Report of the National Eye Institute/Industry workshop on clinical trials in dry eyes. Clao J 21:221–232

32. Yo C (2003) Asian Americans: myopia and refractive surgery. Int Ophthalmol Clin 43:173–187

33. Asano-Kato N, Toda I, Hori-Komai Y, Takano Y, Tsubota K (2002) Risk factors for insufficient fixation of microkeratome during laser in situ keratomileusis. J Refract Surg 18:47–50

34. Albietz J, Lenton L, McLennan S (2002) The effect of tear film and ocular surface management on myopic LASIK outcomes. Adv Exp Med Biol 506(Pt A):711–717

35. Toda I, Asano-Kato N, Hori-Komai Y, Tsubota K (2002) Laser-assisted in situ keratomileusis for patients with dry eye. Arch Ophthalmol 120:1024–1028

36. Toda I, Asano-Kato N, Hori-Komai Y, Tsubota K (2004) Ocular surface treatment before laser in situ keratomileusis in patients with severe dry eye. J Refract Surg 20:270–275

37. Chuck RS, Quiros PA, Perez AC, McDonnell PJ (2000) Corneal sensation after laser in situ keratomileusis. J Cataract Refract Surg 26:337–339

38. Vroman DT, Sandoval HP, Fernandez de Castro LE, Kasper TJ, Holzer MP, Solomon KD (2005) Effect of hinge location on corneal sensation and dry eye after laser in situ keratomileusis for myopia. J Cataract Refract Surg 31:1881–1887

39. Donnenfeld ED, Ehrenhaus M, Solomon R, Mazurek J, Rozell JC, Perry HD (2004) Effect of hinge width on corneal sensation and dry eye after laser in situ keratomileusis. J Cataract Refract Surg 30:790–797

40. Donnenfeld ED, Solomon K, Perry HD et al (2003) The effect of hinge position on corneal sensation and dry eye after LASIK. Ophthalmology 110:1023–1029; discussion 1029–1030

41. Lawrenson JG, Ruskell GL (1993) Investigation of limbal touch sensitivity using a Cochet-Bonnet aesthesiometer. Br J Ophthalmol 77:339–343

42. Muller LJ, Marfurt CF, Kruse F, Tervo TM (2003) Corneal nerves: structure, contents and function. Exp Eye Res 76:521–542

43. Nassaralla BA, McLeod SD, Boteon JE, Nassaralla JJ Jr (2005) The effect of hinge position and depth plate on the rate of recovery of corneal sensation following LASIK. Am J Ophthalmol Ja 139:118–124

44. Nassaralla BA, McLeod SD, Nassaralla JJ Jr (2003) Effect of myopic LASIK on human corneal sensitivity. Ophthalmology 110:497–502

45. Lee KW, Joo CK (2003) Clinical results of laser in situ keratomileusis with superior and nasal hinges. J Cataract Refract Surg 29:457–461

46. Kumano Y, Matsui H, Zushi I et al (2003) Recovery of corneal sensation after myopic correction by laser in situ keratomileusis with a nasal or superior hinge. J Cataract Refract Surg 29:757–761

47. Kim WS, Kim JS (1999) Change in corneal sensitivity following laser in situ keratomileusis. J Cataract Refract Surg 25:368–373

48. Farris RL, Stuchell RN, Mandel ID (1986) Tear osmolarity variation in the dry eye. Trans Am Ophthalmol Soc 84:250–268

49. Kunert KS, Tisdale AS, Stern ME, Smith JA, Gipson IK (2000) Analysis of topical cyclosporine treatment of patients with dry eye syndrome: effect on conjunctival lymphocytes. Arch Ophthalmol 118:1489–1496

50. Kunert KS, Tisdale AS, Gipson IK (2002) Goblet cell numbers and epithelial proliferation in the conjunctiva of patients with dry eye syndrome treated with cyclosporine. Arch Ophthalmol 120:330–337

51. Bron AJ (2001) Diagnosis of dry eye. Surv Ophthalmol 45(Suppl 2):S221–226

52. Hovanesian JA, Shah SS, Maloney RK (2001) Symptoms of dry eye and recurrent erosion syndrome after refractive surgery. J Cataract Refract Surg 27:577–584

53. Lee JB, Ryu CH, Kim J, Kim EK, Kim HB (2000) Comparison of tear secretion and tear film instability after photorefractive keratectomy and laser in situ keratomileusis. J Cataract Refract Surg 26:1326–1331

54. Blades KJ, Patel S (1996) The dynamics of tear flow within a phenol red impregnated thread. Ophthalmic Physiol Opt 16:409–415

55 (2001) Tomlinson A, Blades KJ, Pearce EI. What does the phenol red thread test actually measure? Optom Vis Sci 78:142–146

56. Mainstone JC, Bruce AS, Golding TR (1996) Tear meniscus measurement in the diagnosis of dry eye. Curr Eye Res 15:653–661

57. Lucca JA, Nunez JN, Farris RL (1990) A comparison of diagnostic tests for keratoconjunctivitis sicca: lactoplate, Schirmer, and tear osmolarity. Clao J 16.109–112

58. Korb DR, Greiner JV, Herman J (2001) Comparison of fluorescein break-up time measurement reproducibility using standard fluorescein strips versus the Dry Eye Test (DET) method. Cornea 20:811–815

59. Lee HK, Lee KS, Kim HC, Lee SH, Kim EK (2005) Nerve growth factor concentration and implications in photorefractive keratectomy vs laser in situ keratomileusis. Am J Ophthalmol 139:965–971

60. Lin YY, Carrel H, Wang IJ, Lin PJ, Hu FR (2005) Effect of tear film break-up on higher order aberrations of the anterior cornea in normal, dry, and post-LASIK eyes. J Refract Surg 21:S525–529

61. Goto T, Zheng X, Klyce SD et al (2004) Evaluation of the tear film stability after laser in situ keratomileusis using the tear film stability analysis system. Am J Ophthalmol 137:116–120

62. Goto T, Zheng X, Okamoto S, Ohashi Y (2004) Tear film stability analysis system: introducing a new application for videokeratography. Cornea 23(8 Suppl):S65–70

63. Michaeli A, Slomovic AR, Sakhichand K, Rootman DS (2004) Effect of laser in situ keratomileusis on tear secretion and corneal sensitivity. J Refract Surg 20:379–383

64. Bron AJ, Evans VE, Smith JA (2003) Grading of corneal and conjunctival staining in the context of other dry eye tests. Cornea 22:640–650

65. Feenstra RP, Tseng SC (1992) What is actually stained by rose bengal? Arch Ophthalmol 110:984–993

66. Lee BH, McLaren JW, Erie JC, Hodge DO, Bourne WM (2002) Reinnervation in the cornea after LASIK. Invest Ophthalmol Vis Sci 43:3660–3664

67. Schiffman RM, Christianson MD, Jacobsen G, Hirsch JD, Reis BL (2000) Reliability and validity of the Ocular Surface Disease Index. Arch Ophthalmol 118:615–621

68. Perry HD, Donnenfeld ED (2004) Dry eye diagnosis and management in 2004. Curr Opin Ophthalmol 15:299–304

69. Sobrin L, Liu Z, Monroy DC et al (2000) Regulation of MMP-9 activity in human tear fluid and corneal epithelial culture supernatant. Invest Ophthalmol Vis Sci 41:1703–1709

70. Marsh P, Pflugfelder SC (1999) Topical nonpreserved methylprednisolone therapy for keratoconjunctivitis sicca in Sjögren's syndrome. Ophthalmology 106:811–816

71. Huang B, Mirza MA, Qazi MA, Pepose JS (2004) The effect of punctal occlusion on wavefront aberrations in dry eye patients after laser in situ keratomileusis. Am J Ophthalmol 137:52–61

72. Miljanovic B, Trivedi KA, Dana MR, Gilbard JP, Buring JE, Schaumberg DA (2005) Relation between dietary *n*-3 and *n*-6 fatty acids and clinically diagnosed dry eye syndrome in women. Am J Clin Nutr 82:887–893

73. Tsubota K, Goto E, Shimmura S, Shimazaki J (1999) Treatment of persistent corneal epithelial defect by autologous serum application. Ophthalmology 06:1984–1989

74. Tsubota K, Goto E, Fujita H et al (1999) Treatment of dry eye by autologous serum application in Sjögren's syndrome. Br J Ophthalmol 83:390–395

75. Ogawa Y, Okamoto S, Mori T et al (2003) Autologous serum eye drops for the treatment of severe dry eye in patients with chronic graft-versus-host disease. Bone Marrow Transplant 31:579–583

76. Noda-Tsuruya T, Asano-Kato N, Toda I, Tsubota K (2006) Autologous serum eye drops for dry eye after LASIK. J Refract Surg 22:61–66

Core Messages

- Poor adhesion of the flap leaves a virtual space between the flap and the residual stroma that is supposed to be filled by the epithelial cells.

- The diagnosis of epithelial ingrowth in its initial phase relies entirely in a careful observation of the cornea at the slit lamp after the LASIK surgery.

- Surgical treatment of epithelial ingrowth is very difficult and has a high incidence of recurrence (reports of 10%). Lifting the flap has the danger of spread the cells under the flap or even activates the epithelial cells to grow.

- The mainstay of treatment is observation. If the disease does not progress over time, surgical intervention is not warranted. If progression is observed and documented, then surgical treatment has to be undertaken.

- Several different techniques have been proposed to treat surgically this annoying complication. All of them agree the epithelium has to be cleaned from the stroma, from the undersurface of the flap and from the edges of the wound.

- It is the most frequent complication. Reports in the literature vary from 1 to 10% incidence. However, the incidence of epithelial ingrowth should be declining due to the progress in the LASIK surgical technique, the knowledge of the predisposing factors, and of course, the improvement in microkeratomes and LASIK instruments.

- It is probably the most sight-threatening complication when it progresses uncontrolled after refractive surgery and gets closer to the visual axis.

- Once present, it is a very difficult complication to treat, and confirms the advice of observing its

- progression instead of an early intervention, and the several techniques proposed as a surgical management option.

5.2 Epithelial Ingrowth

Gustavo E. Tamayo

5.2.1 Introduction

There are several reasons why epithelial ingrowth should be considered the most important complication of LASIK surgery:

5.2.2 Etiology of Epithelial Ingrowth

There are several theories as far as etiology of this complication is concerned. Probably the most accepted theory is active proliferation of epithelium at the flap edge and growing under the flap into the interface, a process that starts immediately after surgery. Other theories consider the introduction of epithelial cells under the flap during surgery by the microkeratome blade or with a syringe during the irrigation phase, with the sponge when cleaning or drying, or even with forceps if used.

Regardless of the mechanism of implantation of epithelial cells under the flap, the cells are active epithelial cells, derived apparently from two sources, corneal epithelial cells and/or conjunctival epithelial cells.

Even if there is not a unique theory about the origin of the epithelial cells growing in the interface between the flap and the stroma, there are several well-known risk factors in

5

LASIK surgery; their presence has been associated with epithelial ingrowth:

- Flap striae or folds, as when the flap dislocates after surgery due to trauma or poor adhesion
- Excessive manipulation of the flap with forceps or with sponges. Excessive irrigation or careless surgery with not enough time dedicated to the flap desiccation, resulting in poor adhesion of the flap. This leaves a virtual space between the flap and the residual stroma that is infiltrated by epithelial cells.
- Any type of complication with the creation of the flap can cause growth of the epithelial cells: buttonhole, irregular flaps, decentered flaps, or flaps with an irregular gutter.
- Use of defective microkeratomes with uneven and or irregular advancement, with poor or intermittent suction, blades with non-smooth or sharp borders. All of these can cause irregular stromal bed or irregular junctions between the epithelium of the flap and the remaining epithelium of the cornea, a known trigger for epithelial ingrowth.
- Relifting of the flap, particularly when they are traumatic or difficult, have a higher incidence of epithelial ingrowth.
- Epithelial defects created by the surgery, such as the "fluffy epithelium" caused by some microkeratomes or during the reposition of the flap due to manipulation in patients older than 40 years of age.
- Laser ablation of the corneal epithelium at the border of the flap when the flap is small and the ablation zone is larger creates a gap that could be an open window for the epithelium to enter and grow.
- Surgery over previous surgeries such as LASIK over radial keratotomy cuts.

5.2.3 Clinical Manifestations of Epithelial Ingrowth

One of the problems of epithelial ingrowth is the asymptomatic ingrowth during the initial phase of the problem. Very rarely, patients may complain of photophobia, foreign-body sensation, or red eye. In advanced stages of the disease however, patients may complain of diminished visual acuity or visual symptoms such as glare, haloes, or night visual disturbances that may be attributed to a large growth at the periphery, producing some type of irregular astigmatism or growth of epithelial cells toward the center of the pupil, obstructing light from entering the eye.

Still, the diagnosis of epithelial ingrowth in its initial phase relies entirely in a careful observation of the cornea at the slit lamp after LASIK surgery. Several illumination techniques may be used, such as tangential light or retro-illumination with a dilated pupil, when the aspect of the cornea is suspicious. Careful examination at the gap in the first 24 h after surgery or at the borders of the flap, especially inferiorly with superior hinge or temporal in nasal hinge, should be taken. Corneal topography could help in advanced cases as can pick up the irregular astigmatism. Epithelial ingrowth may appear in two forms:

- As white or grayish small spots or lines at the periphery (Fig. 5.2.1) within 2 mm of the peripheral edge of the flap. It may be diffuse or localized in a cluster. It is usually a benign form of presentation, which remains stationary, without further progression or even disappears over a period of 1–4 months, without any signal or leaving a small and discrete haze at the interface.
- Pearl-like islands of different sizes, elevated white or grayish colonies, sheaths, cysts or elevated strands with delineated borders or without them, adopting a more diffuse form. This is a more aggressive presentation of epithelial ingrowth, usually progressive toward the center of the pupil (Fig. 5.2.2) as well as laterally, sometimes merging with the neighbor cells. These cells eventually involve the affected area of the flap and cause melting and retraction at the periphery. If left untreated, the affected area of the flap may disappear, the keratolysis progresses, and the growth spread over the entire flap.

5.2.4 Classification of Epithelial Ingrowth

Several classifications of epithelial ingrowth have been made. Dr. Arun Gulani presented a very useful one in the 10th European Society Meeting of Cataract and Refractive Surgery in Nice, France:

Grade 1: Epithelium under the flap as a localized island at the periphery. It does not block the red reflex.

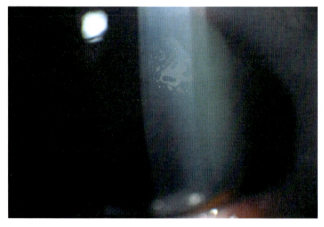

Fig. 5.2.1 Epithelial ingrowth may appear as white or grayish small spots or lines at the periphery. This form is usually a benign form of presentation

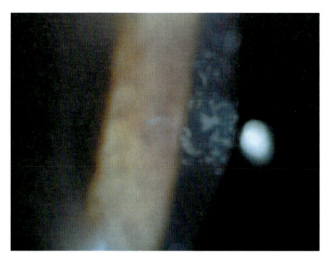

Fig. 5.2.2 A more aggressive presentation of epithelial ingrowth (photo courtesy of Dr. Marcel Avila)

Grade 2: Epithelium grows diffusely at the periphery of the flap, with a faint line in front of it. It distorts red reflex.

Grade 3: Diffuse epithelium under the flap with total blockage of the red reflex.
Another classification from Dr. Jeffrey Machat is useful for defining severity and treatment:

Grade 1: Faintly visible ingrowth 2 mm from the flap edge, with a demarcation line and no involvement of the flap. It is non-progressive and requires observation only.

Grade 2: Epithelial nests of cells within the 2 mm at the periphery of the flap, with no clear demarcation line and some involvement of the flap, which is thickened and gray. It may require treatment in case it progresses.

Grade 3: The epithelial cells grow more than 2 mm from the edge, in whitish nests that approach the visual axis. Flap is involved, thickened, and melted or eroded. This requires urgent treatment.

5.2.5 Management of Epithelial Ingrowth

Surgical treatment of epithelial ingrowth is very difficult and has a high incidence of recurrence (reports of 10%). Lifting the flap introduces the danger of spreading the cells under the flap or even activating epithelial cell growth. That is why the mainstay of treatment is observation. If the disease does not progress over time, then surgical intervention is not warranted. If progression is observed and documented, then surgical treatment has to be undertaken.

Early diagnosis is essential, and careful follow-up is necessary. Slit lamp examination, photos, and fluorescein staining are crucial to elucidate if the epithelial cells are growing and jeopardizing visual acuity. As the treatment is di-

vided into observation and intervention, clinical judgment of when and how to intervene is essential. There are several reasons to perform surgical treatment; careful evaluation of the presence of these situations is necessary to make such an important and difficult decision:

- When epithelial ingrowth progresses toward the visual axis and BCVA is in danger
- When epithelial ingrowth is not progressing, but the cyst forms an elevation that causes irregular and un-correctable astigmatism
- When the flap starts to melt

5.2.6 Prevention of Epithelial Ingrowth

Since the surgical treatment of this condition is complicated and very difficult to perform, and since the disease may turn into a sight-threatening problem with loss of lines of BCVA, the rule that prevention is the best treatment applies in an exact manner to this complication. Recognizing the presence of any of the above-mentioned risk factors is essential in preventing the complication; in many of these situations, bandage contact lens use has been theorized as a way to avoid epithelial cells from going under the flap, since it may act as a frame directing the cells over the flap.

1. Avoid excessive and unjustified manipulation of the flap during LASIK surgery.
2. In the case of an epithelial defect, placement of a bandage contact lens is indicated and careful follow-up is necessary.
3. Avoid relifting of the flap whenever possible, and if needed, careful manipulation and proper surgical technique should be followed. Placement of a bandage contact lens after the flap is repositioned is advised, and the lens must remain in place until epithelization of the gap occurs.
4. The use of modern and well-maintained microkeratomes is advisable as is the use of new and high-quality blades. Theoretically, new femtosecond lasers or disposable microkeratomes to create flaps may have the advantage of producing less epithelial ingrowth.
5. Special care and handling of the flaps in cases of previous surgeries such as radial keratotomies. Evaluate the possibility of surface ablation if indicated. In the case of a flap over radial cuts, extremely careful alignment of the old incisions is mandatory, and a bandage contact lens may be indicated.
6. Avoid small flaps or too-large ablation zones that could hit the epithelium of the remaining cornea. If that is an inevitable situation, then place a bandage contact lens until epithelium heals and closes the gap.
7. Finally, in cases of dislocated flaps or large folds with big gaps between the flap and the rest of the cornea, this is an emergent situation and must be corrected immediately to limit the time for epithelial cell growth. After

the correction has been undertaken, a bandage contact lens is advised.

5.2.7 Surgical Treatment of Epithelial Ingrowth

Once it has been decided to treat surgically this annoying complication, several steps must be followed by the doctor. In general, if it is the first time the ingrowth is going to be treated, then the flap has to be lifted very carefully. Before the epithelium is broken, the border should be determined by inspection through a microscope. If the border is not easily seen, then gentle pressure should be applied to the limbus. The epithelium is then broken only at the junction, and a thin spatula should be used to enter the interface under the flap. Then the flap should be lifted completely (despite some reports suggesting partial lifting). Once the flap is up, the epithelial sheets must be removed by forceps if they detach easily, or by gently scraping with spatula and or sponges. *Care must be taken not to reseed epithelial cells*. One cell is enough for the epithelium to grow back under the flap. Of particular importance is to clean not only the stromal bed, but also the stroma of the flap. Suture of the flap at the end of the cleaning may be important if we consider etiology of the disease, as well as a bandage contact lens until the epithelium closes the wound and no reappearance of cells under the flap observed.

In case of reappearance of the epithelial ingrowths or a very severe form of this complication, some different methods have been proposed to help remove all the epithelial cells that could remain under the flap. Of course, all these methods are only additive therapy; under no circumstances do they replace proper and meticulous cleaning of the cells from the stroma, the undersurface of the flap, and the edges of the wound. Those methods take care of the cells that are not visible under the microscope, and should be applied at the end of a complete manual cleaning of the ingrowth.

The first additive therapy to kill epithelial cells is the application of ethanol (reports from 20 to 50%) with a Merocel sponge after the cleaning, and then removal by careful washing with balanced salt solution.

Another widely used method to clean the "invisible" cells that remain after a careful cleaning is the application of excimer laser in the form of PTK in the undersurface of the flap as well as in the stromal bed. Ten-microns deep has been advocated as the standard PTK application, since deeper ablations may have undesirable refractive effects.

Application of a neodymium-YAG laser directly to the epithelial "nests" before lifting the flap has been advocated for some authors. That way, the flap may not need to be lifted, yet the cells are destroyed by the YAG application. No long-term results have been published.

Cryotherapy on both surfaces is another proposed method to kill those cells that may remain after the manual cleaning. Mitomycin C has also been applied as chemical suppressor of the growth of epithelial cells.

Finally, extensive research has been done on drops that could help to take the cells out of the interface, without the need to lift the flap. Immunotherapy could be the answer to this sight threatening complication.

5.2.8 Conclusion

Epithelial ingrowth is a very important complication of LASIK surgery with a reported incidence of 1–10%. Its management is very complicated; therefore, the main goal in therapy is prevention of its appearance by avoiding flap problems and by careful handling of the flap.

Once is present, two options must be followed by the treating doctor, (1) observation if the epithelium does not progress or jeopardize the visual acuity result of the surgery; and (2) surgical intervention if vision is disturbed or progress of the cells toward the visual axis is documented.

Surgery is difficult and with a high incidence of reappearance. First, a careful cleaning of the surface of the stroma, the underneath surface of the flap, and the borders of the cut must be done. If the disease reappears under the flap, then other additive therapies are advocated to destroy the remaining cells, the most popular being ethanol in varying concentrations and excimer laser in the PTK mode.

> **Take-Home Pearls**
> - Epithelial ingrowth is the most important complication of LASIK surgery because it is the most common: incidence reports of 1–10%. It is vision threatening complication and very difficult to treat.
> - Epithelial ingrowth is associated with the presence of several risk factors, most of them related to lesions of the epithelium, poor handling of the flap, or complications during surgery.
> - The management of epithelial ingrowth is very difficult and has a high incidence of recurrence (10% in some reports). Therefore, the main option is observation and careful monitoring in case its presence is detected under the flap.
> - Surgical treatment of epithelial ingrowth is decided only in this three situations:
>   - When progress over the visual axis is document ed and BCVA is in danger
>   - When the epithelium is elevated and causes symptoms or irregular astigmatism
>   - When there is documented involvement of the flap
> - The surgical treatment of epithelial ingrowth is difficult; prevention is the key factor in its management: use the latest technology in flap production, with careful handling of it. Avoid relifting when possible and use of bandage contact lenses in cases of damage of the epithelium and when the ablation hits the border of the cut. Finally, avoid spaces between the flap and the residual stroma.

Bibliography

Buratto L, Brint S (2000) LASIK: surgical techniques and complications, 2nd edn. Slack, Thorofare, N.J.

Castillo A, Diaz-Valle D, Gutierrez AR et al (1998) Peripheral melt of flap after laser in situ keratomileusis. J Refract Surg 14:61–63

Danjo S, Friend J, Thoft RA (1987) Conjunctival epithelium in healing of corneal epithelial wounds. Invest Ophthalmol Vis Sci 28:1445–1449

Gimbel HV, Penno EE, Van Westenbrugge JA et al (1998) Incidence and management of intraoperative and early postoperative complications in 1000 consecutive laser in situ keratomileusis cases. Ophthalmology 105:1839–1847; discussion 1847–1848

Grayson M (1983) Diseases of the cornea, 2nd edn. Mosby, St Louis

Gulani AC (1993) Epithelial ingrowth. Paper presented at the 10th meeting of the European Society of Cataract and Refractive Surgery. Nice, France

Hardten DR, Lindstrom RL (1998) Management of LASIK complications. Oper Tech Cataract Surg 1:32–39

Haw WW, Manche EE (2001) Treatment of progressive or recurrent epithelial ingrowth with ethanol following laser in situ keratomileusis. J Ref Surg 17:63–68

Machat NJ, Slade SG, Probst LE (1999) The art of LASIK, 2nd edition. Slack, Thorofare, N.J.

Wilson SE (1998) LASIK: management of common complications. Laser in situ keratomileusis. Cornea 17:459–467

Core Messages

- Proven risk factors for ectasia after LASIK:
  - Ectatic corneal disease
  - Forme fruste keratoconus
  - Low residual stromal bed thickness
  - Low preoperative corneal thickness
  - Young patient age
  - High myopia

- Potential risk factors for ectasia after LASIK:
  - Suspicious topographic patterns
  - Chronic trauma (eye rubbing)
  - Family history of ectatic corneal disease
  - Unstable refractions with preoperative best-spectacle acuity worse than 20/20

- Treatments other than LASIK are more suitable for at-risk candidates.

- Effective management strategies for ectasia after LASIK include:
  - Rigid gas permeable contact lenses
  - Intracorneal ring segments
  - Corneal collagen cross-linking
  - Corneal transplantation

- New corneal measurement techniques should facilitate identification of patients at risk for corneal ectasia.

5.3 Corneal Ectasia

J. Bradley Randleman and R. Doyle Stulting

5.3.1 Introduction

Postoperative corneal ectasia, the progressive steepening and thinning of the cornea that reduces uncorrected and often BCVA [63], remains one of the most insidious complications after PRK or LASIK. Since the first reports by Seiler and colleagues in 1998 [68, 69], this complication has been the source of extensive discussion [13, 36, 38, 67], as it has both medical and medico-legal ramifications for patient screening and postoperative management [8].

There have been more than 170 reported cases of ectasia after PRK or LASIK [64]; however, most of these have appeared as case reports, and very few larger series have been reported [3, 5, 35, 50, 59, 63, 64]. From these reports, a variety of risk factors have been proposed, including high myopia, residual stromal bed thickness less than 250 µm, low preoperative corneal thickness, and forme fruste keratoconus. Patients have also developed ectasia without any of these proposed risk factors [3, 5, 35, 42, 53, 75].

Although less common now [64], ectasia still occurs at an unacceptably high frequency. Further, the onset of ectasia may be delayed for years postoperatively, so some individuals who appear to have undergone successful refractive surgery may develop ectasia in the future. Postoperative ectasia can have dramatic consequences and in some instances require corneal transplantation for visual rehabilitation.

The aim of this chapter is to discuss proven and probable risk factors for postoperative ectasia, strategies for avoiding this complication, and management options for visual rehabilitation when postoperative ectasia occurs.

5.3.2 Postoperative Ectasia: What Do We Currently Know?

The estimated incidence of ectasia after LASIK ranges from 0.04% [63] to 0.2% [59] to 0.6% [50]. More than 50% of ophthalmologists who responded to the International Society of Refractive Surgery of the American Academy of Ophthalmology (ISRS/AAO) practice patterns survey in 2004 had at least one case of ectasia in their practice [17]; thus, the true incidence may be higher than currently reported [60]. More than 50% of cases present within the first 12 months [64]; however, its onset can be considerably later [42, 53]. In some instances, ectasia has become manifest 10 or more years after PRK [34, 46, 51].

Corneal refractive surgery by definition alters the shape, thickness, curvature, and tensile strength of the normal cornea. Keratocyte density is greatest in the anterior 10%

5

of the stroma and lowest in the posterior 40% of the stroma [47, 52]; it decreases more significantly in the anterior stroma after PRK and in the posterior corneal stroma after LASIK [20]. Preliminary studies indicate that tensile strength is greatest in the anterior one third and weakest in the posterior two thirds of the corneal stroma [14]. Further, the corneal flap does not contribute to the tensile strength of the cornea after LASIK [11, 68]. Dawson and colleagues [14] have estimated that routine surgery on normal corneas decreases tensile strength by 13% after PRK and 27% after LASIK. Andreassen and colleagues found the elastic modulus of the keratoconic cornea to be 1.6–2.5 (average 2.1) times less than that of a normal cornea [4]. Postoperative ectasia may mimic this altered corneal elastic modulus. Biomechanical modeling approaches utilizing corneal "plasticity" and "viscoelasticity" [18] and factoring corneal parameters such as Young's Modulus, Poisson's ratio, and curvature radius [25] may provide further insight into the ectatic process.

Rather than representing a specific disease entity, postoperative ectasia, like keratoconus, most likely represents an end-stage manifestation of corneal warping that arises from a variety of causes, including preoperatively weak corneas, residual stromal bed too low to maintain structural integrity, trauma, and patients otherwise destined to develop keratoconus. Specific risk factors for the development of postoperative ectasia have been recognized, and screening schemes have been developed to reduce the incidence of postoperative ectasia.

5.3.3 Risk Factors for Postoperative Ectasia

Recognized risk factors for ectasia include corneal ectatic disorders, specific topographic patterns (forme fruste keratoconus), low residual stromal bed thickness, young age, low preoperative corneal thickness, and high myopia (Table 5.3.1).

5.3.3.1 High Myopia

Eyes that developed ectasia have been significantly more myopic than do controls in previous studies [63, 64], and there are many reports of ectasia developing after treatment for extreme myopia (greater than –12 D) [1, 28, 50, 59, 71]. However, ectasia has also been reported in many patients with low myopia and hyperopia; thus, the level of myopia

Table 5.3.1 Defined risk factors for postoperative ectasia

Keratoconus
Pellucid marginal corneal degeneration
Abnormal preoperative topography (forme fruste keratoconus)
Low residual stromal bed thickness
Young age
Low preoperative corneal thickness
High myopia

in itself may be a poor predictor for ectasia, as long as surgeons avoid treating extreme myopia.

5.3.3.2 Preoperative Corneal Thickness

In comparative studies [63, 64], ectasia cases had significantly thinner corneas preoperatively than did controls. Keratoconic corneas are generally thinner than normal corneas are [26, 73]; therefore, low preoperative corneal thickness could be indicative of an abnormal cornea that is destined to develop keratoconus. Alternatively, thinner corneas could be at higher risk for ectasia because there is a higher probability that a thicker than expected corneal flap will result in an extremely low residual stromal bed thickness (RSB) that does not provide sufficient structural integrity to prevent ectasia.

5.3.3.3 Low Residual Stromal Bed Thickness

Ectasia cases have had a significantly lower RSB than controls have had in comparative studies [63, 64], and low RSB has always been suspected to be one of the most significant risk factors for postoperative ectasia. Factors contributing to low RSB include treatment of high refractive errors, excessive flap thickness, and deeper-than-expected stromal ablations. There can be significant variability in the measurement of corneal thickness, flap thickness, and ablation depth measurements [10, 16, 19, 29, 30, 56, 66, 81]. While most of the microkeratome plate markings overestimate average actual flap thickness, flap thickness can vary widely and excessively thick flaps still occur. Additionally, previous studies have found that actual ablation depth is usually greater than estimated ablation depth [10, 19].

A RSB thickness of 250 µm is commonly accepted as the minimum for the safe performance of LASIK; however, ectasia has occurred after LASIK in eyes with a wide range of RSB thicknesses, including those greater than 300 µm, confirmed by intraoperative pachymetry, and after PRK in eyes with RSB greater than 350 µm [34, 46, 61]. Conversely, many eyes that underwent successful LASIK without ectasia had RSB less than 225 µm [63]. Thus, decreasing RSB likely represents a continuum of risk for postoperative ectasia without a definitive safety cutoff.

In the vast majority of published ectasia cases, RSB has been calculated rather than measured. Only 31% of respondents to the ISRS/AAO survey routinely measure flap or residual stromal bed thickness intraoperatively [17]. Using a probability model that accounts for imprecision in corneal thickness, flap thickness, and laser ablation depth measurements, Reinstein and colleagues [65] determined that, depending on the microkeratome used, up to 33% of eyes with attempted RSB thickness of 250 µm could have actual RSB less than 200 µm. Given the known variability in flap thickness that can occur with both mechanical and femtosecond lasers [7, 72], we recommend intraoperative pachymetry for all patients that may at risk for low RSB.

5.3.3.4 Patient Age

Ectasia cases were significantly younger than controls were in recent comparative studies [35, 64], and most reported cases of ectasia without risk factors have been in very young patients. Younger corneas may be more elastic due to decreased collagen cross-linking, making them more susceptible to structural deformation. Additionally, some younger patients may be destined to develop keratoconus in their fourth to sixth decade of life [49, 82] and therefore may not yet exhibit abnormal topographic patterns prior to surgery.

5.3.3.5 Ectatic Corneal Disorders and Abnormal Topographic Patterns

Ectatic disorders, including keratoconus, pellucid marginal corneal degeneration, and defined abnormal topographic patterns (forme fruste keratoconus) [58] are the most significant risk factors for postoperative ectasia, so great diligence should be applied to preoperative topography evaluation. In addition to forme fruste keratoconus, the members of the AAO/ISRS/ASCRS joint committee recommend avoiding LASIK in patients with asymmetric inferior corneal steepening or asymmetric bowtie patterns with skewed steep radial axes above and below the horizontal meridian [8]. Other factors, such as contact lens warping and keratoconjunctivitis sicca can create topographic changes that resemble those of forme fruste keratoconus [15]. These factors may make it more challenging to differentiate normal from abnormal topographies. We therefore recommend repeating topographic examination later in questionable cases, and if available, utilizing multiple technologies, since a variety of imaging systems can provide unique information [57] (Fig. 5.3.1).

5.3.3.6 Other Potential Risk Factors

In addition to the aforementioned risk factors, other factors should be considered, including more subtle topographic abnormalities and high order aberrations, multiple enhancements, chronic trauma (eye rubbing), family history of keratoconus, and refractive instability with preoperative BSCVA worse than 20/20 (Table 5.3.2).

Some patients have very asymmetric topographic patterns in only one eye or subtle changes in both eyes with significant between-eye topographic asymmetry; if patients have suspicious topographic patterns in either eye, then they should currently be excluded from excimer laser corneal refractive surgery bilaterally. Increased high-order aberrations, especially increased coma, may be an early indicator of keratoconus and should be considered [2]. Eye rubbing and trauma can cause or exacerbate keratoconus [31, 39, 83]. Refractive instability with decreased BSCVA may be a sign of progressive changes in the shape of the cornea. The significance of these findings remains undetermined; however, all of these factors should be taken into consideration, especially in borderline cases.

Table 5.3.2 Potential risk factors for postoperative ectasia

Suspicious topography
– Asymmetric bowtie pattern
– Inferior steepening
– Topographic asymmetry between eyes
Chronic trauma (eye rubbing)
Refractive instability
Family history of keratoconus
Preoperative BSCVA worse than 20/20

5.3.3.7 Ectasia Risk Factor Screening: Summary

In order to improve upon our current screening approaches, we propose utilizing screening techniques that takes into account preoperative topography, residual stromal bed thickness, patient age, preoperative corneal thickness, degree of myopia, and the aforementioned potential risk factors in borderline cases.

5.3.4 Prevention of Postoperative Ectasia

5.3.4.1 Utilizing Alternative Treatment Strategies for At-Risk Patients

The best treatment for postoperative ectasia is to avoid its occurrence. Some patients at risk for ectasia after LASIK may be suitable candidates for surface ablation—especially those with normal topographies but thinner corneas, low predicted RSB, or younger age. However, we currently do not advocate performing surface ablation in keratoconus suspects without detailed, patient-specific informed consent. Phakic intraocular lens implantation may also prove beneficial for candidates at risk for ectasia, as lens implantation does not alter the structural integrity of the cornea. These lenses have recently shown promising results in eyes with keratoconus [9, 41].

5.3.4.2 Utilizing New Technology to Identify Abnormal Corneas

Corneal interferometry [33], hysteresis measurements [44], and dynamic corneal imaging [24] may allow identification of at-risk patients with normal topographies but reduced biomechanical integrity preoperatively.

5.3.4.3 Avoiding Retreatment in Corneas with Low residual Stromal Bed Thickness

As corneal thickness measurements taken months after initial LASIK usually overestimate RSB thickness [21, 62], accurate assessment of actual RSB prior to retreatment is critical to avoid excessive ablation of the posterior stroma. This can be avoided by utilizing intraoperative pachymetry measurements prior to laser ablation at the time of retreatment, or by utilizing confocal microscopy [74] or high-speed optical coherence tomography (OCT) [6, 45] prior to retreat-

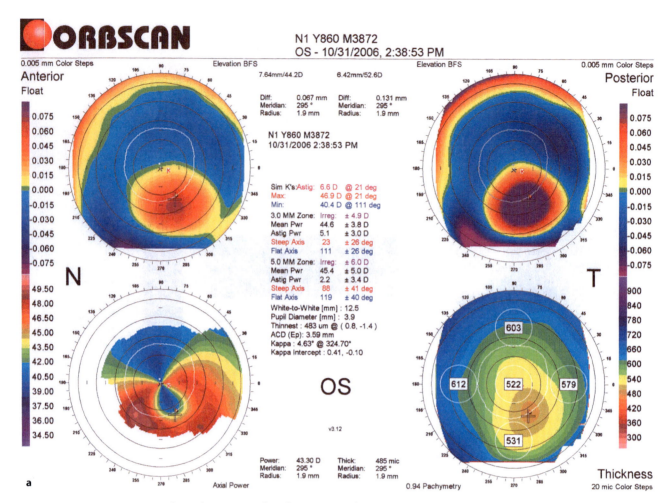

Fig. 5.3.1 Preoperative topographies of a patient with early ectatic corneal disease. **a** Orbscan II image (Bausch & Lomb Surgical, San Dimas, Calif.) of the left eye. The anterior and posterior float values (*upper right* and *left images*, respectively) both demonstrate significant elevations inferiorly. The thickness map (*bottom right*) displays a central thickness of 522 μm and demonstrates an inferior area of thinning corresponding to the areas of elevation on the anterior and posterior float images. The Placido-based keratometric image (*bottom left*) displays a crab-claw pattern, with superior flattening and asymmetric inferior steepening. **b** Pentacam image (Oculus, Lynwood, Calif.) of the same eye. Note the similar appearance in the front and back elevation maps (*upper right* and *left images*, respectively) as compared to the Orbscan II anterior and posterior float maps. The corneal thickness maps are also similar. However, the tangential curvature map displays significant inferior steepening suggestive of keratoconus rather than the Placido-based crab-claw image, suggestive of pellucid marginal corneal degeneration. This patient is at high risk for postoperative ectasia and therefore a poor candidate for corneal refractive surgery

ment, as these instruments can accurately measure residual stromal bed thickness without ever lifting the flap.

5.3.5 Management of Postoperative Ectasia

Some mild ectasia cases have been managed successfully with spectacles or soft contact lenses [35]. There are also reports of reversing early ectasia with intraocular pressure–lowering medications [27]; however, the long-term efficacy of this treatment remains to be determined. All patients with any evidence of early postoperative ectasia should be strongly cautioned to completely avoid eye rubbing, as this may exacerbate the process. Treatment of advanced corneal ectasia includes rigid gas permeable contact lenses, intra-

corneal ring segments, corneal collagen cross-linking, and corneal transplantation (Fig. 5.3.2).

Rigid gas-permeable (RGP) contact lenses are usually necessary and frequently sufficient for visual rehabilitation [63, 76]. In general, fitting strategies for postoperative ectasia are similar to those for keratoconus [12, 48, 76]. Various specific lens styles can be used, including standard aspheric, multicurve, or reverse-geometry lenses either alone or in combination with high oxygen–transmissible soft lenses in a piggyback lens system to improve comfort. The specific fitting parameters should be customized to each case, as postoperative ectatic corneas may present quite dissimilarly.

Recently, intracorneal ring segments (Intacs, Addition Technology, Sunnyvale, Calif.) have been approved for use

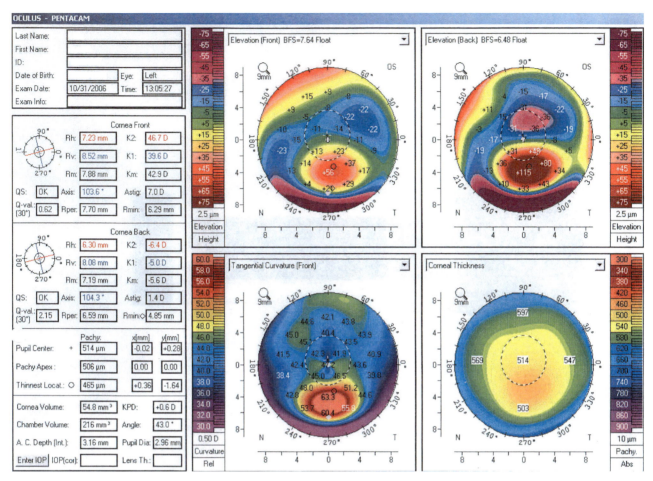

Fig. 5.3.1 b *(continued)*

in keratoconus, and some promising results have been reported when used off-label to treat postoperative ectasia [1, 40, 43, 54, 70]. Techniques reported have varied with regard to wound location and the size, symmetry, and number of Intacs placed; thus, the specific technique that will best stabilize the ectatic cornea remains to be determined.

In addition to the aforementioned treatment strategies, corneal collagen cross-linking may improve the course of postoperative ectasia. Using riboflavin as a photosensitizer, followed by ultraviolet-A exposure, Wollensak and colleagues [79] found that collagen cross-linking halted the progression of keratoconus and in many cases, reversed the ectatic process, as evidenced by a reduction in corneal steepening and refractive error. Further studies have confirmed initial results and evaluated endothelial toxicity [37, 78, 80]. Future work will examine the safety and efficacy of this approach for ectasia after refractive surgery.

Obviously, corneal transplantation should be the final option; however, when patients undergo penetrating keratoplasty for ectasia, their long-term outcomes should be excellent and comparable to those in patients with keratoconus [32, 55]. Recent results with that deep anterior lamellar keratoplasty for keratoconus suggest that this may be another viable surgical option for postoperative ectasia with comparable visual outcomes and significantly reduced rejection risk [22, 23, 77].

5.3.6 Conclusion

Proven risk factors for ectasia after corneal refractive surgery include ectatic corneal disease, forme fruste keratoconus, low RSB, low preoperative corneal thickness, young age, and high myopia. Other factors, such as suspicious corneal topographies, unstable refractions, a family history of ectatic corneal disease, a history of eye rubbing, or an underlying increase in corneal elasticity may also be predictive of corneal ectasia after refractive surgery. There is no single characteristic that identifies all at-risk patients, and we believe that a screening strategy that selectively weighs all of these factors will be more effective than considering any of the factors in isolation. Nevertheless, some patients may still develop postoperative ectasia without any of the aforementioned risk factors.

Alternative surgical options, including surface ablation and phakic intraocular lenses, should be considered for patients at risk for postoperative ectasia. When postoperative ectasia occurs, RGP contact lenses, intracorneal ring segments,

5

Fig. 5.3.2 Treatment algorithm for advanced postoperative ectasia. RGP contact lenses are generally the first treatment attempted and are usually sufficient for visual rehabilitation. When RGP fitting fails, intracorneal ring segments, collagen cross-linking, and RGP lenses can be utilized in a variety of combinations before resorting to corneal transplantation

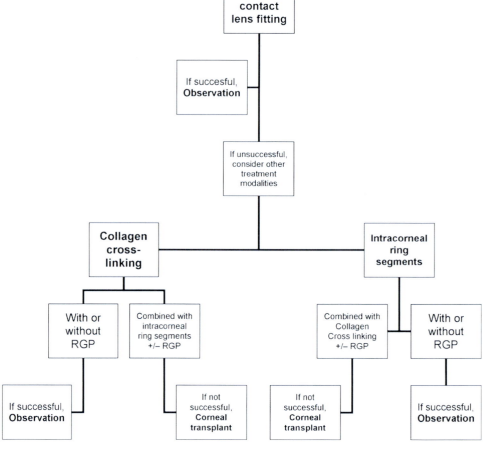

and collagen cross-linking can effectively restore functional visual acuity, and with time, the need for corneal transplantation for postoperative ectasia should significantly diminish.

Take-Home Pearls

■ Diligently analyze preoperative topographic patterns.
■ Measure intraoperative pachymetry in all patients at risk for low RSB.
■ Heightened scrutiny is warranted for younger patients.
■ No single risk factor identifies all at-risk patients.
■ Utilizing risk factors in a combined fashion will improve preoperative screening.
■ Utilize options other than LASIK for at-risk patients.
■ RGP lenses, intracorneal ring segments, and collagen cross-linking in isolation or in combination can effectively rehabilitate most eyes with ectasia.
■ When necessary, corneal transplantation should have a high success rate comparable to grafts performed for keratoconus.

Acknowledgment

The authors were supported in part by Research to Prevent Blindness, Inc., New York,
New York, and the National Institutes of Health Core Grant P30 EYO6360, Bethesda,
Maryland. The authors have no financial interest in any of the products or topics discussed in this chapter.

References

1. Alio J, Salem T, Artola A, Osman A (2002) Intracorneal rings to correct corneal ectasia after laser in situ keratomileusis. J Cataract Refract Surg 28:1568–1574
2. Alio JL, Shabayek MH (2006) Corneal higher order aberrations: a method to grade keratoconus. J Refract Surg 22:539–545
3. Amoils SP, Deist MB, Gous P, Amoils PM (2000) Iatrogenic keratectasia after laser in situ keratomileusis for less than –4.0 to –7.0 diopters of myopia. J Cataract Refract Surg 26:967–977
4. Andreassen TT, Simonsen AH, Oxlund H (1980) Biomechanical properties of keratoconus and normal corneas. Exp Eye Res 31:435–441

5. Argento C, Cosentino MJ, Tytiun A, Rapetti G, Zarate J (2001) Corneal ectasia after laser in situ keratomileusis. J Cataract Refract Surg 27:1440–1448

6. Avila M, Li Y, Song JC, Huang D (2006) High-speed optical coherence tomography for management after laser in situ keratomileusis. J Cataract Refract Surg 32:1836–1842

7. Binder PS (2006) One thousand consecutive IntraLase laser in situ keratomileusis flaps. J Cataract Refract Surg 32:962–969

8. Binder PS, Lindstrom RL, Stulting RD, Donnenfeld E, Wu H, McDonnell P, Rabinowitz Y (2005) Keratoconus and corneal ectasia after LASIK. J Cataract Refract Surg 31:2035–2038

9. Budo C, Bartels MC, van Rij G (2005) Implantation of Artisan toric phakic intraocular lenses for the correction of astigmatism and spherical errors in patients with keratoconus. J Refract Surg 21:218–222

10. Chang AW, Tsang AC, Contreras JE, Huynh PD, Calvano CJ, Crnic-Rein TC, Thall EH (2003) Corneal tissue ablation depth and the Munnerlyn formula. J Cataract Refract Surg 29:1204–1210

11. Chang DH, Stulting RD (2005) Change in intraocular pressure measurements after LASIK the effect of the refractive correction and the lamellar flap. Ophthalmology 112:1009–1016

12. Choi HJ, Kim MK, Lee JL (2004) Optimization of contact lens fitting in keratectasia patients after laser in situ keratomileusis. J Cataract Refract Surg 30:1057–1066

13. Comaish IF, Lawless MA (2002) Progressive post-LASIK keratectasia: biomechanical instability or chronic disease process? J Cataract Refract Surg 28:2206–2213

14. Dawson DG, O'Brien TP, Dubovy SR, Randleman JB, Grossniklaus HE, Edelhauser HF, McCarey BE (2006) Post-LASIK ectasia: histopathology, ultrastructure, and corneal physiology from human corneal buttons and eye bank donors. Presented at the AAO Annual Meeting, Las Vegas

15. De Paiva CS, Harris LD, Pflugfelder SC (2003) Keratoconus-like topographic changes in keratoconjunctivitis sicca. Cornea 22:22–24

16. Dougherty PJ, Wellish KL, Maloney RK (1994) Excimer laser ablation rate and corneal hydration. Am J Ophthalmol 118:169–176

17. Duffey RJ, Leaming D (2005) US trends in refractive surgery: 2004 ISRS/AAO Survey. J Refract Surg 21:742–748

18. Dupps WJ Jr (2005) Biomechanical modeling of corneal ectasia. J Refract Surg 21:186–190

19. Durairaj VD, Balentine J, Kouyoumdjian G, Tooze JA, Young D, Spivack L, Taravella MJ (2000) The predictability of corneal flap thickness and tissue laser ablation in laser in situ keratomileusis. Ophthalmology 107:2140–2143

20. Erie JC, Patel SV, McLaren JW, Hodge DO, Bourne WM (2006) Corneal keratocyte deficits after photorefractive keratectomy and laser in situ keratomileusis. Am J Ophthalmol 141:799–809

21. Flanagan GW, Binder PS (2003) Precision of flap measurements for laser in situ keratomileusis in 4428 eyes. J Refract Surg 19:113–123

22. Fogla R, Padmanabhan P (2006) Results of deep lamellar keratoplasty using the big-bubble technique in patients with keratoconus. Am J Ophthalmol 141:254–259

23. Fontana L, Parente G, Tassinari G (2007) Clinical outcomes after deep anterior lamellar keratoplasty using the big-bubble technique in patients with keratoconus. Am J Ophthalmol 143:117–124

24. Grabner G, Eilmsteiner R, Steindl C, Ruckhofer J, Mattioli R, Husinsky W (2005) Dynamic corneal imaging. J Cataract Refract Surg 31:163–174

25. Guirao A (2005) Theoretical elastic response of the cornea to refractive surgery: risk factors for keratectasia. J Refract Surg 21:176–185

26. Haque S, Simpson T, Jones L (2006) Corneal and epithelial thickness in keratoconus: a comparison of ultrasonic pachymetry, Orbscan II, and optical coherence tomography. J Refract Surg 22:486–493

27. Hiatt JA, Wachler BS, Grant C (2005) Reversal of laser in situ keratomileusis-induced ectasia with intraocular pressure reduction. J Cataract Refract Surg 31:1652–1655

28. Holland SP, Srivannaboon S, Reinstein DZ (2000) Avoiding serious corneal complications of laser assisted in situ keratomileusis and photorefractive keratectomy. Ophthalmology 107:640–652

29. Iskander NG, Anderson Penno E, Peters NT, Gimbel HV, Ferensowicz M (2001) Accuracy of Orbscan pachymetry measurements and DHG ultrasound pachymetry in primary laser in situ keratomileusis and LASIK enhancement procedures. J Cataract Refract Surg 27:681–685

30. Jacobs BJ, Deutsch TA, Rubenstein JB (1999) Reproducibility of corneal flap thickness in LASIK. Ophthalmic Surg Lasers 30:350–353

31. Jafri B, Lichter H, Stulting RD (2004) Asymmetric keratoconus attributed to eye rubbing. Cornea 23:560–564

32. Javadi MA, Motlagh BF, Jafarinasab MR, Rabbanikhah Z, Anissian A, Souri H, Yazdani S (2005) Outcomes of penetrating keratoplasty in keratoconus. Cornea 24:941–946

33. Jaycock PD, Lobo L, Ibrahim J, Tyrer J, Marshall J (2005) Interferometric technique to measure biomechanical changes in the cornea induced by refractive surgery. J Cataract Refract Surg 31:175–184

34. Kim H, Choi JS, Joo CK (2006) Corneal ectasia after PRK: clinicopathologic case report. Cornea 25:845–848

35. Klein SR, Epstein RJ, Randleman JB, Stulting RD (2006) Corneal ectasia after laser in situ keratomileusis in patients without apparent preoperative risk factors. Cornea 25:388–403

36. Koch DD (1999) The riddle of iatrogenic keratectasia. J Cataract Refract Surg 25:453–454

37. Kohlhaas M, Spoerl E, Schilde T, Unger G, Wittig C, Pillunat LE (2006) Biomechanical evidence of the distribution of cross-links in corneas treated with riboflavin and ultraviolet A light. J Cataract Refract Surg 32:279–283

38. Kohnen T (2002) Iatrogenic keratectasia: current knowledge, current measurements. J Cataract Refract Surg 28:2065–2066

39. Krachmer JH (2004) Eye rubbing can cause keratoconus. Cornea 23:539–540

40. Kymionis GD, Siganos CS, Kounis G, Astyrakakis N, Kalyvianaki MI, Pallikaris IG (2003) Management of post-LASIK corneal ectasia with Intacs inserts: one-year results. Arch Ophthalmol 121:322–326

41. Leccisotti A, Fields SV (2003) Angle-supported phakic intraocular lenses in eyes with keratoconus and myopia. J Cataract Refract Surg 29:1530–1536

42. Lifshitz T, Levy J, Klemperer I, Levinger S (2005) Late bilateral keratectasia after LASIK in a low myopic patient. J Refract Surg 21:494–496

43. Lovisolo CF, Fleming JF (2002) Intracorneal ring segments for iatrogenic keratectasia after laser in situ keratomileusis or photorefractive keratectomy. J Refract Surg 18:535–541

44. Luce DA (2005) Determining in vivo biomechanical properties of the cornea with an ocular response analyzer. J Cataract Refract Surg 31:156–162

45. Maldonado MJ, Ruiz-Oblitas L, Munuera JM, Aliseda D, Garcia-Layana A, Moreno-Montanes J (2000) Optical coherence tomography evaluation of the corneal cap and stromal bed features after laser in situ keratomileusis for high myopia and astigmatism. Ophthalmology 107:81–87; discussion 88

46. Malecaze F, Coullet J, Calvas P, Fournie P, Arne JL, Brodaty C (2006) Corneal ectasia after photorefractive keratectomy for low myopia. Ophthalmology 113:742–746

47. Moller-Pedersen T, Ledet T, Ehlers N (1994) The keratocyte density of human donor corneas. Curr Eye Res 13:163–169
48. O'Donnell C, Welham L, Doyle S (2004) Contact lens management of keratectasia after laser in situ keratomileusis for myopia. Eye Contact Lens 30:144–146
49. Owens H, Gamble G (2003) A profile of keratoconus in New Zealand. Cornea 22:122–125
50. Pallikaris IG, Kymionis GD, Astyrakakis NI (2001) Corneal ectasia induced by laser in situ keratomileusis. J Cataract Refract Surg 27:1796–1802
51. Parmar D, Claoue C (2004) Keratectasia following excimer laser photorefractive keratectomy. Acta Ophthalmol Scand 82:102–105
52. Patel S, McLaren J, Hodge D, Bourne W (2001) Normal human keratocyte density and corneal thickness measurement by using confocal microscopy in vivo. Invest Ophthalmol Vis Sci 42:333–339
53. Piccoli PM, Gomes AA, Piccoli FV (2003) Corneal ectasia detected 32 months after LASIK for correction of myopia and asymmetric astigmatism. J Cataract Refract Surg 29:1222–1225
54. Pokroy R, Levinger S, Hirsh A (2004) Single Intacs segment for post-laser in situ keratomileusis keratectasia. J Cataract Refract Surg 30:1685–1695
55. Pramanik S, Musch DC, Sutphin JE, Farjo AA (2006) Extended long-term outcomes of penetrating keratoplasty for keratoconus. Ophthalmology 113:1633–1638
56. Prisant O, Calderon N, Chastang P, Gatinel D, Hoang-Xuan T (2003) Reliability of pachymetric measurements using orbscan after excimer refractive surgery. Ophthalmology 110:511–515
57. Quisling S, Sjoberg S, Zimmerman B, Goins K, Sutphin J (2006) Comparison of Pentacam and Orbscan IIz on posterior curvature topography measurements in keratoconus eyes. Ophthalmology 113:1629–1632
58. Rabinowitz YS, McDonnell PJ (1989) Computer-assisted corneal topography in keratoconus. Refract Corneal Surg 5:400–408
59. Rad AS, Jabbarvand M, Saifi N (2004) Progressive keratectasia after laser in situ keratomileusis. J Refract Surg 20: S718–S722
60. Randleman JB (2006) Post-laser in-situ keratomileusis ectasia: current understanding and future directions. Curr Opin Ophthalmol 17:406–412
61. Randleman JB, Caster AI, Banning CS, Stulting RD (2006) Corneal ectasia after photorefractive keratectomy. J Cataract Refract Surg 32:1395–1398
62. Randleman JB, Hewitt SM, Lynn MJ, Stulting RD (2005) A comparison of 2 methods for estimating residual stromal bed thickness before repeat LASIK. Ophthalmology 112:98–103
63. Randleman JB, Russell B, Ward MA, Thompson KP, Stulting RD (2003) Risk factors and prognosis for corneal ectasia after LASIK. Ophthalmology 110:267–275
64. Randleman JB, Woodward M, Lynn MJ, Stulting RD (2007) Risk assessment for ectasia after corneal refractive surgery. Ophthalmology (in press)
65. Reinstein DZ, Srivannaboon S, Archer TJ, Silverman RH, Sutton H, Coleman DJ (2006) Probability model of the inaccuracy of residual stromal thickness prediction to reduce the risk of ectasia after LASIK part I: quantifying individual risk. J Refract Surg 22:851–860
66. Salz JJ, Azen SP, Berstein J, Caroline P, Villasenor RA, Schanzlin DJ (1983) Evaluation and comparison of sources of variability in the measurement of corneal thickness with ultrasonic and optical pachymeters. Ophthalmic Surg 14:750–754
67. Seiler T (1999) Iatrogenic keratectasia: academic anxiety or serious risk? J Cataract Refract Surg 25:1307–1308
68. Seiler T, Koufala K, Richter G (1998) Iatrogenic keratectasia after laser in situ keratomileusis. J Refract Surg 14:312–317
69. Seiler T, Quurke AW (1998) Iatrogenic keratectasia after LASIK in a case of forme fruste keratoconus. J Cataract Refract Surg 24:1007–1009
70. Siganos CS, Kymionis GD, Astyrakakis N, Pallikaris IG (2002) Management of corneal ectasia after laser in situ keratomileusis with INTACS. J Refract Surg 18:43–46
71. Spadea L, Palmieri G, Mosca L, Fasciani R, Balestrazzi E (2002) Iatrogenic keratectasia following laser in situ keratomileusis. J Refract Surg 18:475–480
72. Talamo JH, Meltzer J, Gardner J (2006) Reproducibility of flap thickness with IntraLase FS and Moria LSK-1 and M2 microkeratomes. J Refract Surg 22:556–561
73. Ucakhan OO, Kanpolat A, Ylmaz N, Ozkan M (2006) In vivo confocal microscopy findings in keratoconus. Eye Contact Lens 32:183–191
74. Vinciguerra P, Torres I, Camesasca FI (2002) Applications of confocal microscopy in refractive surgery. J Refract Surg 18: S378–S381
75. Wang JC, Hufnagel TJ, Buxton DF (2003) Bilateral keratectasia after unilateral laser in situ keratomileusis: a retrospective diagnosis of ectatic corneal disorder. J Cataract Refract Surg 29:2015–2018
76. Ward MA (2003) Contact lens management following corneal refractive surgery. Ophthalmol Clin North Am 16:395–403
77. Watson SL, Ramsay A, Dart JK, Bunce C, Craig E (2004) Comparison of deep lamellar keratoplasty and penetrating keratoplasty in patients with keratoconus. Ophthalmology 111:1676–1682
78. Wollensak G (2006) Crosslinking treatment of progressive keratoconus: new hope. Curr Opin Ophthalmol 17:356–360
79. Wollensak G, Spoerl E, Seiler T (2003) Riboflavin/ultraviolet-a-induced collagen crosslinking for the treatment of keratoconus. Am J Ophthalmol 135:620–627
80. Wollensak G, Wilsch M, Spoerl E, Seiler T (2004) Collagen fiber diameter in the rabbit cornea after collagen crosslinking by riboflavin/UVA. Cornea 23:503–507
81. Yildirim R, Aras C, Ozdamar A, Bahcecioglu H, Ozkan S (2000) Reproducibility of corneal flap thickness in laser in situ keratomileusis using the Hansatome microkeratome. J Cataract Refract Surg 26:1729–1732
82. Zadnik K, Barr JT, Gordon MO, Edrington TB (1996) Biomicroscopic signs and disease severity in keratoconus. Collaborative Longitudinal Evaluation of Keratoconus (CLEK) Study Group. Cornea 15:139–146
83. Zadnik K, Steger-May K, Fink BA, Joslin CE, Nichols JJ, Rosenstiel CE, Tyler JA, Yu JA, Raasch TW, Schechtman KB (2002) Between-eye asymmetry in keratoconus. Cornea 21:671–679

Core Messages

■ Corneal haze and scarring are among the most severe complications of photorefractive keratectomy in patients with high refractive errors and after retreatments.

■ The popularity of LASIK relies on its ability to induce minimal scarring. However, unusual scarring associated with visual loss may occur following LASIK, due to intraoperative or postoperative complications or abnormal wound healing.

5.4 Scarring

Eric E. Gabison and Thanh Hoang-Xuan

5.4.1 Introduction

Scars are areas of fibrosis that replace normal tissue after stromal destruction. Scarring is a natural part of the wound healing process and, with the exception of very minor lesions, every wound, including surgical wounds, results in some degree of scarring. Scar tissue is not identical to the tissue it replaces and is usually of inferior functional quality.

Transparency, regular shape, and a smooth surface are the main properties that allow the cornea to function as the first diopter of the eye. The popularity of LASIK refractive surgery worldwide is largely due to the minimal changes in corneal architecture that it produces. LASIK also gives rapid and stable results. But is LASIK a scarless procedure?

This chapter deals with LASIK-induced changes in corneal structure. Even uncomplicated, asymptomatic LASIK recovery is associated with some structural changes. These may be part of the normal LASIK healing process, or be linked to the patient's medical history, intraoperative complications, or postoperative events.

5.4.2 LASIK: a Scarless Procedure?

After LASIK surgery, it is often difficult to see the interface and the margins of the corneal flap with the slit lamp. While both LASIK and PRK involve central excimer laser photoablation, the corneal fibrotic response to these insults is maximal in the central subepithelial area after PRK and in the subepithelial area of the flap margin after LASIK.

Conflicting data have been published on keratocyte activation status at the flap interface. While several studies using tandem scanning confocal microscopy showed no keratocyte activation either below or above the flap interface, a recent study showed keratocyte activation in the posterior stroma [1–3]. However, histological studies showed no type III collagen accumulation or alpha–smooth muscle actin-positive–activated fibroblasts in this area. This corrobo-

rates clinical reports of no significant scarring in the treated central stroma [4].

5.4.2.1 Flap Margin

Slit lamp biomicroscopy of the flap margin reveals a white reflective circumferential band of fibrosis as early as 3 weeks after LASIK [1].

Confocal microscopy during the first week after surgery reveals a well-defined circular band that, in the following weeks, becomes increasingly reflective as it acquires a more pronounced fibrillar texture. By 2 months, gradual condensation has occurred and the band appears more organized. At 4 and 6 months, the reflectivity of the flap edge falls considerably, leaving a poorly reflective region that, with time, gradually narrows. Histological analysis of the flap margin demonstrates the presence of myofibroblasts in the subepithelial region and basement membrane disruption. Extracellular matrix deposits are shown by the presence of a dichlorotriazinyl aminofluorescein (DTAF)-negative area in the region of the subepithelial flap margin 6 months after LASIK procedures in which the dye is placed in the interface. This fluorescent molecule binds the extracellular matrix (ECM) after topical application, and DTAF negativity of a previously stained area thus reflects the presence of a newly deposited ECM. Immunohistochemistry shows that these deposits contain fibronectin and types III and IV collagen. After LASIK surgery, the subepithelial flap margin region is the only area where pathway activation of the fibrogenic factor TGF-β is detectable, in keeping with clinical observations showing that fibrosis is restricted to this region [1].

LASIK wound healing after femtosecond laser and mechanical microkeratome surgery was recently compared by means of in vivo corneal confocal microscopy. This investigation revealed more fibrotic scarring in the flap margin with the femtosecond laser than with the mechanical microkeratome. The reason is probably that the flap edge produced by tissue ablation with the femtosecond laser leaves an empty space that is filled by an epithelial plug during the first 2 months after surgery. This plug disappears after 2 months, probably by constriction of the wound edges, resulting in a stronger fibrotic response similar to that observed after RK [5]. The low rate of fibrosis observed after LASIK, limited to the flap margin, has been noted by refractive surgeons performing LASIK retreatment. In order to lift the flap, sometimes several years following the initial surgical procedure, the surgeon has to disrupt epithelial and fibrotic connections that have formed in the flap margin; once this has been done, it is much easier to lift the flap [6–8].

5.4.2.2 Flap Interface

After LASIK surgery, the flap interface, as observed by slit lamp biomicroscopy, is usually devoid of visible scars. However, histological examination reveals a periodic acid–Schiff (PAS)-positive extracellular matrix deposited along the lamellar incision, as late as 9 months after the procedure (Fig. 5.4.1). Electron microscopy of treated rabbit eye showed a disorganized extracellular matrix, reflecting slow and incomplete healing 1 year after surgery [9]. This is consistent with reports of traumatic dislocation of LASIK flaps more than a year after surgery [10, 11].

Human postmortem corneas having undergone successful LASIK have been examined by means of transmission electron microscopy [6]. The flap surface showed elongated basal epithelial cells, epithelial hyperplasia, and thickening and undulations of the epithelial basement membrane and Bowman's layer. Findings in, or adjacent to, the wound demonstrated collagen lamellar disarray, with activated and quiescent keratocytes containing small vacuoles. Extracellular matrix abnormalities were also detected, including electron-dense granular material interspersed with randomly ordered collagen fibrils, increased spacing between collagen fibrils, and widely spaced banded collagen. These pathologic alterations in post-LASIK corneas may affect corneal function, as regularity is essential for transparency.

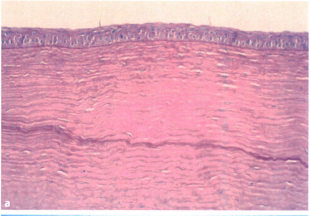

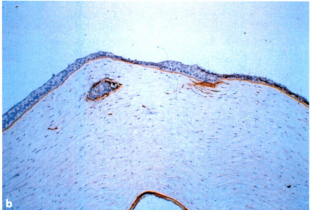

Fig 5.4.1 Extracellular matrix deposition along flap interface after experimental LASIK in a rabbit. **a** PAS-positive staining 9 months after LASIK. **b** Type IV collagen deposition along flap margin and around an island of epithelial ingrowth in the flap interface. (A gift from T. Kato)

5.4.3 Scars Linked to Surgical Complications or Postoperative Trauma

5.4.3.1 Corneal Erosion and Epithelial–Stromal Interaction

Basement membrane disruption has been shown to be the key event responsible for myofibroblastic activation in the anterior stroma, resulting in fibrosis [12, 13]. It is found in RK at the site of the incisions, in PRK in the central cornea, and in LASIK at the flap margin. It induces corneal scarring associated with loss of transparency. Corneal erosion during the LASIK procedure may be linked to excessive ocular dryness or misdiagnosed anterior membrane dystrophy [14]. Epithelial defects may not only alter flap adherence (with a higher threat of displacement or wrinkles) but are also associated with an increased risk of epithelial ingrowth, diffuse lamellar keratitis, and subepithelial fibrosis. A bandage contact lens is then required [15–17].

Experimental studies have evaluated LASIK healing after epithelial removal. Nakamura et al. reported the presence of myofibroblasts and type III collagen in the subepithelial region, corresponding to scar tissue formation [18, 19]. Ivarsen et al. observed temporary changes in corneal reflectivity by means of confocal microscopy, but they found no accumulation of neocollagen and no keratocyte activation [2]. The likely key difference between these studies was probably basement membrane integrity after epithelial removal. Epithelial removal with basement membrane disruption is indeed the main cause of stromal fibrosis.

This raises the question of late postoperative epithelial trauma. Figure 5.4.2 shows corneal slit lamp and confocal microscopy images of a patient with extensive bilateral corneal de-epithelialization due to tear gas exposure 6 months after myopic (unpublished case). Only transient subepithelial opacification associated with fibroblast activation was observed, in spite of extensive epithelial loss and basement membrane disruption. The visual outcome was excellent, probably because of the relatively long interval between LASIK and the corneal insult.

5.4.3.2 Flap Misalignment and Folds

Misplacement of the flap after LASIK can be responsible for folds, which are located beneath Bowman's layer, and irregular epithelial remodeling. This complication leads to a loss of BCVA and must be prevented or treated to avoid abnormal healing and scarring. Flap repositioning, hydration, and stretching may be effective within the first 48 postoperative hours. Once the folds become fixed, epithelial debridement on top of the folds and flap suturing are usually necessary. These flap-lifting procedures place the patient at an additional risk of infection, epithelial erosion, epithelial ingrowth, and DLK, and can potentially trigger an inflammatory response that may lead to the loss of the refractive effect. Irregular astigmatism and decrease in BCVA may then occur [20–22].

Delayed wound healing of the interface after LASIK also places patients at a high risk of traumatic flap displacement.

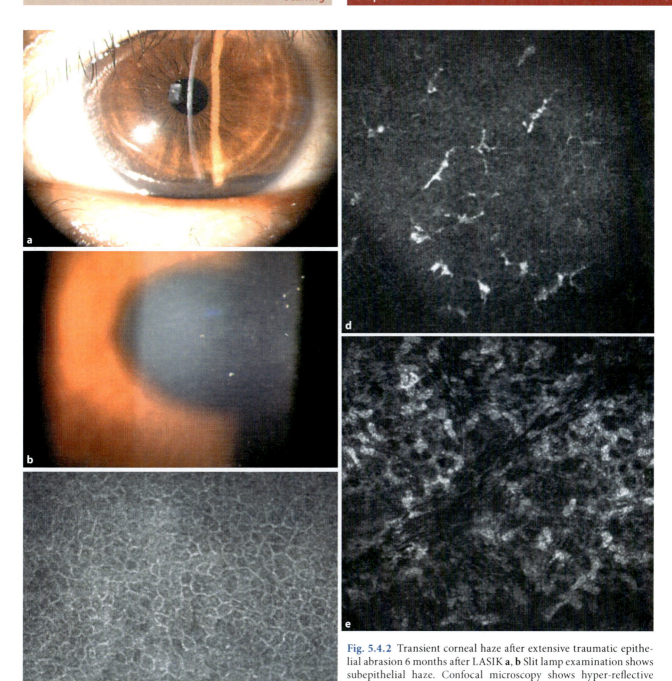

Fig. 5.4.2 Transient corneal haze after extensive traumatic epithelial abrasion 6 months after LASIK **a**, **b** Slit lamp examination shows subepithelial haze. Confocal microscopy shows hyper-reflective epithelial cells (**c**), inflammatory cell infiltration (**d**), and fibroblast activation (**e**)

Scarring, persistent folds, DLK, and epithelial ingrowth may result from this latter complication.

5.4.4 Scars Linked to the Patient's History

5.4.4.1 Abnormal Local Wound Healing

Bilateral Salzmann's-like corneal lesions located at the site of LASIK flap margins have been reported to occur during the first postoperative year. Although the pathogenesis of this complication is uncertain, it is possible that tear hyposecretion, decreased blink rate, and dellen effect that often

5

occur after LASIK could cause the corneal irritation needed to induce Salzmann's nodular degeneration in predisposed patients.

Histological analysis of this type of complication reveals an irregular and thickened epithelium overlying the corneal lesions, and discontinuity of Bowman's layer, replaced by PAS-positive thickened basement membrane–like material. Underlying this basement membrane is a layer of relatively regular, hypocellular, collagen-like connective tissue, displaying hyalinization on trichrome staining, similar to the initial description of Salzmann's nodular degeneration [23].

5.4.4.2 Abnormal General Wound Healing

5.4.4.2.1 Keloids
Conflicting data have been published on the safety and accuracy of LASIK in patients with a history of dermatological keloids. While a history of keloids usually contraindicates PRK, LASIK is generally considered safe in these conditions [24, 25]. While the minimal basement membrane disruption associated with LASIK should prevent abnormal scarring in such patients, abnormal bilateral scars have been reported in a patient for whom LASIK was chosen because of intense corneal haze in his first PRK-treated eye [26]. Although this remains an isolated case, the potential risks should be carefully explained to such patients before surgery.

5.4.4.3 Previous Refractive Surgery
Photorefractive keratectomy used for enhancement of eyes previously treated by myopic LASIK can induce intense corneal scarring after 3–10 months, associated with myopic regression and loss of BCVA [27]. The enhancement procedure of choice is LASIK after lifting the primary flap.

LASIK also appears to be the best procedure to enhance eyes with low haze and residual myopia after PRK, although it is less effective on eyes with severe haze [28–30]. An enhanced tissue response leading to corneal scarring is linked to epithelial basement disruption in a cornea with concomitant or recent injury-mediated stromal activation.

Mechanical and femtosecond LASIK has been used to treat RK-induced hyperopic shift. Although abnormal stromal scarring is a danger in areas involving both the excimer laser and keratotomy treatment zones, the main complication appears to be the reopening of the RK wound, with a risk of epithelial defects or ingrowth [31]. In such cases, PRK with 0.02% mitomycin application has been proposed to correct the refractive error and to prevent major scarring.

5.4.5 Scars Linked to Abnormal Postoperative Inflammation or healing

5.4.5.1 Role of Ultraviolet Light
Excimer laser generates pulses in the UV spectrum at a wavelength of 193 nm, which produces ablative photodestruction of the target tissue. Mutagenicity may be neglect-

ed, but thermal effects, although minimal, exist. The temperature in the cornea immediately adjacent to the excimer laser photoablation can reach 40°C [32]. Therefore, cooling of the ocular surface or the flap interface has been proposed to reduce corneal collagen damage and fibroblast activation. Although UV light has been shown to stimulate wound healing response through corneal fibroblast activation and favor regression of the refractive effect and haze formation after PRK, its effects are minimal after LASIK [33, 34].

5.4.5.2 Diffuse Lamellar Keratitis
DLK, or "Sand of Sahara" syndrome, is a noninfectious disorder characterized by an inflammatory reaction at the flap interface shortly after LASIK. Although many etiologies have been forwarded, the exact cause of DLK is unknown. DLK is thought related to an immunologic or toxic reaction to a contaminant at the lamellar interface, leading to leukocyte migration into the lamellar interface. Predisposing factors include debris or oils derived from the microkeratome, meibomian gland secretions, eyelid debris, antibiotic agents, povidone–iodine solution, and endotoxins derived from gram-negative "biofilms" in sterilizer reservoirs. Other potential factors are problems encountered during or after LASIK surgery, such as epithelial defects [35]. DLK is classified in four stages, with stage 4 being the most severe. The latter is associated with stromal melting, deep flap folds, central haze, hyperopic shift, and irregular astigmatism, leading to a severe reduction in visual acuity. The condition generally improves spontaneously when mild, while topical steroids may be beneficial in more severe cases. Interface scarring on both sides of the lamellar cut and irregular astigmatism may persist after treatment, with a possible decrease in BCVA [22, 36].

5.4.5.3 Epithelial Ingrowth: Fibrosis or Melting?
Epithelial ingrowth is a relatively rare complication of LASIK procedures. While epithelial ingrowth generally produces no symptoms, it can reduce visual acuity by occluding the visual axis or by inducing irregular astigmatism. Two forms of epithelial ingrowth, differing in severity, can be distinguished in central areas of the flap interface. While isolated epithelial nests (not connected to the flap edges) resolve within months with no loss of visual acuity and no need for surgical intervention, progressive epithelial ingrowths forming a continuous sheet with limbal stem cells may disturb interface wound healing, produce unequal remodeling and lead to localized stromal loss. In this latter case, surgical intervention is required to prevent progression or induction of astigmatism and scarring in the area of epithelial ingrowth.

Progressive keratolysis of the flap is the main complication of epithelial ingrowth. The pathogenesis is not completely understood, but epithelial–stromal interactions with protease production may be involved [37]. Figure 5.4.3 shows epithelial ingrowths associated with flap melting.

Treatment consisted of flap lifting and epithelial scraping of the interface. A dense fibrotic scar appeared in the area of epithelial ingrowth, supporting a pathological effect of direct epithelial interaction with the corneal stroma.

Although most epithelial ingrowths in the flap interface occur from the flap margin, they may also arise from the edges of a complicated buttonhole flap. This can lead to a major reduction in visual acuity, particularly because it is close to the visual axis. Transepithelial mitomycin-assisted PRK has been proposed to treat this complication and to prevent intense scarring [38].

Although refractive surgeons generally consider LASIK to be a scarless procedure, it is nonetheless associated with changes in corneal composition. These changes may lead to a loss of transparency due to abnormal healing and scar formation, or may be associated with abnormal recovery of corneal biomechanics. Surgeons and their patients must be aware of these changes in order to prevent or minimize their consequences.

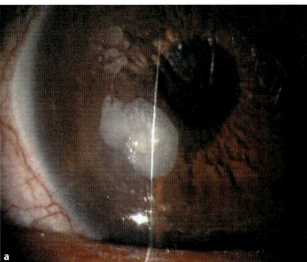

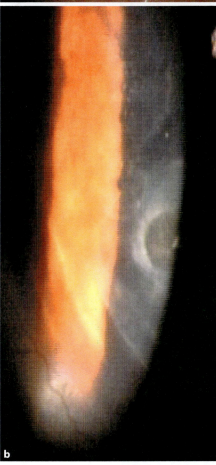

Fig. 5.4.3 Epithelial ingrowth in the LASIK flap interface. **a** Flap melt associated with epithelial ingrowth. **b** Fibrotic scar 2 months following epithelial ingrowth removal

Take-Home Pearls

■ The vast majority of abnormal healing responses following LASIK can be prevented or treated.
■ Proper patient selection, limited flap manipulation to prevent erosions, perfect flap positioning to prevent wrinkles and displacement, and proper treatment of all excessive inflammation or abnormal tissue response such as epithelial ingrowth, are essential to best optimize the visual outcome.

References

1. Ivarsen A, Laurberg T, Moller-Pedersen T (2003) Characterisation of corneal fibrotic wound repair at the LASIK flap margin. Br J Ophthalmol 87:1272–1278
2. Ivarsen A, Laurberg T, Moller-Pedersen T (2004) Role of keratocyte loss on corneal wound repair after LASIK. Invest Ophthalmol Vis Sci 45:3499–3506
3. Ivarsen A, Moller-Pedersen T (2005) LASIK induces minimal regrowth and no haze development in rabbit corneas. Curr Eye Res 30:363–373
4. Philipp WE, Speicher L, Gottinger W (2003) Histological and immunohistochemical findings after laser in situ keratomileusis in human corneas. J Cataract Refract Surg 29:808–820
5. Sonigo B, Iordanidou V, Chong-Sit D et al (2006) In vivo corneal confocal microscopy comparison of IntraLase femtosecond laser and mechanical microkeratome for laser in situ keratomileusis. Invest Ophthalmol Vis Sci 47:2803–2811
6. Kramer TR, Chuckpaiwong V, Dawson DG et al (2005) Pathologic findings in postmortem corneas after successful laser in situ keratomileusis. Cornea 24:92–102
7. Park CK, Kim JH (1999) Comparison of wound healing after photorefractive keratectomy and laser in situ keratomileusis in rabbits. J Cataract Refract Surg 25:842–850
8. Ma XH, Li JH, Bi HS et al (2003) [Comparison of corneal wound healing of photorefractive keratectomy and laser in situ keratomileusis in rabbits]. Zhonghua Yan Ke Za Zhi 39:140–145
9. Kato T, Nakayasu K, Hosoda Y et al (1999) Corneal wound healing following laser in situ keratomileusis (LASIK): a histopathological study in rabbits. Br J Ophthalmol 83:1302–1305
10. Iskander NG, Peters NT, Anderson Penno E, Gimbel HV (2001) Late traumatic flap dislocation after laser in situ keratomileusis. J Cataract Refract Surg 27:1111–1114

5

11. Iskander NG, Peters NT, Penno EA, Gimbel HV (2000) Postoperative complications in laser in situ keratomileusis. Curr Opin Ophthalmol 11:273–279

12. Stramer BM, Zieske JD, Jung JC et al (2003) Molecular mechanisms controlling the fibrotic repair phenotype in cornea: implications for surgical outcomes. Invest Ophthalmol Vis Sci 44:4237–4246

13. Fini ME, Stramer BM (2005) How the cornea heals: cornea-specific repair mechanisms affecting surgical outcomes. Cornea 24(8 Suppl):S2–S11

14. Kenyon KR, Paz H, Greiner JV, Gipson IK (2004) Corneal epithelial adhesion abnormalities associated with LASIK. Ophthalmology 111:11–17

15. Shah MN, Misra M, Wihelmus KR, Koch DD (2000) Diffuse lamellar keratitis associated with epithelial defects after laser in situ keratomileusis. J Cataract Refract Surg 26:1312–1318

16. Harrison DA, Periman LM (2001) Diffuse lamellar keratitis associated with recurrent corneal erosions after laser in situ keratomileusis. J Refract Surg 17:463–465

17. Yavitz EQ (2001) Diffuse lamellar keratitis caused by mechanical disruption of epithelium 60 days after LASIK. J Refract Surg 17:621

18. Nakamura K (2003) Interaction between injured corneal epithelial cells and stromal cells. Cornea 22(7 Suppl):S35–S47

19. Nakamura K, Kurosaka D, Bissen-Miyajima H, Tsubota K (2001) Intact corneal epithelium is essential for the prevention of stromal haze after laser assisted in situ keratomileusis. Br J Ophthalmol 85:209–213

20. Kuo IC, Ou R, Hwang DG (2001) Flap haze after epithelial debridement and flap hydration for treatment of post-laser in situ keratomileusis striae. Cornea 20:339–341

21. Steinert RF, Ashrafzadeh A, Hersh PS (2004) Results of phototherapeutic keratectomy in the management of flap striae after LASIK. Ophthalmology 111:740–746

22. Buhren J, Kohnen T (2003) Corneal wound healing after laser in situ keratomileusis flap lift and epithelial abrasion. J Cataract Refract Surg 29:2007–2012

23. Moshirfar M, Marx DP, Barsam CA et al (2005) Salzmann's-like nodular degeneration following laser in situ keratomileusis. J Cataract Refract Surg 31:2021–2025

24. Cobo-Soriano R, Beltran J, Baviera J (2006) LASIK outcomes in patients with underlying systemic contraindications: a preliminary study. Ophthalmology 113:1124 e1

25. Artola A, Gala A, Belda JI et al (2006) LASIK in myopic patients with dermatological keloids. J Refract Surg 22:505–508

26. Girgis R, Morris DS, Kotagiri A, Ramaesh K (2005) Bilateral corneal scarring after LASIK and PRK in a patient with propensity to keloid scar formation. Eye 21:96–97

27. Carones F, Vigo L, Carones AV, Brancato R (2001) Evaluation of photorefractive keratectomy retreatments after regressed myopic laser in situ keratomileusis. Ophthalmology 108:1732–1737

28. Lazaro C, Castillo A, Hernandez-Matamoros JL et al (2001) Laser in situ keratomileusis enhancement after photorefractive keratectomy. Ophthalmology 108:1423–1429

29. Alio JL, Artola A, Attia WH et al (2001) Laser in situ keratomileusis for treatment of residual myopia after photorefractive keratectomy. Am J Ophthalmol 132:196–203

30. Perez-Santonja JJ, Ayala MJ, Sakla HF et al (1999) Retreatment after laser in situ keratomileusis. Ophthalmology 106:21–18

31. Clausse MA, Boutros G, Khanjian G et al (2001) A retrospective study of laser in situ keratomileusis after radial keratotomy. J Refract Surg 17(2 Suppl):S200–201

32. Berns MW, Liaw LH, Oliva A et al (1988) An acute light and electron microscopic study of ultraviolet 193-nm excimer laser corneal incisions. Ophthalmology 95:1422–1433

33. Nagy ZZ, Toth J, Nagymihaly A, Suveges I (2002) The role of ultraviolet-B in corneal healing following excimer laser in situ keratomileusis. Pathol Oncol Res 8:41–46

34. Nagy ZZ, Hiscott P, Seitz B et al (1997) Clinical and morphological response to UV-B irradiation after excimer laser photorefractive keratectomy. Surv Ophthalmol 42 Suppl 1:S64–S76

35. Mamalis N (2003) Diffuse lamellar keratitis. J Cataract Refract Surg 29:1849–1850

36. Buhren J, Baumeister M, Kohnen T (2001) Diffuse lamellar keratitis after laser in situ keratomileusis imaged by confocal microscopy. Ophthalmology 108:1075–1081

37. Gabison EE, Mourah S, Steinfels E et al (2005) Differential expression of extracellular matrix metalloproteinase inducer (CD147) in normal and ulcerated corneas: role in epithelio–stromal interactions and matrix metalloproteinase induction. Am J Pathol 166:209–219

38. Taneri S, Koch JM, Melki SA, Azar DT (2005) Mitomycin-C assisted photorefractive keratectomy in the treatment of buttonholed laser in situ keratomileusis flaps associated with epithelial ingrowth. J Cataract Refract Surg 31:2026–2030

Refractive Miscalculation with Refractive Surprise

Contents

Core Messages

- Although a refractive surprise due to an error in the sphere is quiet uncommon using excimer technology, its clinical impact may be devastating for the patient and the surgeon.

- There are several sources of mistakes that may cause a refractive surprise: a human source, laser-related condition, laser suite conditions, and the patient's response to surgery.

- Most of the causes that end in a refractive surprise are preventable and must be recognized, understood, and avoided by each refractive surgeon.

- A well-organized facility and an enthusiastic refractive team must be involved in the prevention of the occurrence of these mistakes, supporting the work of the refractive surgeon.

- Corneal wound-healing response is of particular relevance for refractive surgical procedures because it is a major determinant of their efficacy and safety. Unfortunately, these conditions cannot be screened preoperatively and therefore cannot be predicted.

6.1 Sphere

Arturo S. Chayet and Luis F. Torres

6.1.1 Introduction

It is well known that the accuracy of laser-assisted in situ keratomileusis (LASIK) is not absolute, so that residual refractive error may always occur, which may be an under- or an overcorrection. These generally minor defects appear almost immediately after surgery or during the first postoperative week [1–3]. However, a significant refractive surprise due to an error in the sphere is fortunately quiet uncommon in refractive surgery when using excimer laser technology. It probably happens in about 1 in 1,000 cases. The magnitude of the error may depend on the source of the event. Significant under- or overcorrection after LASIK surgery is always frustrating for both the patient and the surgeon [1, 4]. The surgeon must always recognize all the possible causes of the mistake, and base his/her decision of retreatment on a correct evaluation of what went wrong in that particular case, to avoid aggravating the situation [5, 6].

As follows, the most common causes of sphere mistakes after excimer surgery have one of the next sources:

- Human
- Laser
- Laser suite conditions
- Patient

In this chapter, the authors briefly review each of these sources, which may have an affect on the residual spherical error after excimer laser surgery. Some authors have extensively reviewed complications after refractive surgery [7–10].

6.1.2 Refractive Surprise of Human Source

Human mistakes are one of the most common sources of sphere error after surgery. This can be due to several causes.

6.1.2.1 Data Entry Errors

- Typing the wrong number on the keyboard
  This could happen because the person entering the data types too quickly, or can happen due to a bad visualization of the number.
- Getting the wrong number from the patient's chart
  Handwriting can be a problem. We know of a case where the refractive error was +3, but the plus sign was not carefully written, and the surgeon dialed –13. The patient ended up with +15 refraction and later needed a cornea transplant due to ectasia.
- Using the information from a chart of another patient
  The chances of incorrect preoperative data entry into the laser computer database may be lowered when using automated refraction data linked to laser computer software, minimizing the chances of human error and obtaining results that are more consistent [11, 12].

6.1.2.2 Inaccurate Refraction

- Bad refraction technique
  The incorrect use of manifest or cycloplegic refraction for preoperative planning treatment, together with individual factors like patient age, may result in a frank overcorrection. Younger patients with myopia may be overcorrected with their spectacles or contact lenses, so that a surgical plan based upon-

manifest refraction from the preoperative visit, without considering cycloplegic refraction, may end up with a similar error.
- Too much accommodation
  Cycloplegic refraction assessed in younger hyperopic patients may disclose a latent component masked by accommodation that, once treated, cannot be relaxed by the patient's optical system, thus leading to significant overcorrection.
- Inadvertent nuclear sclerosis (progressive myopic shift)
  All ophthalmologic conditions that cause an increased lens power such as osmotic effect (diabetes) or nuclear sclerosis will result in acquired myopia. Obviously, lack of recognition of such conditions will have an affect on the refractive result after excimer treatment [1, 11, 13, 14].

6.1.2.3 Laser Source

Many lasers are now available worldwide [15]. The surgeon must check preoperatively the well functioning of all the components of the excimer that is going to be used. Each laser is subject to a number of steps that must be followed in order to obtain an appropriate calibration. A typical laser checklist includes:

- Evaluation of the optical system for correct functioning
- Fluence testing
- Homogeneity of the beam
- Alignment beams and reticules are concentric with the test ablation
- Eye tracking

6.1.2.3.1 Bad Calibration

The test for fluence and homogeneity is similar for every type of laser. Each laser has a target (generally made from polymethylmethacrylate) to ablate, which acts as the parameter to evaluate fluence and uniformity. For checking fluence, the surgeon must evaluate whether the number of laser pulses for ablating the target falls within the laser manufacturer's approved range. If inadequate, then modifications in voltage and gas must be performed to adjust fluence until optimal conditions.

6.1.2.3.2 Ablation Issues

In order to evaluate how evenly the energy is distributed in the ablated tissue (beam homogeneity) the surgeon must check the appearance of the ablation on the target used for the fluence test. The surgeon must check the regularity in the pattern of ablation, which will be neither symmetrical nor asymmetrical. For example, the central ablation is less than peripheral ablation. All of these variations will result in too much or too little power and hence will influence the visual outcome of every patient. More ablation in the center or more ablation in the periphery will also lead to refractive changes such as hyperopic shift and a myopic shift, respectively [16, 17].

6.1.2.4 Laser Suite Conditions

6.1.2.4.1 Humidity

Surgical and environmental factors may alter tissue hydration and consequently, laser effectiveness. After cutting and lifting the flap, it is necessary to maintain the corneal stroma with a consistent and reproducible hydration level.

Dry Conditions

Drying excessively the stromal surface after flap lifting with microsponges, waiting too long before ablation, and allowing the stromal tissue under high illumination for a long time period are all predisposing factors for stromal dehydration, which will translate clinically in a greater photoablative effect of the laser, leading to overcorrection.

Humid Conditions

Excessive stromal hydration for an inadequate surgical technique or a surgical environment in which the humidity is higher than usual may also lead to undercorrection because the ablative effect of laser pulses becomes less effective, being completely absorbed by humidity.

6.1.2.4.2 Room Air Quality

The cleaner the air, the more tendencies for overcorrection. In general, any particles or gases in the air will decrease the laser beam efficiency [1, 5, 13, 14, 18, 19].

6.1.2.5 Patient Source

6.1.2.5.1 Wound-Healing Response

Corneal wound-healing response is of particular relevance for refractive surgical procedures because it is a major determinant of their efficacy and safety [20]. As this response is usually more intense following PRK than LASIK for the same attempted correction, its modulations are more critical and clinically more important after surface ablation procedures [21]. Preservation of the central corneal epithelium, with subsequent less epithelial–stromal cell interaction and lower rates of keratocyte apoptosis and necrosis may explain the less intense response after LASIK compared with photorefractive keratectomy (PRK), in which disruption of the basement membrane overlying the central cornea exposes anterior stromal keratocytes to the effect of cytokines and growth factors released by the injured epithelial cells, and to factors present in the tear film [21–24]. Epithelial hyperplasia and stromal remodeling are two wound-healing–related processes that make major contributions to refractive accuracy and stability after PRK. In the case of epithelial hyperplasia, the variable number of

activated keratocytes and myofibroblasts producing cytokines that modulate cellular proliferation and differentiation is likely an important determinant of the refractive outcome of surgery in a particular eye [20]. After LASIK, wound-healing responses may also be responsible for an overcorrection. In this surgery, the wound-healing process involves some degree of new-tissue deposition, which is taken into account in the modified algorithm based in the Munnerlyn's formula adopted by all laser systems. Those eyes with absent or reduced wound healing and new-tissue deposition will have an excessive effect from the photoablation, with a consequent overcorrection [1, 4, 13, 14, 21]. Unfortunately, these conditions cannot be screened preoperatively and therefore cannot be predicted.

Take-Home Pearls

- A refractive surprise due to an error in the sphere is quiet uncommon after surface ablation procedures or LASIK.
- The magnitude of the error may depend on the source of the event.
- Human mistakes during data entry into the laser software may cause serious complications after refractive surgery and must be avoided, using automated data systems and a well-organized refractive team. The surgeon must always double check all refractive data before each surgery is performed.
- A complete ophthalmologic examination performed by experienced individuals will lower the chances of possible mistakes due to inaccurate refraction.
- The surgeon must check preoperatively the well functioning of all the components of the excimer, with careful attention to an adequate fluence and homogeneity of the system, ensuring that the number of laser pulses for ablating the target falls within the laser manufacturer's approved range.
- Laser suite conditions must be optimal before, during, and after each surgery. The surgeon must ensure a consistent and reproducible hydration level of the corneal stroma, taking into account all the surgical and environmental factors that may alter laser effectiveness. Corneal wound-healing response is a major determinant of refractive efficacy and safety after surgery. This response is usually more intense after PRK than LASIK. Epithelial hyperplasia and stromal remodeling are two wound-healing–related processes that make major contributions to refractive accuracy and stability after PRK. After LASIK, the wound healing process involves some degree of new-tissue deposition. Those eyes with excessive or reduced wound healing will have an atypical effect from the photoablation, with a consequent suboptimal refractive outcome. Unfortunately, these conditions cannot be screened preoperatively and therefore cannot be predicted.

6

References

1. Balazsi G et al (2001) Laser in situ keratomileusis with a scanning excimer laser for the correction of low to moderate myopia with and without astigmatism. J Cataract Refract Surg 27:1942–1951

2. Chayet AS et al (1998) Laser in situ keratomileusis for simple myopic, mixed, and simple hyperopic astigmatism. J Refract Surg 14(2 Suppl): S175–S176

3. Montes M et al (1999) Laser in situ keratomileusis for myopia of −1.50 to −6.00 diopters. J Refract Surg 15:106–110

4. Magallanes R et al (2001) Stability after laser in situ keratomileusis in moderately and extremely myopic eyes. J Cataract Refract Surg 27:1007–1012

5. Chayet AS et al (1998) Regression and its mechanisms after laser in situ keratomileusis in moderate and high myopia. Ophthalmology 105:1194–1199

6. Zadok D et al (1999) Outcomes of retreatment after laser in situ keratomileusis. Ophthalmology 106:2391–2394

7. Schallhorn SC, Amesbury EC, Tanzer DJ (2006) Avoidance, recognition, and management of LASIK complications. Am J Ophthalmol 141:733–739

8. Sridhar MS et al (2002)Complications of laser-in-situ-keratomileusis. Indian J Ophthalmol 50:265–282

9. Taneri S, Zieske JD, Azar DT (2004) Evolution, techniques, clinical outcomes, and pathophysiology of LASEK: review of the literature. Surv Ophthalmol 49:576–602

10. Wilson SE (1998) LASIK: management of common complications. Laser in situ keratomileusis. Cornea 17:459–567

11. Chayet AS Robledo N (1999) Fully automated refraction in laser refractive surgery using the Nidek COS-2000. J Refract Surg 15(2 Suppl): S257–S258

12. Rodriguez-Zarzuelo G et al (2005) [Refractive surprise after LASIK]. Arch Soc Esp Oftalmol 80:547–549

13. Knorz, M.C et al Laser in situ keratomileusis to correct myopia of -6.00 to -29.00 diopters. J Refract Surg 12:575–84

14. Munnerlyn CR, Koons SJ. Marshall J (1988) Photorefractive keratectomy: a technique for laser refractive surgery. J Cataract Refract Surg 14:46–52

15. Waheed S, Krueger RR (2002) Update on customized excimer ablations: recent developments reported in 2002. Curr Opin Ophthalmol 14:198–202

16. Buratto L2003 Custom LASIK, 1st edn. Slack, Thorofare, N.J., p 805

17. Pettit GH (2006) The ideal excimer beam for refractive surgery. J Refract Surg 22: S969–S9672

18. Argento C et al (2001) Corneal ectasia after laser in situ keratomileusis. J Cataract Refract Surg 27:1440–1448

19. Wilson SE (2000) Cautions regarding measurements of the posterior corneal curvature. Ophthalmology 107:1223

20. Netto MV et al (2005) Wound healing in the cornea: a review of refractive surgery complications and new prospects for therapy. Cornea 24:509–522

21. Mohan RR et al (2003) Apoptosis, necrosis, proliferation, and myofibroblast generation in the stroma following LASIK and PRK. Exp Eye Res 76:71–87

22. Nakamura K et al (2001) Intact corneal epithelium is essential for the prevention of stromal haze after laser assisted in situ keratomileusis. Br J Ophthalmol 85:209–13

23. O'Brien TP et al (1998) Inflammatory response in the early stages of wound healing after excimer laser keratectomy. Arch Ophthalmol 116:1470–1474

24. Stramer BM et al (2003) Molecular mechanisms controlling the fibrotic repair phenotype in cornea: implications for surgical outcomes. Invest Ophthalmol Vis Sci 44:4237–4246

Core Messages

■ Misalignment of the surgical procedure is the major source of refractive surprise in relation to astigmatism.

■ Sources of misalignment include cyclotorsion from the seated to supine position, a physical turning of the patients head, or intentionally placing a cataract incision on a meridian other than the steepest corneal meridian.

■ Any corneal incision for cataract or lens surgery, no matter how small, will alter the corneal structure, and have an influence on the preexisting astigmatism.

■ Refractive cataract surgeons employing a technique to correct astigmatism at the time of surgery (toric IOLs, LRIs, etc.) need to consider the effect of the incision on the remaining astigmatism, otherwise the IOL or LRI will be misaligned.

■ The forces acting to change the corneal structure in a misaligned treatment are flattening (or steepening) and torque. These result in a reduction (or increase) of astigmatism at the intended meridian, and a change in the meridian of the astigmatism.

■ Vector analysis is a useful tool to calculate the effects of a misaligned treatment on the remaining astigmatism.

6.2 Cylinder
Noel Alpins and Gemma Walsh

6.2.1 Introduction

The ultimate goal of modern refractive surgery is to meet, or even exceed, the expectations of the patient. With regard to the spherical component of the correction, this involves obtaining the intended target, which is not necessarily emmetropia. However, concerning the astigmatic component, the universal primary goal is to achieve maximum reduction of astigmatism. The secondary goal is to ensure any remaining cylinder unable to be eliminated from the optical system is optimized toward a more favorable, with-the-rule orientation.

Addressing the correction of astigmatism is crucial for the refractive surgeon, as a large majority of patients have significant preoperative cylinder. Ninety percent of the population has detectable astigmatism, with 25% having more than 1.00 D [1]. An uncorrected astigmatic error of 1.00 D on average will decrease visual acuity to the level of 20/30 or 20/40, depending on its orientation [2]. As well as this blurring of vision, uncorrected astigmatism can also cause distortion, glare, asthenopia, headaches, and monocular diplopia.

Surgical treatments that incorporate astigmatic correction include excimer laser surgery such as photoastigmatic refractive keratectomy (PARK), LASIK, and laser-assisted sub-epithelial keratectomy (LASEK), including epi-LASEK. These procedures have been shown to be effective at correcting low to moderate levels of astigmatism [1, 3, 4]. However, 15–20% of cataract patients also have >1.50 D of astigmatism [5], and with recent advances in technology, the modern cataract surgeon must also consider the treatment of astigmatism as part of the surgical goal. This is particularly true as refractive clear lens exchange surgery is widely becoming more popular, and these patients tend to be young and demanding of excellent visual results. Options for correcting astigmatism at the time of cataract surgery include placing the incision along the steepest corneal meridian [6–8], paired opposite clear corneal incisions along the steepest meridian [9], phakic [10], and pseudophakic [11, 12] toric intraocular lenses (IOLs), limbal relaxing incisions (LRIs) [13], peripheral corneal relaxing incisions (PCRIs) [5], and astigmatic keratotomy (AK) [14].

6.2.2 Misaligned Treatments

In many cases, an astigmatic postoperative surprise is due to the treatment being misaligned with the steepest corneal meridian, otherwise known as "off axis." An unplanned misaligned treatment not only changes the magnitude of the astigmatism in a manner different from that intended, but will also affect the orientation of the astigmatism. A wavefront-guided laser surgery designed to correct higher-order aberrations may in fact induce significant aberrations if misaligned, even if the astigmatic component is minimal. This is noticeable for treatments misaligned by only 2° [15], and the room for error is tightened even further in patients with large pupils of 7 mm or more [16]. With such tight criteria, it is important to understand the causes of misalignment, the forces that act to change the cornea in a misaligned treatment, and how to analyze outcomes of misaligned treatments to improve future results.

6.2.3 Sources of Misalignment

The underlying cause for off-axis treatments may be something as simple as a slight misalignment of the patient's head. However, other factors need to be considered.

6.2.3.1 Cyclotorsion
As the position of the eye changes, it undergoes natural rotational movements around the central axes, known as cyclotorsion. The amount of cyclotorsion depends on the individual and the fixation stimulus, but is usually within 15° of the resting position [15]. In relation to refractive surgery, it is the amount of torsion when the patient moves from the seated position to supine that is important, which is typically between 2 and 7° [15]. Therefore, the meridian of the astigmatism measured by the keratometer or topographer when the patient is seated upright may significantly change as the patient lies down for surgery, resulting in a treatment that may be misaligned by up to 7°. This is well outside the recommended 2° limit for a wavefront-guided ablation.

With such a high level of precision required, many laser machines now incorporate tracking systems to account for cyclotorsion by identifying iris landmarks and rotating the treatment accordingly from the wavefront machine to the laser machine. While off-axis effects are a little more forgiving in cataract surgery, alignment errors can be minimized by marking the corneal meridian for toric IOLs or LRIs with the patient seated in an upright position.

6.2.3.2 The Elusive "Astigmatically Neutral" Incision
The size of the clear corneal incision used to access the anterior chamber for cataract surgery has reduced in recent times. The routine 3-mm incision has moved to sub-2 mm, with the gaining popularity of microincisional cataract surgery (MICS), whether bimanual or coaxial. Many surgeons would claim the incision to be "astigmatically neutral" and therefore do not include it in their surgical calculations. However, while the astigmatism induced by the surgery is certainly reduced with smaller incisions, in reality *there is no such thing as a completely astigmatically neutral incision.* Any incision, no matter how small, will still have an affect on the corneal structure and will alter the astigmatic magnitude and/or direction.

Therefore, a toric IOL or LRI may be placed exactly where the surgeon intended, yet if the effects of the incision are not taken into account and the reference meridian is the preoperative measurement, then the results will still be compromised. The final visual outcome may still be acceptable to the patient depending on how much alignment error occurs [17]. However, if there is a thorough understanding of the forces at play during surgery, a merely acceptable outcome can be optimized to an even better one.

6

6.2.4 Understanding and Analyzing Misaligned Treatments

6.2.4.1 Forces That Act to Change the Cornea

Several forces act to influence the cornea throughout the course of refractive surgery. Flattening (and steepening) of the cornea are the forces most commonly considered, as these are the basic underlying principles of refractive surgery. In a perfect surgery, the cornea is flattened at the steepest meridian (or steepened at the flattest meridian, or a combination of both) to reduce the magnitude of the astigmatism. However, if the treatment is not perfectly aligned and applied off-axis, then another component becomes evident. This component is known as torque, which has two effects on the remaining astigmatism: It acts to increase the magnitude and to rotate the meridian in a clockwise or counterclockwise direction [18]. It is the torque component that is commonly disregarded, yet this is the major source of postoperative surprises in relation to astigmatism. In order for any refractive surgeon (laser or lens) to achieve maximum results, a thorough understanding of these forces is required.

6.2.4.2 Vector Analysis of Outcomes

As astigmatism has both magnitude and direction, it may be represented by vectors, and therefore vector analysis is a simple and effective tool for analyzing the astigmatic outcomes from surgery [2, 18–20]. The target-induced astigmatism vector (TIA) is the astigmatic change the surgery was intended to induce, and the surgically induced astigmatism vector (SIA) is the astigmatic change actually induced by the surgery. The various relationships between the SIA and TIA can determine whether too much or too little treatment was applied, and whether the treatment was aligned effectively or not.

The amount of misalignment is the angle of error (AE) and is described by the angle subtended between the SIA and TIA. The AE is positive if the SIA lies in a counterclockwise (CCW) direction to the axis of the TIA, and similarly the AE is negative if the SIA lies in a clockwise (CW) direction relative to the TIA. In a misaligned treatment the SIA acts to change the cornea in two ways: A proportion of the induced change will act to rotate the astigmatic meridian (through the effect of torque), and the remaining proportion will act to flatten the cornea at the intended meridian. This latter change is known as the flattening effect (FE) measured in diopters, and is dependent on the AE: FE $=$ SIA cos 2(AE).

It can be seen from the above formula that the FE is equal to the SIA when the AE is 0, and the treatment is perfectly aligned. The effective proportion of flattening achieved is the flattening index (FI) and is equal to the FE divided by the TIA. The relationship between the amount of misalignment and the amount of flattening is seen in Fig. 6.2.1. This model assumes a full correction of astigmatism is achieved (i.e., SIA = TIA). It is seen that the FI is reduced as the AE increases. When the treatment is misaligned by 30°, the ef-

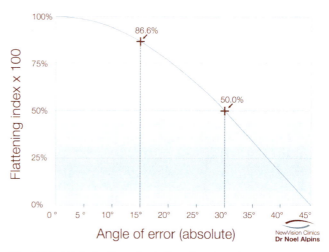

Fig. 6.2.1 (Alpins) effect of misaligned astigmatism treatment on flattening index when SIA = TIA

fective proportion of flattening at the intended axis is reduced by half, with the other half being the torque effect. When the misalignment is 45°, there is no flattening effect at all, and the only force acting to change the cornea is torque. If the misalignment is greater than 45°, then there is a negative flattening effect (i.e., the cornea is steepened).

It is a common misconception to regard a misaligned treatment as causing an undercorrection in the magnitude of the astigmatism. However, this is not strictly correct. An over or under correction is determined by the correction index (CI), which is the ratio of SIA to TIA. The CI is equal to 1 if a full correction of astigmatism occurs. If the CI is greater than 1, then an overcorrection has occurred, and similarly a CI of less than 1 indicates an undercorrection. In a misaligned treatment, the magnitude of the SIA is in fact unaffected as it is independent from the AE, and therefore the CI is also unaffected. Instead, a misaligned treatment results in a shift of the orientation of the existing astigmatism (through the effect of torque). The effect of the misaligned treatment on the remaining astigmatism magnitude and axis can be seen in Figs. 6.2.2 and 6.2.3.

Example: Let us look at an example to demonstrate. This form of analysis applies for both laser and incisional surgery, so we use a general example that can be used for all refractive surgery. A patient scheduled for refractive surgery has 2.00-D corneal astigmatism at a 25° meridian. The surgeon performs uncomplicated surgery that was thought aligned correctly, but postoperatively the corneal astigmatism is measured again and found to be 1.00 D at 63°. Why did this happen?

A polar diagram is a simple way to represent astigmatism as it appears on the eye. This is seen in Fig. 6.2.4, in which the preoperative value of 2.00 D at 25° is represented by the light blue line, and similarly, the dark blue line represents the postoperative value of 1.00 D at 63°. The TIA represents the amount of astigmatic change the surgeon wants to induce. A reduction of astigmatism may be achieved either by flattening the cornea at 25° or by steepening the cor-

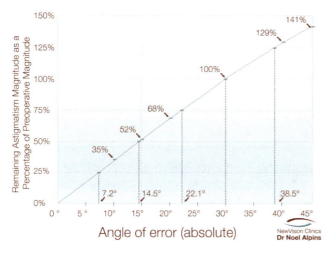

Fig. 6.2.2 (Alpins) effect of misaligned astigmatism treatment on remaining astigmatism magnitude

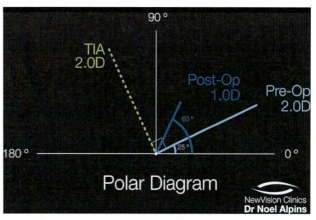

Fig. 6.2.4 Polar diagram displaying the pre and post-operative status as it appears on the eye. The TIA is the intended astigmatic treatment and is perpendicular to the preoperative value

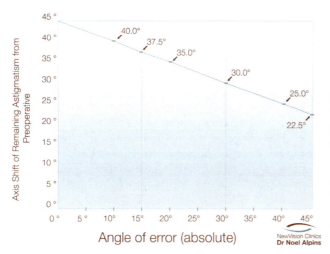

Fig. 6.2.3 (Alpins) effect of misaligned astigmatism treatment on remaining astigmatism axis

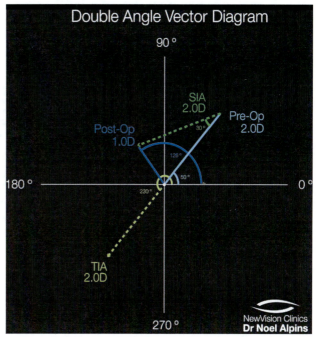

Fig. 6.2.5 DAVD to allow analysis of the outcome. All the angles have been doubled without altering the magnitudes. This allows calculation of the SIA vector

nea at the perpendicular meridian of 115°. However, as the TIA always represents a steepening force, it is displayed on the polar diagram at the perpendicular meridian of 115° as seen in Fig. 6.2.4. In this example, the magnitude of the TIA is equal to that of the preoperative value as the surgery was intended to achieve a full correction of astigmatism.

To allow analysis of the results, the polar diagram (which represents the situation as it appears on the eye) must be converted to a mathematical construct. This is easily done by doubling all the angles to create a double-angle vector diagram (DAVD) as seen in Fig. 6.2.5. The magnitudes remain unchanged; the angles are simply doubled.

The SIA is the vector joining from the pre- to the post-operative values. This vector may be moved to the origin without changing the magnitude or the angle as seen in Fig. 6.2.6. The SIA and TIA in this example are equal in length, indicating a full correction of astigmatism and a correction

index of 1. Therefore, even though the amount of flattening and thus the reduction in astigmatism magnitude at the intended meridian was less than expected, there has not been an undercorrection of astigmatism magnitude. The angle between the SIA and TIA may then be easily measured at 30°. A line is drawn perpendicularly between these two vectors to give the FE, which in this case is 86.6%—the length of the TIA. This represents almost a 15% loss of flattening effect at the intended meridian.

In order to represent this in "real" terms on the eye, the DAVD is converted back to a polar diagram by simply halving the angles, again leaving the magnitudes unchanged, as shown in Fig. 6.2.7. The angle between the SIA and TIA (i.e., the AE) is now 15°. It is therefore easily seen that the treatment was actually applied 15° off axis in a CW direction.

Thus by vector analysis, the loss of flattening effect at the intended placement of the astigmatism treatment (whether incision or ablation) is around 15% when the treatment is 15° off axis from the intended meridian. This relation-

ship between the AE and FI correlates with Fig. 6.2.1. The remaining 13.4% of the SIA acted as torque to rotate the remaining astigmatism. Figures 6.2.2 and 6.2.3 display the effect of misalignment on the remaining astigmatism magnitude and axis. It can be seen from these graphs that a misalignment of 15° in this example reduces the magnitude of the astigmatism by approximately 50% and shifts the meridian by 37.5°. This correlates with our example in which the astigmatism was reduced by half and rotated from 25 to 63°. It is important to note in this example that this reduction is just a scalar comparison of pre- and postoperative astigmatism magnitudes.

6.2.4.3 Practical Use in the Clinical Setting

Imagine the surgery in the above example was cataract surgery, and the surgeon was to perform LRIs at the time of cataract surgery to correct the astigmatism. If the incision were not taken into account, the LRI would be centered around 25°, based on the assumption that the preoperative value of 2.00 D at 25° had not changed. In fact, the effect of the cataract incision has changed the astigmatism to 1.00 D at 63°. The LRI would therefore have been misaligned by almost 40°. Similarly, if a toric IOL were implanted at the preoperative meridian of 25° to correct 2.00 D of cylinder, then a postoperative surprise would have occurred, as the real astigmatism correction should have been 1.00 D at 63°.

Therefore, if a surgeon assumes the incision is neutral and does not place the incision along the corneal meridian, then the misalignment will change both the meridian and magnitude of the astigmatism that is being treated. The amount of change will obviously not only depend on the amount of misalignment, but also on the amount of induced flattening by the incision. Each surgeon will achieve a certain average value of corneal flattening depending on the incision size used and the orientation of the incision at the limbal meridian. Due to the ovoid shape of the cornea, incisions placed vertically have a greater flattening effect than do those placed temporally, as they are slightly closer to the centre of the cornea. Each surgeon ideally should track the data from previous cases to calculate their own average amount of flattening for each site of placement.

Software is now available with some toric IOLs to allow the surgeon to calculate the effect of the incision on the astigmatism and incorporate this into the surgical plan, but the same result is obtained by simple vector analysis.

6.2.4.4 Calculating the Effect of the Incision

A patient scheduled for right-eye cataract surgery has 2.00-D astigmatism at 30° measured by keratometry. The surgeon intends to use a temporal (0°) clear corneal incision for cataract extraction, and then use LRIs to correct the remaining astigmatism. Thus, the incision will be deliberately off axis by 30°, so what will this do to the remaining astigmatism? From analyzing the previous data, the surgeon knows the average flattening induced by his temporal incisions is approximately 0.50 D. Therefore, he would ex-

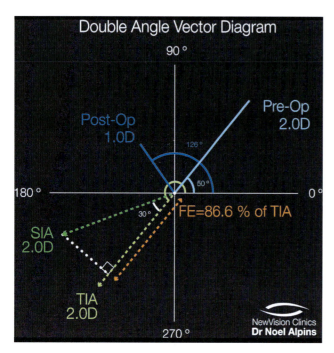

Fig. 6.2.6 DAVD, in which the SIA has been moved to the origin without altering the angle subtended or the magnitude. This allows calculation of the FI

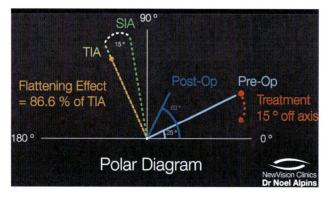

Fig. 6.2.7 Polar diagram representing the analysis as it would appear on the eye. The angles have been halved without altering the magnitudes. The AE subtended by the SIA and TIA is 15°, so it is easy to see the treatment was misaligned by this amount

pect the TIA vector (which is always perpendicular to the incision as it represents a steepening force) to be 0.50 D at 90°. This is represented on the polar diagram in Fig. 6.2.8.

Again, we need to convert this to a mathematical construct, so we double all angles, without altering the magnitudes to create a double angle vector diagram in Fig. 6.2.9. The preoperative angle of 30° now becomes 60°, and similarly, the TIA vector has doubled from 90 to 180°. This TIA vector may be moved to the end of the preoperative value without altering either the 180° angle or the magnitude as displayed in Fig. 6.2.9.

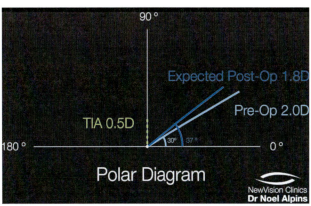

Fig. 6.2.10 Polar diagram representing the expected outcome as it would appear on the eye. All angles have been halved without altering the magnitudes. By simple measurement, the predicted postoperative astigmatism following the temporal cataract incision is 1.80 D at 37°

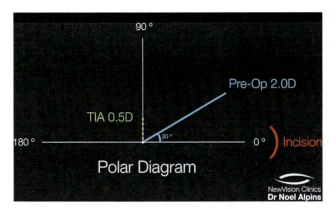

Fig. 6.2.8 Polar diagram representing the preoperative situation as it appears on the eye. The incision is at 180° and is expected to induce approximately 0.50-D flattening. Therefore, the expected TIA is perpendicular to this (as the TIA represents a steepening force)

The expected postoperative value may now be estimated simply by drawing a line from the head of the TIA to the origin. Measuring the length and angle subtended by this line gives a value of 1.80 D at 74°. To determine how this will appear on the eye, we create another polar diagram by halving all angles. This is seen in Fig. 6.2.10, in which the expected postoperative value is 1.80 D at 37°. Therefore, following a temporal incision, this surgeon should center the LRI around 37°, instead of the preoperative value of 30°.

Take-Home Pearls

■ If marking the limbus, do so prior to surgery, with the patient in the seated position before he/she lies down. This way it will match the preoperative keratometry or topography meridian where the patient is also seated. This meridian may actually change by 2–7° as the patient lies down due to cyclotorsion of the eyes.

■ If a treatment is applied exactly at the steepest corneal meridian, then the magnitude of the astigmatism is reduced, and the meridian of any remaining astigmatism remains unchanged.

■ If a treatment is applied in a direction other then the steepest corneal meridian (i.e., a misaligned, off-axis treatment), then the magnitude of the astigmatism is either reduced or increased, *and* the meridian of the remaining astigmatism is changed in the opposite direction of the misaligned incision due to the force of torque.

■ Many cataract surgeons place all incisions temporally or superiorly regardless of where the steepest meridian lays, but then orientate the toric IOL or LRI with the preoperative corneal meridian without accounting for any change in magnitude or direction from the incision. This results in a compro-

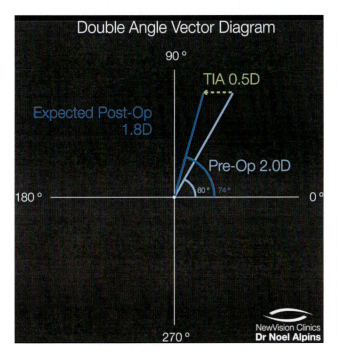

Fig. 6.2.9 DAVD to allow analysis of the expected outcome. The angles have been doubled without altering the magnitudes, and the TIA vector has been moved to the tip of the preoperative value. This allows calculation of the expected postoperative value

mised result with incomplete astigmatism reduction.

■ Use vector analysis or special software to calculate the effect of the incision on the remaining astigmatism magnitude and meridian prior to performing surgery to tighten results from toric IOLs or LRIs.

6

References

1. Febbraro JL, Aron-Rosa D, Gross M et al (1999) One year clinical results of photoastigmatic refractive keratectomy for compound myopic astigmatism. J Cataract Refract Surg 25:911–20
2. Alpins N, Stamatelatos G (2003) Vector analysis applications to photorefractive surgery. Int Ophthalmic Clinics 43:1–27
3. Yang CN, Shen EP, Hu FR (2001) Laser in situ keratomileusis for the correction of myopia and myopic astigmatism. J Cataract Refract Surg 27:1952–1960
4. Partal AE, Rojas MC, Manche EE (2004) Analysis of the efficacy, predictability, and safety of LASEK for myopia and myopic astigmatism using the Technolas 217 excimer laser. J Cataract Refract Surg 30:2141–2144
5. Wang L, Misra M, Koch DD (2003) Peripheral corneal relaxing incisions combined with cataract surgery. J Cataract Refract Surg 29:712–722
6. Alpins NA (1994) What type of cataract surgeon are you? OSN USA edn., 15 January 1994
7. Matsumoto Y, Hara T, Chiba K, Chikuda M (2001) Optimal incision sites to obtain an astigmatism-free cornea after cataract surgery with a 3.2 mm sutureless incision. J Cataract Refract Surg 27:1617–1619
8. Borasio E, Mehta JS, Maurino V (2006) Surgically induced astigmatism after phacoemulsification in eyes with mild to moderate corneal astigmatism. J Cataract Refract Surg 32:565–572
9. Qammar A, Mullaney P (2005) Paired opposite clear corneal incisions to correct preexisting astigmatism in cataract patients. J Cataract Refract Surg 31:1167–1170
10. Dick HB, Alio J, Bianchetti M et al (2003) Toric phakic intraocular lens. Ophthalmology 110:150–162
11. Rushwurm I, Scholz U, Zehetmayer M et al (2000) Astigmatism correction with a foldable toric intraocular lens in cataract patients. J Cataract Refract Surg 26:1022–1027
12. Sun XY, Vicary D, Montgomery P, Griffiths M (2000) Toric Intraocular Lenses for Correcting Astigmatism in 130 eyes. Ophthalmology 107:1776–1781
13. Kaufmann C, Peter J, Ooi K et al (2005) Limbal relaxing incisions versus on-axis incisions to reduce corneal astigmatism at the time of cataract surgery. J Cataract Refract Surg 31:2261–2265
14. Oshika T, Shimazaki J, Yoshitomi F, et al (1998) Arcuate keratotomy to treat corneal astigmatism after cataract surgery: a prospective evaluation of predictability and effectiveness. Ophthalmology 105:2012–2016
15. Chernyak DA (2004) Cyclotorsional eye motion occurring between wavefront measurement and refractive surgery. J Cataract Refract Surg 30:633–638
16. Bueeler M, Mrochen M, Seiler T (2004) Maximum possible torsional misalignment in aberration-sensing and wavefront-guided corneal ablation. J Cataract Refract Surg 3019–25
17. Bartels MC, Saxena R, van den Berg TJTP, et al (2006) The influence of incision-induced astigmatism and axial lens position on the correction of myopic astigmatism with the Artisan toric phakic intraocular lens. Ophthalmology 113:1110–1116
18. Alpins NA (1997) Vector analysis of astigmatism changes by flattening, steepening, and torque. J Cataract Refract Surg 23:1503–1513
19. Alpins NA (2001) Astigmatism analysis by the Alpins method. J Cataract Refract Surg 27:31–49
20. Alpins NA, Goggin M (2004) Practical astigmatism analysis for refractive outcomes in cataract and refractive surgery. Survey of Ophthalmology 49:109–122

Optical Aberrations

7

Contents

Core Messages

- Night vision complaints can complicate corneal photorefractive corrections and are related to the altered corneal optical properties after surgery.

- Improvement of laser algorithms, energy delivery improvements, and active trackers have significantly improved the optical results of refractive surgery and minimized visual complaints of the treated patients over the last few years.

- The introduction of wavefront aberrometry in the clinical practice offered a better understanding of the optical results of corneal photorefractive surgery, and may be a useful tool to achieve the so-called supervision in the future.

7.1 Optical Implications of Corneal Photorefractive Surgery
Vikentia J. Katsanevaki

7.1.1 Introduction

Photorefractive procedures are performed in anatomically normal corneas to reduce ametropias and patient dependence on corrective spectacles and contact lenses.

The optical factors affecting visual performance are diffraction, uncorrected refractive errors, and high-order aberrations. The latter term describes deviations after the negation of cylinder and sphere as described by the refractive error. High-order aberrations are directly related to the pupil size, as is contrast sensitivity.

Night vision complaints, ghosting, and phenomena such as starburst and glare were reported at rates of 10–60% [1, 2] in the early days of photorefractive corrections, when treatments were attempted at 3.5–4 mm, with no blend zone between the treated area and the peripheral cornea.

The importance of treatment zones and their matching with pupil size, the limits of attempted correction in terms of aimed corneal refractive change as well the laser ablation profile, and the energy delivery have been recognized as important factors for optimum postoperative corneal optical performance in order to prevent optical complications after photorefractive corrections.

With the years of experience, currently used laser algorithms not only maximized the treatment zones, but also attempt overablation of the peripheral cornea in order to blend the principal curvature of the optical zone smoothly into the curvature of the peripheral cornea.

Despite the above-mentioned improvements in the latest-generation lasers, peer-reviewed literature suggests corneal photorefractive surgery induces higher-order aberrations, affecting contrast sensitivity [3] as a result of either changes of the corneal shape or by surface microirregularities caused by the treatment.

In the clinical setting, there is evidence that in uncomplicated treatments, functional vision is mainly affected by the changes of the corneal shape, whereas surface microirregularities, although present, are clinically insignificant.

Even when high-contrast visual acuity remained unaffected or even improved after the surgery, low-contrast visual acuity was shown decreased as compared with baseline after treatment of low myopia [4]. Data suggest that after the surgery, high-contrast visual acuity may increase because of reduced minification by the spectacles, but the altered corneal optical quality (due to its altered shape) may affect functional vision. In other words, treated patients may have subjective visual complaints regardless of unaffected Snellen acuity.

7.1.2 Night Visual Complaints: Role of the Mesopic Pupil Size

Central corneal flattening after myopic corrections affects the corneal natural asphericity, turning natural prolate corneal surface to oblate. Similarly, hyperopic corrections alter the corneal shape in a reverse way. Shape changes causing spherical, coma, and astigmatic aberrations are directly related to the pupil size and worsen as light levels decrease.

Higher treatments alter shape more than do lower treatments, and larger pupils unmask more of this altered contour. Small optical zones, large pupils, and high myopic corrections are directly related to increases in spherical

aberrations and as previously proposed [5], 6.00 D should probably be the upper limit of allowed correction in patients with pupil size up to 7 mm.

The correlation of pupil size to night vision complaints has been recently questioned. Pop and Payete presented a comprehensive evaluation of night vision complaints in nearly 1,500 laser-assisted in situ keratomileusis (LASIK) procedures. They reported 5% rate of night vision complaints at 1 year after treatment. One of the major findings of the above-mentioned study was that the pupil size is probably not related to the night vision complaints [6].

One of the main weaknesses in this study, as well as in other studies that come to the same conclusion, is that they analyze their data using the manufacturer's specified treatment zone. However, the pupil size–treatment zone disparity may not be accurate, as previous studies have shown that the higher the attempted correction, the smaller the effective zone [7, 8] (Fig. 7.1.1). Furthermore, as shown by clinical experience, symptomatic patients report a dramatic decrease of symptoms when their pupils are pharmacologically constricted.

It seems it is not only the actual pupil size, but also its combination with the level of attempted correction that plays a role in the night vision complaints after the surgery.

According to current consensus, preoperative measurement of pupil size remains the standard of care. Even with the use of the latest-generation lasers, care should be taken with patients with both large mesopic pupils and high (>6.00 D) attempted corrections, as they seem to be at higher risk for postoperative poor vision in mesopic conditions.

7.1.3 Clinical Assessment of Symptomatic Patients

The recent evolution of wavefront and other higher-order aberration analyzers in the clinical practice gave new insight into human optics, especially for eyes after photorefractive corrections (Fig. 7.1.2). These analyzers use the refractive deviation of many points of light passing into the eye through the entrance pupil, imaged as an aberration pattern on the retina. The wavefront error is defined as the difference between the actual wavefront (leading edge of propagating rays) and the ideal wavefront in the place of the eye's exit pupil.

Wavefront analyzers are valuable diagnostic tools in evaluating symptomatic patients after photorefractive corrections.

In a recent study, Chalita et al. have shown correlation of double vision with total and horizontal coma, glare with spherical and total aberrations, and starburst with spherical aberrations [9]. In a similar study, Tuan et al. used wavefront-derived optical metrics and found marked similarities of calculated point spread functions with patients drawings elicited by testing with a Fenthoff muscle light, while using their best-corrected distance vision [10].

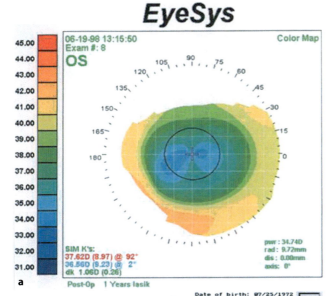

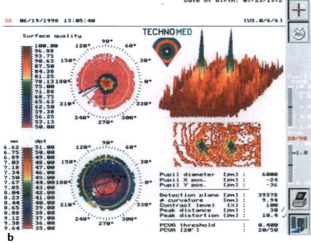

Fig. 7.1.1 **a** Corneal topography of a symptomatic eye with no line loss 1 year after correction of −8.00 D. The correction that was attempted at 6-mm optical zone resulted in a small effective zone. **b** Corneal ray tracing image of the same eye visualizes the effect of small effective zone for a simulated pupil of 6 mm. Low refractive homogeneity of the central cornea results in poor mesopic visual performance and predicted corneal acuity of 20/50

The results of these studies demonstrate the diagnostic capability of the wavefront system in predicting visual symptoms and complaints of patients with high-order aberrations.

7.1.4 Management of Symptomatic Patients

Corneal surface irregularities, decentered ablations, or small treatment zone diameters are possible complications of excimer laser refractive surgery, and their management is discussed in depth in the related chapters of this textbook.

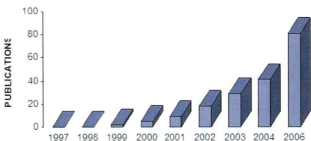

LITERATURE SEARCH:LASIK + aberrations

Fig. 7.1.2 Since the introduction of wave front analyzers in the clinical practice, there has been increasing awareness of the optical effects of photorefractive surgery on optical performance

The evolution of the used laser platforms introducing large treatment zones and active trackers minimized the incidence of such important complications; however, the problem of managing those patients remains an issue in the everyday routine of a busy refractive surgeon.

Corneal topography has historically played an important role in the clinical evaluation of patients reporting visual symptoms after photorefractive corrections. The unique topographic patterns of those eyes introducing irregular astigmatism necessitated the development of customized surgical techniques for their treatment.

Before the introduction of topographic-guided ablations, the management of these eyes included numerous surgical approaches of surgeon-guided, customized treatments: arcuate keratotomies [11], diagonal ablations [12], and masked ablations with different masking agents [13, 14] are only some of the different primitive surgical modalities for the correction of gross aberrations after complicated photorefractive treatments. However, all these techniques were proved to have limited success in only a minority of the treated patients and are currently abandoned.

Topography-driven treatments gave a reasonably effective surgical tool for the management of those eyes combining videokeratography and subsequent topography-based, ablation-customized patterns. Cited manuscripts [15–20] exploring this approach appeared in the literature in the late 1990s, and new studies keep being published in peer-reviewed literature. Clinical data suggest that this modality works clinically; however, the results also show that despite the clinical improvement of the reported series, there is considerable undercorrection especially in highly irregular corneas.

The main drawbacks of this technology are the missing direct link between the corneal topography and the laser treatment, as well as the questionable ability of the clinically used topographic systems to provide accurate captures of highly irregular corneas (Fig. 7.1.3). It is not only the probable underestimation of corneal irregularities by corneal topographers, but also as Roberts [21, 22] emphasized the limitations of measuring aspherical surfaces such

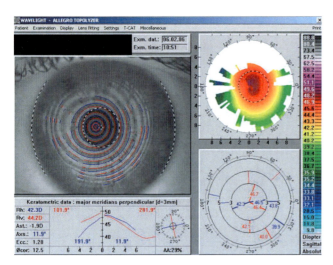

Fig. 7.1.3 Corneal topography of a patient referred for management of line loss and significant visual complaints after hyperopic correction. Due to highly distorted cornea, capture of a reliable corneal topography was not feasible excluding patient for a topographic-guided treatment (notice the small number of data points on the map). Wavefront capture of this eye was not possible

as the human cornea, using spherically biased (axial) computerized reconstructions.

Clinical experience showed that much like corneal topographers, wavefront analyzers also have limitations in measuring highly aberrated eyes [9, 23], and that the calculated refraction even in the successful captures of those eyes does not correlate well with manifest refraction. As shown by the study of Chalita et al., wavefront refraction has poor correlation with manifest and cycloplegic refraction in post-LASIK eyes. As opposed to 85% matching when examining virgin eyes, the mean match percentage in a post-LASIK group of 105 eyes was only 51%, suggesting that the remaining 49% would represent the high-order aberrations affecting the vision [9].

Furthermore, any customized photorefractive correction based on wavefront-guided data requires much deeper tissue excision; thus, corneal anatomical limitation can be another drawback for this kind of retreatments.

Despite the theoretical advantage of the wavefront-guided treatments over the topography guided corrections, the similar inherent problems of both modalities, as well as the unquestionable dramatic effect of a previously complicated correction on the eye's optics, still keeps topography-guided approach in the top list of surgical modalities for the management of previous decentered ablations.

However, a medical general rule is "prevention is the best cure." New generation laser systems minimize, if not eliminate, the incidence of decentered ablations and have minimized night vision complaints of conventional treatments. Preliminary results from wavefront-guided treatments in virgin eyes suggest that this modality may further reduce night vision complaints and optical disturbances after photorefractive corrections. Further improvement of clinically used imaging systems and probably real-time abla-

tion-capturing combinations may enable us in the future to achieve "super" postoperative optics, even in highly aberrated eyes.

Take-Home Pearls

- Careful patient selection remains mandatory for optimal visual results following photorefractive corrections.
- Even with the use of latest generation lasers caution should be paid in patients with both large mesopic pupils and high (>6.00 D) attempted corrections as these seem to be at higher risk for postoperative poor vision and night vision complaints.

References

1. Gartry DS, Kerr Muir MG, Marshall J (1991) Photorefractive keratectomy with an argon fluoride excimer laser: a clinical study. J Refract Corneal Surg 7:420–435
2. O' Bart DP, Lohmann CP, Fitzke FW et al (1994) Discrimination between the origins and functional implications of haze and halo at night after photorefractive keratectomy. J Refract Corneal Surg 10(Suppl):S281
3. Yamane N, Miyata K, Samejima T et al (1004) Ocular high order aberrations and contrast sensitivity after conventional laser in situ keratomileusis. Invest Ophthalmol Vis Sci 45:3986–3989
4. Holladay JT, Dudeja DR, Chang J (1999) Functional vision and corneal changes after laser in situ keratomileusis determined by contrast sensitivity, glare testing and corneal topography. J Cataract Refract Surg. 25:663–669
5. Hiatt AJ, Grant CN, Boxer Waxler BS (2005) Establishing analysis parameters for spherical aberration after Wavefront LASIK. Ophthalmology 112:998–1002
6. Pop M, Payete Y (2004) Risk factors for night vision complaints after LASIK for myopia. Ophthalmology 111:3–10
7. Holladay JT, Janes JA (2002) Topographic changes in corneal asphericity and effective optical zone size after laser in situ keratomileusis. J Cataract Refract Surg 28:942–7
8. Boxer Wachler BS, Huynh VN, El Shiaty AF et al (2002) Evaluation of corneal functional optical zone after laser in situ keratomileusis. J Cataract Refract Surg 28:948–953
9. Chalita MR, Chavala S, Xu, Krueger RR (2004) Wavefront Analysis in post LASIK eyes and its correlation with visual symptoms, refraction and topography. Ophthalmology 111:447–453
10. Tuan KM, Chernyak D, Fedman ST (2006) Predicting patients' night vision complaints with wavefront technology. Arch Ophth 141:1–6
11. Pallikaris IG, Siganos DS, Katsanevaki VJ (1998) LASIK complications and their management. In: Pallikaris IG, Siganos DS (eds) LASIK. Slack, Thorofare, N.J., pp 257–274
12. Alkara N, Genth U, Seiler T (1999) Diametral ablation: a technique to manage decentered photorefractive keratectomy for myopia. J Refract Surg 15:436–440
13. Alio JL, Artola A, Rodriguez-Mier FA (2000) Selective zonal ablation with excimer laser for the correction of the irregular astigmatism induced by refractive surgery. Ophthalmology 107:662–673
14. Pallikaris IG, Katsanevaki VJ (2000) Management of eccentric ablations. In: McRae SM, Krueger RR, Applegate RA (eds) Customized corneal ablation: the quest for supervision. Slack, Thorofare, N.J., pp 293–298

15. Alessio G, Boscia F, La Tegola MG, Sborgia C (2001) Topography-driven excimer laser for the retreatment of decentralized myopic photorefractive keratectomy. Ophthalmology 108:1695–1703

16. Alessio G, Boscia F, La Tegola MG, Sborgia C (2001) Corneal interactive programmed topographic ablation customized photorefractive keratectomy for correction of postkeratoplasty astigmatism. Ophthalmology 108:2029–2037

17. Knorz MC, Jendritza B (2000) Topographically guided laser in situ keratomileusis to treat corneal irregularities. Ophthalmology 107:1138–1143

18. Knorz MC, Neuhann T (2000) Treatment of myopia and myopic astigmatism by customized laser in situ keratomileusis based on corneal topography. Ophthalmology 107:2072–2076

19. Alessio G, Boscia F, La Tegola MG, Sborgia C (2000) Topography-driven photorefractive keratectomy: results of corneal interactive programmed topographic ablations software. Ophthalmology 107:1578–1587

20. Kymionis GD, Panagopoulou SI, Aslanides IM, Plainis S, Astyrakakis N, Pallikaris IG (2004) Topographically supported customized ablation for the management of decentered laser in situ keratomileusis Am J Ophthalmol 137:806–811

21. Roberts C (1994) Characterization of the inherent error in a spherically-biased corneal topography system in mapping a radially aspheric surface. J Refract Corneal Surg 10:103–116

22. Roberts C (1995) Analysis of the inherent error of the TMS-1 topographic modeling system in mapping a radially aspheric surface. Cornea 14:258–265

23. Mrochen M, Krueger RR, Bueeler M, Seiler T (2002) Aberration sensing and wavefront guided laser in situ keratomileusis: management of decentered ablation. J Refract Surg 18:418–429

Core Messages

■ Night vision disturbances are among the most important complaints after refractive surgery. They vary from patient to patient, limiting normal activities such as night driving.

■ No established gold standard clinical test exists to quantify night vision disturbances. Subjective questionnaires are the most commonly used method.

■ Night vision disturbances are multifactorial, caused by different factors. The existence of significant levels of higher-order aberrations after refractive surgery is one of these key factors.

■ The use of optimized aspherical ablations may prevent, or reduce, spherical aberration after keratorefractive surgery.

■ The topography-guided refractive surgery is the best method for minimizing higher-order aberrations that occur in symptomatic post-refractive surgery patients.

7.2 Night Vision Disturbances after Refractive Surgery

César Albarrán, David Piñero, and Jorge L. Alió

7.2.1 Introduction

A number of photorefractive surgery patients, with none or minimal residual spherocylindrical error and good vision measured by means of high-contrast visual acuity or contrast sensitivity, are not fully satisfied with their post-surgery quality of vision due to disturbances occurring at night, such as glare or halos. The expression "night vision" points to a large illumination range divided into two zones, scotopic (from 10^{-6} to 10^{-3} cd/m^2) and mesopic (from 10^{-3} to 3 cd/m^2). This wide range of illumination is one of the main sources of visual complaints in patients after uncomplicated LASIK surgery. Thus, in a recent study, the most common subjective visual complaint in patients seeking consultation after refractive surgery was blurred far vision (59%), followed by night vision disturbances (43.5%).

The terminology of night vision is confusing, since there is a wide range of symptoms affecting the quality of vision at low illumination levels, which are all described as "night vision disturbances" or "night vision complaints." Night vision disturbances involve glare, halos, starburst, and ghosting.

Glare is the inability of looking at a light source, which appears too bright for the patient, making it difficult to see a sharp image of objects.

Halos are perceived as globes of illuminated fog surrounding light sources. This pattern is typically perceived when looking at street lamps or car lamps at night.

Starburst image refers to a radial scatter of light from a point source, like fine light filaments radiating from the light source.

Ghosting is a double perceived image seen even monocularly.

Starburst and ghosted images are related to refractive surgery, whereas glare and halos are often experienced by myopes wearing glasses and/or contact lenses, without having undergone refractive surgery.

Apart from the former disturbances, some post-photorefractive surgery patients may also experience some loss in contrast under dim lighting conditions, especially when passing from photopic to mesopic or scotopic illuminations.

In the following figure, we can see a comparison of the affect on night driving with vision disturbances (glare in 7.2.1b, halos in 7.2.1c, starbursts in 7.2.1d, ghosting in 7.2.1e, and contrast loss in 7.2.1f), compared with driving without night vision disturbances (in 7.2.1a):

7

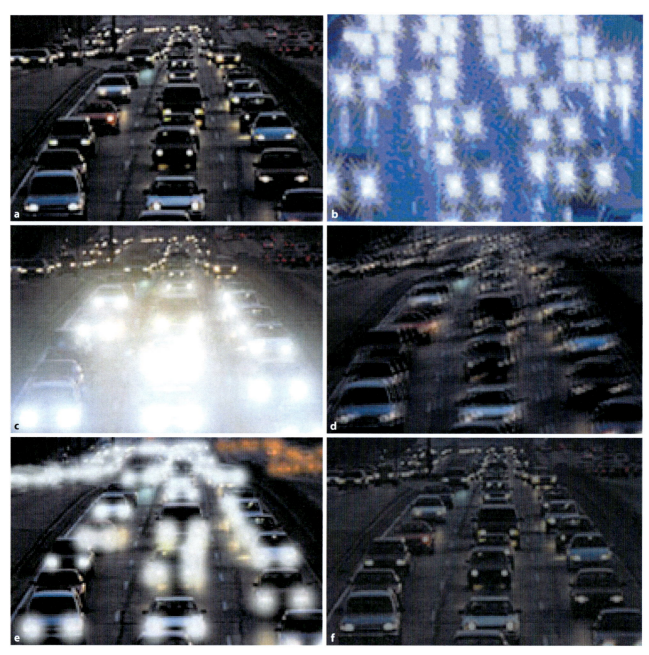

Fig. 7.2.1 Night driving with vision disturbances

7.2.2 Incidence and Measurement

According to some studies, 30% of patients operated by photorefractive keratectomy (PRK) report night vision disturbances to be worse than before surgery, glare and halos being the most frequent complaints. After LASIK, almost 12% of patients experience night vision problems, starburst being the major complaint, followed by halos. Other studies reported no differences in night vision disturbances 1 year after PRK or LASIK.

Night vision symptoms appear to significantly affect night driving, with almost 30% of patients experiencing worsening in their driving capabilities after photorefractive surgery.

In the immediate post-surgery recovery, the vast majority of LASIK patients experience some night vision disturbances, which may even last a few weeks, depending on a number of factors, such as residual refractive error, corneal swelling, and reorganization of the corneal architecture, neural adaptation, ablation diameter, profile, and pupil size, among others. A recent study with LASIK patients evaluated for a 12-month period revealed that overall night vision complaints considerably decreased from 25.6% at 1 month to 4.7% at 12 months postoperatively. This decrease in subjective night vision complaints can be compared with the case of multifocal intraocular lenses. Although halos do not actually disappear, the patients become more tolerant, and the neural adaptation process makes the unwanted images less noticeable.

As for contrast sensitivity and night vision, LASIK induces significant reductions under mesopic conditions only at high spatial frequencies, whereas the low spatial frequencies remain in the same level as in non-operated eyes.

No established gold standard clinical test exists to quantify night vision disturbances, even though several procedures have been proposed. This leads to a dependence on the prevalence and extent of night vision complaints on the chosen methodology, which results in a wide difference of prevalence reports in night vision disturbances. The main reason for this lack of normative methodology goes back to the fact that night vision disturbances are subjective experiences, which may not be easily described by some patients.

The case of cerebral spinal fluid measurement is different because gold standard tests are recognized, such as FACT or VCTS-1000. The most used measurement method for night vision disturbances is the subjective questionnaire, in which patients are asked about their symptoms, which are rated on a given scale. Photos can be used in questionnaires to rate disturbances by comparing several snaps with increasing degrees of the patient's visual symptom. Another simple method to perform a subjective quantification consists of asking the patient to look at a light spot after dark adaptation and drawing any perceived disturbances (halos, starburst, etc.) using a grid (the Amsler chart can be used for this purpose). In addition, there are computer-based methods like Glare & Halos (Tomey AG), which is used to measure the extent of glare and halo. A computer screen is used to show a white, circular light source of 15 mm in diameter with 56-cd/m^2 luminance against a 0.01-cd/m^2 background luminance. The operator controls a cursor that is moved from the periphery toward the halo source in the center of the monitor until the patient indicates that the cursor touches the outer perimeter of the halo. The halo area is then calculated in square degrees (sq deg) by the computer software.

7.2.3 Etiology

The causes for night vision disturbances are undoubtedly multifactorial, including (1) the wound healing process, (2) light scattering, (3) pupil size, (4) amount of correction, (5) ablation diameter and profile, (6) quality of the ablation, (7) quality of the flap, and (8) the individual patient's subjective neural processing and plasticity adaptation to new vision.

The "simple" fact of performing an ablation in a living tissue such as the cornea, which involves a wound-healing process, may lead to night vision complaints. Rays of light being refracted by a healthy human cornea with a well-organized equidistant collagen fibril structure interact in a coherent way, resulting in the reduction and even the elimi-nation of scattered light by destructive interference. Wound healing after excimer laser treatment leads to corneal haze and edema, disturbing this well-organized pattern of collagen fibrils, forming a three-dimensional array of diffraction gratings that causes light scattering. This scattered light is responsible for loss in contrast sensitivity, starburst, glare, and halo effects, and is observed in patients with cataract or keropathy, when the loss of transparency of the optical media of the eye leads to light scattering.

Preoperative large pupil size was the first parameter to be proclaimed as the cause of night vision disturbances after photorefractive surgery. Pupil size has two contradictory effects on the optical quality of any optical system–a larger pupil causes some image degradation in an optically aberrated system, but it also results in less diffraction and higher contrast in a diffraction-limited optical system. The effect of pupil dilation on optical aberrations is believed to be much greater after standard laser refractive surgery.

Early studies reported a high incidence of glare, haze, and halo symptoms 1 month after surgery in patients with large pupils. However, recent evidence suggests that large pupil size is not so critical than previously thought, at least with the latest generation of excimer lasers. Recent studies have reported no statistical correlation between the preoperative pupil size and the development of night vision complaints and visual functions such as visual acuity or contrast sensitivity. Some studies, however, have found that poor visual quality is associated with large pupils in the early postoperative period, but not 6 months after surgery. Other authors have found that scotopic pupil size is not predictive of some night vision disturbances such as halos and glare, but may play an important role in others, such as ghosting and starburst. On the other hand, there are some patients with very small pupils, even less than 4 mm, who have experienced night vision problems. Hence, most current refractive surgeons believe that the role of pupil size has been overrated in patients with low myopia who are treated with larger optical zone ablations.

When patients with night vision disturbances have their pupil size pharmacologically reduced, they report a dramatic reduction in their symptoms. Although the actual role of pupil size in night vision disturbances after photorefractive surgery is still debated, we cannot entirely deny its importance, which is almost coupled with other factors. Recent peer-reviewed literature cites a large pupil size coupled with a small optical zone as a dominant factor leading to increased night vision disturbances. Thus, even though pupil size seems to be a poor predictor for night vision disturbances when considered in isolation. It is a better predictor when coupled with the optical zone treatment, which is considered one of the main factors involved in night vision disturbances after LASIK.

Early PRK was performed using an optical zone of 3–4.5 mm in diameter, but a high incidence of night vision complaints was soon reported, which was reduced by extending the ablation to a 6-mm optical zone. In modern LASIK procedures, multiple regression analyses would predict that an eye with –6.00 D of myopia has a 4% chance of having night vision disturbances at 12 months postoperatively, using a 6.5-mm optical zone treatment. However, this chance would decrease to 1.8% if a 7-mm zone is used. Thus, since correcting high myopia, using small optical zones would result in a higher chance of night vision complaints, it is recommended to avoid the reduction of the optical zone size to minimize corneal depth ablation in high myopic patients.

Some authors proposed that a 1-mm difference between the optical zone and the pupil size should be maintained to lower the incidence of night vision disturbances. Consequently, many surgeons recommend avoiding LASIK surgery in patients whose pupil size is greater than the possible treatment optical zone. This seems obvious since if the measured pupil diameter is greater than the ablation zone, then two focal points are generated by the cornea, one by the central ablated zone and the second by the peripheral untreated cornea, causing degradation in the image quality because there are two overlapped images in the retina, in focus and out of focus.

The amount of attempted correction has also been proposed as an important factor affecting night vision. It is related to the amount of ablated tissue. The higher the preoperative refraction, the higher the amount of ablated tissue, and so the higher the distortion in the well-organized collagen fibril structure, resulting in a higher light scattering. However, the amount of attempted correction is also related to the size of the optical zone treatment, the higher the myopic correction, the smaller the effective size of the treated area. Studies about the relationship of the amount of refraction to be corrected and the effective size of the optical zone treatment state that, even setting the same laser adjustment for an optical zone of 6.5 mm, an ablation of $-10\,D$ results in a 25% less effective treatment size zone than does a -1.00-D ablation.

The ablation profile is an important factor. A blend zone that smoothes the transition between the treated and the untreated cornea helps to minimize night vision complaints. This may be due to achieving a larger treatment area and a more gradual transition at the edge of ablation. The blend adjustment in photorefractive surgery has shown to reduce spherical aberration of operated eyes, which can also be one of the reasons for a decrease in night vision complaints. Hence, the newer ablation algorithms not only attempt to maximize the optical zone, but also achieve a smoother transition zone to blend the principal curvature of the optical zone into the curvature of the peripheral untreated cornea. Recent studies reveal that 74% of patients perceived more glare with an eye operated on with a single ablation zone than with an eye operated on with a blend transition zone. The only negative feature of using a blend zone is an increase of about 20% in the required ablation depth.

Wavefront technology has an important role in the reduction of night vision complaints. Higher-order aberrations have been observed to increase after both PRK and standard LASIK and may be responsible for night vision problems. Since optical aberrations generally increase with increasing pupil sizes, aberrations can misdirect light into the eye and can result in symptoms such as glare and haze affecting night vision, when the pupil dilates. Improvement in ablation profiles to reduce higher-order aberrations, especially coma and spherical aberration, can reduce these complaints and improve the quality of vision and increase satisfaction in postoperative patients.

The qualities of the flap and stromal bed are also important parameters to be taken into account. Halos, starburst, and ghosting can occur when the corneal flap does not adhere correctly to the eye after it is replaced. In such cases, there can be areas in the cornea in which the imperfect adherence can act as a sort of plane–parallel plate, creating a double image or ghosting.

In summary, refractive surgeons should not rely solely on the pupil size as the predictor of night vision problems since recent literature finds little or no correlation with night vision complaints, at least with modern laser algorithms that optimize optical and transition zone sizes.

Neural plasticity must be considered as a factor for night vision complaint acceptance, and patience must be considered, in some cases, as the best method to treat some night vision disturbances.

7.2.4 Treatment

As it has been pointed before, one of the main causes of night vision disturbances, such as halos or glare, after refractive surgery using the excimer laser is the induction of higher-order aberrations with the surgery itself. These aberrations make the retinal image more distorted, with a clear lack of focus. From all the aberrometric components, the primary spherical aberration and coma are annoying errors that occur more frequently in the eye after refractive surgery. The coma aberration is related to decentered treatments, where an asymmetry is present in the cornea. This is one complication that can be seen in some cases after refractive surgery, and it could be due to a lack of fixation from the patient, a wrong selection of the point of centration, or a poor control of the fixation of the patient by the surgeon. This produces an enlargement of the image light distribution along an axis, generating a comet-like image of a point light object.

In uncomplicated eyes after refractive surgery, the most frequent aberration is the spherical aberration. The primary spherical aberration is a higher-order aberration corresponding to the fourth order of the Zernike decomposition. This error is due to the difference of refractive power between the central and the peripheral area of the optical ocular system (between the ablated and the non-ablated area), where all the light rays passing through the system do not focus at the same point. Several light rays will be focused in front of the retinal plane, whereas others will be focused behind it. This phenomenon generates a concentric circle of blurred light around the focused point or halo. The halo generated is more significant with higher aperture of the system (the pupil diameter), because the aberrated peripheral area has a greater impact on the retinal image. Obviously, this optical situation induces significant disturbances and discomfort in the patient, especially under scotopic conditions.

The ablation shape performed by the excimer laser in order to compensate a refractive error, following the Munnerlyn's equation or algorithms derived from it, unavoidably induces positive spherical aberration. This effect is produced by the flattening of the corneal curvature, without taking into account the preoperative aspherical shape of the cornea. There is a significant reduction of the central refractive power of the optical ocular system but an increment in the periphery (Fig. 7.2.2a, b). This effect is magnified when the degree of myopia to correct is larger because the refractive difference between center and periphery is

more acute, as commented before. New ablation profiles, using aspherical geometry, have been developed in order to achieve a minimizing algorithm for not inducing positive spherical aberration with myopic ablations. This new technology has shown effective results and promising new applications. However, the problem is how to solve former cases with high degrees of spherical aberration caused by the use of classic ablation profiles.

On the other hand, the ablation for the compensation of hyperopia is peripheral. The laser removes tissue in a concentric peripheral area in order to achieve an increase of the central corneal curvature. Then, in an opposite situation, with this kind of ablation an increase of the negative spherical aberration is produced. Therefore, there will be a significant difference in refractive power between the cen-

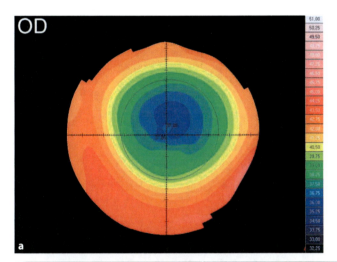

Fig. 7.2.2 Corneal topography and aberrometry after a myopic LASIK, performed with a classic ablation profile. **a** Corneal topography. The difference in curvature can be clearly seen between the central and the peripheral area. **b** Corneal aberrometry. *Top left*, total wavefront map. To the *right* of the image the decomposition, in components, of the total wavefront is shown. From *left to right* and from *top to bottom*, the astigmatism map, the spherical aberration map, the coma map and, the residual higher-order error map can be seen. All maps are calculated for a pupil of 6 mm. The spherical aberration map shows a greater deformation of the wavefront in a peripheral concentric area

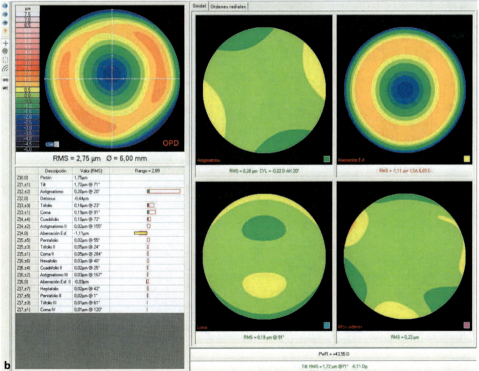

tral and the peripheral area of the cornea. Specifically, the central area of the ocular optical system has greater refractive power than the peripheral (Fig. 7.2.3a, b). Obviously, this also induces the presence of a disturbing halo, which is magnified under scotopic conditions (larger pupil size). As for myopia, it has also been designed with algorithms with aspherical ablation profiles in order to avoid the induction of spherical aberration. As for myopia, the problem is how to solve former cases with high degrees of spherical aberration caused by the use of classic ablation profiles.

We must take into account other factors–more difficult to analyze–that contribute to the induction of spherical aberration. Some of these factors could be the loss of efficiency when the laser ray meets the peripheral cornea, the epithelial healing, or the biomechanical response of the corneal structure.

7.2.4.1 Optimized Ablation Profiles

The optimized ablation profiles have become a standard way to proceed when refractive surgery with excimer laser is performed. It is a method for minimizing the induction of spherical aberration inherent in ablation profiles based on classic algorithms (such as the Munnerlyn equation).

It is well known that the anterior corneal surface is not spherical. There is a progressive flattening of the cornea toward the periphery. It is an aspherical surface. Therefore, it makes no sense to use an ablation profile based on the generation of a spherical surface. A profile like this will theoretically create a spherical cornea in the optical zone, but with a significant abrupt transition step between ablated and nonablated areas (oblate profile). New designs of the ablation

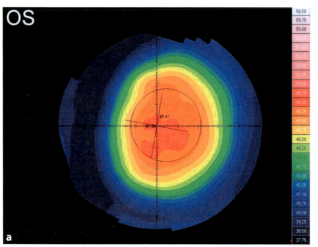

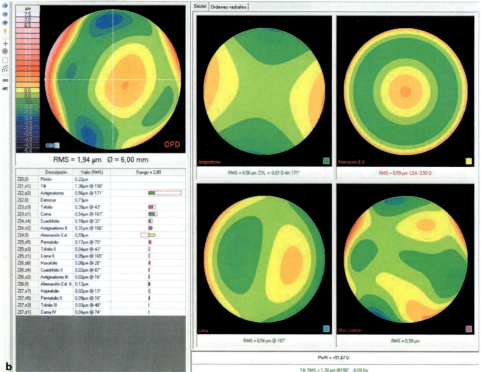

Fig. 7.2.3 Corneal topography and aberrometry after a hyperopic LASIK, performed with a classic ablation profile. **a** Corneal topography. The difference in curvature can be clearly seen between the central and the peripheral area. **b** Corneal aberrometry. *Top left,* total wavefront map. To the *right* of the image the decomposition, in components, of the total wavefront is shown. From *left to right* and from *top to bottom,* the astigmatism map, the spherical aberration map, the coma map, and the residual higher-order error map can be seen. All maps are calculated for a pupil of 6 mm. The spherical aberration map shows a greater deformation of the wavefront in a central area

have been developed in order to avoid this effect. These designs are aspherical and they try to reproduce the physiologic prolateness of the cornea, providing a gradual and progressive transition between ablated and non-ablated zones.

Nowadays, there are several commercially available refractive surgery platforms with specific software for generating aspherical ablation profiles (Fig. 7.2.4a, b). Different studies have proved the efficacy and safety of these kinds of treatments. Examples of these commercially available systems are the following: CATz from Nidek, CRS-Master from Zeiss, ORK-CAM from Schwind, Custom-Q from Wavelight, etc.

7.2.4.2 Customized Ablation Profiles

The use of an optimized aspherical profile is a first level of customization, because we are taking into account the prolateness of the cornea. However, when we talk about customized treatments, we are usually referring to tailored treatments with a high level of customization. In these cases, the distribution of the excimer laser energy is asymmetric in order to ablate more tissue from specific corneal areas. The final objective is to decrease the optical aberrations to a physiological level. This way, the patient will reach a high quality of vision increasing the level of satisfaction.

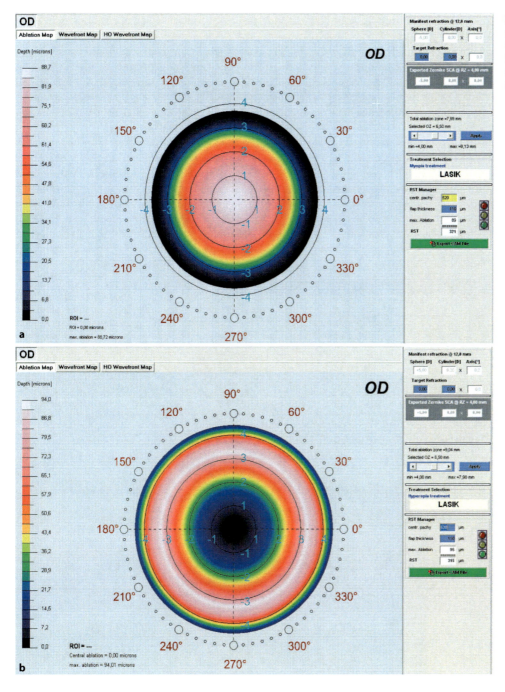

Fig. 7.2.4 Aspherical profile designed by means of the ORK-CAM software from Schwind. **a** Myopic aspherical ablation profile. **b** Hyperopic aspherical ablation profile

7

Several studies have showed the applicability and the benefits of using these customized systems.

There are two methods for customizing the ablation, ocular and corneal customization. For ocular customization, it is necessary to measure the aberrations of the entire ocular optical system, taking into account the cornea and the lens. With these data and the corneal topography, an ablation for minimizing the second- and the higher-order aberrations could be designed.

This approach is less effective in patients with large amounts of corneal aberrations due to previous refractive surgery, whether uncomplicated classic algorithms or following surgical complications during LASIK, corneal scars, or wounds. One explanation for this fact is the inability of some wavefront sensors or aberrometers to accurately measure high levels of aberrations. This is especially true for wavefront sensors that subdivide the wavefront and take the measurements simultaneously. Crowding or superimposing of the light spots associated to different parts of the wavefront is produced when we are analyzing a highly aberrated eye. In such cases, the reliability of the measurements is reduced. In addition, with some kind of sensors it is assumed that the slope of the wavefront in each portion analyzed is locally flat. This approach induces significant errors in the final calculated results. Then, it is a better option in highly aberrated corneas to retreat using ablation based on corneal customization or topography guided. In these cases, we must take into account that the anterior corneal surface is the aberrated element, normally by a previous surgical procedure,

and additionally this surface supposes the greatest refractive contribution to the total refractive power. There are different topography systems, with specific software, that calculate and show the aberrations associated to the anterior corneal surface. The elevation data from topography is transformed into aberration components by means of the decomposition of Zernike polynomials. Nowadays, several topography systems have the option of providing the corneal aberrometry as the CSO system (CSO) or Keratron (Optikon).

One of the commercially available software for the calculation of customized ablations is the ORK-CAM software from Schwind (Schwind Eye-Tech-Solutions, Kleinostheim, Germany). This tool allows us to design and program different kinds of customized ablations by previously loading the topography data from the CSO. The treatment designed is loaded in the Esiris excimer laser machine (Schwind) in order to perform the treatment. This laser is a flying-spot system with a para-Gaussian spot of 0.8 mm of diameter, and it is combined with a very fast eye-tracker system with a frequency of 330 Hz. For these customized systems, the use of small spots for ablating small selective corneal areas is crucial, as well as an ultrafast eye-tracker system in order to avoid the improper orientation of the laser beam and the inadequate ablation of some zones.

The procedure for calculating ORK-CAM ablations is very simple: the corneal topography is acquired and exported, and then the file created is imported to the ORK-CAM software. Some clinical data must be introduced: the age of the patient, the subjective spherocylindrical refraction, the

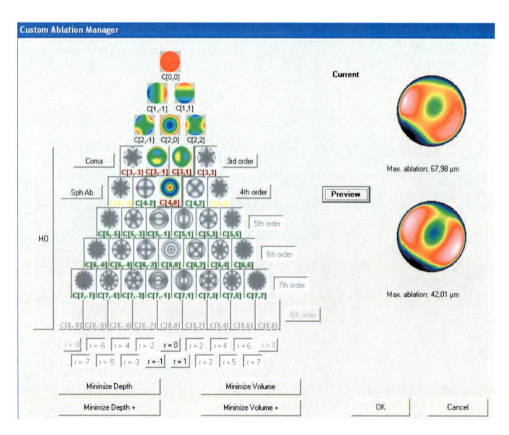

Fig. 7.2.5 Selection in the ORK-CAM software (Schwind) of the Zernike components for treatment during the ablation design process. We observed that the correction of the combination primary coma and spherical aberration is highly effective and very satisfying for the patient in almost 100% of cases

central corneal pachymetry, and the flap pachymetry. An ablation profile is generated with all these data, and this can be modified by the specialist to reach the best adequate profile for a specific case. The optical zone could be modified according to the pachymetry. Additionally, specific terms from the Zernike decomposition could be chosen for the treatment (Fig. 7.2.5). Modifying the optical zone and the number of Zernike terms treated, the ablation profile could be customized in order to get the more appropriate profile according to the corneal shape and the refractive error.

In the following section, we show the results obtained by us with this surgical option in patients with high levels of positive spherical aberration. These results are extracted from a paper submitted for publication in the journal *Ophthalmology*.

A total of 40 eyes (27 patients) previously operated with a primary spherical aberration coefficient (Z_4^0) equal or higher than 0.5 underwent LASIK surgery using the excimer laser Esiris and a topographic-guided customized ablation designed by means of the ORK-CAM software. All of them complained of night vision disturbances or lack of visual quality with and without optical correction of the residual error.

Figure 7.2.6 shows a summary of the refractive results obtained with this procedure. No complications occurred during and after the surgery. The efficacy and safety levels achieved were excellent, 0.87±0.23 and 1±0.25 respectively.

We found a statistically significant reduction of the primary spherical aberration 3 months after surgery ($p < 0.001$) (Fig. 7.2.7). This reduction was significantly greater

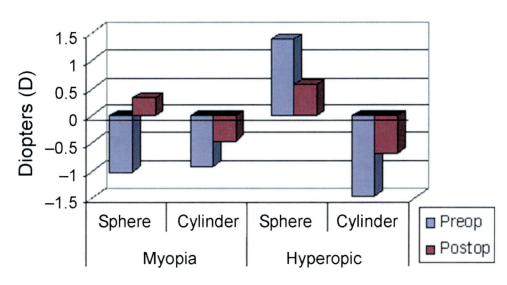

Fig. 7.2.6 Summary of the refractive outcomes obtained in patients with high levels of primary spherical aberrations and treated with a topographic-guided ablation designed with the ORK-CAM system (Schwind). We divided the results in myopic and hyperopic patients

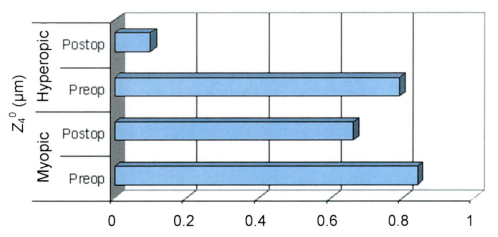

Fig. 7.2.7 Changes in the primary spherical aberration coefficient after refractive surgery with corneal customization. We divided the results in myopic and hyperopic patients

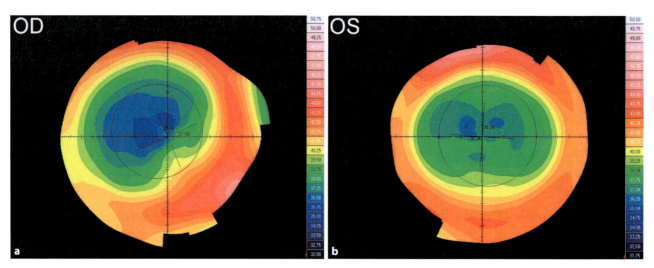

Fig. 7.2.8 Clinical case: preoperative corneal topography obtained by the CSO system. **a** Right eye, **b** left eye

in the hyperopic patients. This is logical because the ablation itself for correcting the hyperopia induces a compensation of the positive spherical aberration because the ablation is ring shaped and concentric. However, the myopic ablation itself produces positive spherical aberration, making the efficacy of the ablation not so effective.

Concerning the negative spherical aberration, we have few cases (12 eyes) with high levels of this defect, and all of them are myopes. In these cases, after the treatment, there is a very slight reduction of the primary spherical aberration, and it is not statistically significant. No clear improvement of the visual quality was observed, and it seems that improvements in the algorithms for these cases are necessary. Anyway, we must take into account that the number of eyes treated is small and a larger sample is necessary for obtaining firm conclusions.

7.2.4.3 Example of Topographic-Guided Customization

Patient underwent LASIK surgery 1 year ago for correction of moderate myopia in both eyes. He complains of lack of clarity in his vision and difficulties with night driving. He has worn glasses for driving, but it felt awkward.

These are the results of the ophthalmologic examination. Preoperative exam (06/02/2006):

■ Uncorrected visual acuity (UCVA): OD (right eye), 0.7; OS (left eye), 0.9
  Subjective refraction and best-corrected visual acuity (BSCVA):
  – OD, +1.00 –1.00 × 45°; BSCVA, 1
  – OS, +1.25 –0.50 × 150°; BSCVA, 1
■ Corneal topography: see Fig. 7.2.8a, b
■ Corneal asphericity (*Q*) over the central 4.5 mm: OD, 1.70; OS, 1.24

■ Corneal aberrations (Fig. 7.2.9a, b): significant level of primary spherical aberration
  – Z4^0: OD, 0.82 μm; OS, 0.68 μm
  – Primary coma root mean square (RMS): OD, 0.52 μm; OS, 0.34 μm
  – Residual higher-order RMS: OD, 0.37 μm; OS, 0.32 μm
  – Strehl ratio: OD, 0.11; OS, 0.14
■ Scotopic pupil (Procyon): OD, 6.75 mm; OS, 6.82 mm
■ Biomicroscopy: LASIK both eyes, anterior segment OK
  Surgery (08/03/2006):
■ Treatment plan: see Fig. 7.2.10a, b. The correction of the primary coma and spherical aberration is programmed in the right eye, whereas in the left eye the correction of the primary spherical aberration is only programmed. In addition, in both eyes the spherocylindrical error was planned for correction.
■ The lift of the flap and the laser retreatment is performed with the following parameters:
  – Optical zone: OD, 7 mm; OS, 7 mm
  – Total ablation diameter: OD, 7.92 mm; OS, 7.98 mm
  Three months postoperatively (12/06/2006):
■ UCVA: OD, 0.95; OS, 1.00
■ Subjective refraction and BSCVA:
  – OD: +0.50 –0.50 × 110°; BSCVA, 0.95
  – OS, +0.50 spherical; BSCVA, 1.00
■ Corneal topography: see Fig. 7.2.11a, b
■ *Q* over the central 4.5 mm: OD, 0.94; OS, –0.20
■ Corneal aberrations (Fig. 7.2.12a, b): no significant level of higher-order aberrations
  – Z4^0: OD, 0.37 μm; OS, 0.17 μm
  – Primary coma RMS: OD, 0.10 μm; OS, 0.33 μm
  – Primary residual higher-order RMS: OD, 0.33 μm; OS. 0.32 μm
  – Strehl ratio: OD, 0.13; OS, 0.15

7

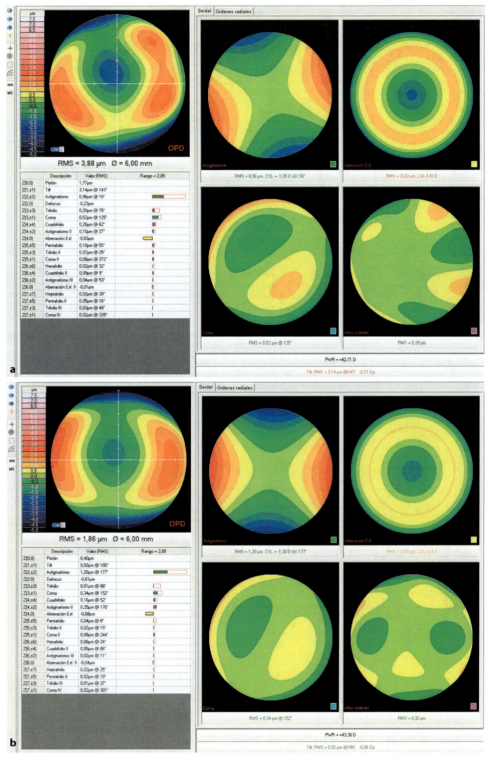

Fig. 7.2.9 Clinical case: preoperative corneal aberrometry obtained by the CSO system. **a** Right eye: significant level of primary coma and spherical aberration. **b** Left eye: significant level of primary spherical aberration, although smaller than to corresponding right eye

- Biomicroscopy: LASIK both eyes without problems, anterior segment OK

An improvement in UCVA and quality of vision was observed. Reducing the positive spherical aberration increased the corneal asphericity and provided the cornea with a more prolate shape. The patient is satisfied, reporting a significant subjective improvement.

7

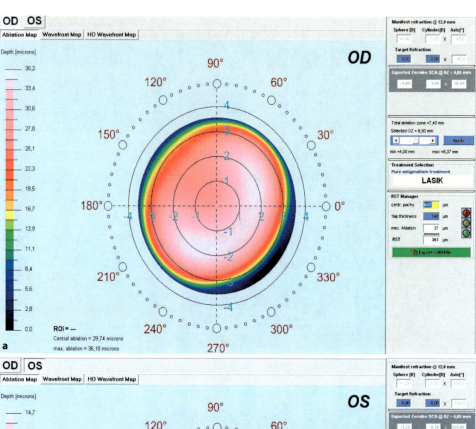

a

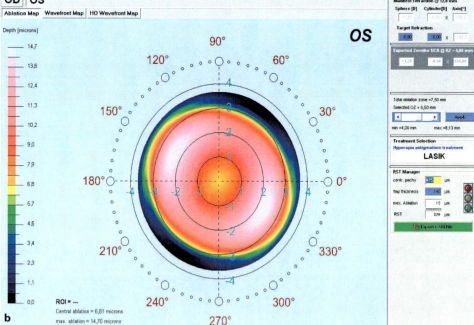

b

Fig. 7.2.10 Clinical case: ablation profiles obtained by the ORK-CAM software. **a** Right eye: correction of the primary coma and spherical aberration. **b** Left eye: correction of the primary spherical aberration; it can be seen that the ablation is circular and peripheral in order to reduce the excessive refractive power of that area

Take-Home Pearls

■ One of the most common subjective complaints after refractive surgery with the excimer laser is night vision disturbances.

■ These night vision disturbances include glare, halos, starburst, and ghosting, and they could dramatically affect common tasks such as night driving.

■ The generation of these night vision disturbances is multifactorial, including the wound healing process, pupil size, and amount of correction or the existence of significant levels of higher-order aberrations.

■ The use of the optimized aspherical ablation profiles is a way of preventing the induction of significant amounts of spherical aberration.

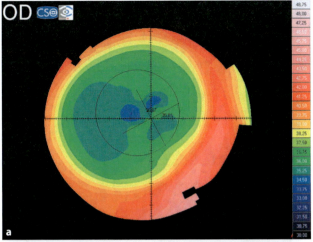

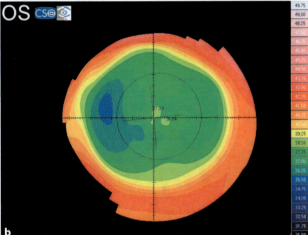

Fig. 7.2.11 Clinical case: postoperative corneal topography obtained by the CSO system. The widening of the optical zone can be seen with the non-ablated area out from the pupillary area. **a** Right eye, **b** left eye

- Cases with very high levels of spherical aberrations could be corrected by means of a topography-guided ablation, which attempts to distribute the laser energy in order to ablate specific tissue areas.
- The correction of positive spherical aberration with the ORK-CAM system from Schwind seems to be more effective in hyperopic eyes.

Bibliography

Albarran-Diego C, Munoz G, Montes-Mico R, Rodriguez A, Alio JL (2006) Corneal aberration changes alter hyperopic LASIK: a comparison between the VISX Star S2 and the Asclepion-Meditec MEL 70 G Scan excimer lasers. J Refract Surg 2:34–42

Carones F, Vigo L, Scandola E (2006) Wavefront-guided treatment of symptomatic eyes using the LADAR6000 excimer laser. J Refract Surg 22:S983–S989

Carones F, Vigo L, Scandola E (2003) Wavefront-guided treatment of abnormal eyes using the LADARVision platform. J Refract Surg 19:S703–S708

El-Danasoury A, Bains HS (2005) Optimized prolate corneal ablation: case report of the first treated eye. J Refract Surg 21(5 Suppl):S598–S602

Gatinel D, Malet J, Hoang-Xuan T, Azar DT (2004) Corneal asphericity change after excimer laser hyperopic surgery: theoretical effects on corneal profiles and corresponding Zernike expansions. Invest Ophthalmol Vis Sci 45:1349–1359

Gatinel D, Malet J, Hoang-Xuan T, Azar DT (2002) Analysis of customized corneal ablations: theoretical limitations of increasing negative asphericity. Invest Ophthalmol Vis Sci 43:941–948

Hersh PS, Fry K, Blaker JW (2003) Spherical aberration after laser in situ keratomileusis and photorefractive keratectomy. Clinical results and theoretical models of etiology. J Cataract Refract Surg 29:2096–2104

Hori-Komai Y, Toda I, Asano-Kato N, Ito M, Yamamoto T, Tsubota K (2006) Comparison of LASIK using the NIDEK EC-5000 optimized aspheric transition zone (OATz) and conventional ablation profile. J Refract Surg 22:546–555

Jankov MR, Panagopoulou SI, Tsiklis NS, Hajitanasis GC, Aslanides M, Pallikaris G (2006) Topography-guided treatment of irregular astigmatism with the wavelight excimer laser. J Refract Surg 22:335–344

Kanjani N, Jacob S, Agarwal A, Agarwal A, Agarwal S, Agarwal T, Doshi A, Doshi S (2004) Wavefrontand topography-guided ablation in myopic eyes using Zyoptix. J Cataract Refract Surg 30:398–402

Kermani O, Schmiedt K, Oberheide U, Gerten G (2003) Early results of Nidek customized aspheric transition zones (CATz) in laser in situ keratomileusis. J Refract Surg 19(2 Suppl):S190–S194

Koller T, Iseli HP, Hafezi F, Mrochen M, Seiler T (2006) Q-factor customized ablation profile for the correction of myopic astigmatism. J Cataract Refract Surg 32:584–589

Lin DY, Manche EE (2004) Custom-contoured ablation pattern method for the treatment od decentered laser ablations. J Cataract Refract Surg 30:1675–1684

Llorente L, Barbero S, Merayo J, Marcos S (2004) Total and corneal optical aberrations induced by laser in situ keratomileusis for hyperopia. J Refract Surg 20:203–216

Manns F, Ho A, Parel JM, Culbertson W (2002) Ablation profiles for wavefront-guided correction of myopia and primary spherical aberration. J Cataract Refract Surg 28:766–74

Mantry S, Yeung I, Shah S (2004) Aspheric ablation with the Nidek EC-5000 CXII with OPD-Scan objective analysis. J Refract Surg 20(5 Suppl):S666–S668

Marcos S, Cano D, Barbero S (2003) Increase in corneal asphericity after standard laser in situ keratomileusis for myopia is not inherent to the Munnerlyn algorithm. J Refract Surg 19:S592–S596

Mastropasqua L, Toto L, Zuppardi E, Nubile M, Carpineto P, Di Nicola M, Ballone E (2006) Photorefractive keratectomy with aspheric profile of ablation versus convencional photorefractive keratectomy for myopia correction: six-month controlled clinical trial. J Cataract Refract Surg 32:109–116

Mrochen M, Donitzky C, Wullner C, Loffler J (2004) Wavefront-optimized ablation profiles: theoretical background. J Cataract Refract Surg 30:775–785

Reinstein DZ, Neal DR, Vogelsang H, Schroeder E, Nagy ZZ, Bergt M, Copland J, Topa D (2004) Optimized and wavefront guided corneal refractive surgery using the Carl Zeiss Meditec platform: the WASCA aberrometer, CRS-Master, and MEL80 excimer laser. Ophthalmol Clin North Am 17:191–210

Sarkisian KA, Petrov AA (2002) Clinical experience with the customized low spherical aberration ablation profile for myopia. J Refract Surg 18(3 Suppl):S352–S356

7

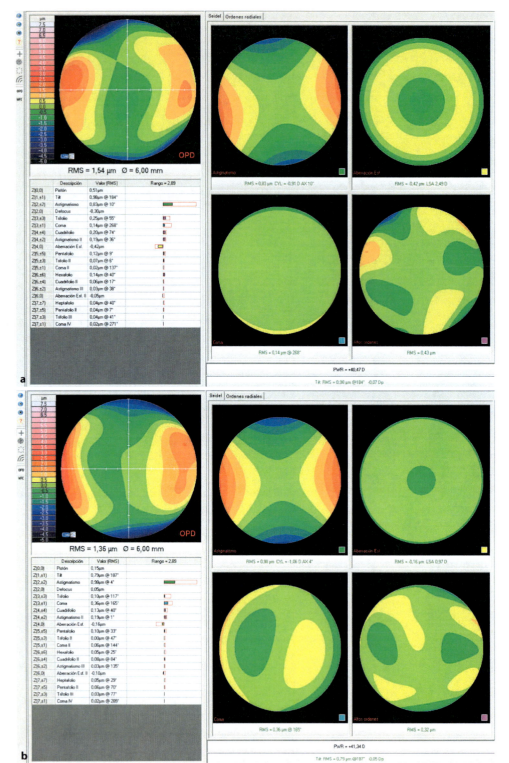

Fig. 7.2.12 Clinical case: postoperative corneal aberrometry obtained by the CSO system. Physiologic levels of higher order aberrations. **a** Right eye, **b** left eye

Vinciguerra P, Camesasca FI, Calossi A (2003) Statistical analysis of physiological aberrations of the cornea. J Refract Surg 19 (Suppl):S265–S269

Vinciguerra P, Munoz MI, Camesasca FI (2002) Reduction of spherical aberration: experimental model of photoablation. J Refract Surg 18(3 Suppl):S366–S370

Yeung IY, Mantry S, Cunliffe IA, Benson MT, Shah S (2004) Higher order aberrations with aspheric ablations using the Nidek EC-5000 CXII laser. J Refract Surg 20(5 Suppl):S659–S662

Yoon G, Macrae S, Williams DR, Cox IG (2005) Causes of spherical aberration induced by laser refractive surgery. J Cataract Refract Surg 31:127–135

Core Messages

■ Prevention is easier (and more effective) than treatment.

■ The accurate centration technique is important: Intraoperative vigilance is needed even with eye tracking.

■ Thorough understanding of laser technology and calibration is essential to prevent errors.

■ Be certain to exclude abnormal wound healing as a cause.

■ Do not rush re-treatment.

7.3 Decentration

Jonathan H. Talamo

7.3.1 Description of the Problem

7.3.1.1 Definition of Centration

Decentration of ablation effect after laser vision correction or other refractive surgical procedures can occur when the effect of surgery results in an unintentional, asymmetric alteration of the eye's optical system, which results in increased higher-order aberrations and causes what was often described in the past as irregular astigmatism. In order to describe decentration after keratorefractive or lenticular refractive surgery, it is important to first define a Take-Home point for the center of the eye's optical system. As described in the classic paper by Uozato in Guyton in 1987 [1], corneal refractive surgical procedures can be centered by using either the corneal light reflex or the pupil center, which represents the line of sight (the line connecting the fixation point with the pupil center, and corresponds to the chief ray of the bundle of light rays passing through the pupil and reaching the fovea) [2]. While there remains some controversy as to which approach is correct (some surgeons advocate for centration based on patient fixation rather that pupil center for patients with large angle kappa measurements), the consensus at this time is that all procedures (corneal or lenticular) should be performed with the goal of centration over the physiologic pupil. Additionally, it is now widely recognized that for astigmatic or wavefront-derived custom laser treatments, the eye should not only be centered with respect to the x–y-axis, but also with respect to the cyclotorsional position of the globe in the upright position, as there may be shifts in this parameter when moving the patient from the upright position used for clinical testing to the supine orientation needed during laser treatment [3]. The major exception to this approach is, of course, the treatment of decentered prior treatments, which is the subject of this chapter. Due to space considerations, we cover only decentration of laser vision-correction procedures.

7.3.1.2 Centering Technique

For the purposes of this chapter, we discuss technique primarily with respect to laser vision-correction procedures, but such an approach can be viewed as valuable for any corneal or lenticular procedure. As the best treatment for decentered laser treatments remains prevention, we first discuss appropriate centering technique.

To most accurately center a corneal laser treatment over the pupil, the patient should be fixating on a target, with a physiologic pupil with the head and eye in an orthogonal position with respect to the laser optics, and fixating on a target that is coaxial with the examiner's sighting eye through the surgeon microscope [4]. To ensure appropriate orientation to the globe from a cyclorotational perspective during treatment, the limbus should be marked at the slit lamp with the patient fixating a target coaxial with the microscope's optics. Generally, marks at 3 and 9, or 6 and 12 o'clock are most helpful. With the advent of wavefront-sensing devices with iris or limbal registration techniques, it may not be necessary in many instances to manually mark the globe, as these devices will allow transmission of information to the excimer laser's eye-tracking system that enable automatic cyclorotational centering, but it is still advisable to mark in case these functions fail to perform during surgery.

Another important consideration for centration is the position of the pupil centroid. As lighting conditions vary, the pupil's centroid shifts along with changes in diameter [5]. If wavefront-capture occurs under dimly lit conditions and centration during surgery under bright illumination, then the pupil centroid may shift, usually nasally. This phenomenon may lead to a decentration of the laser treatment with respect to the pupil centroid in mesopic lighting conditions, under which symptoms such as glare, halo, and starburst, are most pronounced following surgery. Although no data yet exist to prove clinical significance of such an approach, it may be important to control ambient lighting during surgery to mimic mesopic conditions whenever possible if the eye-tracking system being used does not correct for pupil centroid shifts.

7.3.2 Causes of Decentration or Decentration-Like Effect (Pseudo-Decentration)

It is important to distinguish a truly decentered laser ablation from other etiologies (pseudo-decentration), as the appropriate treatment may vary. The various entities that may lead to decentration or pseudo-decentration are discussed below.

7.3.2.1 Misalignment of Reference Point: Static or Dynamic

As discussed above, improper alignment of the pupil/line of sight, cyclorotational axis of the globe, and pupil centroid may all lead to decentration. While it is crucial for the surgeon to be certain such alignment is present at the initiation of treatment, it is also critical to maintain alignment during photoablation. It is common for the globe or head to drift off center or cyclorotate during surgery. Tense or sedated patients are particularly apt to allow the chin to drift down toward the chest during surgery, with a corresponding Bell's response to maintain fixation on the target light inside the laser microscope. The presence of an eye-tracking function will not protect against a decentration effect: The tracking function will continue to work in a two dimensional x–y-plane while parallax is introduced between the laser optics and the corneal dome, resulting in an asymmetric distribution of laser energy with respect to the pupil center. No excimer laser system yet exists to correct for this phenomenon, so it is critical to monitor patient position during surgery and verbally encourage the best compliance possible. If the patient is unable to control eye movement during photoablation, then the globe can be manually fixated with a toothed fixation ring or microkeratome suction ring with a low vacuum setting to regain control of the situation. This is not ideal, but better than allowing the ablation to proceed. If the surgeon cannot gain control over the tendency toward excessive eye or head movement, then it is better to stop the procedure and try again later.

7.3.2.2 Uneven Uptake of Laser Energy

Uneven corneal hydration may lead to a decentration of ablation effect due to uneven uptake of excimer laser energy despite appropriate ocular alignment during surgery. The corneal topographic appearance in this setting is often that of an asymmetric, peninsula-shaped area of reduced ablation effect (Fig. 7.3.1). Central islands can also occur, but these are more distinctive and hard to mistake for a decentration. To avoid such problems, it is critical to minimize the amount of fluid on the surgical field. For surface ablation procedures, this is easily accomplished by placing a cellulose sponge drain or similar material on the globe if excess moisture is present. If alcohol is used to remove the epithelium, then it is important to irrigate the cornea to remove excess alcohol prior to removing the epithelium and to dry the surface to be ablated in a uniform fashion. During epi-LASIK or LASIK procedures with blade microkeratomes, large amounts of balanced salt solution are sometimes used for irrigation as the instrument is passed across the cornea, so it is critical in these settings to dry the stromal bed to be treated quickly and uniformly. When performing all-laser LASIK with a device such as the IntraLase femtosecond laser, it is not necessary to use a larger amount of moisture to mobilize the corneal flap, and fluid should be used sparingly during flap dissection/lifting.

Another cause of uneven laser energy uptake is the presence of localized corneal scarring or, in the case of surface ablation, residual corneal epithelium within the ablation zone. Corneal scars ablate at a slower rate than normal stroma and can result in a pseudo-decentration effect similar to that seen with uneven hydration.

7.3.2.3 Uneven Emission of Laser Energy

Much like the situation described above for corneal dehydration, pseudo-decentration can occur if the distribution of laser energy is uneven. While flying spot lasers using a small beam profile (1 mm) to deliver energy via a pattern of many overlapping pulses tend to have a fairly homogeneous energy profile, broad-beam excimer lasers can develop an irregular beam profile usually detectable by calibration devices. This most commonly occurs when solutions used during surgery are splashed up into the laser microscope and coat the laser optics. For such systems, the laser optics should be carefully inspected between cases and, where possible, frequent external calibration using a test ablation in plastic.

7.3.2.4 Asymmetric or Abnormal Wound Healing

If evidence suggestive of decentration is present, then the presence of abnormal wound healing should be excluded. Epithelial ingrowth often creates the appearance of localized corneal flattening, which may seem to shift the position of ablation effect (Fig. 7.3.2) Stromal tissue melting of the flap or deeper tissue may result in the appearance of localized flattening or steepening depending upon its location. Careful clinical examination should be performed to ensure that a laser treatment that appears decentered by topography is in fact not due to problems related to corneal would healing, as the correct treatment will differ.

Rarely, corneal ectasia may create the appearance of decentration. To rule out this unlikely but serious cause of pseudo-decentration, analysis of corneal shape with Orbscan (Bausch & Lomb, Rochester, N.Y.) or Pentacam (Oculus, Heidelberg, Germany) technology is essential prior to proceeding with additional laser treatment. Optical coherence tomography (OCT) may also become useful, but the ability of this technology to detect more than qualitative evidence of ectasia is limited at present.

7.3.3 Clinical Manifestations of Decentration

7.3.3.1 Symptoms

The most common symptoms of decentered laser treatments include:

- Blurred vision
- Ghosting
- Poor vision in low light
- Glare or halo, often asymmetric around point sources of light

Because symptoms associated with decentered laser ablations increase as the pupil dilates, patient complaints often relate to lighting conditions. During the early weeks or months after surgery, such symptoms may be explained away as normal, but one should be particularly suspicious of complaints that lateralize to one eye or the other.

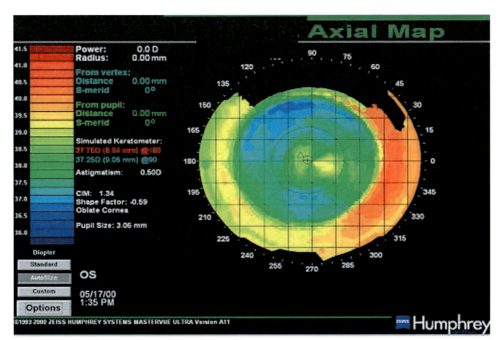

Fig. 7.3.1 "Peninsula" of decreased effect following myopic photorefractive keratectomy. This axial topographic map shows a ablation that is well centered over the physiologic pupil, but with differential flattening effect

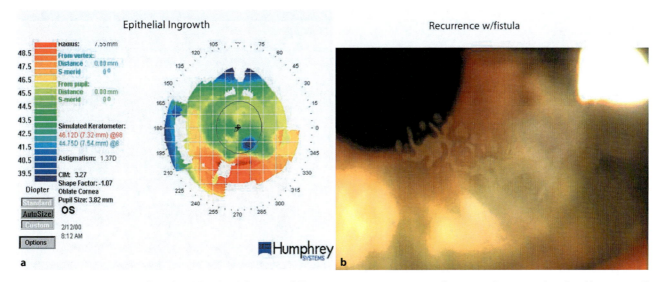

Fig. 7.3.2 Epithelial ingrowth–induced localized flattening following LASIK. **a** Asymmetric flattening after LASIK, but the ablation is well centered over the physiologic pupil. **b** This area of flattening corresponds to epithelial ingrowth visible at the slit lamp

7.3.3.2 Signs

The most common clinical signs of decentration include:

- Decreased uncorrected and BCVA
- Visual acuity results that vary with ambient lighting
- Difficult refraction or wavefront capture
- Scissors reflex during retinoscopy suggestive of irregular astigmatism

- Significantly increased higher order aberrations of the ocular wavefront versus before surgery, especially horizontal or vertical coma [6] (Figs. 7.3.3, 7.3.4).
- Abnormal corneal topography

When analyzing corneal topography, it is important to distinguish between true ablation decentration (Figs. 7.3.3, 7.3.4) and pseudo-decentration (Fig. 7.3.2), as the treat-

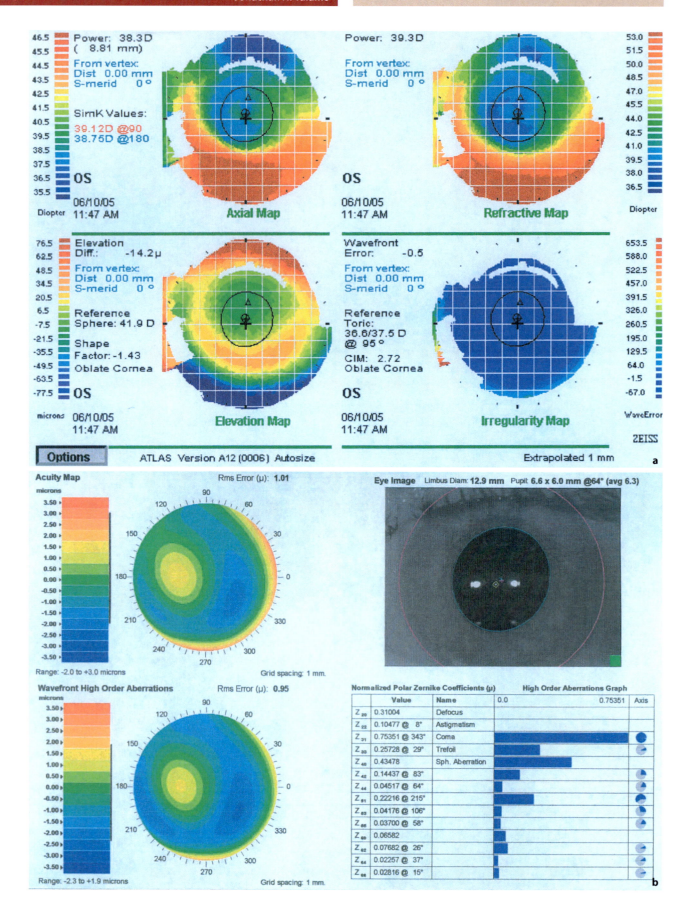

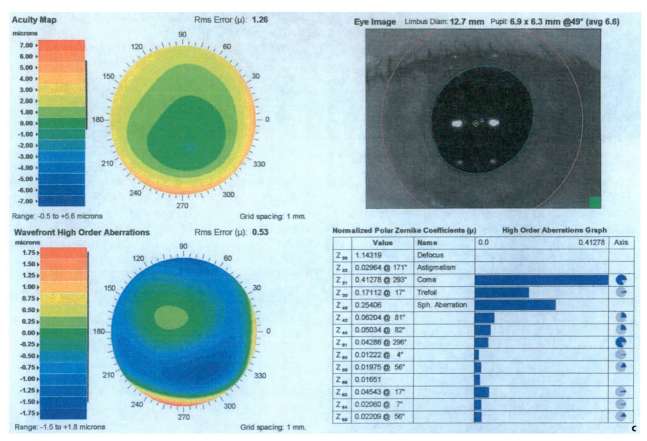

Fig. 7.3.3 Higher-order aberrations (HOA) after ablation decentration and wavefront guided retreatment. This patient sustained a superotemporally decentered myopic ablation and overcorrection after LASIK (**a**) and complained of vertical light scatter and ghosting at night. Uncorrected visual acuity was 20/60, improving to 20/25 with +2.00 sphere on manifest or cycloplegic refraction. Note the significant reduction in total HOA (44%), coma (44%), and spherical aberration (42%) when comparing before (**b**) and after custom hyperopic/astigmatic laser retreatment (**c**). After retreatment, UCVA was 20/25 and 20/15 with a manifest refraction of −.25 −.50 × 120

ments may vary if the problem is due to abnormal wound healing. The most powerful tool for doing this is the difference map function on topography devices, which allows analysis of surgically induced changes in corneal curvature. Without a difference map, it is very difficult to quantify the degree of decentration. Axial maps are useful, but some investigators feel tangential corneal topography is the most sensitive means for evaluating such changes [7]. Reliable and reproducible patient fixation is important to allow meaningful analysis of topographic changes, as small shifts in fixation can create the appearance of decentration where none exists.

After conventional photoablation treatments using spherocylindrical treatments, topographic decentrations of 1 mm or greater are widely considered to be clinically significant [8], although differences in BCVA have been demonstrated if topographic decentration exceeds 0.5 mm [7]. However, as pointed out above, if a patient exhibits symptoms of decentration despite the lack of significant decentration with corneal topography measurements, then increased higher-order aberrations may be responsible, hence the importance of wavefront analysis for all patients with persistent or unusual visual symptoms after refractive surgery.

For custom ablations, the allowable degree of lateral translation error in the x–y-plane to prevent degradation of wavefront correction effect is less forgiving, ranging from 0.2 to 0.07 mm for small (3 mm) and large pupils, respectively [9]. This degree of control is difficult to maintain during photoablation, which may be one reason why reductions in higher-order ocular aberrations are not consistently seen after photoablation, and why patients with larger pupils could be more likely to develop symptoms after lesser degrees of ablation decentration. Furthermore, if one is contemplating laser retreatment with a wavefront driven ablation, then great care should be taken to ensure that patient fixation is optimized and eye movement minimized during subsequent surgery.

7.3.4 Prevention of Decentration

The well-known Revolutionary Era scientist–politician Benjamin Franklin was notably known to say, "An ounce of prevention is worth a pound of cure." This dictum holds firm when it comes to the management of decentered refractive surgical procedures. While medical and surgical treatments do exist, the physical effects of a significantly decentered laser ablation are difficult to reverse completely. Fortunately, there are many precautions the surgical team can take, and serious decentrations are quite rare with current laser technology.

Preoperative data should be carefully scrutinized before surgery to ensure that the data being utilized are for the correct patient, correct eye, and correct axis. Furthermore, if custom ablation is being performed, then it is essential to validate the quality and reproducibility of both the raw and processed wavefront or topographic data. If inaccurate custom data is entered because the ocular wavefront was distorted by a dry eye, eye movement [9], or excessive accommodation, an asymmetric ablation may be delivered, resulting in the appearance and effect of a decentration even if treatment is appropriately centered on the pupil.

The role of patient education should not be underestimated. If patients understand ahead of time what is expected of them during surgery and what they will experience, it will be easier for them to cooperate fully during treatment by maintaining fixation and a stable head position under the laser. A prepared patient is a less anxious and more cooperative patient, and as such, it is worth the time for the surgeon and operating room staff to ensure that the patient is as prepared as possible when he or she is readied for surgery. Many surgeons use small doses of anxiolytic medications such as diazepam or alprazolam by mouth prior to surgery to aid in patient relaxation. While helpful in low doses, an over-sedated patient may be less cooperative and it may be difficult to control involuntary Bell's response of the globe that often occurs in this situation.

Calibration of laser centering and tracking devices is also of paramount importance to prevent decentered laser treatments. Even the most cooperative patient may end up with a bad result if the excimer laser being used for treatment is allowed to slip out of calibration. All laser systems have both internal and external means for calibrating these functions, and it is important to follow manufacturers' instructions religiously in this regard.

Once in the operating room, positioning of the patient, head, and eye are critical to provide for proper alignment of laser photoablation as energy strikes the cornea. Ideally, the globe should be positioned so that the corneal apex is orthogonal (or very close to orthogonal) to the incident laser beam. The corneal limbus should be marked in the upright position to avoid off-axis astigmatic ablation [3], which can be considered a decentration of sorts. If manual centering of the laser's optical path is used, then care should be taken to avoid parallax error by following manufacturer's instructions for each laser's microscope. If an automated eye-tracking system is utilized, then it is important to activate the tracking function with the eye in the correct position (i.e., with the patient fixating on the appropriate target within the laser microscope).

7.3.5 Medical Treatment of Decentration

Symptoms of decentered laser ablations can often be treated with medical intervention alone. If the degree of disability is mild, then correction of the residual refractive error with spectacles or soft contact lenses is often sufficient to minimize or eliminate the increased ghosting or glare that may be worst under mesopic lighting conditions.

Miotic agents are also useful adjuncts. Alpha agonists such as Alphagan P (Allergan, Irvine, Calif.) cause a transient, mild pupillary miosis of 1–2 mm lasting 2–3 h in duration, which is often enough to minimize mesopic symptoms while driving at night or at the movies. Tachyphylaxis is a problem with these agents, and the duration of effect may decrease with prolonged or frequent usage, so patients should be encouraged to use these drugs sparingly to maintain good effect. More pronounced symptoms might require the use of dilute (0.5–1%) pilocarpine, a much more potent muscarinic agent. Many patients, however, experience a decline in visual function when the pupil is less than 2 mm in diameter, limiting pilocarpine's utility in this situation. When used three times daily, a permanent miotic effect can be maintained, but chronic usage of this drug has attendant complications, such as a high incidence of allergic reaction as well as increased risk of iris cyst formation and retinal detachment.

When decentration is profound (generally greater than 1 mm from the pupillary center), significant irregular astigmatism with decreased spectacle corrected visual acuity often result. Rigid gas permeable (RGP) contact lenses can be helpful in this setting, restoring visual acuity and minimizing irregular astigmatism and its symptoms. For patients whose corneal thickness is insufficient to allow further photoablation, RGP lens fitting may be the only option short of lamellar or penetrating corneal transplantation. While patients who have a history of RGP lens use may tolerate this type of treatment, most laser–vision correction patients are poorly disposed toward this type of solution to the problem.

7.3.6 Surgical Treatment of Decentration

Decentered ablations may be treated using manual calculations and laser offsets to administer trans-epithelial PRK and phototherapeutic keratectomy (PTK) ablations (usually based on interpretation of corneal topography) [10–12], custom ablations mathematically derived and programmed into a laser from corneal topography [12,13] or ocular wavefront data [14]. Astigmatic keratotomy (AK) and single Intacs segments have been used as well, but with unpredictable results (Jonathan H. Talamo, 2006, personal communication). With the arrival of reliable ocular aberrometry to measure the ocular wavefront, surgical therapy for laser decentration has become greatly simplified for all but the most severe cases. In the United States, wavefront or topography guided re-treatment of decentered laser ablations is an off-label, non–US Food and Drug Administra-

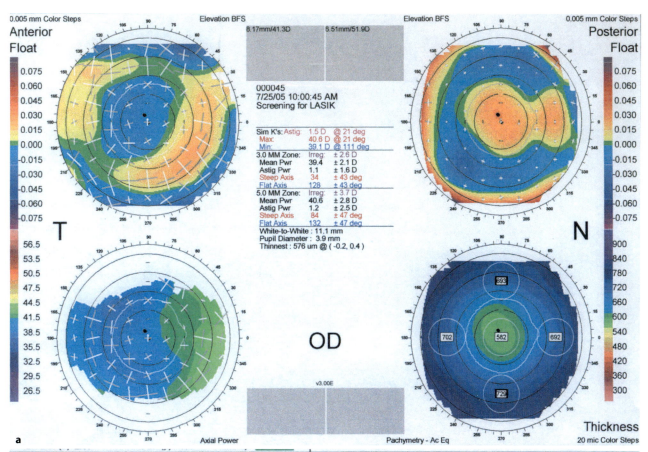

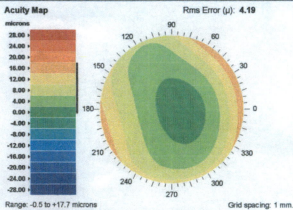

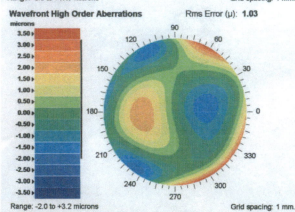

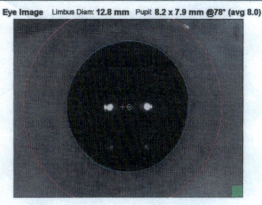

a

Acuity Map   Rms Error (µ): **4.19**

microns

28.00
24.00
20.00
16.00
12.00
8.00
4.00
0.00
-4.00
-8.00
-12.00
-16.00
-20.00
-24.00
-28.00

Range: -0.5 to +17.7 microns   Grid spacing: 1 mm.

Eye Image   Limbus Diam: **12.8 mm**   Pupil: **8.2 x 7.9 mm @78° (avg 8.0)**

Wavefront High Order Aberrations   Rms Error (µ): **1.03**

microns

3.50
3.00
2.50
2.00
1.50
1.00
0.50
0.00
-0.50
-1.00
-1.50
-2.00
-2.50
-3.00
-3.50

Range: -2.0 to +3.2 microns   Grid spacing: 1 mm.

Normalized Polar Zernike Coefficients (µ)   **High Order Aberrations Graph**

	Value	Name	0.0	0.83513	Axis
Z_{20}	3.66623	Defocus			
Z_{22}	1.73987 @ 22°	Astigmatism			
Z_{31}	0.83513 @ 0°	Coma			
Z_{33}	0.45320 @ 63°	Trefoil			
Z_{40}	0.14371	Sph. Aberration			
Z_{42}	0.10828 @ 113°				
Z_{44}	0.11685 @ 75°				
Z_{51}	0.15720 @ 212°				
Z_{53}	0.03982 @ 17°				
Z_{55}	0.20848 @ 63°				
Z_{60}	0.17270				
Z_{62}	0.07302 @ 108°				
Z_{64}	0.05119 @ 36°				
Z_{66}	0.05005 @ 18°				

b

7

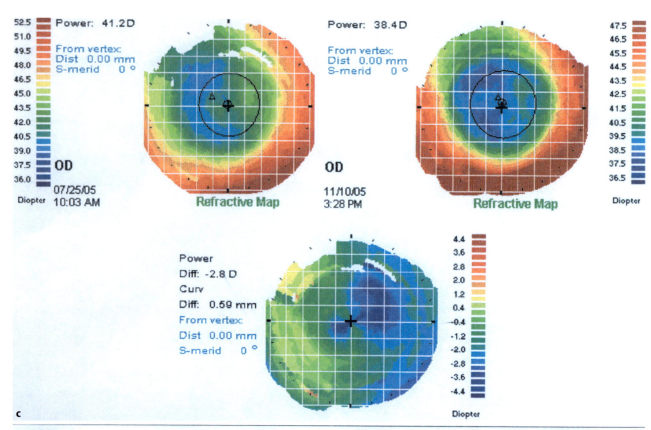

Power: 41.2D

From vertex:
Dist 0.00 mm
S-merid   0 °

OD

07/25/05
10:03 AM

Diopter

Refractive Map

Power: 38.4D

From vertex:
Dist 0.00 mm
S-merid   0 °

OD

11/10/05
3:28 PM

Refractive Map

Diopter

Power
Diff: -2.8 D
Curv
Diff: 0.59 mm
From vertex:
Dist 0.00 mm
S-merid   0 °

Diopter

c

Acuity Map   Rms Error (μ): **1.51**

microns

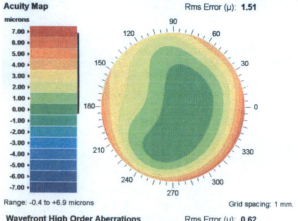

Range: -0.4 to +6.9 microns   Grid spacing: 1 mm.

Eye Image   Limbus Diam: **12.8 mm**   Pupil **7.8 x 7.6 mm @58° (avg 7.7)**

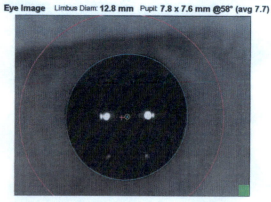

Wavefront High Order Aberrations   Rms Error (μ): **0.62**

microns

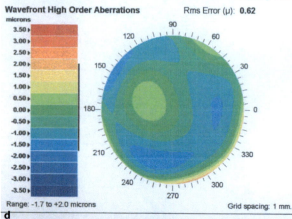

Range: -1.7 to +2.0 microns   Grid spacing: 1 mm.

d

Normalized Polar Zernike Coefficients (μ)   **High Order Aberrations Graph**

	Value	Name	0.0	0.43414	Axis
Z_{20}	1.31767	Defocus			
Z_{22}	0.40864 @ 170°	Astigmatism			
Z_{31}	0.43414 @ 324°	Coma			
Z_{33}	0.16501 @ 66°	Trefoil			
Z_{40}	0.32775	Sph. Aberration			
Z_{42}	0.12823 @ 69°				
Z_{44}	0.01555 @ 7°				
Z_{51}	0.14482 @ 240°				
Z_{53}	0.05755 @ 98°				
Z_{55}	0.09951 @ 61°				
Z_{60}	0.06409				
Z_{62}	0.03599 @ 151°				
Z_{64}	0.03818 @ 9°				
Z_{66}	0.03886 @ 59°				

Fig. 7.3.4 Corneal topography after ablation decentration and wavefront-guided retreatment. This patient complained of significant glare disability and monocular/ghosting due to temporal ablation decentration with respect to the pupil center seen on Orbscan testing after LASIK for approximately –5.00 D (a). UCVA was 20/40, and BCVA 20/25, with a manifest refraction of –.25 –.75 × 94. Wavefront analysis showed a profound degree of horizontal coma (b). Eight months after wavefront-guided custom retreatment, UCVA improved

to 20/25 and 20/20, with manifest refraction using plano –0.50 × 80 and complete resolution of glare/ghosting symptoms. As expected, ablation centration as assessed by corneal topography also improved dramatically (c, upper right) when compared with preoperative topography (c, upper left). The pTake-Homential flattening achieved nasally by custom retreatment is depicted in the difference map (c, below center). Wavefront sensing showed reduction in horizontal coma of almost 50% (d)

---

tion (FDA)-approved procedure, and appropriate informed consent should be obtained.

Most decentrations symptomatic enough to require laser retreatment are displaced 0.75 mm or more from the pupil center. In general, wavefront guided re-treatment is the preferred method, as this approach allows the higher order ocular aberrations induced by the decentered corneal optics to be treated with less likelihood of a large residual refractive error than if topography is used.

If the decentration is very severe or there are significant corneal opacities, then wavefront sensing may not be possible, but for the vast majority of cases it is the preferred treatment modality (Figs. 7.3.3, 7.3.4).

Prior to laser re-treatment of decentered ablations, it is important to exclude other causes of visual symptoms and to demonstrate refractive stability. In particular, ocular surface dysfunction from dry eye and blepharitis should be treated aggressively, as symptoms may be magnified and the ability to measure the ocular wavefront compromised by an unstable tear film. Careful slit lamp biomicroscopy should be performed to exclude the presence of incipient cataract, and if the patient has undergone recent intraocular surgery (such as phakic intraocular [IOL] implantation or refractive lensectomy patients undergoing planned bioptics procedures), then the presence of cystoid macular edema (CME), posterior capsular opacification or IOL sublux-

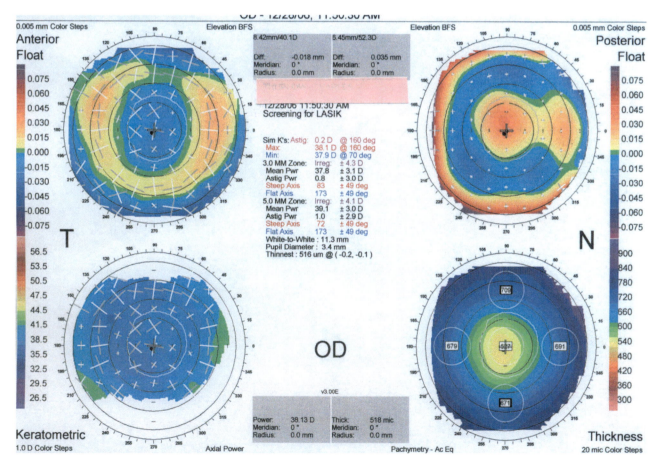

Fig. 7.3.5 Custom contoured ablation for irregular corneas. This figure depicts the ability of the VISX excimer laser system to program and precisely decenter topography-derived, custom-programmed photoablation (using C-CAP software) with respect to the pupil

center after capture by an active eye-tracking system. Intentional decentration allows application of asymmetric ablations to improved corneal topographic symmetry

ation should be excluded. A hard contact lens over-refraction is crucial to demonstrate a reduction in symptoms to the patient and to confirm that the etiology is corneal.

Wavefront measurements must be reproducible and of sufficient quality to reliably calculate a custom treatment. If imaging is not possible with one type of aberrometer, then it may be easier with another. It is important to maximize the pupil diameter during measurement, since the diameter of the custom ablation will only be as wide as the captured wavefront (6 mm or greater is usually sufficient). As wavefront-guided laser systems using Hartmann-Shack (VISX, Alcon, Bausch & Lomb), Tserning (Wavelight), and Scanning Slit-Skiascopy (Nidek) are all available, it may be worth imaging with more than one system if data is difficult to capture. Where possible, it is very useful to cut a "test lens" in polymethylmethacrylate (PMMA; available with the VISX CustomVue System) and have the patient test his or her vision in a trial frame with an over-refraction to establish (1) if improvement in symptoms occur, and (2) if the target spherical equivalent is accurate.

When calculating wavefront-guided custom treatments, it is important to be mindful of tissue-removal depth requirements. In general, wavefront-derived re-treatments require significantly greater tissue ablation depths than either conventional spherocylindrical or primary custom treatments. To avoid insufficient residual stromal bed thickness in a LASIK patient, it may often be necessary to re-treat with surface ablation. Single application, low dose intra-operative topical Mitomycin C (0.01–0.02% for 12–15 s) is useful in this setting (also off-label, non-FDA approved in the United States).

For the unusual cases where wavefront guided re-treatment cannot be performed, topography can be used to generate a custom ablation algorithm (Fig. 7.3.5). As noted above, additional refractive surgery is often indicated to adjust further the spherical equivalent to a level compatible with comfortable uncorrected vision.

While dramatic progress has been made in both the diagnosis and therapy of decentered corneal laser ablations over the 14 years the excimer laser has been in widespread use, surgical correction remains a challenging problem. As technology and surgeon skill continue to improve, perhaps decentration will become even more infrequent and treatment less complex.

Take-Home Pearls

- The best defense is a good offense–have a system for preventing decentration.
- Leave enough stromal tissue after primary treatment to re-treat unexpected problems, as there are no good surgical options for a decentered ablation in a too-thin cornea.
- Do not overlook medical treatment options.
- Before re-treatment, clearly establish refractive stability and that the etiology of symptoms is corneal.

- Wavefront-guided re-treatments, when possible, offer the simplest and most accurate method of surgical correction.
- Informed consent should underscore off-label nature of any surgery.

References

1. Uozato H, Guyton DL (1987) Centering corneal surgical procedures. Am J Ophthalmol 103:264–275
2. Fry GA (1969) Geometrical optics. Chilton, Philadelphia, p 110
3. Smith EM, Talamo JH (1995) Evaluation of ocular cyclotorsion using a Maddox double-rod technique. J Cataract Refract Surg 21:402–403
4. Uozato H, Guyton DL, Waring GO (1992) Centering corneal surgical procedures. In: Waring GO (ed) Refractive keratotomy for myopia and astigmatism. Mosby-Year Book, St. Louis, pp 491–505
5. Porter J, Yoon G, Lozano D et al (2006) Aberrations induced in wavefront-guided laser refractive surgery due to shifts between natural and dilated pupil center locations. J Cataract Refract Surg 32:21–32
6. Mrochen M, Kaemmerer M, Mierdel P et al (2001) Increased higher order aberrations after laser refractive surgery: a problem of subclinical decentration. J Cataract Refract Surg 27:362–369
7. Azar DT, Yeh, PC (1997) Corneal topographic evaluation of decentration in photorefractive keratectomy: treatment displacement vs intraoperative drift. Am J Ophthalmol 124:312–320
8. Doane JF, Cavanaugh TB, Durrie DS et al (1995) Relation of visual symptoms to topographic ablation zone decentration after excimer laser photorefractive keratectomy. Ophthalmology 102:42–47
9. Bueeler M, Mrochen M, Seiler T (2003) Maximum permissible lateral decentration in aberration sensing and wavefront guided corneal ablation. J Cataract Refract Surg 29:257–263
10. Talamo JH, Wagoner MD, Lee SY (1995) Management of ablation decentration following excimer photorefractive keratectomy. Arch Ophthalmol 113:706–707
11. Lafond G, Bonnet S, Solomon L (2004) Treatment of previous decentered excimer laser ablation with combined myopic and hyperopic ablations. J Refract Surg 20:139–148
12. Tamayo GE, Serrano MG (2000) Early clinical experience using custom excimer laser ablations to treat irregular astigmatism. J Cataract Refract Surg 26:1442–1450
13. Lin DY, Manche EE (2004) Custom contoured ablation pattern method for the treatment of decentered laser ablations. J Cataract Refract Surg 30:1675–1684
14. Mrochen M, Krueger RR, Bueeler M et al (2002) Aberration sensing and wavefront-guided laser in situ keratomileusis: management of decentered ablation. J Refract Surg 18:418–429

Core Messages

- Corneal irregularity is the most frequent complication of corneal refractive surgical procedures.

- Corneal topography and corneal aberrometry are both important in understanding the challenge of corneal irregularity.

- Macro- and micro-irregular components may appear individually or associated, depending on the case.

- A comprehensive approach and grading of the clinical characteristics and impact of the symptoms in the patient's quality of life are important in the management of each case.

- Consecutive approaches can successfully treat most of the cases, avoiding corneal grafting.

7.4 Corneal Irregularity

Jorge L. Alió

7.4.1 Concept

Corneal irregularity is one of the most frequent complications that appears as a consequence of refractive surgery. Corneal irregularity leads to unacceptable visual symptoms and the loss of best-corrected vision. Until recently, its role in corneal refractive surgery outcomes has been misdiagnosed and underestimated in its frequency. Recently, with the massive use of aberrometers, most corneal refractive surgery cases end with a different profile than normal at the anterior corneal surface, changing the aberrometry pattern of the cornea [1]. The consequence of this is a change in the visual perception and in vision quality. To a certain extent, the neuroprocessing role of the brain is able to compensate these changes. However, when the corneal optical dysfunction reaches high levels, such as with the loss of best-corrected vision, a complication is difficult to solve. In this situation, an adequate clinical examination and surgical expertise can lead to the correction of the irregularity with restoration of acceptable or normal levels of vision [1, 2].

Corneal irregularity, also called irregular astigmatism, appears when the principal meridians of the anterior corneal surface are not 90° apart, without a progressive transition from one meridian to another. This optical system is impossible to correct by conventional spherical or cylindrical lenses. The refraction in different meridians conforms to a non-geometric plane, and the refractive rays have no planes of symmetry [3].

Corneal irregularity causes a variety of unpleasant symptoms in patients. It can be studied with modern examination techniques to lead an adequate therapeutic decision-making process in the benefit of the disabled patient.

7.4.2 Symptoms

The irregular or aberrated cornea causes visual distortion with night and/or day glare. Patients refer halos, dazzling, monocular diplopia, or polyopia, either in night or daylight conditions. A decrease in best-corrected vision is also perceived by most patients.

The subjective feeling that a patient may refer to depend, largely, on the ocular dominance, the severity of the irregularity, and the type of corneal aberrations that are more abnormally deviated.

7.4.3 Clinical Examination and Classification

When studying an eye, in which previous corneal refractive surgery has caused corneal irregularity, we should trace the previous history of the eye, knowing which type of corneal refractive surgery has been performed. In the case of lamellar surgery, if possible, the physician should know details about flap construction and flap complications that might have occurred, the preoperative BSCVA of the patient, and the changes in the quality of life. The recording of these data in the initial examination is important to avoid potential later masquerades related to medical legal issues that frequently change the clinical subjective symptoms reported by the patient. Previous medical reports and adequate clinical documents to support previous patients' history are mandatory at this stage. Then, a complete ocular examination should be performed including UCVA, BCVA, pinhole visual acuity, cycloplegic refraction, retinoscopy, keratometry, ultrasonic pachymetry, corneal topography, corneal aberrometry, and global aberrometry examination. Pupil size in high- and low-mesopic conditions, if possible, should also be recorded. Best-overcorrected vision over a rigid contact lens is important to ascertain the role of corneal irregularity in cases where other problems, such as corneal opacity, may play a role in visual loss. Other visual findings that could be related to loss of best-corrected vision, such as lens changes and macular problems, should be also highlighted in a medical examination.

Clinically, corneal irregularity will present a typical retinoscopy pattern with spinning and in-scissoring of the red pupil retinoscopy reflex. On keratometry, the mires and rings will appear distorted. Modern corneal topography shows certain patterns and numerical indexes of corneal irregularity that can be useful for the follow up (Fig. 7.4.1a, b). However, today the most useful clinical examination technique is corneal aberrometry (Fig. 7.4.1c). Corneal aberrometry is a mathematical transformation of the corneal topography data that can obtain up to 8.5 mm of the cornea diameter, is independent of pupil size, analyses the anterior corneal surface–usually the one affected by the previous refractive surgery–and can be analyzed by different mathematical approaches such as the Zernike polynomials, the Seidel equations, or Fourier analysis [1, 2, 4, 5].

Global wavefront examination with the pupil in mydriasis should also be performed in moderate or severe cases of

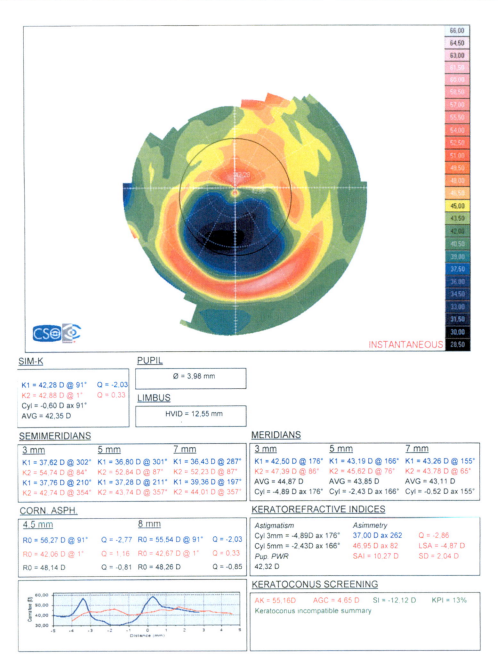

Fig. 7.4.1 a The different appearance that the same case may have on corneal topography, instantaneous map (**a**), axial (**b**), corneal aberrometry (**c**), and the different components of the Seidel aberrations. The clinicians should be aware of these differences, so as not to have misunderstandings in the clinical interpretation of the topography. Corneal aberrometry represents the numerical optical value of the corneal topography and indeed is the most important examination tool for the understanding of irregular astigmatism

corneal irregularity, even though it cannot be recorded in most instances. However, global aberrometry is affected by the intraocular aberrations and can be masqueraded by residual accommodation [6] (Fig. 7.4.2a–d).

Other examination techniques, such as ray tracing [7], in which a laser beam is delivered parallel to the optical axis of the retina sequentially through different pupil locations, can be useful. The ray-tracing technique is able to analyze separately the corneal, intraocular, and global aberrations.

Based on this clinical information, other auxiliary clinical examination techniques can be used. The most relevant of them are anterior segment optical coherence tomography (OCT), very high frequency (VHF) ultrasound bioimaging of the anterior segment of the eye and corneal confocal microscopy.

Diagnostic imaging techniques such as anterior segment OCT and VHF ultrasound are, at this moment, capable of globally analyzing the corneal profile. The VHF ultrasound

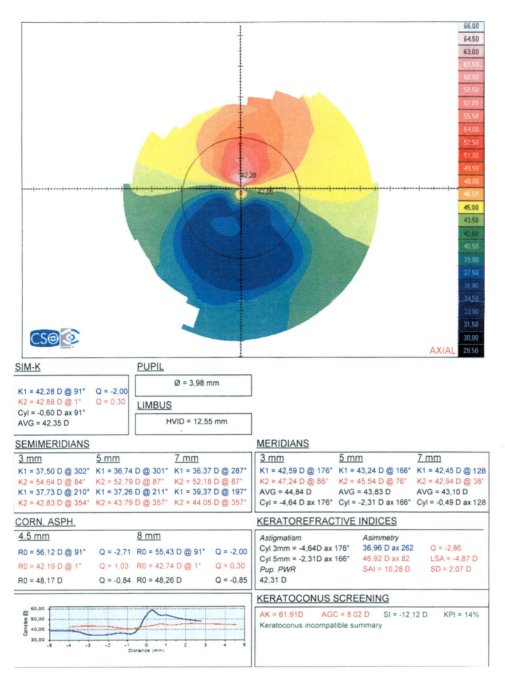

Fig. 7.4.1 b *(continued)*

technique (Artemis II, Ultralink, Canada) is a highly efficient technology that can precisely detect and measure irregularities in a corneal flap and can measure topographical differences in corneal thicknesses at different meridians of the cornea, creating pachymetry maps of different types for the epithelium, residual stroma, and total cornea. This is important in difficult cases where data on the type of complication that the patient suffered from during surgery are lacking. Similar information, even though less precise, is offered today by anterior segment OCT (Visante, Carl-Zeiss, Germany). Corneal confocal microscopy is relevant in measuring light scattering, and analyzing the degree of

corneal scarring that is present at the central cornea, which is important in certain cases.

7.4.4 Clinical Classification of Corneal Irregularity

7.4.4.1 Macro-Irregular and Micro-Irregular Patterns

When the main reason for visual disability is a steeper or flatter area of a cornea larger than 2 mm, the case can be classified as macro-irregular [1]. When a disperse irregularity, not specifically creating a well-defined elevated or

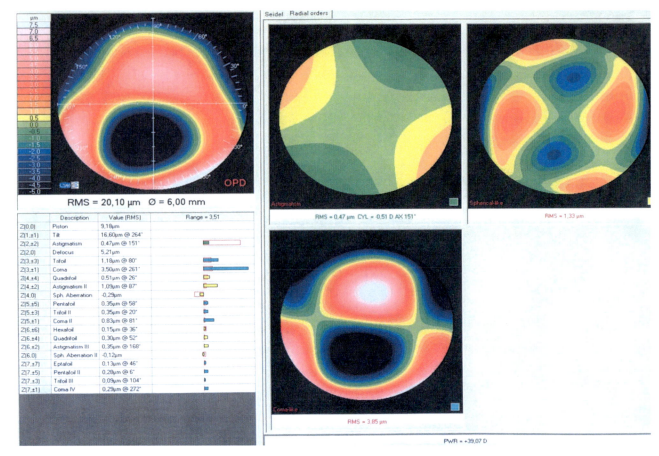

Fig. 7.4.1 c *(continued)*

flatter area of the cornea, then the case can be termed as micro-irregular. This initial classification is obtained from the corneal topography map and has important clinical implications in the therapeutic decision-making process for the case. Also, mixed patterns with a macro-irregular area associated to some degree of micro-irregularity are frequently present.

Typical macro-irregular patterns are those caused by decentrated ablations. Micro-irregular patterns are found frequently in cases with flap complications.

7.4.4.2 Measuring Corneal Irregularity by Higher-Order Aberration Analysis

Probably the most specific way to analyze and grade corneal irregularity is the mathematical transformation of the topography analyzed by corneal aberrometry. In the normal eye, more than 90% of the eye aberrations are derived from the cornea, and the proportion is larger when corneal irregularity is present [7]. This makes corneal aberrometry a very precise and comprehensive method to analyze globally the optical profile of the anterior corneal surface. The Zernike decomposition of this analysis, precisely the measurement of the higher-order aberrations from the third to the eighth order from the maximum area of the anterior

corneal surface, offers us global data about the irregularity. This information will be very important in the decision of how to treat such cases [5].

7.4.4.3 Clinical Classification

We have defined a scale to classify corneal irregularity in four grades, based on (1) patient symptoms, (2) loss of lines of BCVA, (3) quality-of-life changes, and (4) objective data such as aberrometry. This classification is displayed in Table 7.4.1. In order to have an adequate classification and grading of the corneal irregularity, it is mandatory to treat corneal irregular astigmatism. It is also important to observe changes induced in the cornea from therapeutics and surgeries performed on the patient. In medical legal terms, it is also important to offer objective data about how severe the corneal irregularity is and how much the patient's life is affected by the problem.

7.4.5 Correction and Treatment of Corneal Irregularity

No surgical correction should be attempted prior to 6 months of follow-up of the case from the causing surgery.

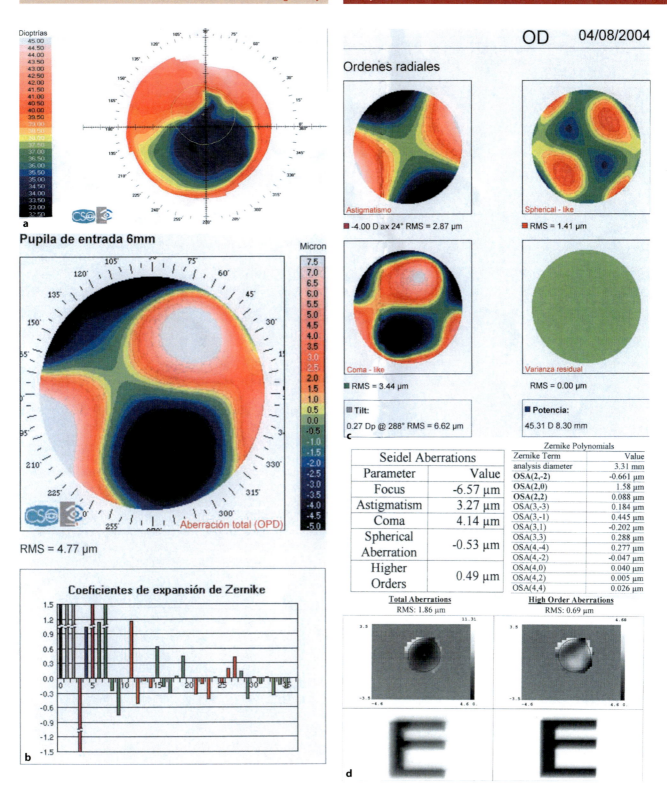

Fig. 7.4.2 The limitations of total aberrometry in understanding corneal irregular astigmatism. **a** A severe decentered myopic ablation. **b** Very severe increase in global corneal aberrations. **c** Very high coma and spherical aberration that this decentration causes, when ana-lyzed with the Seidel aberrations. **d** The same case when analyzed by global aberrometry (COAS aberrometry, for a 5-mm pupil). Global aberrometry shows a much lower amount of aberrations than does the corneal aberrometry map

Table 7.4.1 Grading of irregular astigmatism

Grade	Signs and symptoms
1	Mild symptoms at night or daylight conditions
	Loss of 1–2 lines of BCVA
	Useful vision for reading, driving and walking
	No disability for normal life, but with discomfort
	No monocular diplopia
	Ray tracing abnormal. Distortion = 2–8 µm
	Aberrometry: RMS = 2–3 µm
2	Moderate disability
	Loss of 3–4 lines of BCVA
	Reading and driving partially affected, especially in dim-light conditions
	Some patients prefer not to use the eye
	Moderate monocular diplopia
	Ray tracing affected. Distortion = 8–14 µm
	Aberrometry: RMS = 3–6 µm
3	Severe disability. Eye not useful for visual performance
	Loss of >5 lines of BCVA
	Patients prefer not to use the eye
	Reading and driving affected, all light conditions
	Severe Monocular diplopia or polyopia
	Ray-tracing disaster. Distortion > 14 µm
	Aberrometry: RMS > 6 µm
4	Eye not useful, legally blind
	BCVA = 20/200 or less
	Aberrometry, ray tracing, and topography not possible to capture due to the severity of irregularities

In many mild cases, corneal irregularity improves with time, thanks to the role of the corneal epithelium remodeling. Visual symptoms somehow are improved by neuroprocessing, and for this reason, some cases become less symptomatic with time. This time interval is also important, as some changes related to the corneal wound-healing process may need time to improve or to worsen and an adequate perspective on the case cannot be obtained prior to this time in many cases.

7.4.5.1 Contact Lens Adaptation

During this waiting period, contact lenses can be very helpful in relieving the patient's symptoms, as the patient accepts that this is a temporary solution. Corneal contact lens adaptation is not easy in these cases due to (1) lack of patient motivation, (2) frequent concomitant existence of ocular surface syndrome related to the previous corneal surgery (especially following LASIK), (3) prior patient history of contact lens intolerance, and (4) intolerance related to the corneal surgical process. All types of contact lenses can be used in these patients: hard (PMMA), gas permeable (silicon fluoromethacrylate and silicon acrylate), hybrid (Sinergicon Soft Perm CibaVision), and hydrophilic. Preoperative corneal topography, fluorescein pattern, and topographic pattern of the corneal irregularity should be used to select the trial contact lens. Some companies manufacture customized contact lenses depending on the corneal topography for severely disabled corneal irregularity. These types of contact lenses are becoming very helpful when available, also in mild cases.

When adapting contact lenses, the diameter of the lens should depend on the choice of the diameter of the flap. The lens should lean on the zone not affected by the previous refractive surgery (or to the corneal periphery). In cases of incisional surgery, such as RK, toric hydrophilic lenses and Soft Perm are preferred because these lenses have larger diameters, and they rest on the scleral ring, avoiding the corneal periphery usually affected by the healing effect of the incision and poor stability of the lens [8]. Contact lens adaptation should be performed by a contact lens specialist, as these are very demanding cases. Adequate follow-up should be offered during the waiting period in cases in which visual disability is high enough not to allow normal patient behavior with glasses and contact lenses.

7.4.5.2 Wavefront-Guided Excimer Laser Surgery: Global Wavefront versus Corneal Wavefront

Global wavefront analysis has a limited value in the understanding and correction of the irregular cornea. The reasons for these limitations are the following:

(1) Most wavefront sensors cannot measure highly aberrated corneas; (2) in moderate- or low-corneal irregularity, global wavefront analysis is restricted to pupil size; and (3) most of the global wavefront sensors limit their analysis to 1 mm inside the pupil diameter, which further limits the knowledge of the corneal irregularity. In many instances, corneal irregularity is outside these limits and cannot be rightly understood. Conversely, corneal wavefront analysis can measure up to 8 or 8.5 mm of diameter of the cornea (Fig. 7.4.1c, 7.4.2a–d), is not limited by pupil size, and measures a much larger amount of points, which renders much more accurate information on the corneal irregularity. Corneal wavefront analysis can be obtained almost in any

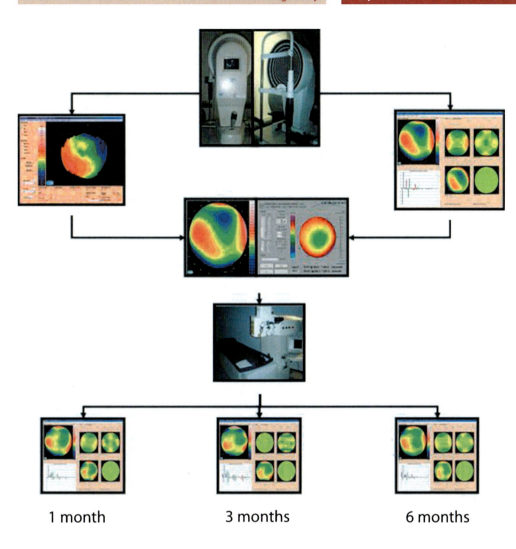

Fig. 7.4.3 Process to correct irregular astigmatism (decentrated myopic ablation) based on the use of corneal aberrometry. Corneal topography is mathematically converted into corneal aberrometry, and an adequate treatment map is created. The treatment is adjusted to pupil size, corneal pachymetry. and other clinical parameters. When a treatment happens, an immediate improvement is observed, which is followed by a further improvement that is continuing up to the sixth month

1 month   3 months   6 months

case of corneal irregularity, even in highly aberrated corneas. Corneal wavefront analysis is a mathematical analysis of corneal topography by measuring the abnormality of the anterior corneal surface. As most of the corneal irregularity following refractive surgery comes from problems in the anterior surface of the cornea, corneal wavefront analysis comes to be much more useful than any other tool in the analysis that helps in planning the treatment of an irregular cornea (Figs. 7.4.3, 7.4.4).

Corneal wavefront analysis is not interfered by accommodation or intraocular aberrations and offers adequate, specific, and precise information about the corneal problem as a larger number of points are studied on the cornea. This allows information that is much more precise to build the customized program required for the correction of such cases. Macro-irregular patterns can be analyzed and treated based on this information, and to some extent, the micro-irregular component. The use of corneal topography to guide excimer laser surgery has been used in several investigations, which have concluded that the macro-irregular components can be rightly treated by topography-guided treatments [10–12]. Recently, corneal wavefront de-

rived from corneal topography using the CSO topographer (Florence, Italy), converting the elevation data in terms of Zernike and Seidel polynomials to quantify the corneal wavefront aberrometry, have been reported [13]. The RMS was used as a measure of the optical quality before and after customized corneal wavefront analysis.

To correct an irregular cornea using corneal wavefront analysis, we capture and analyze corneal aberration up to the seventh Zernike order, and we process these data with the software of Esiris-Schwind technology (Frankfurt, Germany), which transforms corneal aberration data into an adequate ablation profile. In correcting the irregular cornea, especially in severe cases, software that enables the surgeon to take an active part in the decision-making process, selecting the best solution for each patient based on corneal pachymetry, mesopic pupil size, and total ablation thickness, is important. The specific surgical criteria with which to choose the optical zone, transition zones, and the exclusion of specific aberrations from the treatment might be decided by the surgeon. Using this surgeon's corneal wavefront–guided methods, total higher-order aberrations can be reduced significantly, increasing the BCVA and decreas-

Fig. 7.4.4 The evolution of the case treated by corneal aberrometry guided excimer laser ablation (the Esiris-Schwind technology), with the evolution of corneal topography (**b**), corneal aberrometry (**c**) and PSF and high and low contrast simulation charge derived from the corneal aberrometry. This figure corresponds to the following clinical case:

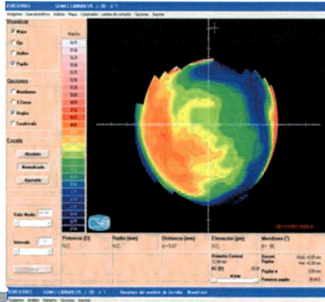

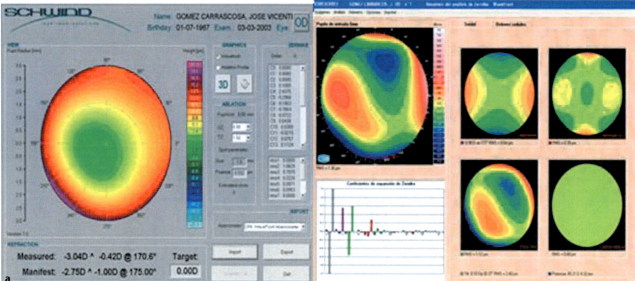

Patient history

- A 33-year-old white male came to our clinic with an ocular history of refractive surgery in both eyes. He complained of poor quality of vision, ghost images, and halos, especially at night in his right eye. He had his first standard LASIK treatment in March 2000. His previous ocular history was:
  - BCVA OD: 1.00
  - Rx OD: −3.75 −1.00 cyl × 115°
- After we examined the patient his ocular history was as follows:
  - UCVA OD: 0.60
  - BCVA OD: 0.70
  - Rx OD: −1.75 −0.75 × 170°
  - Pachymetry: 482 µm
  - Slit lamp examination: within normal limits

- 1-month postoperative evaluation:
  - Patient reported that vision in his OD improved, and he did not perceive ghost images.
  - UCVA OD: 0.80
  - BCVA: 0.80
  - Rx OD: −0.50 cyl × 30°
- 3-month postoperative evaluation:
  - UCVA OD: 0.90
  - BCVA: 1.00
  - Rx OD: −0.50 cyl × 180°
- 6-month postoperative evaluation:
  - UCVA OD: 1.00
  - BCVA: 1.00
  - Rx OD: −0.50 cyl × 180°

Corneal Topography

Pre op

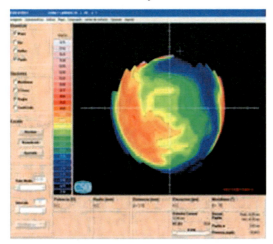

1 month post op

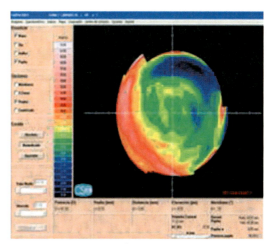

3month post op

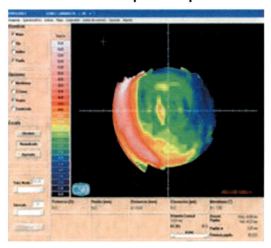

3month post op

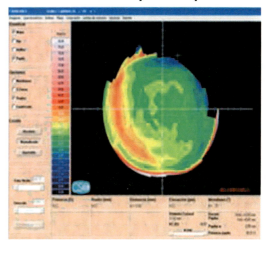

Fig. 7.4.4 b *(continued)*

ing patients' symptoms [13] (Fig. 7.4.4a–d). As it is demonstrated in other chapters of this book, corneal wavefront–guided methods are especially valuable in the correction of hyperopic and myopic decentrations, and to enlarge the optical zone in symptomatic patients with night vision problems related to optical zone treatment.

7.4.5.3 Masking Solutions

The use of a viscous masking agent during the ablations of an irregular cornea aims to protect the valleys between the irregular corneal peaks, leaving these peaks of pathology exposed to laser treatment. Of the different masking agents that have been evaluated, methylcellulose is the most commonly used and is available in different concentrations. However, it turns white during ablation due to its low boil-

ing point, and thus was not ideal for treatment [14]. Other attempts to improve irregular astigmatism with a masking substance were made by Pallikaris and colleagues, applying their PALM technique to smooth the corneal surface. However, this technique was abandoned due to its lack of reproducibility [15]. Alió and coworkers described a new technique using sodium hyaluronate 0.25% as the masking solution, so called excimer laser assisted by sodium hyaluronate (ELASHY). The physical characteristics of sodium hyaluronate confer important rheological properties to the product, and the photoablation rate is similar to that of corneal tissue, forming a stable and uniform coating on the surface of the eye, filling depressions on the cornea and effectively masking tissues to be protected against ablation by the laser pulses in PTK mode. They performed a prospective clinically controlled study performed on 50 eyes

Zernike Analysis

Pre op   RMS sph 0.39
RMS coma 1.12

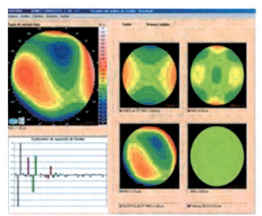

1 month   RMS sph 0.36
RMS coma 0.83

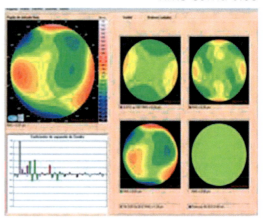

3 month   RMS sph 0.57
RMS coma 0,9

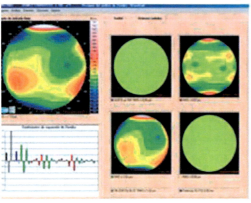

6 month   RMS sph 0.34
RMS coma 0,63

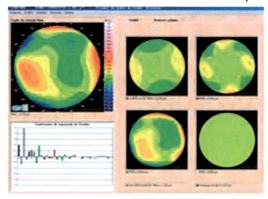

Fig. 7.4.4 c *(continued)*

of 50 patients with induced irregular astigmatism [17–19]. The safety index was equal to 1.1, and the efficacy index was 0.74. The ray-tracing parameters improved, and most of the patients (89.3%) subjectively noted improvement of the visual acuity and disappearance of the visual aberrations that previously impaired their quality of vision.

The clinical indications for this procedure include irregular astigmatism caused by irregularity in flap or on stromal base, induced by LASIK [16].

7.4.6 Corneal Excision (Superficial Lamellar Keratectomy)

Corneal excision has been successfully used to eliminate superficial corneal irregularities after flap complications and severe decentrations. Automatic mechanical methods have been used for this purpose successfully [17]. Corneal excision can be safely performed, leaving corneal thickness reduced up to 320 μm successfully without creating corneal ectasia [17]. Mechanical microkeratomes usually leave a rough surface that requires at least 30–40 μm of ELASHY. Recently, the use of femtosecond laser technology may allow a more precise calculation of the excised corneal thickness, with more successful outcomes. Up to this moment, there is no adequate knowledge about the limit of corneal thickness compatible with adequate recovery of best-corrected vision. All these cases will be left with a residual ametropia that should be corrected with a phakic IOL, usually a toric design. It is advisable to complete the corneal excision with a 30-μm masking solution excimer laser ablation in PTK mode (ELASHY) as the smoothness of the corneal surface is increased. Superficial lamellar keratectomy or corneal incisions should be used as a last resource prior to corneal lamellar grafting.

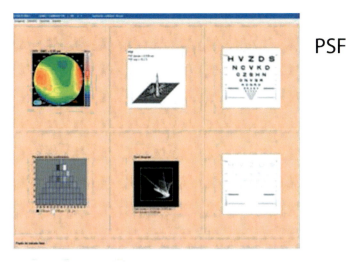

PSF

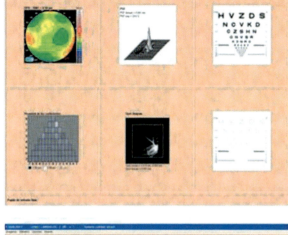

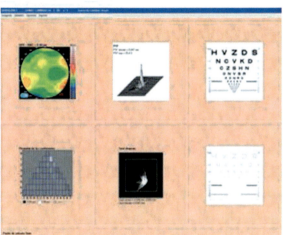

Fig. 7.4.4 d *(continued)*

7.4.7 Non-Laser Corneal Surgery

7.4.7.1 Automated Anterior Lamellar Keratoplasty

This technique was originally designed to treat superficial stromal disorders, but it has also been used in the treatment of difficult cases of irregular astigmatism, with variable results [18]. The surgeon performs PTK or a microkeratome or femtosecond laser lamellar resection to 250- to 400-µm stromal depth, followed by transplantation of a donor lamella of the same dimension and thickness on to the recipient bed. It is a good option for patients with thin corneas, and with the preservation of the Descemet's membrane, the complications of rejection should be minimized. Results seem to be better if lenticules are over 300 µm. Visual recovery is fast, occurring between 2 and 4 months. Sutures are removed during the third month, and astigmatism can be retreated with LASIK or better surface ablation techniques. Although complications are rare, some epithe-

lial invasion has been observed with thin tissues that have been inadequately sutured.

7.4.7.2 Deep Anterior Lamellar Keratoplasty

Deep anterior lamellar keratoplasty (DALK) is an alternative surgical technique in which optically abnormal corneal tissue is substituted by a normal donor cornea, leaving untouched the corneal endothelium and Descemet's membrane of the recipient cornea. This allows a large decrease in the risk of immunological rejections. The technique has been made popular by Melles and Terry, but it has been practiced by only a few ophthalmologists due to technical surgical difficulties and the limitations in visual recovery that is associated with DALK [19].

Apparently, the presence of residual corneal stroma over the Descemet's membrane and the irregular surface left by the handmade surgery creates a wound-healing surface and optical irregularities that are responsible for the limited visual functional outcome in some cases of DALK. Although the clinical results of DALK vary with the indication, the final visual acuity averaged 20/25 [18]. However, about a third of these patients still needed hard contact lens fitting to achieve this result. DALK is therefore reserved for those patients who suffer from post-refractive surgery irregular astigmatism who cannot be managed with other forms of treatment, or from astigmatism combined with scarring, near or within the optical axis.

7.4.7.3 Penetrating Keratoplasty

Penetrating keratoplasty (PK) is the first option in the management of irregular astigmatism associated with full-thickness corneal opacities. However, it may also be indicated in a clear cornea (after trauma or previous surgery) as a last resort, when all other treatments have failed. The difficulty lies in deciding when PK is the only solution, which may spare both the patient and the surgeon frustration and energy invested in ineffective attempts with milder techniques.

Although a lamellar keratoplasty has a much lower risk of rejection, this is counterbalanced by a greater technical complexity and the above-discussed difficulties in effectively eliminating all irregularity. PK provides, at least, a corneal "brand new start." As long as topography-guided laser ablation is not widely available and time tested, PK will remain an option for some irregular astigmatism, even in the absence of significant leukoma.

Take-Home Pearls

- Astigmatism is defined as irregular if the principal meridians are not 90° apart, usually because of an irregularity of the corneal curvature, and cannot be completely corrected with a spherocylindrical lens.
- The most common clinical symptoms of induced irregular astigmatism are decreased in best-corrected vision and visual distortion, together with night and/or day glare.
- Clinically, irregular astigmatism will present with a typical retinoscopy pattern, the most common being spinning and scissoring of the red reflex.
- The most recent and sophisticated technique in examination is the application of wavefront examination (aberrometers), especially corneal wavefront analysis.
- Corneal wavefront – guided excimer laser surgery, superficial corneal excision either mechanical, femto
- second or controlled by masking solution, anterior lamellar corneal graft techniques or PK can be used orderly to solve moderate to severe cases of corneal irregularity.

References

1. Alió JL, Belda JI, Patel S (2004) Treating irregular astigmatism and keratoconus. Highlights of Ophthalmology International, Miami 2004, pp 1–14
2. Alió JL, Belda JI (2004) Practical Guidelines for the correction of irregular astigmatism and keratoconus. In: Alió JL, Belda JI, Patel S (eds) Treating irregular astigmatism and keratoconus, Highlights of Ophthalmology International, Miami 2004, pp 335, 342
3. Goggin M, Alpins N, Schmid LM (2000) Management of irregular astigmatism. Curr Opin Ophthalmol 11:260–266
4. Alió JL, Shabayek MH (2006) Corneal higher order aberrations: a method to grade keratoconus. J Refract Surg 22:539–545
5. Caliz A, Montes-Mico R, Belda JI, Alió JL (2004) Corneal aberrometry as a guide for the correction of irregular astigmatism. In: Treating irregular astigmatism and the keratoconus. Highlights of Ophthalmology International, El Dorado, Republic of Panama
6. Boyd BF, Agarwal A, Alió JL, Krueger RR, Wilson SE (2003) Wavefront analysis, aberrometers and corneal topography. Highlights of Ophthalmology International, El Dorado, Republic of Panama
7. Berny F (1968) Formation des images retienes: Determination de l'aberration spherique due system de l'œil. Ph.D. thesis, University of Paris
8. Alió JL, Belda JI, Artola A, García-Lledó M, Osman A (2002) Contact lens fitting in the correction of irregular astigmatism after corneal refractive surgery. J Cataract Refract Surg 28:1750–1757
9. Cáliz A, Montes-Micó R, Belda JI, Alió JL (2004) Corneal aberrometry as a guide for the correction of Irregular astigmatism. In: Alio JL, Belda JI (eds) Treating irregular astigmatism and keratoconus. Highlights of Ophthalmology International, El Dorado, Republic of Panama, pp 121–133
10. Alió JL, Belda JI, Osman AA, Shalaby AMM (2003) Topography-guided laser in situ keratomileusis (TOPOLINK) to correct irregular astigmatism after previous refractive surgery. J Refract Surg 19: 516–527
11. Alió JL, Artola A, Rodríguez-Mier FA (2000) Selective zonal ablations with excimer laser for correction of irregular astigmatism induced by refractive surgery. Ophthalmology 107:662–673
12. Knorz MC, Jendiritza B (2000) Topography guided laser in situ keratomileusis to treat corneal irregularities. Ophthalmology 107:1138–1143
13. Alio JL, Galal A, Montalban R, Piñero D (2006) Corneal wavefront guided LASIK retreatments for correction of highly aberrated corneas following refractive surgery. J Refract Surg (in press)
14. Thompson V, Durrie DS, Cavanaugh TB (1993) Philosophy and technique for excimer laser phototherapeutic keratectomy. J Refract Corneal Surg 9:81–85
15. Pallikaris IG, Katsanevaki VJ, Ginis HS (2004) The PALM technique for the treatment of corneal irregular astigmatism. In: Alio JL, Belda JI (eds). Treating irregular astigmatism and keratoconus. Highlights of Ophthalmology International, El Dorado, Republic of Panama, pp 97–101
16. Artola A, Alió JL, Bellot JL, Ruiz JM (1993) Protective properties of viscoelastic substances (sodium hyaluronate and 2% hydroxymethyl cellulose) against experimental free radical damage to the corneal endothelium. Cornea 12:109–114
17. Alió J.L, Javaloy J, Merayo J, Galal A (2004) Automated superficial lamellar keratectomy augmented by excimer laser masked PTK in the management of severe superficial corneal opacities. Br J Ophthalmol 88:1289–1294

18. Alió JL, Uhah J, Barraquer C, Bilgihan K, Anwar M, Melles GRJ (2002) New techniques in Lamellar keratoplasty. Curr Opin Ophthalmol 13:224–229

19. Melles GRJ, Lander F, Rietveld FJR et al (1999) A new surgical technique for deep stromal, anterior lamellar keratoplasty. Br J Ophthalmol 83:327–333

Chapter 8

Optic Neuropathy and Retinal Complications after Refractive Surgery

8

J. Fernando Arevalo, Reinaldo A. Garcia,
Rafael A. Garcia-Amaris, and Juan G. Sanchez

Contents

Core Messages

- It is important to adopt preventive measures for optic neuropathy after LASIK.

- Vitreoretinal stress is induced at the posterior vitreous base during a posterior vitreous detachment after LASIK.

- Macular diseases may be a relative contraindication to LASIK in:
  - Patients with high myopia and lacquer cracks
  - Patients with angioid streaks and traumatic choroidal ruptures

- Macular hole may develop in myopic eyes after LASIK or photorefractive keratectomy.

- LASIK may be associated with uveitis.

- LASIK may be a safe and efficient option for treating refractive errors in eyes with previous retinal detachment surgery.

- Cryopexy, laser retinopexy, pneumatic retinopexy, or vitrectomy without a scleral band tend not to change the shape or length of the globe and should be preferred to repair RRD.

- Prophylactic treatment of vitreoretinal pathology before LASIK does not guarantee the prevention of post-LASIK vitreoretinal complications.

- It is very important to inform patients LASIK only corrects the refractive aspect of myopia, and vitreoretinal complications after LASIK although infrequent may occur.

- Reasons for poor VA after surgery for RRD post-LASIK include delayed referral to a vitreoretinal specialist.

8.1 Introduction

The prevalence of myopia in the United States ranges from 25 to 46.4% of the adult population [35–63]. In Asian populations, these proportions may be much higher and in African and Pacific island groups, much lower. The market for refractive surgery has a very large potential for people with low (less than –5.00 D) and moderate myopia (–5.01 to –10 D), and most patients fall into one of these two groups [63].

Refractive surgery has been accepted for correcting ametropias; however, this procedure may lead to complications. Hofman et al. [26], Sanders et al. [55], and Feldman et al. [20] have described cases of retinal detachment (RD) after radial keratotomy. Rodriguez and Camacho [45] reported on 14 eyes (12 patients) that had either asymptomatic or symptomatic retinal breaks, subclinical and clinical rhegmatogenous retinal detachment (RD), or both, 7 after automated lamellar keratoplasty (ALK), and 7 after radial keratotomy (RK). Rodriguez et al. [46], Barraquer et al. [11], and Ripandelli et al. [44] have reported retinal detachments af-

8

ter clear-lens extraction for myopia correction. Ruiz-Moreno and associates [48] reported the results of a clinically controlled study to investigate the rate of retinal detachment after implantation of phakic anterior chamber intraocular lenses (IOLs). The implantation of a phakic anterior chamber IOLs, as a correcting procedure, for severe myopia was followed by a 4.8% incidence of retinal detachment.

Laser-assisted in situ keratomileusis (LASIK) has become one of the most popular options for the correction of low to moderate myopia worldwide [41, 68]. However, complications including optic neuropathy [13], undercorrection and overcorrection [10], flap displacement [29], epithelial ingrowth [37], flap melting [5], keratitis [65], retinal tears [32], RDs [49], retinal phlebitis [29], corneoscleral perforations [3], retinal hemorrhages [3], macular hemorrhages [68], macular holes [15], serous macular detachments [60], choroidal neovascular membranes [3], reactivation of ocular toxoplasmosis [9], and irregular astigmatism have been reported.

The objective of this chapter is to review optic neuropathy and retinal complications that may occur after refractive surgery with an emphasis on LASIK.

8.2 Optic Neuropathy after LASIK

8.2.1 History and Mechanism of Optic Nerve Damage

Anterior ischemic optic neuropathy (AION), in most cases, is due to either arteriosclerosis or temporal arteritis. There are also large varieties of systemic, local vascular, and ocular disorders that can produce anterior ischemic optic neuropathy. The relationship between AION and LASIK was first reported by Lee et al. [30], with four cases of optic neuropathy and an onset of visual loss ranging from the day of surgery to 3 days after LASIK. Since that report, some studies have described the relationship between LASIK and the compromise of vascular supply of the posterior ciliary arteries such as in optic nerve ischemia (Fig. 8.1) [14], cilioretinal artery occlusion associated with ischemic optic neuropathy [1], appearance or progression of visual field defects in ocular hypertensive patients and normal tension glaucoma [13, 66], and choroidal infarcts [27].

Can all these conditions be explained by the same pathophysiology principle? In 1975, Hayreh [23] explained in detail that partial occlusion of the posterior ciliary arteries (due to any cause) is responsible for the development of AION because they supply the lamina cribosa, the prelaminar, and retrolaminar regions of the optic nerve. Anterior ischemic optic neuropathy, glaucoma, and low-tension glaucoma are manifestations of ischemia of the optic nerve head and retrolaminar optic nerve due to interference with posterior ciliary artery circulation because of an imbalance between perfusion pressure in the posterior ciliary arteries and intraocular pressure. If the process is sudden, then it produces anterior ischemic neuropathy with infarctions of the optic nerve head and retrolaminar region. If the pro-

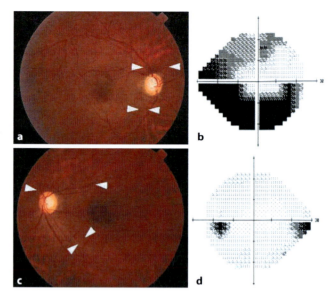

Fig. 8.1 A 39-year-old man had loss of vision on day one after bilateral LASIK. He described a hazy quality of vision in both eyes immediately after LASIK. His medical history had no other risk factors for optic neuropathy. Examination revealed a visual acuity of 20/20 in both eyes, normal color vision, increased cupping of the optic nerve, and a relative afferent pupillary defect in the right eye (RE). **a** Fifty-degree fundus photo of the RE shows diffuse loss of retinal nerve fiber layer (RNFL) at the superior pole of the disc and early wedge defects in the RNFL at the inferior pole of the disc (*arrows*). **b** Visual field shows a dense inferior nerve fiber bundle–type scotoma and a moderate superior nerve fiber bundle–type scotoma corresponding to the disc and RNFL defects in the RE. **c** Fifty-degree fundus photo of the left eye (LE) shows diffuse loss of RNFL at the superior pole of the disc and a wedge defect in the inferotemporal RNFL corresponding to the notch in the inferior neuroretinal rim (*arrows*). **d** Visual field shows an early inferior nerve fiber bundle–type scotoma corresponding to loss of superior RNFL in the LE (modified and reprinted from [14], with permission from the American Academy of Ophthalmology)

cess is chronic (as in glaucoma and low tension glaucoma), it produces slow degeneration of neural tissue in the optic nerve head and retrobulbar region, resulting in cupping of the optic disc and cavernous degeneration of the retrolaminar optic nerve.

When imbalance is produced between perfusion and intraocular pressure, by either lowering perfusion pressure or raising intraocular pressure, the susceptibility of intraocular blood vessels to obliteration varies considerably. The optic disc circulation is the first to compromise, then the peripapillary choroid, and finally the rest of the choroid. This explains the frequent presence of anterior ischemic optic neuropathy without a chorioretinal lesion. However, since a chorioretinal artery arises from a posterior ciliary artery, a cilioretinal artery occlusion may be associated with AION as described in the case reported by Ahmadieh and Javadi [1]. Finally, in AION the visual fields defects can be extremely variable and mimic many ocular and neurologic conditions. In fact, nerve fiber bundle defects with an arcuate scotoma may be seen in AION and simulate a glaucomatous defect as in the case reported by Weiss et al. [66] and Bushley et al. [13] after LASIK. Therefore, occlusion of the supply of one of the small subdivisions of the posterior ciliary arteries could involve a sector of the prelaminar, lamina cribosa, and retrolaminar regions of the optic nerve [23].

In LASIK, the creation of a corneal lamellar flap requires placement of a suction ring on the anterior segment of the eye, which transiently elevates the intraocular pressure (IOP) to levels exceeding 65 mmHg [67]. Experimental studies in animal eyes have found that the IOP can increase to between 80 and 230 mmHg during this vacuum phase, with the microkeratome. Other studies have suggested that an even greater increase in IOP of 140–60 mmHg may occur during the lamellar cut itself [30].

IOP elevation during LASIK may cause deterioration in perfusion of the retina and optic nerve head, posterior displacement of the lamina cribrosa, and a decline in ocular perfusion pressure of the posterior ciliary arteries. Although this IOP elevation is temporary, the potential for ischemic or pressure-induced damage to the optic nerve head and the retinal nerve fiber layer exists [67]. Therefore, LASIK-induced damage to the optic nerve could be ischemic because of transient interruption of blood flow in the short posterior ciliary arteries when the IOP is greater than the arterial perfusion pressure. Although less probable, LASIK related optic neuropathy could be due to barotrauma, with compression of the ganglion cells, nerve fiber layer, and lamina cribrosa. This would lead to posterior cupping of the optic nerve and damage to the nerve fibers, with resultant visual defect.

8.2.2 Optic Neuropathy Risk Factors

Optic neuropathy after LASIK surgery is an extremely rare, though an important vision-threatening complication because the visual acuity and visual field loss may be permanent. Furthermore, ophthalmologists should be aware of the potential for an acute anterior or retrobulbar optic neuropathy after LASIK, and should perform a comprehensive eye examination before and immediately after LASIK surgery to identify risk factors and promptly treat any complications.

Risk factors for ischemic optic neuropathy include personal and family history of glaucoma, previous optic neuropathy, severe cardiovascular disease such as hypertension or a tendency toward systemic arterial hypotension (congestive heart failure, myocardial ischemia, anesthesia and surgical or nonsurgical shock), any tendency towards elevated IOP or glaucoma, structural changes in optic disc such as "structural small disk at risk" and optic nerve head drusen, and finally, systemic conditions such as diabetes, hyperlipidemia, and factor V Leiden heterozygosity [13, 23, 30, 36].

Hayreh has suggested that nocturnal arterial hypotension is an important risk factor for the development and progression of non-arteritic anterior ischemic optic neuropathy (NA-AION). Potent antihypertensive drugs, when used aggressively and/or given at bedtime, are emerging as an important risk factor for nocturnal hypotension, and there is some evidence that NA-AION may be occurring as an iatrogenic disease in some individuals [25].

8.2.3 Clinical Findings

At the onset of optic neuropathy after LASIK, the patient can present postoperative visual acuity and color vision deterioration, relative afferent pupillary defect, variable swelling of the disc, and optic nerve-related visual field defects. Deep cupping of the optic nerve, focal changes in the neuroretinal rim, and decreased thickness of the retinal nerve fiber layer can be seen 2 or 3 months after the onset of AION, and sometimes as soon as 6 weeks [14, 23, 30].

8.2.4 Management

Treatment options in AION are controversial. Steroid treatment for the NA-AION has its advocates. A number of reports suggest that systemic corticosteroids given during the very early stages of the disease may help to improve visual function in some patients [22, 24]. Hayreh has found definite evidence of a significant visual improvement with steroids in a small group of patients, particularly those with incipient NA-AION, treated early [22–24].

Surgical treatment including optic nerve fenestration was advocated for AION until the completion of the Ischemic Optic Neuropathy Decompression Trial (IONDT). This study conclusively showed no effect of the surgical procedure [38]. Optic neurotomy has been advocated recently for NA-AION [62]. In this procedure, a radial cut is made through the entire thickness of the optic nerve head; this procedure not only cuts thousands and thousands of nerve fibers in the optic nerve head, but also cuts the blood vessels supplying the optic nerve head, both of which are bound to produce more loss of vision without any beneficial effect [25].

8.2.5 Prevention

Because there is no real treatment for this condition, it is extremely important to adopt preventive measures. Prevention should include (1) avoiding any sudden fall in systemic arterial blood pressure (hypotensive anesthesia, congestive heart failure), (2) improving systemic circulatory hemodynamics by medical therapy, (3) preventing any sudden rise in intraocular pressure (angle closure and intraocular surgery such as cataract extraction), and (4) keeping intraocular pressure as low as possible by medical means [23, 24, 37, 59].

Patients with personal or family history of AION, systemic diseases, or ophthalmic risks such as a small optic nerve, glaucoma, a family history of glaucoma, as well as glaucoma suspects should be cautioned of LASIK associated visual field loss prior to the procedure. For many of these patients, photorefractive keratectomy, intrastromal corneal ring segments, or continued use of contact lens or eyeglasses may offer satisfactory vision without subjecting the optic nerve to the small but real risk of pressure-associated visual field loss [66].

8.3 Retinal Detachments and Retinal Breaks

Several studies have been reported in the literature regarding retinal detachments after LASIK [32, 39, 64]. Ozdamar et al. [39] have reported a case of bilateral retinal detachment associated with giant retinal tear after LASIK. Stulting and associates [64] reported a case of rhegmatogenous RD after LASIK for the correction of myopia. Ruiz-Moreno and coworkers [49] reported 4 RDs (an incidence of 0.25%) in myopic eyes after LASIK and a mean best-corrected visual acuity (BCVA) of 20/45 after retinal surgery. Aras et al. [2] described 10 RDs (an incidence of 0.22%) in myopic eyes after LASIK. Farah and coworkers [19] recently reported four eyes that had early rhegmatogenous RDs within 3 months LASIK for correction of high myopia. Although no cause–effect relationship between LASIK and retinal detachment can be stated from their study, the authors' cases suggest that LASIK may be associated with retinal detachment, particularly in highly myopic eyes.

We have previously reported a 2-year follow-up of 29,916 eyes after LASIK for the correction of ametropias (myopes and hyperopes).The incidence at 24 months of vitreoretinal pathology in our study was 0.06%, including 14 rhegmatogenous retinal detachments (RRDs) [32]. The incidence of RRD after LASIK in our previous studies ranges between 0.04 and 0.05% [4, 32].

For our latest analyzed data [6], we reviewed the medical records and obtained follow-up information on all patients in our files with RRD after LASIK for the correction of myopia at five institutions. A total of 38,823 LASIK procedures (eyes) were performed during the study period (5 years) by five experienced refractive surgeons. The mean age of the patients that had LASIK was 36 years. Patients underwent surgical correction of myopia ranging from –0.75 to –29 D (mean, –6.00 D). Patients were scheduled to be seen during the first postoperative day, at 3 months, at 12 months, and yearly thereafter. Patients were followed for a mean of 48 months after LASIK (range, 6–60 months).

Five vitreoretinal surgeons and 33 eyes (27 patients) that developed RRD after LASIK for the correction of myopia participated in the study (Fig. 8.2). The clinical findings, frequency of RRD after LASIK, characteristics (fundus drawings of the 33 eyes were evaluated), and surgical outcomes of 31 eyes (two patients refused surgery) are presented. Patients with RRD after LASIK were included in the study independent on the length of follow-up. Final visual acuity (VA) was defined as the BCVA at last follow-up examination, ranging from 3 to 34 months (mean, 14 months) after vitreoretinal surgery to repair RRD after LASIK.

LASIK was performed on patients with no history of prior refractive surgery, keratoconus, prior cataract surgery,

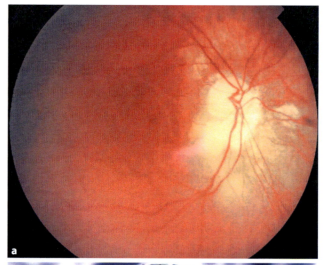

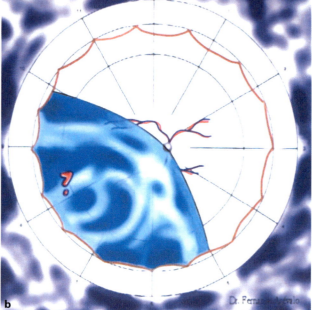

Fig. 8.2 a Fundus photograph of a subtotal inferotemporal retinal detachment (macula off) after LASIK. **b** Retinal drawing of the same case with partial posterior vitreous detachment, a horseshoe retinal tear at 8 o'clock, and a retinal hole at the same location

proliferative diabetic retinopathy, or collagen vascular disease. Preoperative examinations included a very thorough dilated fundoscopy with scleral depression and treatment of any retinal lesion predisposing for the development of a RRD. We found 33 eyes (27 patients) that developed RRD after LASIK for the correction of myopia. Our 27 patients had an average age of 37.8 (16–60) years old. Eighteen patients (66.6%) were male. In our series, 9% (3/33) of eyes that developed a RRD had some kind of enhancement after LASIK. The left eye was affected in 18 (54.5%) cases. No patient had a history of any other ocular surgery after LASIK. The frequency of rhegmatogenous retinal detachments determined in our study is 0.08% (33/38,823).

RRDs occurred between 12 days and 60 months (mean, 16.3 months) after LASIK. Eyes that developed a RRD had from –1.50 to –16 D of myopia (mean, –8.75 D) before LASIK. Retinal detachments were managed with vitrectomy, cryoretinopexy, scleral buckling, argon laser retinopexy, and pneumatic retinopexy techniques. Vitreoretinal surgery to repair RRD after LASIK was performed at a mean of 56 days (range, 1 day to 18 months) after the onset of visual symptoms. The mean follow-up after retinal surgery was 14 months (range, 3–34 months) and 38.7% of the 31 eyes (two patients refused surgery) had a final BCVA of 20/40 or better. Final VA was better than 20/200 in 77.4% of eyes. Poor VA (20/200 or worse) occurred in 22.6% of eyes. Reasons for poor VA included the development of proliferative vitreoretinopathy (PVR) (n = 5), epiretinal membrane (n = 1), chronicity of RRD (n = 1), new breaks (n = 1), displaced corneal flap (n = 1), and cataract (n = 1).

Final VA after RRD surgery improved two lines or more in 51.6% (16/31) of eyes. The anatomic success at final follow-up with one surgery was 87.1% (27/31). Three eyes required from one to three reoperations with pars plana vitrectomy and silicone oil injection, and one eye required argon laser retinopexy to seal new retinal breaks. The anatomic success at final follow-up including reoperations was 90.3% (28/31). Information regarding VA after LASIK and before the development of RRD was available in 24 eyes, 45.8% (11/24) of eyes lost two or more lines of VA after vitreoretinal surgery.

Recently, Ruiz-Moreno et al. [47] studied the incidence of retinal disease observed in 9,239 consecutive eyes (5,099 patients) after refractive surgery (including LASIK). Retinal detachment occurred at a mean 24.6 +/–20.4 months after LASIK in 11 eyes (0.36%).

8.3.1 Retinal Detachment Characteristics and Retinal Breaks Distribution

Fundus drawings of the 33 eyes were evaluated [6] (Fig. 8.2b). Eight detachments were total, and 25 were subtotal. Of the 25 subtotal RRDs, 12 had the macula off and, 13 were macula on RRD. Of the 25 subtotal RRDs, 15 involved predominantly inferior quadrants, and 10 were predominantly superior RRDs. An RRD involved more than one quadrant in 10 out of 25 subtotal RRDs. The inferotemporal quadrant was involved in 14 of the subtotal RRDs in our series, the inferonasal quadrant was involved in 9, the superotemporal in 8, and superonasal in 7. The mean number of retinal breaks per RRD was 4.3 (range, 0–40), including 98 holes, 41 horseshoe tears, two retinal dialyses, and one giant retinal tear. One hundred one (71.1%) retinal breaks were located temporally (61 inferotemporal), and 41 (28.9%) were located nasally (28 inferonasal). The vitreous status was available from 27 of our cases, 17 (62.9%) had posterior vitreous detachment (PVD), and 10 (37.1%) had no PVD. Seven (22.5%) of our RRD cases had a retinal break associated to lattice degeneration. Six (19.3%) of our cases had proliferative vitreoretinopathy (PVR) grade C (Fig. 8.3).

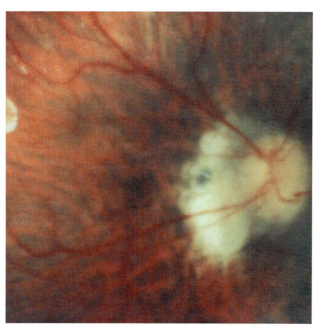

Fig. 8.3 Postoperative fundus photograph of a myopic eye that developed a rhegmatogenous retinal detachment with proliferative vitreoretinopathy (PVR) after laser in situ keratomileusis. Vitrectomy and silicone oil injection were successfully performed

The long interval between the onset of symptoms and RRD surgery may be responsible for some of the factors (including a 19.3% rate of PVR) that contributed to poor final VA in more than 20% of our cases. In some of our patients, there may have been some delay in the referral to the vitreoretinal specialist due to a belief that the visual symptoms were related to a refractive or corneal problem after LASIK. In addition, other factors related to high myopia (including myopic degeneration and amblyopia) might also influence the final functional results, regardless of our high anatomic success rate.

Recently, Chan and coworkers [16] described the characteristics of a large number of eyes (60) with substantial myopia (mean myopia, –9.5±5.8 D) with pre-LASIK retinal examinations (14 eyes had documented lattice degeneration or small retinal breaks) and characteristics of post-LASIK retinal breaks and RRD. Many of those eyes developed complex vitreoretinal complications (53.3% with two or more breaks, 26.7% eyes with three or more breaks, 30% with bilateral conditions, 8.3% with total RD, 8.3% with PVR, 6.7% with giant tears, and 5% with extensive retinal dialysis). Forty percent developed vitreoretinal complications within 6 months after LASIK. Distributions of retinal breaks in this study are comparable to those found in similar myopic eyes not involved with LASIK in the young adult category.

The authors concluded that in this study, retinal breaks, tears, and holes were distributed relatively evenly between the superior and inferior quadrants. The reason for this even distribution is unknown, but vitreoretinal stress induced at the posterior vitreous base during a posterior vitreous detachment will more likely lead to retinal breaks and RD in the temporal rather than in the nasal quadrants.

8.4 Serous Macular Detachment

Singhvi et al. [60] reported a case of bilateral serous macular detachment after LASIK. They conclude that the possible mechanism of occurrence of central serous corioretinopathy (CSCR) after LASIK includes the generation of shockwaves due to the mechanical force of suction of the microkeratome ring, leading to alterations in the fragile submacular vessels or the retinal pigmented epithelial (RPE). Preexisting macular pathology, such as RPE atrophy could be a new contraindication to LASIK for hypermetropia with possible development of CSCR.

8.4.1 Macular Hemorrhage, Lacquer Cracks, and Choroidal Neovascular Membranes

Kim and Jung [28] reported one eye that lost greater than two lines of preoperative best-corrected vision due to macular hemorrhage. Luna et al. [33] have reported a case of bilateral macular hemorrhage after LASIK. One day after surgery the patient's uncorrected visual acuity was in the 20/50 range, and by 17 days after surgery his visual acuity had declined to 20/200 range. Fundus examination showed multifocal subretinal macular and posterior pole hemorrhages. Fluorescein angiography showed some macular lesions compatible with lacquer cracks. Principe et al. [43] reported the first case of unilateral macular hemorrhage after uncomplicated, bilateral, simultaneous LASIK with femtosecond laser flap creation in a patient without macular pathology. In this case, the IOP is only raised to approximately 35–40 mmHg during flap creation because this technique does not use a mechanical microkeratome.

In conclusion, macular hemorrhage may occur after LASIK, even in the absence of previously identified risk factors, such as high myopia, preexisting CNV, lacquer cracks, and sudden changes in intraocular pressure associated with microkeratome-assisted flap creation.

We were the first to describe a CNV after LASIK [32]. A 48 year-old Hispanic hyperopic (+3.50 D OD and +4.00 D OS) man was seen on December of 1997 at our institution because of visual loss OS 2 years after a LASIK procedure. On examination, visual acuity was 20/400, and biomicroscopy was unremarkable. Dilated fundoscopy and fluorescein angiography showed a juxtafoveal CNV membrane (CNVM) with subretinal fluid. A pars plana vitrectomy and a temporal retinotomy were performed to remove the CNVM from the subretinal space, and air was instilled into the vitreous cavity. Topical steroids and cycloplegics were prescribed. Eight months later, his visual acuity OS was Counting fingers and fundoscopy showed a juxtafoveal retinal pigment epithelium defect.

Ruiz-Moreno et al. [50, 51] have reported an incidence of 0.1% CNV after LASIK and one case after photorefractive keratectomy (1/5,936). Saeed et al. [54] reported one case of CNV after LASIK in a patient with low myopia. The incidence seems to be very low; however, the appearance and treatment of CNV was followed by a significant decrease of visual acuity.

Recently Maturi et al. [34] and Ruiz-Moreno et al. [53] have reported two letters describing the characteristics and potential mechanisms of a macular lacquer crack (one with subsequent development of subfoveal CNV) in myopic patients corrected by LASIK. Lacquer cracks often lead to poor visual outcomes because of CNV and macular atrophy in pathologic myopia. The risk of developing lacquer cracks in highly myopic patients corrected by LASIK, though uncommon, must be kept in mind.

Scupola et al. [57] and Arevalo et al. [7] have recently reported success in stabilizing or improving vision in patients with subfoveal CNV from pathologic myopia after LASIK with photodynamic therapy (PDT) with verteporfin. Scupola et al. [57] reported a case of CNV after LASIK following penetrating keratoplasty (PK). Photodynamic therapy was performed and 1 year later VA was stable at 20/200. Arevalo et al. [7] reported the management of subfoveal CNV in highly myopic eyes after LASIK with PDT. Five cases of CNV after LASIK for the correction of myopia (mean, 13.3 D; range, –8.00 D to –16.25 D) treated with single or multiple sessions of PDT with verteporfin were presented (Fig. 8.4). Two cases improved VA (two to five lines) after PDT, two cases remained the same, and one case lost four lines of VA. VA improved or remained the same in 80% of cases (4/5 eyes). Photodynamic therapy with verteporfin seems to increase the chance of stabilizing or improving vision in patients with subfoveal CNV after LASIK in high myopes at least with a short period of follow-up (mean, 9.4 months; range, 3–13 months).

Choroidal neovascularization is related to myopia itself and its incidence varies from 4 to 11% in patients with high myopia. In addition, lacquer cracks have been found to be associated to CNV in up to 82% of cases with myopia [53]. Theoretically, when a break in Bruch's membrane occurs, it allows the progression of the neovascular complex under the retina. The increase in IOP to levels over 60 mmHg during suction, with the microkeratome suction ring up to 4 mm posterior to the limbus may exert traction and compression posteriorly. In addition, we have to consider that the excimer laser is responsible for a shock wave that is transmitted to the eye. These mechanisms may open the gap in Bruch's membrane even more. We believe that in patients with high myopia and lacquer cracks, LASIK should be considered contraindicated and some other method of refractive surgery offered.

8.4.2 Macular Hole

Chan and Lawrence [15] have recently reported three eyes of three myopic patients that developed a macular hole in one eye after bilateral LASIK or PK. The macular hole formed between 4 to 7 weeks after LASIK in case 1 (a 48-

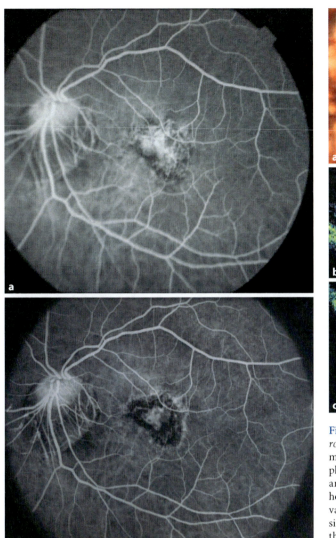

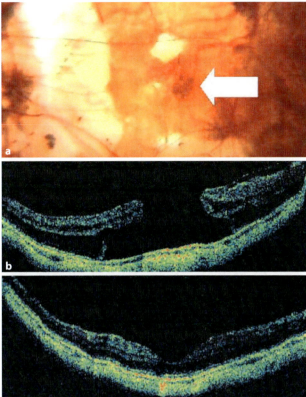

Fig. 8.5 a Retinal examination revealed a stage 4 macular hole (*arrow*) in the left eye associated with a posterior pole retinal detachment, and a BCVA of counting fingers. b Optical coherence tomography (OCT) image showing features of both foveal retinal detachment and retinoschisis. c OCT after vitrectomy reveals a closed macular hole with a BCVA of 20/150. (Reprinted with permission from Arevalo et al [2005] Vitreoretinal surgery for macular hole after laser assisted in situ keratomileusis for the correction of myopia. Br J Ophthalmol 89:1423–1426)

Fig. 8.4 a Subfoveal choroidal neovascular membrane (CNV) after LASIK was diagnosed with fluorescein angiography (FA). b The CNV was treated with two sessions of photodynamic therapy (PDT) with verteporfin 6 months apart. After the last PDT treatment, the CNV was totally closed, with a small central area of staining and no leakage on FA

year-old woman), and within 2 months after LASIK in case 2 (a 36-year-old woman). In case 3 (a 45-year-old man), the macular hole was found 9 months after PK. A vitrectomy closed the macular hole of case 1 with final BCVA of 20/25 and case 2 with 20/30, whereas case 3 declined further surgery. The authors conclude that macular hole may develop in myopic eyes after LASIK or PK. and that vitreoretinal interface changes may play a role.

Ruiz-Moreno et al. [52] reported a case, and recently our group [8] reported on 20 eyes (19 patients) that developed a macular hole in one eye after bilateral LASIK for the correction of ametropia (Fig. 8.5). The macular hole formed between 1 to 83 months after LASIK (mean, 12.1 months). Eighteen percent of patients were female. All eyes were my-

opic. Posterior vitreous detachment was not present before and was documented after LASIK on 55% of eyes. A vitrectomy closed the macular hole on all 14 eyes that underwent surgical management. These twenty eyes reflect an incidence of 0.02% (20/83,938), and represent the largest series of macular hole after LASIK to date.

How could the excimer laser or the microkeratome cause a macular hole? What is the pathophysiology? When the suction ring induces an increase in IOP and after that it is suddenly released, the anterior segment is rapidly drawn into a vacuum chamber with its shape changed rapidly, and all structures posterior to the suction ring are also compressed and decompressed in sequence. This type of "trauma" is in some ways analogous to what happens in a closed-eye injury. A mechanism for development of peripheral retinal tears or macular disease could be anterior–posterior compression and expansion. The eye elongates along the anterior–posterior axis, and the diameter of the globe may increase. At the same time, because the eye is a closed system, the eye is constricted in the equatorial plane (Fig. 8.6a). As

8

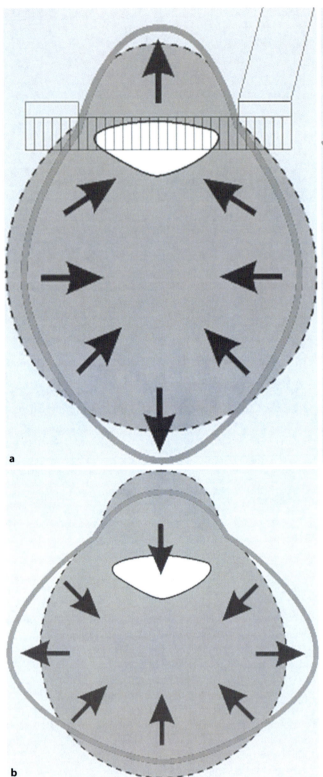

a

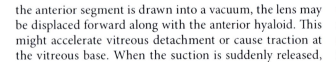

b

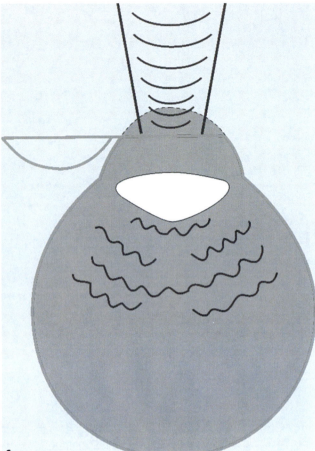

c

Fig. 8.6 The following changes may cause acute vitreoretinal traction at the vitreous base and posterior pole. **a** When the suction ring is in place, the eye deforms along the anterior–posterior axis, and the diameter of the globe may increase. At the same time, because the eye is a closed system, the eye must contract along the horizontal axis, and equatorial diameter may decrease. **b** When the suction stops, and the suction ring is released, decompression leads to a dynamic overshoot with equatorial elongation and anterior–posterior contraction. **c** In addition, the excimer laser–induced shock wave may play a role in the development of posterior vitreous detachment. (Reprinted from [5], with permission from the American Society of Cataract and Refractive Surgery and the European Society of Cataract Refractive Surgeons)

the anterior segment is drawn into a vacuum, the lens may be displaced forward along with the anterior hyaloid. This might accelerate vitreous detachment or cause traction at the vitreous base. When the suction is suddenly released,

decompression leads to a dynamic overshoot with equatorial expansion and shortening in the anterior–posterior dimension (Fig. 8.6b). These events may cause acute vitreoretinal traction at the vitreous base and posterior pole.

In addition, when the excimer laser light ablates tissue, energy is released anteriorly as a plume of ablated tissue and is thrown into the air in front of the cornea. Certainly, such a powerful force might also be associated with backward force into the vitreous. Posteriorly, energy is transmitted in the form of a shockwave (Fig. 8.6c). The effect of shockwaves and posteriorly radiated energy on the vitreous integrity is unknown.

8.5 Uveitis

Anterior uveitis after LASIK for the correction of ametropia is infrequent, with an incidence of 0.18%, or an annual incidence of 0.06% (60 per 100,000 eyes) according to data reported by Suarez et al. [65]. This number is much higher than the annual incidence of anterior uveitis in the general population (0.008% or 8 cases per 100,000 people). The authors concluded that uveitis may be due to uveal trauma during surgery with disruption of normal anterior chamber–associated immune deviation, decreased anti-inflammatory cytokines, and increased proinflammatory cytokines.

Lin and Tsai [30] recently reported a case of retinal phlebitis with cystoid macular edema in both eyes 8 weeks after LASIK. Their patient experienced blurred vision and demonstrated focal whitish patches in the parafoveal and juxtafoveal areas and lack of foveal reflex in both eyes. Visual acuity returned to normal, and the whitish fundus patches decreased in number and size in both eyes after the patient was treated with oral corticosteroids. They conclude that the shockwaves induced for LASIK may cause mechanical stress to the retina, resulting in structural damage and intraocular inflammation.

Barbara et al. [9] have reported a case of reactivation of ocular toxoplasmosis in a patient who underwent bilateral LASIK. The posterior segment examination revealed an old toxoplasmosis scar in the retinal periphery of the right eye. Uncorrected visual acuity improved postoperatively, and the patient was satisfied. However, 52 days after the procedure, he complained of loss of visual acuity in his right eye. Examination revealed signs of anterior uveitis, vitreitis, and active chorioretinal lesion satellite of the old toxoplasmosis scar. The patient was treated with a multidrug regiment with resolution of the vitreous and lesion activity. The authors conclude that toxoplasmosis reactivation may develop after LASIK.

In eyes with uveitis, LASIK should be performed when the inflammation is quiescent to avoid severe postoperative inflammation. However, patients and clinicians should be aware of possible signs and symptoms of intraocular inflammation after LASIK [65].

8.6 LASIK after Retinal Detachment Surgery

Belda et al. [12], Sforza and Saffra [58], and Sinha et al. [61] have recently described 16 patients with a previously placed encircling scleral buckle for a retinal detachment who had LASIK to correct myopia. In all patients, the uncorrected VA improved, and the myopic spherical equivalent decreased after the procedure. However, scarred conjunctiva in such cases (12.5%, 2/16) may prevent generation of optimal suction for the microkeratome. Long-term follow-up is necessary to determine the safety of LASIK in these eyes.

Barequet et al. [10] evaluated the safety and efficacy of LASIK for correction of myopia in nine eyes with previous retinal detachment surgery. LASIK was performed in

130±123 months following retinal detachment surgery. The postoperative LASIK follow-up was 14.8±12.5 months. No significant intraoperative, postoperative, or retinal complications were observed. The mean preoperative spherical equivalent refraction was –9.00±3.00 D, uncorrected visual acuity (UCVA) was 0.06±0.02, and best spectacle-corrected visual acuity (BSCVA) was 0.64±0.16. At the end of follow-up, the mean spherical equivalent refraction was 0.65±0.88 D, mean UCVA was 0.57±0.14, and mean BSCVA was 0.72±0.19. Therefore, LASIK was found to be a safe and efficient option for treating refractive errors in eyes with previous retinal detachment surgery.

8.7 Corneoscleral Perforations

In our series [3], two eyes suffered corneoscleral perforations with the surgical microkeratome when a corneal flap was being performed (one of them developed a vitreous hemorrhage and the other one later developed a retinal detachment).

A 24 year-old Hispanic myopic (–5.00 D OD and –4.25 D OS) woman was seen at our institution because of visual loss OD immediately after a LASIK procedure. According to the refractive surgeon, he had omitted to place a spacing plate into the microkeratome when a corneal flap was being performed. An ocular perforation occurred with corneal and iris wounds, loss of the crystalline lens, vitreous loss, and the development of vitreous hemorrhage. A thorough anterior vitrectomy was performed with suture of the corneal and iris wounds with 10-0 nylon. Oral and topical steroids were prescribed. Thirteen months later, her visual acuity was 20/25[-1] with a contact lens.

In our second case, a 38 year-old Hispanic myopic (–20 D OD and –15 D OS) woman was seen at our institution because of visual loss OS after a LASIK procedure. According to the refractive surgeon, a corneal perforation had occurred with the microkeratome when a corneal flap was being performed. She had undergone crystalline lens remnants aspiration and an anterior vitrectomy one week later. On examination, a sutured (10-0 nylon) corneal wound with Descemet's folds is seen on biomicroscopy. Dilated fundoscopy does not show details of the retina due to media opacities. Diagnostic B-scan ultrasound shows an inferior retinal detachment. A vitrectomy is performed with a 360° circumferential scleral band, endolaser, and SF_6. Topical steroids and cycloplegics were prescribed. Three months later, she developed a retinal tear in the fellow eye (also treated with LASIK), which was managed with an argon laser retinopexy. Six months later, her visual acuity OS was hand motions due to corneal scarring and a recurrent inferior rhegmatogenous retinal detachment.

Some cases of LASIK-induced corneal perforation have been treated by applying a therapeutic soft contact lens with topical antibiotics, oral carbonic anhydrase inhibitors, and eye patching. However, we believe that it is important to mention that LASIK-induced corneal perforations can be very severe, and sutures may be necessary. In addition, severe cases may be associated to posterior segment damage as demonstrated in our report. [3] The incidence of vitreoretinal complications (vitreous hemorrhage and retinal detachment after corneoscleral perforations) during LASIK determined in our study is 0.006% (2/29,916).

We recommend that refractive surgeons be meticulous in properly assembling the microkeratome to create a corneal flap during LASIK. The use of currently available disposable microkeratomes may help to avoid this complication in the future.

8.8 Displacement of Corneal Cap during Vitrectomy

In one of our cases, a dislocated corneal flap occurred from corneal epithelial debridement during vitrectomy 69 months after LASIK. A similar case has been previously reported by Chaudhry and Smiddy [18]; their case underwent vitreous surgery only 4 months after LASIK.

Displacement of a corneal flap after LASIK is a serious complication. Possibilities include losing the cap, epithelial ingrowth, interface particles, and striae in the flap (trauma to the flap may affect the final refractive status). Displacement of the corneal flap has been described after corneal epithelial debridement during a scleral buckling procedure, and vitrectomy.

Recommendations for vitreoretinal surgeons when treating an eye with a history of LASIK include avoiding debridement of the corneal epithelium. However, if it is necessary, start corneal debridement nasally and advance temporally (most cases have a nasal hinge). If a displaced corneal flap occurs, then initial management includes repositioning of the flap, followed by patching and topical steroids. Refractory cases may require suture fixation. A bandage contact lens may be useful if striae develop. If striae persist, it is an indication to elevate and reposition the flap.

8.9 Final Considerations

The incidence of vitreoretinal pathology after LASIK in our study was 0.06% (annual incidence 0.02%) [3]. This number is much lower than the incidence of RRD in myopes in general [55]. This finding may be explained by the fact that refractive surgery patients in the institutions involved underwent preoperative examinations, including a very thorough dilated indirect fundoscopy with scleral depression and treatment of any peripheral retinal lesion predisposing for the development of a RRD before LASIK. In this study extensive lattice degeneration, flap tears, atrophic holes, and retinal tufts were prophylactically treated regardless of symptoms. Such indication is justified by the fact that vitreoretinal surgery causes changes in corneal shape thus damaging the refractive surgeon's results. We suggest that cryopexy, argon laser retinopexy, pneumatic retinopexy, or vitrectomy without a scleral band be performed when appropriate because they tend not to change the shape or

length of the globe. Another option in case of scleral buckling procedures is to remove the explants early, as suggested by Rodriguez and Camacho [45], after being sure all breaks have sealed, and that no retinal detachment is present anywhere in the fundus.

Lin and Tseng [32] have recently published a study to determine the efficacy and safety of prophylactic laser photocoagulation for retinal breaks in myopic patients undergoing LASIK. Retinal breaks were identified and treated in 39 eyes (2.02%) of 32 patients (3.2%). During a mean 19-month follow-up, none of the patients developed RRD except for one in a patient without retinal breaks who sustained ocular trauma 19 months after LASIK.

Chan et al. [17] suggested that pre-LASIK retinal examination might predict locations of certain post-LASIK retinal lesions (breaks, retinal detachment) that may develop in highly myopic eyes with pre-LASIK vitreoretinal pathology (lattice, breaks), but prophylactic treatment of vitreoretinal pathology before LASIK does not guarantee the prevention of post-LASIK vitreoretinal complications.

Based on published data, we cannot determine whether prophylactic treatment is indicated. Currently, it is not possible to determine scientifically whether peripheral retinal lesions should be treated in a way different from standard practice just because a patient is to undergo LASIK. Most practitioners suggest that patients scheduled for LASIK be carefully examined with indirect ophthalmoscopy and scleral depression under pupillary dilatation to detect any myopic peripheral lesion that requires treatment before LASIK is performed. One could argue that this is prudent in myopes whether they undergo LASIK; given the potential of the procedure to exacerbate preexisting pathology, it might be wise to treat such pathology more aggressively.

Another important factor to take into consideration when we evaluate our state of knowledge in this area is duration of follow-up. Patients described with vitreoretinal pathology after LASIK have been followed up for relatively short duration (0.5–3 years). It is reasonable to expect that the incidence of RRD in the initial cohort of patients that had LASIK will rise with time. It is possible LASIK-induced trauma might accelerate vitreous liquefaction, and over the years these patients might have a higher incidence of retinal detachments and other vitreoretinal problems. It is equally likely that with the current practice patterns, we ophthalmologist would be unaware of this.

Macular diseases may be a relative contraindication to LASIK. Patients with high myopia and lacquer cracks in the macula are at high risk to develop macular hemorrhage or CNV after the IOP is raised with the suction ring during the procedure. Patients with angioid streaks and traumatic choroidal ruptures are in the same category of risk. Stage 1 macular holes may progress due to traction in the posterior pole during LASIK. In addition, eyes that are at risk of needing vitreoretinal surgery in the future have a relative contraindication to LASIK. On the other hand, in eyes with stable macular disease (scars), LASIK may be performed depending on the refractive surgeon criteria if the patient is aware and accepts his visual acuity limitations.

In summary, serious complications after LASIK are infrequent. It is very important to inform patients that LASIK only corrects the refractive aspect of myopia. Vitreoretinal complications in these eyes will occur and only careful and large prospective studies in patients can determine if the procedure exacerbates myopic pathology. Such studies will need to be performed using careful prospective examinations including, determination of risk factors, echography of the vitreous, indirect ophthalmoscopy and scleral depression and possible photography and angiography of the macula region to determine whether the LASIK procedure itself can exacerbate pathologic changes in the myopic eye. In addition, our latest study shows that results may be not as good as expected after RRD surgery. Reasons for poor VA include the development of epiretinal membrane, proliferative vitreoretinopathy, chronicity of RRD, new retinal breaks, and cataract formation. Final VA may be limited by myopic degeneration, amblyopia, or delayed referral to a vitreoretinal specialist.

Take-Home Pearls

- Because there is no real treatment for optic neuropathy after LASIK, it is extremely important to adopt preventive measures.
- Vitreoretinal stress induced at the posterior vitreous base during a posterior vitreous detachment after LASIK may lead to retinal breaks and RRD.
- Preexisting macular pathology in hypermetropia, such as RPE atrophy, might be associated with the development of CSCR or subretinal fluid after LASIK.
- Macular diseases may be a relative contraindication to LASIK:
  - Patients with high myopia and lacquer cracks in the macula are at high risk to develop macular hemorrhage or CNV after the IOP is raised with the suction ring during the procedure.
  - Patients with angioid streaks and traumatic choroidal ruptures are in the same category of risk.
- Macular hole may develop in myopic eyes after LASIK or photorefractive keratectomy. Fortunately, vitrectomy is successful in closing the macular hole.
- In eyes with uveitis, LASIK should be performed when the inflammation is quiescent to avoid severe postoperative inflammation.
- LASIK was found to be a safe and efficient option for treating refractive errors in eyes with previous retinal detachment surgery. However, scarred conjunctiva in such cases may prevent generation of optimal suction for the microkeratome.
- To avoid corneoscleral perforations, we recommend refractive surgeons be meticulous in properly assembling the microkeratome to create a corneal flap during LASIK or use a disposable microkeratome.
- Vitreoretinal surgeons when treating an eye with a history of LASIK should avoid debridement of the corneal epithelium.

- Cryopexy, laser retinopexy, pneumatic retinopexy, or vitrectomy without a scleral band tend not to change the shape or length of the globe and should be preferred to repair RRD.
- Prophylactic treatment of vitreoretinal pathology before LASIK does not guarantee the prevention of post-LASIK vitreoretinal complications.
- At the time, it is not possible to scientifically determine whether peripheral retinal lesions should be treated in a way different from standard practice just because a patient is to undergo LASIK; however, given the potential of the procedure to exacerbate pre-existing pathology, it might be wise to treat such pathology more aggressively.
- It is very important to inform patients that LASIK only corrects the refractive aspect of myopia, and that vitreoretinal complications after LASIK although infrequent may occur.
- Reasons for poor VA after surgery for RRD post-LASIK include delayed referral to a vitreoretinal specialist.

References

1. Ahmadieh H, Javadi MA (2005) Cilioretinal artery occlusion following laser in situ keratomileusis. Retina 25:533–537
2. Aras C, Ozdamar A, Karacorlu M et al (2000) Retinal detachment following laser in situ keratomileusis. Ophthalmic Surg Lasers 31:121–125
3. Arevalo JF, Ramirez E, Suarez E et al (2000) Incidence of vitreoretinal pathologic conditions 24 months after laser-assisted in situ keratomileusis (LASIK). Ophthalmology 107:258–262
4. Arevalo JF, Ramirez E, Suarez E et al (2000) Retinal detachments after laser-assisted in situ keratomileusis (LASIK) for the correction of myopia. Retina 20:338–341
5. Arevalo JF, Ramirez E, Suarez E et al (2001) Rhegmatogenous retinal detachment in myopic eyes after laser in situ keratomileusis, frequency, characteristics, and mechanism. J Cataract Refract Surg 27:674–680
6. Arevalo JF, Ramirez E, Suarez E et al (2002) Retinal detachment in myopic eyes after laser in situ keratomileusis. J Refract Surg 18:708–714
7. Arevalo JF, Ruiz-Moreno JM, Fernandez CF et al (2004) Photodynamic therapy with verteporfin for subfoveal choroidal neovascular membranes in highly myopic eyes after laser in situ keratomileusis. Ophthalmic Surg Lasers Imaging 35:58–62
8. Arevalo JF, Mendoza AJ, Velez-Vasquez W et al (2005) Full-thickness macular hole after lasik for the correction of myopia. Ophthalmology 112:1207–1212
9. Barbara A, Shehadeh-Masha'our R, Sartani G, Garzozi HJ (2005) Reactivation of ocular toxoplasmosis after LASIK. J Refract Surg 21:759–761
10. Barequet IS, Levy J, Klemperer I et al (2005) Laser in situ keratomileusis for correction of myopia in eyes after retinal detachment surgery. J Refract Surg 21:191–193
11. Barraquer C, Cavelier C, Mejia LF (1994) Incidence of retinal detachment following clear-lens extraction in myopic patients: retrospective analysis. Arch Ophthalmol 112:336–339

8

12. Belda JI, Ruiz-Moreno JM, Perez-Santonja JJ et al (2003) Laser in situ keratomileusis to correct myopia after scleral buckling for retinal detachment. J Cataract Refract Surg 29:1231–1235

13. Bushley DM, Parmley VC, Paglen P. Visual field defect associated with laser in situ keratomileusis. Am J Ophthalmol 2000 May;129:668–671

14. Cameron BD, Saffra NA, Strominger MB (2001) Laser in situ keratomileusis-induced optic neuropathy. Ophthalmology 108:660–665

15. Chan CK, Lawrence II FC (2001) Macular hole after laser in situ keratomileusis and photorefractive keratectomy. Am J Ophthalmol 131:666–667

16. Chan CK, Arevalo JF, Akbatur HH et al (2004) Characteristic of sixty myopic eyes with pre-laser in situ keratomileusis retinal examination and post-laser in situ keratomileusis retinal lesions. Retina 24:706–713

17. Chan CK, Tarasewicz DG, Lin SG (2005) Relation of pre-LASIK and post-LASIK retinal lesions and retinal examination for LASIK eyes. Br J Ophthalmol 89:299–301

18. Chaudhry NA, Smiddy WE (1998) Displacement of corneal cap during vitrectomy in a post-LASIK eye. Retina 18:554–555

19. Farah ME, Hofling-Lima AL, Nascimento E (2000) Early rhegmatogenous retinal detachment following laser in situ keratomileusis for high myopia. J Refract Surg 16:739–743

20. Feldman RM, Crapotta JA, Feldman ST et al (1991) Retinal detachment following radial and astigmatic keratotomy. Refract Corneal Surg 7:252–253

21. Guell JL, Muller A (1996) Laser in situ keratomileusis (LASIK) for myopia from –7 to –18 diopters. J Refract Surg 12:222–228.

22. Hayreh SS. Anterior ischaemic optic neuropathy III (1974) Treatment, prophylaxis, and differential diagnosis. Br J Ophthalmol 58:981–989

23. Hayreh SS (1975) Anterior ischemic optic neuropathy, 1st edn. Springer, Berlin Heidelberg New York

24. Hayreh SS (1996) Acute ischemic disorders of the optic nerve: pathogenesis, clinical manifestations and management. Ophthalmol Clin North Am 9:407–442

25. Hayreh SS (2000) Ischaemic optic neuropathy. Indian J Ophthalmol 48:171–94, review; erratum, 48:317

26. Hofman RF, Starling JC, Hovland KR (1985) Case report: retinal detachment after radial keratotomy surgery. J Refract Surg 1:226

27. Jain RB, Chopdar A (2003) LASIK induced choroidal infarcts. Br J Ophthalmol 87:649–50

28. Kim HM, Jung HR (1996) Laser assisted in situ keratomileusis for high myopia. Ophthalmic Surg Lasers 27:508–511

29. Lee AG (2002) LASIK-induced optic neuropathy. Ophthalmology 109:817; author reply 817

30. Lee AG, Kohnen T, Ebner R et al (2000) Optic neuropathy associated with laser in situ keratomileusis. J Cataract Refract Surg 26:1581–1584

31. Lin JM, Tsai YY (2005) Retinal Phlebitis after LASIK. J Refract Surg 21:501–504

32. Lin SC, Tseng SH (2003) Prophylactic laser photocoagulation for retinal breaks before laser in situ keratomileusis. J Refract Surg 19:661–665

33. Luna JD, Reviglio VE, Juarez CP (1999) Bilateral macular hemorrhage after laser in situ keratomileusis. Graefes Arch Clin Exp Ophthalmol 237:611–613

34. Maturi RK, Kitchens JW, Spitzberg DH et al (2003) Choroidal neovascularization after LASIK. J Refract Surg 19:463–464

35. McCarty CA, Livingston PM, Taylor HR (1997) Prevalence of myopia in adults: implications for refractive surgeons. J Refract Surg 13:229–234

36. Mulhern MG, Condon PI, O'Keefe M (1997) Endophthalmitis after astigmatic myopic laser in situ keratomileusis. J Cataract Refract Surg 23:948–950

37. Najman-Vainer J, Smith RJ, Maloney RK (2000) Interface fluid after LASIK: misleading tonometry can lead to end-stage glaucoma. J Cataract Refract Surg 26:471–472

38. Optic Neuropathy Decompression Group (2000 Ischemic Optic Neuropathy Decompression Trial: twenty-four-month update. Arch Ophthalmol 118:793–798

39. Ozdamar A, Aras C, Sener B et al (1998) Bilateral retinal detachment associated with giant retinal tear after laser-assisted in situ keratomileusis. Retina 18:176–177

40. Pallikaris IG, Siganos DS (1994) Excimer laser in situ keratomileusis and photorefractive keratectomy for correction of high myopia. J Refract Corneal Surg 10:498–510

41. Pallikaris IG, Papatzanaki ME, Siganos DS (1991) A corneal flap technique for laser in situ keratomileusis. Arch Ophthalmol 109:1699–1702

42. Perez-Santonja JJ, Sakla HF, Abad JL et al (1997) Nocardial keratitis after laser in situ keratomileusis. J Refract Surg 13:314–317

43. Principe AH, Lin DY, Small KW et al (2004) Macular hemorrhage after laser in situ keratomileusis (LASIK) with femtosecond laser flap creation. Am J Ophthalmol 138:657–659

44. Ripandelli G, Billi B, Fedeli R et al (1996) Retinal detachment after clear lens extraction in 41 eyes with high axial myopia. Retina 16:3–6

45. Rodriguez A, Camacho H (1992) Retinal detachment after refractive surgery for myopia. Retina 12:S46–S50

46. Rodriguez A, Gutierrez E, Alvira G (1987) Complications of clear lens extraction in axial myopia. Arch Ophthalmol 105:1522–1523

47. Ruiz-Moreno JM, Alió JL (2003) Incidence of retinal disease following refractive surgery in 9,239 eyes. J Refract Surg 19:534–547

48. Ruiz-Moreno JM, Alió JL, Perez-Santonja JJ et al (1999) Retinal detachment in phakic eyes with anterior chamber intraocular lenses to correct severe myopia. Am J Ophthalmol 127:270–275

49. Ruiz-Moreno JM, Perez-Santoja JJ, Alió JL (1999) Retinal detachment in myopic eyes after laser in situ keratomileusis. Am J Ophthalmol 128:588–594

50. Ruiz-Moreno JM, Artola A, Ayala MJ et al (2000) Choroidal neovascularization in myopic eyes after photorefractive keratectomy. J Cataract Refract Surg 26:1492–1495

51. Ruiz-Moreno JM, Perez-Santonja JJ, Alió JL (2001) Choroidal neovascularization in myopic eyes after laser-assisted in situ keratomileusis. Retina 21:115–120

52. Ruiz-Moreno JM, Artola A, Perez-Santonja JJ et al (2002) Macular hole in a myopic eye after laser in situ keratomileusis. J Refract Surg 18:746–749

53. Ruiz-Moreno JM, Montero J, Alio JL (2003) Lacquer crack formation after LASIK. Ophthalmology 110:1669–1671

54. Saeed M, Poon Wallace, Goyal S et al (2004) Choroidal neovascularization after laser in situ keratomileusis in a patient with low myopia. J Cataract Refract Surg 30:2632–2635.

55. Sanders DR, Hofman RF, Salz JJ (1986) Refractive corneal surgery. Slack, Thorofare, N.J., p 388

56. Schepens CL (1983) Retinal detachment and allied diseases. Saunders, Philadelphia, p 47

57. Scupola A, Mosca L, Balestrazzi A et al (2003) Choroidal neovascularization after laser-assisted in situ keratomileusis following penetrating keratoplasty. Graefes Arch Clin Exp Ophthalmol 241:682–684

58. Sforza PD, Saffra NA (2003) Laser in situ keratomileusis as treatment for anisometropia after scleral buckling surgery. J Cataract Refract Surg 29:1042–1044

59. Shaikh NM, Shaikh S, Singh K, Manche E (2002) Progression to end-stage glaucoma after laser in situ keratomileusis. J Cataract Refract Surg 28:356–359

60. Singhvi A, Dutta M, Sharma N et al (2004) Bilateral serous macular detachment following laser in situ keratomileusis. Am J Ophthalmol 138:1069–1071

61. Sinha R, Dada T, Verma L et al (2003) LASIK after retinal detachment surgery. Br J Ophthalmol 87:551–553

62. Soheilian M, Koochek A, Yazdani S, Peyman GA (2003) Transvitreal optic neurotomy for nonarteritic anterior ischemic optic neuropathy. Retina 23:692–697

63. Sperduto RD, Seigel D, Roberts J et al (1983) Prevalence of myopia in the United States. Arch Ophthalmol 101:405–407

64. Stulting RD, Carr JD, Thompson KP et al (1999) Complications of laser in situ keratomileusis for the correction of myopia. Ophthalmology 106:13–20

65. Suarez E, Torres F, Vieira JC et al (2002) Anterior uveitis after laser in situ keratomileusis. J Cataract Refract Surg 28:1793–1798

66. Weiss HS, Rubinfeld RS, Anderschat JF (2001) Case reports and small case series: LASIK-associated visual field loss in a glaucoma suspect. Arch Ophthalmol 119:774–775

67. Whitson JT, McCulley JP, Cavanagh HD et al (2003) Effect of laser in situ keratomileusis on optic nerve head topography and retinal nerve fiber layer thickness. J Cataract Refract Surg 29:2302–2305

68. Zaldivar R, Davidorf JM, Oscherow S (1998) Laser in situ keratomileusis for myopia from −5.50 to −11.50 diopters with astigmatism. J Refract Surg 14:19–25

Contents

Core Messages

- In this chapter, the authors illustrate the types of potential complications that can arise from the use of the femtosecond laser:

- To compare the similarities and differences of the available flap making technologies
- To discuss, where these technologies are similar, the unique complications that arise from the microkeratome versus the femtosecond laser
- To provide the reader knowledge of the current state of the art of flap making as well as its strengths and weaknesses

9.1 Complications and Management with the Femtosecond Laser

*Karl G. Stonecipher, Teresa S. Ignacio¹,
and Kody G. Stonecipher*

9.1.1 Introduction

As one noted ophthalmic surgeon Dr. John Kearney put it, "…if you never cut, then you will never cry." Complications in surgery are the antithesis to success. In a series by Siga-

---

¹ Dr. Ignacio's contribution to this book chapter was limited to data collection and analysis. All data contributed by Dr. Ignacio is intended to supplement the knowledge of physicians and other health care professionals involved in patient care.

nos et al., over 95% of the complications were related to flap creation in laser refractive surgery. In this chapter, the authors detail complications and the management of various complications related to the femtosecond laser. Risks and benefits of mechanically created flaps and femtosecond laser created flaps have been published in multiple papers [1–5]. The authors have reviewed a total of 19,852 cases (13,721 microkeratome cases and 6,131 femtosecond laser cases) to review the incidence of postoperative complications in a refractive surgical practice from one surgeon (Karl G. Stonecipher). When appropriate, the comparison rates to mechanical keratomes were utilized. As with any new technology, there are complications unique to that technology, and these are covered as well. The complications are divided into sight-threatening, potential sight-threatening, and non–sight-threatening complications. This division allows for distinction of the severity of the complication based on outcomes related to the complication.

9.1.2 Sight-Threatening Complications

9.1.2.1 Infections
To date in a review of 6,131 cases, we have not seen a postoperative infection with femtosecond laser-assisted in situ keratomileusis (LASIK). Additionally, in a report by Binder et al., in 1,000 cases followed prospectively, no infections were noted [6]. Management in such cases would be directed toward the pathogen or suspected pathogen.

9.1.2.2 Vitreoretinal Complications

9.1.2.2.1 Macular Hemorrhage
Vitreoretinal complications have been reported with mechanical keratomes [7]. There were no vitreoretinal complications in this series treated with the femtosecond laser. There is only one reported case of macular hemorrhage in over 1,000,000 cases treated with the femtosecond laser [8].

9.1.3 Potential Sight-Threatening Complications

9.1.3.1 Diffuse Lamellar Keratitis
Diffuse lamellar keratitis (DLK) has been reported following either mechanical or femtosecond related keratectomies [9]. The etiology appears to be multifactorial in published papers reviewing the syndrome [7, 9–13]. The first paper reporting this syndrome was by Smith and Maloney in 1998 [14]. The most commonly used classification system grades DLK in four stages [9]. Stage 1 is defined as the presence of white granular cells in the periphery of the flap. Stage 2 is progression to white granular cells in the center of the flap. Stage 3 is condensation of more dense clumped cells in the central visual axis, with relative clearing in the periphery.

Stage 4 is defined as severe lamellar keratitis with stromal melting and scarring.

DLK related to laser-treated flaps has been mostly seen to start in the periphery and has been reported to occur 2–7 days after flap creation. The cause is unknown; however, it has been thought related to excessive manipulation of the flap edge and high–side-cut energy settings. Transition from the 10- to 60 kHz platform has allowed the surgeon to program lower energy settings. However, decreasing side-cut energy does not conclusively prove DLK etiology is energy related, as DLK has been reported even in low-energy settings.

In a review of 6,131 femtosecond LASIK cases, DLK stages 1–2 were present in 0.08% of cases. To date, no cases of stages 3 or 4 have been seen in this series. All cases were managed with aggressive topical corticosteroids, and no postoperative complications were observed. Lifting the flap and irrigating underneath will be necessary for management of stages 3 or 4 DLK in addition to aggressive postoperative corticosteroids and possible systemic oral corticosteroids.

As mentioned, causes of DLK are multifactorial. The importance of identifying causal relationships and prevention is key to the management of this complication. Pretreatment with topical antibiotics and corticosteroids has reduced the incidence of DLK in this series of 6131 cases from 0.08% to 0.04%. Pretreatment may reduce the inflammatory components of the tear film thereby reducing the reactionary patterns associated with DLK.

9.1.3.2 Central Toxic Keratopathy
Central toxic keratopathy is the acute onset of a dense central or paracentral focal inflammation with scarring characterized by loss of overlying tissue and an associated "lacquer" or "mud crack" appearance [15, 16]. The incidence in a series of over 6,131 cases is 0.016%. Treatment is aggressive early intervention with lifting, floating, and irrigation underneath the flap, followed by topical corticosteroids.

9.1.3.3 Flap Slippage
The definition of a slipped flap is one that has moved significantly enough to affect postoperative best-corrected visual acuity (BCVA) compared to that of the patient's preoperative level. Most of these are related to traumatic dislocations but other etiologies include medication related and postoperative dry eye–related flap slippage. The reported incidence of flap slippage with the mechanical keratome has been reported to be as high as 1.1–2.0% [7, 17]. In the reviewed series, the use of the femtosecond laser reduced the incidence of slipped flaps by 50% compared with that of the mechanical keratome.

Management includes relifting and refloating the flap. Rarely, suturing of the flap is necessary.

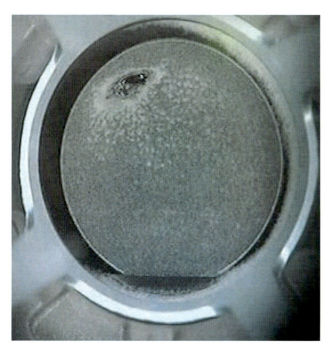

Fig. 9.1.1 In the peripheral edge of the flap at the 10- to-11 o'clock position, we see evidence of gas trapped between the docking cone and the surface epithelium

9.1.3.4 Partial or Buttonhole Flaps without Excimer Laser Ablation

The reviewed series of 19,582 cases contained no partial flaps with the femtosecond laser. The reason for this is if suction loss occurs, then the suction ring can be reapplied, and the procedure repeated without incident. However, with the mechanical keratome, partial flaps or buttonhole flaps occurred with an overall incidence of 0.11%, which did not allow the procedure to be completed. The management of these microkeratome-related complications was to replace the flap, wait on average 6 months, and retreat the patient with either surface photorefractive keratectomy or re-cutting of the flap at a deeper depth when the etiology was identified.

9.1.3.5 Vertical (Epithelial) Gas Breakthrough

In the prospective evaluation of the femtosecond laser, the surgeon had only had one incidence of this complication, but it occurred peripherally related to a previous scar, and the flap was lifted and the patient treated at the initial surgical intervention without complication. This complication appears to be most commonly seen in the creation of thin flaps (programmed at 90 μm). If a significant vertical gas breakthrough is seen between the glass cone and the epithelium, then the surgeon must stop the procedure and not wait for the side cut to finish. If the side cut is completed, then it is recommended that the flap not be lifted and the surgeon treats the patient later either with photorefractive

keratectomy or cut at least 40 μm deeper than the original flap intended depth. It will also be prudent to save the cone used and return to the manufacturer as well as have the femtosecond laser system serviced to check the z-calibration. This comprises a complete investigation of the probable cause of the incident (Fig. 9.1.1).

9.1.3.6 Epithelial Defects or Loose Epithelium

Epithelial defects or loose epithelium is a complication more commonly seen with the mechanical keratome versus the femtosecond laser [2, 18]. Even newer mechanical keratome designs have reported epithelial slides in as high as 2.6% of the population [17] Epithelial preservation is a major factor related to healing and other subsequent postoperative complications such as DLK, epithelial ingrowth, and enhancements [2]. In this series, epithelial slides were reported in 0.45% of mechanical keratectomies and only 0.016% with the femtosecond laser, which is a fourfold reduction. Management of perioperative epithelial issues may include cessation of the case, bandage lens application and its associated potential risks for complications, and management of the associated risks such as DLK and epithelial ingrowth.

9.1.3.7 Decentration

In the series of 19,582 cases reported, no significant decentrations were seen that did not allow excimer laser ablations either with the mechanical keratome or the femtosecond laser. However, it can occur if the suction ring is not placed properly. They have been reported and have been related to decentered placement of the suction ring. If this happens, then replace the flap back or do not lift the flap and wait to intervene at another surgical episode once refractive stabilization and healing has occurred. The suggested wait time is around 3–6 months.

9.1.3.8 Flap Striae and Flap Edema

Flap striae can be divided into two subcategories, visually significant and visually insignificant. Visually significant striae result from a true flap movement or slippage. Visually significant striae are defined as those that affect postoperative BCVA. These may be traumatic or pathophysiologic in origin. Management includes relifting and refloating the flap. Rarely, placement of suture/s may be necessary. In this case series, I (Karl G. Stonecipher) have not seen a case of visually significant striae after femtosecond laser treatment, with the exception of those related to postoperative day 1 flap slippage. (Please refer to the section of flap slippage regarding management of this finding.) Visually insignificant striae or microstriae (VIMS) are defined as striae that are observed objectively by the examiner but do not interfere with BCVA. VIMS are more likely to be seen in patients of higher myopic preoperative refractions, which have been observed in this case series after femtosecond and microkeratome LASIK [24]. Monitoring of VIMS is the treatment of choice, but thorough examination to determine if the quality of vision is affected by this finding is imperative. Patient subjective complaints may warrant intervention similar to that of visually significant striae. Flap edema is a localized swelling of the flap related to the surgical insult itself. It is usually limited to a 24- to 72-h postoperative course, which is normal. The treatment is standard corticosteroids prescribed postoperatively as is antibiotic prophylaxis. However, should flap edema persist, then toxic etiologies should be ruled out and managed appropriately. This should be differentiated from interface flap edema syndrome, which is fluid in the interface with increased intraocular pressure usually related to corticosteroid responsiveness [7, 22] Management is directed at treatment of the rise in intraocular pressure and cessation of corticosteroids.

9.1.3.9 Interface Haze

In the reported series, no interface haze has been noted in either the mechanical keratome or femtosecond keratome group. Rarely, in both groups, the authors have seen a reticulated haze that was visually insignificant that occurred at 2–3 months, without major subjective complaints or objective findings. In these rare isolated cases, a 2- to 3-week intervention of topical corticosteroids has resulted in resolution.

9.1.3.10 Femtosecond Lasers in Previous Refractive Surgery

The femtosecond laser has been used by the surgeon in this series (Karl G. Stonecipher) for a variety of previous refractive surgeries such as radial keratotomy (RK), automated lamellar keratoplasty (ALK), penetrating keratoplasty (PKP), photorefractive keratotomy (PRK), and LASIK. The use of the femtosecond laser in these patients is an off-label use of the device. The femtosecond laser pass will follow the path of least resistance, notably old incisional scars and previous flap planes. Caution in those patients with previous mechanical flaps, radial incisions, and astigmatic incisions are suggested. With the mechanical flap's meniscus architecture and the planar flap made by the femtosecond laser, surgeons can encounter multiple planes and irregular flaps if the femtosecond laser flap cuts through the previously made flap. With PKP enhancements, it is recommended that the flap diameter be adjusted to 0.5 mm less than the trephination diameter to avoid the graft–host interface. PRK patient enhancements have not resulted in any issues with this series of patients reported.

9.1.4 Non–Sight-Threatening Complications

9.1.4.1 Enhancements

To date in the series of 13,721 microkeratome cases versus 6,131 femtosecond laser cases with the same surgeon, enhancement rates after at least 1-year follow-up were 4.2 and

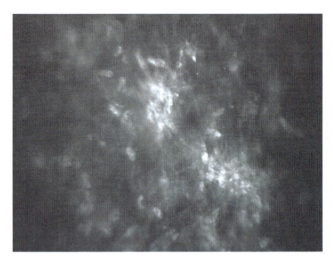

Fig. 9.1.2 Confocal microscopy of a patient with active TLSS illustrates the underlying activated keratocytes

1.6%, respectively. Enhancements rates have been dropping over the course of time related to excimer laser technological advancements, as well as the way in which the flap is created with improvements in enhancement rates favoring those patients receiving flaps created by the femtosecond laser [2, 3, 19, 20].

Enhancements are routinely performed after refractive stability, which usually occurs between the 3- and 6-month visits. Most surgeons prefer to lift the previously made flap and treat the residual stromal bed as long as enough tissue remains to treat without fear of keratectasia. In those cases where residual stromal bed thickness is in question, many surgeons are resorting to surface photorefractive keratectomies as an option with prophylactic administration of topical mitomycin C and oral vitamin C to reduce the risk of postoperative haze or scarring.

9.1.4.2 Transient Light Sensitivity Syndrome

Transient light sensitivity syndrome (TLSS) is a complication unique to the femtosecond laser and has not been seen as a complication related to the mechanical microkeratome. It was initially reported in 2001, when higher energies were used in earlier femtosecond laser keratome platforms. The documentation, incidence, and treatment of TLSS have been reported at 0.17 and 0.4% in two separate series [4, 5]. The incidence significantly decreased after the introduction of lower raster bed and side-cut energies. TLSS presents in patients between 6 and 12 weeks after surgery, with good visual acuity with delayed onset of photophobia. As the name implies, it is transient and resolves with aggressive corticosteroid intervention over a short course of 2–3 weeks. Objective findings are absent; however, confocal analysis has shown increased keratocytic activity. In my personal experience (Karl G. Stonecipher), the 60-kHz platform and even lower applied energies have significantly decreased this complication (Fig. 9.1.2).

9.1.4.3 Anterior Chamber Bubbles

Anterior chamber bubbles are another unique complication associated with the femtosecond laser, which occurs with an incidence of 0.2%; however, to date it has not resulted in an interruption of treatment of any patient in this prospective series of 6,131 cases. One hypothesis is that the bubbles created from photodisruption track reversely through Schlemm's canal and into the anterior chamber. It has been reported to interfere with certain eye trackers on different excimer laser platforms, but treatment has only been interrupted by 1 day, allowing for bubble reabsorption or resolution with routine intervention [22, 23].

9.1.4.4 Rainbow Glare

Rainbow glare is a rare phenomenon whereby patients report the perception of a spoke-like spectrum of light in the peripheral field of vision. The incidence in this series is 0.016%. Rainbow glare can be observed when looking at extremely bright, point-like light sources with a dark background. There are no clinical findings and no effect on visual acuity; however, the potential diffractive effects may be bothersome to patients. Observation and monitoring is the management for these patients since the symptom eventually resolves in time.

9.1.5 Opaque Bubble Layer

The intraoperative finding of opaque bubble layer (OBL) is more of a nuisance than a complication with the femtosecond laser. It is unique to the femtosecond laser and not seen with mechanical keratomes. It is a term used to describe the collection of the gas bubbles in the interlamellar space above and below the planar flap. OBL is directly related to the photodisruptive mechanism of the femtosecond laser. Delaying immediate treatment with the excimer laser results in its resolution by allowing the bubbles to dissipate. Interference with the laser tracking or iris registration has been noted in some cases and management involves waiting to allow for resolution.

9.1.5.1 Early or Hard Opaque Bubble Layer

This occurs when the pulses initially placed in the cornea have no space available, and the water vapor and carbon dioxide produced have nowhere to go. Early or hard OBL can block subsequent pulses and lead to uncut or poorly cut tissue, making flap lifts more difficult. Appropriate management includes changing laser settings to reduce OBL (Fig. 9.1.3).

9.1.5.2 Late Opaque Bubble Layer

The produced gases can also travel into the intralamellar spaces after their placement. The main cause of this type of OBL is the result of poor separation of the corneal tissue, and it appears more transparent and patchy. Again, lifts

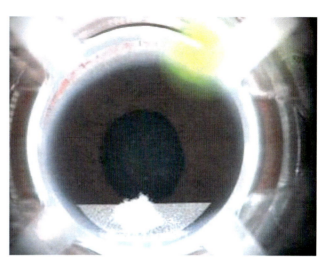

Fig. 9.1.3 Early or hard OBL is seen at the initial flap creation and appears opaque in comparison to the normal raster pattern

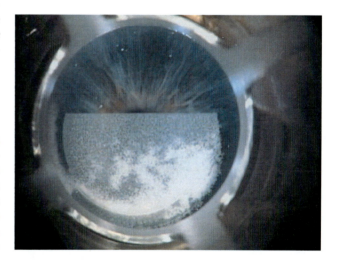

Fig. 9.1.4 Late OBL has a notably diffuse pattern and appears later in the stage of flap creation

can be more difficult with late OBL. Management includes changing laser settings to reduce OBL (Fig. 9.1.4).

9.1.6 Suction Loss

Loss of suction with the mechanical keratome usually results in a devastating flap complication, and this has already been covered previously. Loss of suction with the femtosecond laser keratome is resolved by replacement of the suction ring on the patient and re-docking into the patient interface to subsequently repeat the treatment at the same time if the suction loss occurred outside the visual axis. If the suction loss occurred at the visual axis, then there are several options to treat. One can re-treat on a different day or one can also opt to do surface ablation.

9.1.5 Difficult Lifts

Difficult lifts are flaps that require more dissection to free the residual adhesions not separated by the original raster pattern. Rarely will difficult lifts be encountered in varying anatomy of patients; however, they may be related to raster bed energies and the distance of spot and line separation. Adjusting the laser settings can improve difficult flap lifts.

9.1.6 Conclusion

Since the introduction of the femtosecond laser for patient use in 2002, several technological advances have been implemented have reduced flap creation times and allowed for reduced energy levels. Many of the complications reported have been eliminated or reduced to lower levels with these changes. With new technology, new complications can arise. Fortunately, with femtosecond technology, these complications are not sight threatening. In fact, the comparative series showed roughly a fourfold reduction in over all complications and enhancement rates. With tools such as the femtosecond laser, flap creation is taken to a new level.

> **Take-Home Pearls**
>
> ■ The femtosecond laser platform continues to improve its ability to make a consistently planar and predictably uniform flap.
> ■ In a large series of 19,852 cases, a roughly fourfold reduction in flap complications was seen overall comparing favorably to the femtosecond technology over the microkeratome.
> ■ Unique to the femtosecond laser platform are the complications of transient light sensitivity, anterior chamber bubble formation, vertical gas breakthrough, the opaque bubble layer, and rainbow glare; however, all of these issues are not sight-threatening complications if managed appropriately.

References

1. Binder PS (2004) Flap dimensions created with the IntraLase FS laser. J Cataract Refract Surg 30:26–32
2. Kezirian GM, Stonecipher, KG (2004) Comparison of the IntraLase femtosecond laser and mechanical keratome for laser in situ keratomileusis. J Cataract Surg 30:804–811
3. Durrie DS, Kezirian GM (2005) Femtosecond laser versus mechanical keratome flaps in wavefront guided laser in situ keratomileusis: prospective contralateral eye study. J Cataract Refract Surg 31:120–126
4. Montes-Mico R, Rodriguez-Galietero A, Alió JL (2007) Femtosecond laser versus mechanical keratome LASIK for Myopia. Ophthalmology 114:62–68
5. Stonecipher KG, Dishler JG, Ignacio TS, Binder PS (2006) Transient Light Sensitivity after femtosecond laser flap creation: clinical findings and management. J Cataract Refract Surg 32:91–94
6. Binder, PS (2006) 1,000 LASIK flaps created with the IntraLase FS laser. J Cataract Refract Surg 32:962–969
7. Knorz M (2002) Flap and interface complications in LASIK. Curr Opin in Ophthalmol 13:242–245
8. Principe A, Lin D, Small K, Aldave A (2004) Macular hemorrhage after LASIK with femtosecond laser flap creation. AJO 138:657–659
9. Linebarger EJ, Hardten DR, Lindstrom RL (2000) Diffuse lamellar keratitis: diagnosis and management. J Cataract Refract Surg 26:1072–1077
10. Lazaro C, Perea J, Aria A (2006) Surgical-glove-related diffuse lamellar keratitis alter LASIK: long-term outcomes. J Cataract Refract Surg 32:1702–1709
11. Holland J, Mathias R, Morck D, Chiu J, Slade S (2000) Diffuse lamellar keratitis related to endotoxins released from sterilizer reservoir biofilms. Ophthalmology 107:1227–1234
12. Whitby JL, Hitchins V (2002) Endotoxin levels in steam and reservoirs of tabletop steam sterilizers. J Refract Surg 18:51–57
13. Yuhan K, Nguyen L, Boxer-Wachler B (2002) Role of instrument cleaning and maintenance in the development of DLK. Ophthalmology 109:400–404
14. Smith R, Maloney R (1998) Diffuse lamellar keratitis: a new syndrome in lamellar refractive surgery. Ophthalmol 105:1721–1726
15. Frankel GE, Cohen PR, Sutton GL, Lawless MA, Rogers CM (1998) Central focal interface opacity after laser in situ keratomileusis. J Refract Surg 14:571–576
16. Parolini B, Marcon G, Panozzo GA (2001) Central necrotic lamellar inflammation after laser in situ keratomileusis. J Refract Surg 17:110–112
17. Lichter H, Russell G, Waring GO (2004) Repositioning the laser in situ keratomileusis flap at the slit lamp. J Refract Surg 20:166–169
18. Vivien M, Tham B, Maloney R (2000) Microkeratome complications of laser in situ keratomileusis. Ophthalmol 107:920–924
19. Tanzer DJ, Schallhorn S, Brown MC et al (2005) Comparison of femtosecond vs. Mechanical microkeratome in wavefront guided LASIK. Data presented at the American Society of Cataract and Refractive Surgery Symposium; Washington, D.C.
20. Tran D, Sarayaba M, Bor Z, et al (2005) Randomized prospective clinical study comparing induced aberrations with IntraLase and Hansatome flap creation in fellow eyes. Potential impact on wavefront-guided laser in situ keratomileusis. J Cataract Refract Surg 31:97–105
21. Galal A, Artola A, Belda J, Rodriguez-Prats J, Claramonte P, Sanchez A, Ruiz-Moreno O, Merayo J, Alió J (2006) Interface corneal edema secondary to steroid-induced elevation of intraocular pressure simulating diffuse lamellar keratitis. J Refract Surg 22:441–447
22. Kim A, Myrowitz E, Pettinelli D, Stark W, Chuck R (2006) Appearance of gas bubbles in the anterior chamber after femtosecond laser flap creation. Data presented at the 2006 ARVO meeting, Fort Lauderdale, Fla.
23. Lifshitz T, Levy J, Klemperer I, Levinger S (2005) Anterior chamber gas bubbles after corneal flap creation with a femtosecond laser. J Cataract Refract Surg 31:2227–2229
24. Steinert R, Ashrafzadeh A, Hersh P (2004) Results of phototherapeutic keratotomy in the management of flap striae after LASIK. Ophthalmol 111:740–746

- Corneal curvature does not carry the same significance with a laser-created flap, and thus there is much less risk of a buttonhole with a laser-created flap versus a blade-created flap.

- If the surgeon recognizes preoperatively the presence of a stromal defect and either does not do the case or is very delicate with this situation intraoperatively, then the chance of a problem will be minimized.

- It is also important when making a thin flap to remember that you may need to enhance this patient's vision someday. If the goal is to be able to lift the laser-created flap, then it is important to realize that if the flap was made to thin the risk of lifting and tearing the flap is greatly increased.

- Delicate, continual, slight, downward motion dissection of the flap interface, where the number of "swipes" is customized to each situation based on interface resistance will minimize this risk.

- The surgeon and patient will enjoy unparalleled flap-creation safety with the femtosecond laser.

9.2 Management of a Perforated Femtosecond Laser–Created Flap

Vance Thompson

9.2.1 Introduction

Perforation of a flap in an elective corneal refractive surgery procedure such as LASIK has traditionally been one of the most feared complications in mechanical microkeratome flap creation [1–4]. The reason for this fear is the uniquely organized collagen fibrils that give the cornea optical clarity become disorganized and irregular in the corneal scar-formation process [5–7]. If the resultant scar is in or near the visual axis, then the reduction in image quality and visual acuity can be quite profound. Refractive surgeons do everything in their power in an attempt to minimize the risk of this dreaded complication. One of the main reasons that femtosecond technology has brought so much inner peace to flap creation during LASIK is the fact that flap perforation should be extremely rare. Increased safety and accuracy are the main beauties of transitioning from mechanical metal blade microkeratome–created flaps to femtosecond laser–created flaps [8–10]. That being said, there are certain situations that the surgeon needs to be aware of both preoperatively and intraoperatively to minimize the risk of flap perforation, even with the increased safety provided by the femtosecond laser. The purpose of this chapter is to discuss these special situations.

9.2.2 Preoperative Patient Selection Issues

9.2.2.1 Steep Corneas and the Risk of a Buttonhole

It is felt that flap thickness can vary with mechanical microkeratome technology, based on corneal curvature [11]. Steep corneas are at increased risk of perforation with a microkeratome blade–created flap. That is why it is recommended with mechanical microkeratome technology that certain adjustments be made to minimize the chance of a buttonhole in a steep cornea, namely go for a lesser diameter and a thicker flap. We consider a cornea with a curvature of 46 or greater steep and at risk for buttonhole after mechanical microkeratome flap creation. Corneal curvature does not carry the same significance with a laser–created flap, and thus there is much less risk of a buttonhole with a laser-created flap versus a blade-created flap [12]. Adjustments based on corneal curvature do not need to be made with a laser-created flap as they do with a blade created flap.

9.2.2.2 Presence of a Stromal Defect Preoperatively

One situation that needs to be carefully evaluated is the presence of a corneal stromal defect. A laser-created flap has intrastromal gases (mainly carbon dioxide and water) that are under a certain amount of pressure; these gases tend to diffuse toward the path of least resistance. If there is a stromal defect, then the gases can diffuse through this defect and accumulate between the focusing lens of the laser and the cornea and thus block the laser from creating a flap, or cause an irregular dissection.

Femtosecond laser has been shown to be safe after previous, well-healed radial keratotomy [13]. One needs to be careful though since the gases can dissect through the incisions and block the ablation, especially in the presence of an epithelial plug (Fig. 9.2.1). Whenever there is a preexisting corneal stromal defect and the patient wishes to have a femtosecond-created flap, the informed consent needs to include this discussion with the patient's acceptance of the fact that the procedure may not be able to be completed if this occurs. If the flap cannot be completed because of this issue, I like to let the partially laser-dissected stromal interface heal for 6 months and then perform either blade flap LASIK or photorefractive keratectomy (PRK). A phakic lens implant could also be an option for patients where flap creation was not completed. With proper patient selection though, this should be an extremely rare event.

9.2.3 Intraoperative Issues

9.2.3.1 Flap Creation and Lifting

When creating a laser flap, it is important to achieve full applanation, with the focusing lens of the laser and the area of the cornea where the flap is to be created. If only partial applanation is achieved in the area of the desired flap, then there will be a gap between the focusing lens and the cornea, and a thinner, more fragile flap will be created. That is

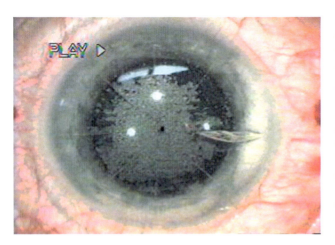

Fig. 9.2.1 This patient had radial keratotomy 5 years earlier, with an extension of the interface gases into the incision, which did not quite break through. The case was completed successfully

why it is so important to achieve full applanation over the area of desired flap creation. The other situation to be aware of is when there is a preexisting stromal defect and the laser flap goes well, the flap lift can be an issue. Laser-created flaps have a slightly increased resistance to lifting due to some collagen fibrils not having been cut by the laser. Some liken this to a slight Velcro-like feel in the interface when lifting the flap. You do not simply lift a laser-created flap; often, your first need is to dissect the residual small stromal attachments and then lift. It is during this dissection of the interface step that if the surgeon is applying upward pressure on the flap and there is a stromal defect that the dissection instrument can go right through the flap and potentially increase the magnitude of the preexisting corneal defect and scar.

Whether there is a preexisting stromal defect or not, the proper maneuver to dissecting a laser-created flap is the same maneuver a surgeon uses in a lamellar dissection of a cornea, namely slight, downward pressure during the dissection, which puts minimal stress on the flap.

9.2.4 Thin-Flap LASIK

More and more surgeons are trying to make flaps as thin as possible [14]. The reasons for this include the goal of minimizing the risk of future ectasia by maximizing the amount of "untouched" posterior corneal tissue through the creation of a thin flap. In our center, we commonly make our flaps 110-μm thick. In general, the first 50 μm of this flap are epithelium only. This means that the stromal aspect of the flap is only 60 μm thick. One can see that if the flap is not handled delicately, the surgeon can perforate the flap with the dissecting instrument. That is why it is important during the lifting procedure for the surgeon to have a feel for how much resistance to lifting the flap is present dur-

ing the dissection of the interface. If there is minimal resistance, then the surgeon can take a larger swipe underneath the flap and potential dissect the whole interface in one to three "swipes" and then lift the flap. However, if there is a good deal of resistance, then this maneuver could tear the flap. It may take 10–15 or more swipes in the situation of much flap interface resistance, with the surgeon focusing on slight, downward pressure, to avoid undue stress on the flap. The amount of "downward-pressure" dissection of the interface is dependent on the resistance at the interface for proper flap management, especially with thin-flap LASIK.

It is also important when making a thin flap to remember that you may need to enhance this patient's vision someday. If the goal is to be able to lift the laser-created flap, then it is important to realize that if the flap was made too thin, then the risk of lifting and tearing the flap is greatly increased. That is why my flaps are typically 110 μm. That is thin enough to preserve posterior corneal tissue, yet thick enough to withstand the pressure of a properly lifted flap. If one is trying a year later to lift a flap that was made at 80 μm of thickness (roughly 50 μm of epithelium and 30 μm of stroma), then the risk of flap perforation or tear is increased.

9.2.5 Management of a Perforated Flap

In general, if this dreaded complication occurs in surgery, then the best course of action is to reposition the partial flap (if necessary), sit the patient up and explain to the patient (and any family members) what just occurred. The best management is to allow the cornea to heal for 6 months minimum and then return for PRK, blade-flap LASIK, or a phakic implant. Many flap perforations can heal well and result in a good visual outcome if managed properly [15–17].

Since the laser gases created during the laser flap want to follow the path of least resistance, I am very cautious when considering the performance a laser flap in a previous blade- or laser-flap complicated case. The reason is the gases want to travel along the previously created tissue plane and come to the surface and settle between the focusing lens of the laser and the cornea and block the creation of a smooth flap. In the situation of a previous flap complication (blade or laser), I am more comfortable with PRK in lower corrections, or phakic implant in higher corrections. If the well-educated patient desires a laser flap be created in his or her previous blade-flap complication situation and is fully aware that the risk of the gases rising to the surface and blocking the flap creation is present, I will attempt a laser flap in special situations. For instance, if a very thin, partial-blade flap occurred more than 6 months ago, then I will consider attempting a deeper laser flap if the corneal thickness allows, but if any gases start toward the surface, then I stop and come back in 6 months with a PRK or phakic implant procedure.

9.2.6 Conclusion

Prevention is always the best philosophy when it comes to complications management in any surgery. In the LASIK procedure, this is of critical importance in flap creation. If the surgeon recognizes preoperatively the presence of a stromal defect and either does not do the case or is very delicate with this situation intraoperatively, then the chance of a problem occurring will be minimized. Other factors that help to prevent femtosecond laser–created flap perforation are (1) not attempting too-thin flaps, which can be quite risky to lift in an enhancement situation; (2) focusing on full applanation of the tissue to be lasered; (3) not trying to make flaps too thin, remembering that the epithelium is 50 μm thick and very fragile; and (4) being careful of femtosecond flaps after previous incisional corneal surgery.

The femtosecond laser has brought an increased amount of safety and predictability to flap creation. Even with this increase in accuracy and safety, the surgeon needs to be aware of preoperative and intraoperative situations in which his or her technique can minimize the risk of flap perforation. Delicate, continual, slight, downward motion dissection of the flap interface where the number of swipes is customized to each situation based on interface resistance will minimize this risk. If flap perforation does occur, then conservative management can still provide the patient with the eventual outcome of quality vision. By respecting the principles outlined in this chapter, the surgeon and patient will enjoy unparalleled flap creation safety with the femtosecond laser.

Take-Home Pearls

■ Even though the IntraLase femtosecond laser has become the safest and most accurate way to make a flap, it is still imperative to realize that quality surgical technique and flap management are important to prevent the risk of flap perforation.

References

1. Liu Q, Gong XM, Chen JQ et al (2005) Laser in situ keratomileusis induced corneal perforation and recurrent corneal epithelial ingrowth. J Cataract Refract Surg 31:857–859
2. Leung AT, Rao SK, Cheng AC et al (2000) Pathogenesis and management of laser in situ keratomileusis flap buttonhole. J Cataract Refract Surg 26:358–362
3. Schallhorn SC, Amesbury EC, Tanzer DJ (2006) Avoidance, recognition, and management of LASIK complications. Am J Ophthalmol 141:733–739
4. Epstein AJ, Clinch TE, Moshirfar M et al (2005) Results of late flap removal after complicated laser in situ keratomileusis. J Cataract Refract Surg 31:503–510
5. Davison PF, Galbavy EJ (1986) Connective tissue remodeling in corneal and scleral wounds. Invest Ophthalmol Vis Sci 27:1478–1484
6. Ishizaki M, Shimoda M, Wakamatsu K et al (1997) Stromal fibroblasts are associated with collagen IV in scar tissues of alkali-burned and lacerated corneas. Curr Eye Res 16:339–348
7. Carlson EC, Wang IJ, Liu CY et al (2003) Altered KSPG expression by keratocytes following corneal injury. Mol Vis 9:615–623
8. Stonecipher K, Ignacio TS, Stonecipher M (2004) Advances in refractive surgery: microkeratome and femtosecond laser flap creation in relation to safety, efficacy, predictability, and biomechanical stability. J Cataract Refract Surg 30:804–811
9. Kezirian GM, Stonecipher KG (2004) Comparison of the IntraLase femtosecond laser and mechanical keratomes for laser in situ keratomileusis. J Cataract Refract Surg 30:804–811
10. Durrie DS, Kezirian GM (2005) Femtosecond laser versus mechanical keratome flaps in wavefront-guided laser in situ keratomileusis: prospective contralateral eye study. J Cataract Refract Surg 31:120–126
11. Flanagan GW, Binder PS (2003) Precision of flap measurements for laser in situ keratomileusis in 4428 eyes. J Refract Surg 19:113–123
12. Binder PS (2004) Flap dimensions created with the IntraLase FS laser. J Cataract Refract Surg 30:26–32
13. Munoz G, Albarran-Diego C, Sakla HF et al (2006) Femtosecond laser in situ keratomileusis after radial keratotomy. J Cataract Refract Surg 32:1270–1275
14. Kymionis GD, Tsiklis N, Pallikaris AI et al (2006) Long-term results of superficial laser in situ keratomileusis after ultrathin flap creation. J Cataract Refract Surg 32:1276–1280
15. Jin GJ, Merkley KH (2006) Laceration and partial dislocation of LASIK flaps 7 and 4 years postoperatively with 20/20 visual acuity after repair. J Refract Surg 22:904–905
16. Sharma N, Ghate D, Argarwal T et al (2005) Refractive outcomes of laser in situ keratomileusis after flap complications. J Cataract Refract Surg 31:1334–1337
17. Jabbur NS, Myrowitz E, Wexler JL et al (2004) Outcome of second surgery in LASIK cases aborted due to flap complications. J Cataract Refract Surg 30:993–999

Chapter 10

Corneal Haze after Refractive Surgery

10

David Fahd, José de la Cruz, Sandeep Jain,
and Dimitri Azar

Contents

Core Messages

■ Loss of corneal clarity (haze) after refractive surgery can be a serious condition, leading to decrease in VA, myopic regression and irregular astigmatism.

■ Most cases of post-PRK haze are clinically insignificant and self-limiting.

■ In addition to haze post-PRK, haze can also be seen after LASIK, epi-LASIK, and LASEK.

■ Haze is due to abnormal collagen deposition and decreased corneal refractility.

■ Grading, as described by Fantes et al., is necessary for proper management.

■ Adequate follow-up postoperatively can detect and help prevent development of haze.

■ MMC can adequately prevent and treat haze after refractive surgery.

10.1 Introduction

The number of refractive surgery procedures performed has increased dramatically over the last 20 years. Photorefractive keratectomy (PRK) was the first technique to employ ophthalmic excimer laser for the correction of refractive error. It can be effectively used to correct moderate myopia, astigmatism, and hyperopia by surface ablation. One of the common side effects of corneal surface excimer laser ablation is haze; however, significant haze is seen in less than 5% of the cases [1]. Laser in situ keratomileusis (LASIK) has become the most common refractive surgery performed today, and is associated with a considerably less incidence of corneal haze compared to PRK.

10.2 Definition of Haze

Different definitions of haze include (1) a decrease in tissue transparency, (2) a marginal loss of corneal clarity, and (3) a subepithelial stromal opacity [2].

Haze can be completely asymptomatic. It can also lead to starbursts and visual loss or, more seriously, to a stromal reaction that induces refractive regression, increases corneal surface irregularity, and leads to irregular astigmatism. Haze is often accompanied by myopic regression.

The assessment of haze magnitude in clinical studies is subjective. Different studies report different incidences following PRK. Clinically *insignificant* corneal haze is present in most eyes after PRK and may last for 1–2 years after surgery. Clinically *significant* haze only occurs in a small percentage of eyes, usually less than 0.5–4%, depending on the level of correction and other factors. Lohmann et al. worked on developing an objective method of haze assessment in 1992 and reported an incidence of 4% at 6 months [3]. In 1998, Moller-Pedersen et al. used the confocal microscope to assess haze and reported an incidence of 3% at 12 months [4]. These results and others are summarized in Table 10.2.1.

Table 10.2.1 Subepithelial haze at 6 to 12 months post-treatment with PRK (stages according to Fantes et al. [5])

Study	Time of examination (months)	0 (%)	0.5–1 (%)	2 (%)	3 (%)	4 (%)
el Danasoury 1999	6	41.7	54.2	4.2	0	0
el Danasoury 1999	12	54.2	37.5	4.2	0	0
el Maghraby 1999	12	83	83	13	0	3
SUMMIT	6	45.6	44.1	5.9	4.4	0

From: Shortt AJ, Allan BDS (2006) Photorefractive keratectomy (PRK) versus laser-assisted in-situ keratomileusis (LASIK) for myopia. Cochrane Database of Systematic Reviews, issue 2, article no. CD005135. doi:10.1002/14651858.CD005135.pub2

Table 10.3.1 Haze staging (stages according to Fantes et al. [5])

Stage	Description of image by slit lamp
0	No haze, completely clear cornea
0.5	Trace haze seen with careful oblique illumination
1	Haze not interfering with visibility of fine iris details
2	Mild obscuration of iris details
3	Moderate obscuration of the iris and lens
4	Complete opacification of the stroma in the area of the scar, anterior chamber is totally obscured

10.3 Grading System

Fantes et al. [5] described five stages of corneal haze ranging from 0 (no haze) to 4 (total obscuration of anterior chamber). (See Table 10.3.1 for a full description of stages.)

Two types of haze are observed after PRK, the typical transitory haze and the late haze [6]:

Typical transitory haze: This is more common; however, it is rarely associated with clinical symptoms. It is noted between 1 and 3 months postoperatively, and disappears within the first year after surgery.

Late haze: Initially, the eye is normal. Between 2 to 5 months postoperatively haze appears. Though less common, this type of haze may severely compromise vision. The result is a decrease in the corneal transparency and myopic regression. It usually resolves over time; however, it may stay longer and may persist for up to 3 years.

10.4 Course

Typically, corneal haze appears a few weeks after surgery, plateaus, and then decreases slowly and becomes visually insignificant over time [7]. Different authors report different time courses: Winkler von Mohrenfels et al. initially noted subepithelial haze 3–4 weeks postoperatively as a diffuse zone of altered light reflex. Haze then increased progressively to a maximum at 3 months, and then slowly re-

gressed [8]. Mohan et al. reports that it tends to peak 6–9 months after PRK, and then gradually diminishes over time–taking years to resolve in some patients [9]. Rajan et al., in a study published in 2006, described it as increasing during the first months post up reaching a maximum between 3 and 6 months after surgery, and thereafter declining [10]. In the article by Netto et al., also published in 2006, haze was noted to begin 2 weeks after PRK, and peak at 4 weeks postoperatively [11].

10.5 Pathophysiology

Haze is the end stage of a cascade of events secondary to corneal epithelial and stromal injury (Fig. 10.5.1). Many different molecular growth factors, cytokines, and chemokines (interleukin-1, tumor necrosis factor-α, chondroitin sulfate proteoglycans, and others) interplay to promote regeneration instead of fibrosis after wounding [6]. Surgical trauma leads to disruption of the basement membrane and apoptosis/necrosis of the surrounding corneal cells. This will result in keratocyte activation and further transformation into fibroblasts. These fibroblasts then migrate centripetally to the site of injury. Their role is multiple, namely, they (1) lay down the extracellular matrix, (2) they transform into myofibroblasts, (3) they cause stromal edema, and (4) they lead to an irregularity of the stromal surface.

In normal clear corneas collagen types I and VI are arranged in a repeating-orthogonal arrangement [12]. In contrast, postoperatively, fibrillar Type IV collagen, normally not present in this region of the corneal stroma, increases. In addition, Type I and III fibrillary collagen molecules become arranged in a non-orthogonal pattern. These two changes are thought to lead to the development of subepithelial haze observed clinically postoperatively. Myofibroblasts, highly contractile cells with reduced transparency attributed to decreased intracellular crystallin production [13], invade the stroma. The extracellular matrix is also altered in the anterior stroma. The integrity of the epithelial membrane is necessary for proper wound healing and prevention of haze development; hence, the presence of an intact epithelial barrier immediately after laser ablation has an important role in curbing subepithelial haze and myofibroblast differentiation [2]. Haze is seen when

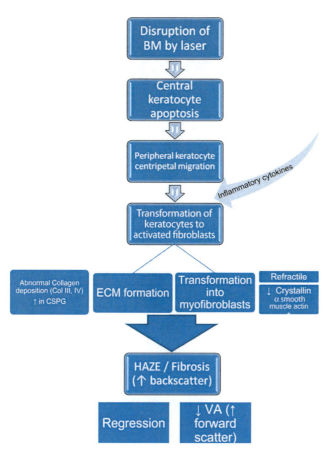

Fig. 10.5.1 Pathophysiology of haze development. CSPG: chondroitin sulfate proteoglycan, ECM: extracellular matrix, VA: visual acuity, Col: collagen

light from highly reflective myofibroblasts within the photoablated region is scattered randomly, forward and backward [14, 15].

Late apoptosis may have a role in disappearance of myofibroblasts and haze over time [11]. Disappearance of haze is correlated with disappearance of myofibroblasts and remodeling of disorganized stromal collagen.

10.6 Risk Factors

In order to prevent haze occurrence after refractive surgery, many studies have been conducted to assess the possible risk factors. These risk factors include depth of ablation [16], diameter of ablation [10, 17], slope of wound surface over the entire area of ablation [18], volume of stromal tissue removed [19], level of correction [11], length of time required for corneal healing, irregularity of postoperatively stromal surface [11], basement membrane integrity, Bowman's layer ablation, and tear fluid transforming growth factor (TGF)-β levels [20].

Depth of ablation: The depth of ablation, together with the diameter of ablation and the attempted error of correction, are contributing factors to the volume of tissue removed. Braun-

stein et al. noted in 1996 that there is a significant increase in light scatter and haze in patients with ablation depths greater than 80 μm compared with those with ablation depths less than 80 μm [16]. The study, conducted on 34 patients, found a significantly higher amount of haze in patients with ablation depths greater than 80 μm. Conversely however, O'Brart et al., in a study on 33 patients, found that increasing the depth of ablation has no significant influence on haze [21].

Slope of wound surface over the entire area of ablation: Corbett et al., on a review of 100 patients, found that the factor with greatest apparent influence on the development of haze and regression was the slope of the wound surface over the entire area of the ablation. Tapering the wound edge provided no additional benefit and to night vision problems. [18]

Diameter of ablation and volume of tissue removed: Different authors have attempted to correlate the diameter of ablation and the volume of stromal tissue removed with haze, as mentioned before. Objective measures of haze were less with 6 mm compared with 4- and 5-mm treatments ($p < 0.001$) [10, 17]. An important regulating factor for haze postoperatively, according to Moller-Pedersen et al., is the increased volume of stromal tissue removed [19].

High levels of correction: It is well known and established that haze rarely occurs in eyes that have lower levels of myopic correction (<6.00 D) treated with PRK [11]. Incidence of clinically significant haze after PRK increases with higher levels of myopic corrections, as refractive error goes beyond −6.00 D [22–26].

Irregularity of postop stromal surface: There is an increase in the irregularity of the ablated surface as the depth of the ablation increases [27]. Surface ablation disturbs the stroma and increases its irregularity. Haze post-PRK is proportional to the stromal surface irregularity remaining after ablation [11]. Studies on rabbits suggest that PRK smoothing reduces haze after PRK, and demonstrates conclusively that haze and myofibroblast density increase as surface irregularity is artificially increased [9]. In a study on 80 human eyes, Vinciguerra et al. noted that there is a clinical correlation between the irregularity of the ablated surface after PRK and the incidence of corneal haze; haze decreased when PRK included a stromal PTK-smoothing procedure [28, 29].

Tear fluid TGF-β levels: Long et al., in a search to find a method to predict which patients will develop haze postoperatively, found that those who had a higher degree of TGF-β1 in tears on day 1 Postoperatively had a greater incidence of haze after 1 month [20].

Other factors: Removal of the epithelial basement membrane, ablation of Bowman's layer, and length of time required for epithelial defect healing have also been ascribed as risk factors for haze development. In addition the surgical method and the type of laser used influence haze incidence. Haze is more common in PRK than in the other surgical models. Its incidence is less with the use of small flying spot laser as compared to the use of the old, broadbeam lasers [30].

10.7 Clinical Assessment

Haze can be measured by different methods, some of which are widely used and some of which have been abandoned. Table 10.7.1 summarizes the different techniques that have been used. These methods can be divided into subjective and objective methods of assessment.

Subjective assessment is carried out via slit lamp biomicroscopy. It is graded from 1 to 4 as described in Table 10.3.1. Figure 10.7.1 shows the different stages of haze as seen by a slit lamp. Though this method is easy and does not require any additional equipment, and it is very subjective and not reproducible, with high intrasession (4%) and day-to-day variation (7%) [31].

Objective measures use additional equipment, either mounted on the slit lamp or as stand-alone machines to measure haze. These can be further subdivided into "reflected-light methods" that measure forward light scatter and those that measure backward light scatter. Backward scatter is defined as scattering of light toward the origin of the incident light. Forward scatter is when light is scattered toward the retina.

Using the law of conservation of energy and basic physics, the following formula can be generated. This formula forms the basis of the rationale of scattered light measurement:

incident white light = reflected light + light absorbed by haze + scattered light + transmitted light.

The value of the incident white light is known and constant. Reflected light of the cornea is constant and is equal to 2% [32]. Since haze appears white–and from basic physics, white is obtained when all incident light is reflected–then absorbed light by haze can be considered to be equal to zero. The light that is transmitted goes to the retina. Simplifying the above equation will lead to the conclusion that scattered + transmitted light should remain constant as long as the incident white light is constant. Haze is inverse-

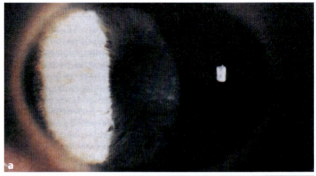
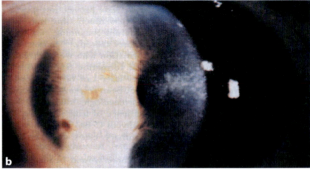
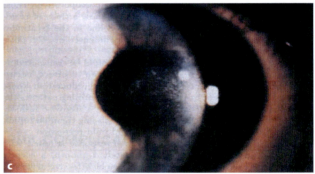

Fig. 10.7.1 Stages of haze. **a** Trace haze, **b** mild haze, **c** moderate haze. (From: Thompson V, Seiler T, Hardten DR [2007] Photorefractive keratectomy (PRK). In: Azar DT (ed), Gatinel D and Hoang-Xuan T (associate eds) Refractive surgery, 2nd edn. Elsevier, Dordrecht, pp 223–237

Table 10.7.1 Objective methods to measure haze

Mechanism	Method	Advantage(s)	Disadvantage(s)
Slit lamp biomicroscope	Subjective grading	Easy, no special tools required	Subjective, low reproducibility
Opacity lensometer	Two-color scattering response	Better than slit lamp	Poor discrimination of low haze
Scheimpflug -EAS1000	Backward light scatter	Subjective measure	Small magnification
TSPC-3 hazemeter	Backward light scatter	Can objectively measure subtle changes, more magnification, wide area of coverage	Not reflective of forward scattered light
van den Berg stray light meter	Forward light scatter	More reflective of retinal image quality	Not practical
Confocal microscope	Backward light scatter	High magnification, good resolution	Cannot be used clinically

ly proportional to backward scatter and directly proportional to forward scatter.

Following is a description of the different machines that have been developed and used to assess corneal haze.

■ **Reflected light**
- *Scheimpflug anterior eye segment analysis system EAS-1000 [33]*

This is the method of choice and the first method that was developed. It can measure mild-to-moderate corneal haze well, but severe haze cannot be adequately quantified [32]. It uses a charge coupled device camera mounted on the slit lamp to measure reflected light and assess corneal haze. Limitations to this technique include [32]:
- Only a narrow area of the cornea is covered.
- There is a lack of sensitivity in measuring low grades of haze.
- Photographic processing is required (which may increase result variability).
- There is possibly a background scatter light from the lens contamination.
- It is impossible to focus on the entire depth of the cornea in a single image.
- The magnification is too small for a detailed analysis of the corneal subepithelial region.
- Zero calibration is not confirmed in the background area.
- *TSPC-3 hazemeter [32]*

This is a modification of the EAS-1000 system, which can objectively measure subtle changes in haze levels. It has good detail assessment and has 6.25-times more magnification than does the EAS-1000 system. A xenon flashlight source and a charge-coupled device camera are used. The light source generates a vertical slit beam of 7×0.08 mm, which is projected perpendicularly onto the cornea. The charge-coupled device camera is placed 45° to the plane of the slit light and focuses on the entire depth of the cornea by using the Scheimpflug principle. The flashlight power can be set to 50, 100, or 200 W by changing the electrical current, thus enabling coverage of a very wide range of scattering (haze) intensity by simply altering light illuminance. The image is then captured and digitized. Latex microsphere solution is used for calibration. Advantages include the ability to cover a wide area of the cornea and the ability to obtain results without the need for photographic processing.
- *Confocal microscope*

The basis of the confocal microscope is the focusing of the illumination and observation systems on the same point. This dramatically improves the axial and lateral resolution of the microscope and enables it to reach a magnification of ×600 [34]. This method can measure corneal haze quantitatively and objectively, and it is considered to be the gold standard for haze quan-

tification. The amount of backscattered light given in intensity-units or in intensity-thickness-units can be used to assess and monitor the relative transparency of the corneal stroma and provide an estimate of corneal haze [35–39]. Changes in the appearance of the corneal stroma, keratocytes, and corneal nerves can be visualized over time at high resolution. This method can also be used to characterize cellular changes associated with the wound healing response. Sublayer thickness can also be measured, allowing for in vivo monitoring of subepithelial haze depth after excimer PRK.

■ **Forward scattered light**
(Van den Berg straylight meter)

The forward scattering in the eye is what reduces the contrast of the retinal image and thus influences contrast sensitivity. This is more likely to affect retinal image quality and visual acuity measurements. Two light sources are directed towards the cornea and the flickering patch of straylight formed on the cornea is measured. Though more accurate and more reflective of actual haze magnitude, this technique is not widely used clinically because of its impracticality in the clinical setting

10.8 Preventive Measures

10.8.1 Mitomycin C

MMC (mitomycin C) is an antibiotic derived from *Streptomyces caespitosus*. Its alkylating properties enable it to cross-link DNA between adenine and guanine, thereby inhibiting DNA and RNA replication and protein synthesis. Although its actions are exerted primarily during the late G1 and S phases, it is non–cell-cycle specific. Rapidly dividing cells are more sensitive to its action, and therefore it may inhibit proliferation of corneal epithelial cells, stromal cells, endothelial cells, conjunctival cells, and Tenon capsule fibroblasts [40–42]. It has chemotherapeutic properties that induces keratocyte apoptosis and may lead to myofibroblast death by inducing apoptosis and necrosis. This results in myofibroblast differentiation blockade [43]. It is directly responsible for triggering corneal cell apoptosis and/or necrosis in vitro. The death of some keratocytes in the anterior stroma typically results in proliferation and activation of remaining keratocytes. It has been used to modulate scarring in different areas of ophthalmology: topical application has improved the results of glaucoma surgery, pterygium excision, and treatment of conjunctival and corneal intraepithelial neoplasia. Modulation of wound healing with the use of MMC was first suggested by Talamo in 1991 [44]; since then, intraoperative MMC has been used to prevent haze formation after PRK for high myopia [45–47].

The usual concentration of MMC is 0.02% applied to the corneal surface for 2 min, followed by copious irrigation with balanced salt solution [48]. Initially, application was

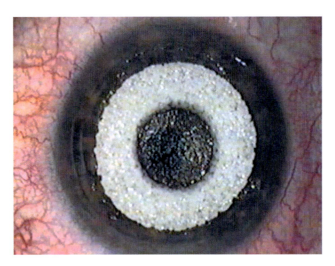

Fig. 10.8.1 MMC application using a ring-shaped sponge.

done using a circular sponge disc; however, the higher recurrence of haze in the periphery led to Azar and Jain [49] proposing the use of rings instead of discs (Fig 10.8.1).

MMC has higher efficacy in preventing haze formation than in treating it after it has formed [48, 50]. This is more pronounced in PRK patients with a spherical equivalent correction between –6.00 and –10 diopters [43].

MMC is far from being perfect. In some cases, haze may recur after its application, which may lead to secondary astigmatism. In addition, there might be a progressive decrease in keratocyte density thus and decreased collagen production leading to late corneal melting and keratectasia. Another problem is that, in the presence of previously existing corneal opacification, MMC may not completely eliminate haze due to an eventual persistence of myofibroblast cells.

10.8.2 Vitamin C

Oral ascorbic acid (Vitamin C) supplementation might have a prophylactic effect in decreasing haze development after PRK [51]. However, this is not widely accepted due to the difference in results after its prescription postoperatively. It works by preventing UV damage produced by excimer laser and reducing keratocyte activation.

10.8.3 Use of Epithelial Sheets Postoperatively

Hayashida et al. reported on the use of tissue engineered epithelial cell sheets after laser ablation by PRK [2]. Post-keratectomy wound healing was enhanced after the application of tissue-engineered corneal epithelial cell sheets directly after excimer laser ablation. The PRK wound-healing surface area was reduced to just a circumferential margin similar to the flap margin in LASIK.

10.9 Control and Treatment

A variety of therapeutic regimens have been used to prevent corneal haze after PRK, including topical corticosteroids, nonsteroidal anti-inflammatory drugs, plasmin inhibitors, antimetabolites, interferon-α and growth factors. Unfortunately, use of these pharmaceuticals results minimal reduction, if any, in corneal haze after PRK [52, 53].

Increasing the ablation zone size from 4 to 6 mm and using MMC intraoperatively have been shown to improve the refractive outcomes and reduce corneal haze after PRK [10, 17, 54, 55].

Different studies report that treatment with MMC proved effective in preventing the recurrence of fibrosis when combined with superficial keratectomy. In all cases, there was an improvement of corneal clarity [54, 55]. Although better results are obtained after using MMC as a preventive measure, Epstein et al. reported that the majority of PRK could be retreated successfully by a PRK retreatment with MMC or by PTK [56].

Raviv et al. describes a technique for eliminating haze and myopic regression [55] by removing the subepithelial haze using a no64 blade or a pterygium burr. A MMC-soaked sponge is then placed on the cornea for 2 min, followed by copious irrigation of the cornea and conjunctiva with a balanced salt solution. A pressure patch or a bandage contact lens is then applied, and the patient is given antibiotics and steroids four times daily for 1 week. The steroid drops are then tapered over 1–3 months.

Horgan et al. reported on the use of PTK to treat stromal irregularity after PRK in porcine corneas [57]. Another report by Serrao reports its use to treat 10 human patients [58].

10.10 Conclusion

Though refractive surgery is safe and very prevalent, it is not without complications. The most common complication of PRK is haze. Despite the high incidence of mild haze, it is clinically significant in less than 5% of cases and resolves on its own. The most prevalent method of assessment is slit lamp subjective assessment; however, the gold standard is confocal microscopy. Care should be taken in selecting patients and assigning them to different refractive surgery models. In the case of high myopic patients to be treated by PRK, MMC should be administered before completion of the procedure. In the event of development of clinically significant haze and visual compromise, a repeat MMC procedure or a repeat PTK/PRK is the way to go.

Take-Home Pearls
- Haze postoperatively should be graded.
- Fantes grades ≤ 2 requires only observation.
- For more advanced stages, treatment that is more aggressive is necessary.

■ Steroids are used effectively in humans, though not found to be beneficial in animal trials. Topical steroids four times daily for 1 week is the first line treatment in stage 2 or more haze post-refractive surgery.

■ MMC can adequately prevent and treat haze after refractive surgery. Though it is more effective as a preventive measure, PRK retreatment with MMC can retreat the majority of cases.

References

1. Lohmann CP et al (1992) Corneal light scattering after excimer laser photorefractive keratectomy: the objective measurements of haze. Refract Corneal Surg 8:114–21

2. Hayashida Y et al (2006) Transplantation of tissue-engineered epithelial cell sheets after excimer laser photoablation reduces postoperative corneal haze. Invest Ophthalmol Vis Sci 47:552–557

3. Hersh PS, Abbassi R(1999) Surgically induced astigmatism after photorefractive keratectomy and laser in situ keratomileusis. Summit PRK-LASIK Study Group. J Cataract Refract Surg 25:389–398

4. El-Maghraby A et al (1999) Randomized bilateral comparison of excimer laser in situ keratomileusis and photorefractive keratectomy for 2.50 to 8.00 diopters of myopia. Ophthalmology 106:447–457

5. Fantes FE et al (1990) Wound healing after excimer laser keratomileusis (photorefractive keratectomy) in monkeys. Arch Ophthalmol 108:665–675

6. Netto MV et al (2005) Wound healing in the cornea: a review of refractive surgery complications and new prospects for therapy. Cornea 24:509–522

7. Stephenson CG et al (1998) Photorefractive keratectomy: a 6-year follow-up study. Ophthalmology 105:273–281

8. Winkler von Mohrenfels C, Reischl U, Lohmann CP (2002) Corneal haze after photorefractive keratectomy for myopia: role of collagen IV mRNA typing as a predictor of haze. J Cataract Refract Surg 28:1446–1451

9. Mohan RR et al (2003) Apoptosis, necrosis, proliferation, and myofibroblast generation in the stroma following LASIK and PRK. Exp Eye Res 76:71–87

10. Rajan MS et al (2006) Effects of ablation diameter on long-term refractive stability and corneal transparency after photorefractive keratectomy. Ophthalmology 113:1798–1806

11. Netto MV et al (2006) Stromal haze, myofibroblasts, and surface irregularity after PRK. Exp Eye Res 82:788–797

12. Chen C et al (2000) Measurement of mRNAs for TGFss and extracellular matrix proteins in corneas of rats after PRK. Invest Ophthalmol Vis Sci 41:4108–4116

13. Jester JV et al (1999) The cellular basis of corneal transparency: evidence for "corneal crystallins." J Cell Sci 112:613–622

14. Moller-Pedersen T et al (1998) Confocal microscopic characterization of wound repair after photorefractive keratectomy. Invest Ophthalmol Vis Sci 39:487–501

15. Moller-Pedersen T et al (1998) Neutralizing antibody to TGF-beta modulates stromal fibrosis but not regression of photoablative effect following PRK. Curr Eye Res 17:736–747

16. Braunstein RE et al (1996) Objective measurement of corneal light scattering after excimer laser keratectomy. Ophthalmology 103:439–443

17. O'Brart DP et al (1995) The effects of ablation diameter on the outcome of excimer laser photorefractive keratectomy. A prospective, randomized, double-blind study. Arch Ophthalmol 113:438–443

18. Corbett MC et al (1996) Effect of ablation profile on wound healing and visual performance 1 year after excimer laser photorefractive keratectomy. Br J Ophthalmol 80:224–234

19. Moller-Pedersen T et al (1998) Corneal haze development after PRK is regulated by volume of stromal tissue removal. Cornea 17:627–639

20. Long Q et al (2006) Correlation between TGF-beta1 in tears and corneal haze following LASEK and epi-LASIK. J Refract Surg 22:708–712

21. O'Brart DP et al (1994) Excimer laser photorefractive keratectomy for myopia: comparison of 4.00- and 5.00-millimeter ablation zones. J Refract Corneal Surg 10:87–94

22. Lipshitz I et al (1997) Late onset corneal haze after photorefractive keratectomy for moderate and high myopia. Ophthalmology 104:369–373; discussion 373–374

23. Hersh PS et al (1997) Results of phase III excimer laser photorefractive keratectomy for myopia. The Summit PRK Study Group. Ophthalmology 104:1535–1553

24. Shah S, Chatterjee A, Smith RJ (1998) Predictability of spherical photorefractive keratectomy for myopia. Ophthalmology 105:2178–2184; discussion 2184–2185

25. Siganos DS, Katsanevaki VJ, Pallikaris IG (1999) Correlation of subepithelial haze and refractive regression 1 month after photorefractive keratectomy for myopia. J Refract Surg 15:338–342

26. Kuo IC, Lee SM, Hwang DG (2004) Late-onset corneal haze and myopic regression after photorefractive keratectomy (PRK). Cornea 23:350–355

27. Taylor SM et al (1994) Effect of depth upon the smoothness of excimer laser corneal ablation. Optom Vis Sci 71:104–108

28. Vinciguerra P et al (1998) A method for examining surface and interface irregularities after photorefractive keratectomy and laser in situ keratomileusis: predictor of optical and functional outcomes. J Refract Surg 14(2 Suppl):S204–S206

29. Vinciguerra P et al (1998) Effect of decreasing surface and interface irregularities after photorefractive keratectomy and laser in situ keratomileusis on optical and functional outcomes. J Refract Surg 14(2 Suppl):S199–S203

30. Pallikaris IG et al (1999) Photorefractive keratectomy with a small spot laser and tracker. J Refract Surg 15:137–144

31. Olsen T (1982) Light scattering from the human cornea. Invest Ophthalmol Vis Sci 23:81–86

32. Soya K, Amano S, Oshika T (2002) Quantification of simulated corneal haze by measuring back-scattered light. Ophthalmic Res 34:380–388

33. Sasaki K et al (1990) The multi-purpose camera: a new anterior eye segment analysis system. Ophthalmic Res 22(Suppl 1):3–8

34. Jalbert I et al (2003) In vivo confocal microscopy of the human cornea. Br J Ophthalmol 87:225–326

35. Nagel S, Wiegand W, Thaer AA (1995) [Corneal changes and corneal healing after keratomileusis in situ. In vivo studies using confocal slit-scanning microscopy]. Ophthalmologe 92:397–401

36. Nagel S et al (1996) [Light scattering study of the cornea in contact lens patients. In vivo studies using confocal slit scanning microscopy]. Ophthalmologe 93:252–256

37. Slowik C et al (1996) Assessment of corneal alterations following laser in situ keratomileusis by confocal slit scanning microscopy. Ger J Ophthalmol 5:526–531

38. Moller-Pedersen T et al (1997) Quantification of stromal thinning, epithelial thickness, and corneal haze after photorefractive keratectomy using in vivo confocal microscopy. Ophthalmology 104:360–368

39. Ciancaglini M et al (2001) Morphological evaluation of Schnyder's central crystalline dystrophy by confocal microscopy before and after phototherapeutic keratectomy. J Cataract Refract Surg 27:1892–1895

40. Lee JS, Oum BS, Lee SH (2001) Mitomycin C influence on inhibition of cellular proliferation and subsequent synthesis of type I collagen and laminin in primary and recurrent pterygia. Ophthalmic Res 33:140–146

41. Watanabe J et al (1997) Effects of mitomycin C on the expression of proliferating cell nuclear antigen after filtering surgery in rabbits. Graefes Arch Clin Exp Ophthalmol 235:234–240

42. Pinilla I et al (1998) Subconjunctival injection of low doses of mitomycin C: effects on fibroblast proliferation. Ophthalmologica 212:306–309

43. Carones F et al (2002) Evaluation of the prophylactic use of mitomycin-C to inhibit haze formation after photorefractive keratectomy. J Cataract Refract Surg 28:2088–2095

44. Talamo JH et al (1991) Modulation of corneal wound healing after excimer laser keratomileusis using topical mitomycin C and steroids. Arch Ophthalmol 109:1141–1146

45. Akarsu C, Onol M, Hasanreisoglu B (2003) Effects of thick Tenon's capsule on primary trabeculectomy with mitomycin-C. Acta Ophthalmol Scand 81:237–241

46. Oguz H (2003) Mitomycin C and pterygium excision. Ophthalmology 110:2257–2258; author reply 2258

47. Gambato C et al (2005) Mitomycin C modulation of corneal wound healing after photorefractive keratectomy in highly myopic eyes. Ophthalmology 112:208–218; discussion 219

48. Netto MV, Chalita MR, Krueger RR (2007) Corneal haze following PRK with mitomycin C as a retreatment versus prophylactic use in the contralateral eye. J Refract Surg 23:96–98

49. Azar DT, Jain S (2001) Topical MMC for subepithelial fibrosis after refractive corneal surgery. Ophthalmology 108:239–40

50. Bedei A et al (2006) Photorefractive keratectomy in high myopic defects with or without intraoperative mitomycin C: 1-year results. Eur J Ophthalmol 16:229–234

51. Stojanovic A, Ringvold A, and Nitter T (2003) Ascorbate prophylaxis for corneal haze after photorefractive keratectomy. J Refract Surg 19:338–343

52. O'Brart D.P et al (1994) The effects of topical corticosteroids and plasmin inhibitors on refractive outcome, haze, and visual performance after photorefractive keratectomy. A prospective, randomized, observer-masked study. Ophthalmology 101:1565–1574

53. Rajan MS et al (2204) Effect of exogenous keratinocyte growth factor on corneal epithelial migration after photorefractive keratectomy. J Cataract Refract Surg 30:2200–2206

54. Majmudar PA et al (2000) Topical mitomycin-C for subepithelial fibrosis after refractive corneal surgery. Ophthalmology 107:89–94

55. Raviv T et al (2000) Mytomycin-C for post-PRK corneal haze. J Cataract Refract Surg 26:1105–1106

56. Epstein D et al (1994) Excimer retreatment of regression after photorefractive keratectomy. Am J Ophthalmol 117:456–461

57. Horgan SE et al (1999) Phototherapeutic smoothing as an adjunct to photorefractive keratectomy in porcine corneas. J Refract Surg 15:331–333

58. Serrao S, Lombardo M, Mondini F (2003) Photorefractive keratectomy with and without smoothing: a bilateral study. J Refract Surg 19:58–64

10

Complications of LASEK

David P.S. O'Brart

Contents

Core Messages

■ LASEK is safe and effective, but sight-threatening complications may occur.

■ Most complications are avoidable.

11.1 Introduction

Laser epithelial keratomileusis (LASEK) was described independently by Camellin [1], Azar [2], and Shah [3]. It combines elements of photorefractive keratectomy (PRK) and laser in situ keratomileusis (LASIK). In contrast to PRK, in which the central corneal epithelium is completely debrided, in LASEK a hinged epithelial flap is fashioned, using a dilute solution of alcohol (15–20%) applied for 20–30 s to loosen the epithelial attachment (Fig. 11.1). After laser ablation, the intact epithelial sheet is replaced over the ablated stromal surface, and a bandage contact lens is used to keep it in place during the immediate and early phase of wound healing. The aim of replacing an intact epithelial sheet over the ablated surface is to attempt to speed visual recovery, reduce postoperative pain, and lessen epithelial/stromal wound-healing responses. The creation of an epithelial flap rather than a deeper partial thickness stromal flap as in LASIK avoids intralamellar flap associated complications such as wrinkling, free and incomplete flaps, epithelial ingrowth, flap melt, interface debris, diffuse lamellar keratitis and ectasia [4].

Comparative studies have reported few differences in medium and long-term refractive and visual outcomes between PRK, LASEK, and LASIK for low- and moderate-hyperopic and low-, moderate- and even relatively high-my-

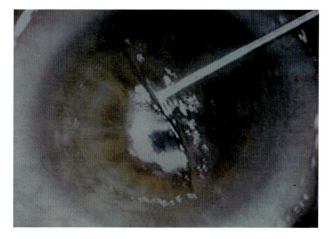

Fig. 11.1 Creation of an intact epithelial flap using a microhoe after administration of 15% alcohol for 20 s

opic corrections [5–12]. In terms of early postoperative recovery, results comparing PRK and LASEK have been conflicting. While Leccisotti [5] demonstrated no differences, Autrata and Rehurek [6] and Lee [7] in prospective bilateral studies found less postoperative pain and faster visual recovery after LASEK. In contrast, Litwak et al. [8] found more pain and slower epithelial healing after LASEK, although they exposed the epithelium to 20% alcohol for 45 s, which would result in the death of virtually all cells in the flap [9]. In the only reported comparative study of hyperopic corrections, Autrata and Rehurek [10] reported less pain, faster visual recovery, and quicker refractive stability with LASEK compared with PRK.

Published studies of LASEK outcomes over the past 6 years have been very encouraging [6, 10–16]. In a review article, the cumulative reported safety index (mean postoperative best spectacle corrected visual acuity [BSCVA]/mean preoperative BSCVA) of 11 peer-reviewed papers was 1, with only a single eye of nearly 1,500 studied, losing two or more lines of BSCVA due to a macular cyst unrelated to the LASEK procedure [11]. Reported predictability was excellent with 83% of eyes within ±0.50 D of the intended correction at 6 months, with an efficacy index (mean postoperative uncorrected visual acuity [UCVA]/ mean preoperative BSCVA) of 0.947 [11]. In the author's consecutive case series (unpublished data) of 376 myopic eyes (mean preoperative spherical equivalent [SEQ], –4.92 D; range, –1.25 to –10.75 D) treated with a Schwind ESIRIS flying-spot excimer laser over the past 4 years and reaching 6-month follow-up, 89% were within ±0.50 D, and 98% within ±1.00 D of the intended correction, with an efficacy index of 0.952 and a safety index of 1.04. Similarly, in 70 consecutively treated hyperopic eyes (mean preoperative SEQ, +2.32 D; range, 0 to +5.00 D), 86% were within ±0.50 D and 100% within ±1.00 D of the intended correction at 12 months, with an efficacy index of 0.95 and a safety index of 1.06 [16].

While such outcomes are encouraging, they are the result of two decades of increasing knowledge of laser tissue interactions and corneal wound-healing responses, access to advanced technologies, and meticulous attention to detail in regards to preoperative patient education and counseling, preoperative evaluation, operative procedures, and postoperative care. A thorough knowledge of potential complications both sight threatening and non–sight threatening, their prevention and management is vital in order to minimize adverse events postoperatively (Table 11.1.1). This is particularly important considering the elective nature of keratorefractive procedures and extremely high patient expectations.

11.2 Intraoperative Complications

11.2.1 Alcohol Escape

The LASEK procedure is typically painless. Patients should be warned, however, that if alcohol should escape underneath the LASEK well and onto the conjunctival surface, ocular pain/discomfort will be experienced. Alcohol escape should be avoided in order to facilitate a painless procedure, and because it may cause limbal epithelial stem cell damage, which may delay epithelial wound healing, and conjunctival epithelial cell damage, which will increase postoperative inflammation. In order to avoid this problem, the surgeon must guide the patient to limit movement when the well is place on the cornea and when the patient experiences an ocular pressure sensation and loss of visual clarity, movement is limited as much as possible. Firm, but not excessive, pressure should be used when applying the well to the corneal surface. Should alcohol escape occur, the ocular surface should be irrigated immediately with a balanced saline solution, the bulbar conjunctiva and corneal surface dried with a LASIK spear, and the alcohol well reapplied.

Table 11.1 Complications of LASEK

Intraoperative
Alcohol escape
Poor flap creation
Free flap

Early (hours/days)
Pain
Delayed epithelial healing
Slow visual recovery
Sterile infiltrates
Infectious keratitis[a]

Early (days/weeks)
Corneal melt[a]
Corticosteroid intraocular pressure response[a]
Corneal erosion
Delayed visual recovery
Herpes simplex keratitis[a]
Delayed infectious keratitis[a]

Medium (weeks/months)
Overcorrection/undercorrection
Subepithelial corneal haze[a]
Recurrent erosion syndrome
Night vision disturbances
Ptosis

Late (months/years)
Overcorrection/undercorrection
Corneal scarring[a]
Recurrent corneal erosion syndrome
Ectasia[a]

[a] Potential sight-threatening complications

11.2.2 Poor Epithelial Flap

With administration of 15–20% alcohol for 20–25 s, the creation of an intact epithelial flap with an adequate hinge is usually straightforward [16, 17] (Fig. 11.1). In some eyes, however, the epithelium may be particularly adherent. In the author's experience, this tends to occur in patients who have undergone excessive long-term contact lens wear. This was similarly noted by Claringbold, who also identified young men and postmenopausal women as having more adherent epithelium [14]. Camellin, in his series, reported difficulty in obtaining an intact epithelial flap in 12% of eyes [1]. We reported adherent and incomplete epithelial flaps in 4% of high myopic [17] and 6% of hyperopic eyes [16]. If it is not possible to obtain an intact epithelial flap, then the procedure can be easily converted to a PRK technique by mechanically debriding the epithelium with the knowledge that the patient might experience more postoperative pain and a slightly slower visual recovery [5–8, 10, 11].

11.2.3 Free Flap

Occasionally, it may be difficult to fashion an adequate epithelial hinge, and a free epithelial flap can occur. In such cases, the flap may still be repositioned over the ablated stromal surface. Care should be taken to ensure the flap is placed basal epithelial–side down. Once a free flap has been repositioned, a bandage contact lens can then be inserted in the usual manner to keep it in place.

11.3 Early Postoperative Complications (Hours/Days)

11.3.1 Pain

While some comparative studies report less postoperative pain after LASEK compared with PRK [6, 7], others have shown no differences [5]. Camellin reported that over 60% of his patients experienced no pain after surgery [18].According to the author's experience, is the majority of individuals do experience some discomfort/pain after LASEK during the first 2–18 h, and some may report considerable pain. Most practitioners prescribe oral analgesics for 2–3 days after the procedure, both opiate and non-opiate. Some benefit has also been found from the use of topical non-steroidal anti-inflammatory agents [19]. Considerable pain relief without any detrimental effects on visual and refractive recovery has been demonstrated with the use of topical anesthetic administration after PRK [20]. In the author's practice great benefit is found, with no detrimental effects, with the use of topical preservative free anesthetic drops (Benoxinate 0.4%) in a limited dosage (maximum of 1 drop every 2–3 h for the first 18 h, a maximum of 10 drops in total) for acute pain control after LASEK.

11.3.2 Delayed Epithelial Healing

In the author's experience, epithelial closure is usually complete in myopic LASEK corrections within 3–4 days [17] and hyperopic corrections, which have a larger overall ablation diameter (9 mm), within 3–7 days [16]. Kornilovsky reports closure at 4 days [21], Camellin 4–5 days [1, 18], and Lee 3.68±0.69 days [7] in myopic corrections. Taneri reported a closure rate of 78% at 3 days and 99% at one week [13]. Most practitioners typically remove the bandage contact lenses between 3 and 4 days or when epithelial closure is complete. Delayed epithelial closure beyond 5–7 days is unusual, and such patients need to be carefully monitored because of the risks of underlying stromal melt, the ongoing risk of infection, and the possible development of corneal haze. Signs of stromal infiltration should alert the practitioner to the possibility of a potentially sight-threatening complication (infection and/or melt). Conditions predisposing to delayed epithelial closure include dry eye problems, preservative toxicity, drug allergy (topical antibiotics), and limbal stem cell anomalies.

Preoperatively, it is important to exclude dry eye problems, as this may exacerbate epithelial healing problems following surgery. Patients with overt dry eye problems do not make good candidates for laser refractive surgery and should not be treated. Those with mild and moderate dry eye symptoms and signs can be treated preoperatively with punctal plugs, topical cyclosporine eye drops, and aggressive treatment of concurrent lid disease, if present. If satisfactory resolution occurs, then keratorefractive surgery may be possible provided there is no associated manifest connective tissue problem. If delayed epithelial healing occurs in the presence of dry eye, punctual plugs should be inserted.

Preservative toxicity/drug allergy should be suspected in cases of delayed epithelial healing and in the presence of a history of previous intolerance to contact lens solutions, continuing conjunctival injection and punctate epithelial erosions. In eyes where epithelial closure is delayed beyond 4–5 days, the use of preservative free-medications is advisable.

Patients with limbal stem cell deficiencies and conjunctival cicatrizing conditions are not candidates for keratorefractive surgery and should be excluded preoperatively.

11.3.3 Slow Visual Recovery

After LASEK, patients typically notice an immediate improvement in unaided postoperative visual performance, provided an intact epithelial flap has been obtained and successfully replaced. It is not uncommon for some patients to experience a reduction in visual acuity after the first 24 h, as epithelial cells damaged by alcohol swell and die.

The flap can also slough off in some eyes at this stage. Patients should be warned before hand of this early visual impairment. Vision begins to return once epithelial closure has occurred. We have documented that even in high myopic corrections, 90% of eyes have an UCVA of 20/40 or better and 70% of 20/30 or better by one week [17]. Visual recovery is generally faster with low myopic corrections and in younger patients. In hyperopic LASEK corrections, visual recovery is slower, with less than 50% of patients achieving an UCVA of 20/40 or better by one week [16]. This is due to slower epithelial regeneration (larger flap diameter, generally older patients) and myopic overcorrection during the first few weeks and months following surgery [16]. Hyperopic patients need to be informed that although functional unaided near vision may be achieved during the first few weeks, satisfactory levels of unaided distance visual acuity may take weeks/months.

Slow visual recovery during the early postoperative phase is usually due to delayed or irregular epithelial healing. Predisposing causes include dry eye, preservative toxicity, drop allergy, infection, preexisting ocular surface anomalies. Prevention is better than cure, and it is mandatory that all patients have a comprehensive ophthalmic examination by an experienced practitioner with a thorough knowledge of anterior segment disease so that preexisting conditions are adequately treated prior to surgery and unsuitable patients excluded.

11.3.4　Sterile Infiltrates

Punctate sterile epithelial infiltrates may develop during the first few weeks after LASEK. They may occasionally be the result of preservative toxicity/drug allergy. They can be treated by increasing the frequency of the topical corticosteroid administration. It is the author's preference to use preservative-free preparations in these cases.

Occasionally, anterior stromal infiltration may occur. Infectious keratitis needs to be excluded, and eyes with an associated overlying epithelial defect must be assumed infected and treated appropriately. Where the overlying epithelium is closed, such eyes may be treated by increasing the frequency of topical corticosteroid medication, while maintaining antibiotic cover and keeping the patient under careful observation until the infiltrates have resolved.

11.3.5　Infectious Keratitis

Infectious keratitis is fortunately a very rare event after LASEK. As the infectious process commences at the epithelial level in LASEK and not intrastromally as in LASIK, it should be easier to manage [22]. It has been reported in only one case due to *Staphylococcus haemolyticus* as early as 2 days [23], and in one case as late as 4 weeks due to *Mycobacterium chelonae* [24]. It is a site-threatening complication and needs to be treated promptly and appropriately with microbiological investigations and targeted intensive topical antimicrobial therapy.

In order to minimize potential risks, patients must be examined preoperatively for signs of active lid margin disease and treated appropriately with systemic tetracyclines and lid hygiene before undergoing laser refractive procedures. Most practitioners advocate the use of topical antibiotic therapy until epithelial closure is complete. Common regimens include the use of an aminoglycoside, such as tobramycin, which covers gram-negative organisms including *Pseudomonas*, and/or a fluoroquinolone, which cover both gram-positive and gram-negative species. Preferred agents include Ofloxacin and fourth-generation fluoroquinolones such as gatifloxacin, and moxifloxacin.

11.4　Early Postoperative Complications (Days/Weeks)

11.4.1　Slow Visual Recovery

By 1 month, 70–80% of myopic eyes after LASEK achieve an UCVA of 20/20 or better [5–9, 11–15, 17, 18]. Occasionally, visual recovery may take longer (up to 3–4 months). This can be due to epithelial irregularity because of delayed epithelial healing (as discussed above). Such patients need to be carefully monitored to exclude the presence of sight-threatening complication such as corneal haze, melt, and steroid-induced raised intraocular pressure.

In hyperopic corrections, visual recovery is slower, with less than 40% of eyes achieving an UCVA of 20/20 or better due to myopic overcorrection that may take several months to settle, especially in high-order (greater than +4.00 D) corrections [16].

11.4.2　Intraocular Steroid Pressure Response

Although randomized clinical studies indicate little benefit from their usage [25], many practitioners still advocate the use of topical corticosteroid preparations during the first few days/weeks after LASEK to minimize the risks of corneal haze development. Fluorometholone 0.1% (FML) is often the preferred agent, as reduced ocular penetration reduces the risk of associated complications such as elevated intraocular pressure, increased risk of infection, and cataract formation [26, 27]. It is essential to monitor patients using corticosteroid eye drops to check for an intraocular pressure response if they are used for longer than 10 days. Patients should be examined every 2 weeks while receiving steroid eye drops. With FML, steroid-induced glaucoma has been reported in up to 3% of cases [26]. Should intraocular pressure problems occur, the medication should be terminated where possible. Topical anti-glaucomatous medications, in the first instance preservative-free Timoptol 0.25% twice daily (unless contraindicated), should be prescribed. Preservative-free Aproclonidine 1% thrice daily is useful if the pressure is greater than 30 mmHg. Systemic acetazolamide may occasionally be required. The intraocular pressure usually returns to normal levels a week to 10 days after cessation of steroid eye drops.

11

11.4.3 Recurrent Corneal Erosion Syndrome

Fifteen to 20% of patients undergoing LASEK and PRK report "dryness" and discomfort on opening their eyes when waking in the morning [28]. Such symptoms are typical of mild recurrent corneal erosion syndrome, occuring during the first few months, and then usually resolving. In persistent cases or where symptoms become problematic or when the patient wakes up in the middle of the night with ocular pain, the use of topical lubricant ointments such as Lacrilube at night for 6 weeks, is useful in alleviating and resolving symptoms. In those with preexisting lid disease, systemic tetracyclines are a useful adjunctive treatment, possibly due to inhibition of metalloproteinase-9 [29]. In persistent cases, it may be necessary to carry out a peripheral anterior stromal puncture procedure. This is performed outside the optical zone in order to avoid scar formation across the visual axis, and as the epithelium overlying the area of stromal ablation is typically firmly adherent. In the author's experience in 6 years of performing LASEK, anterior stromal puncture has been necessary in six eyes of four patients (<0.05%) when symptoms have persisted after 9 months. In all cases, it has resulted in improvement/resolution of symptoms.

Such cases tend to occur in low order myopic corrections (typically less than –4.00 D) and are more common in myopes rather than hyperopes due to the width of the stromal ablation. Patients should be warned preoperatively about such symptoms. Prior to alcohol administration, it is useful to test the adherence of the epithelium with a LASIK sponge. If the epithelium moves and wrinkles due to an underlying basement membrane epithelial dystrophy, then the procedure should ideally be performed without alcohol administration, it is unnecessary in these eye to achieve a satisfactory epithelial flap, and it might increase the risk of subsequent epithelial instability problems.

11.4.4 Corneal Melt

Corneal melting is a rare occurrence. Cases have been reported in the presence of collagen vascular diseases such as systemic lupus erythematosus (SLE) [30], and it is important to exclude such patients preoperatively. Although some practitioners regard collagen vascular diseases as a relative contraindication to refractive laser surgery, the presence of active systemic disease and past ocular involvement must be absolute contraindications. If corneal melt should occur, then associated dry eye problems must be treated adequately and promptly and infectious keratitis excluded. Expert subspecialist ophthalmic medical management is required with intensive topical preservative-free corticosteroid and systemic immunosuppressive therapy. Further surgical interventions such as amniotic membrane grafting and keratoplasty may be necessary [30].

11.4.5 Herpes Simplex Keratitis

Patients with recurrent herpes simplex keratitis are not candidates for routine refractive laser surgery. Phototherapeutic keratectomy can be useful in selected cases, but reactivation can occur [31], and such eyes require prophylactic systemic antivirals (acyclovir). Any eye with an unexplained corneal scar preoperatively must be regarded as suspicious, and a full history must be taken. In patients that develop labial herpes simplex during the early/medium postoperative period, it is recommended to prescribe systemic prophylactic acyclovir.

11.4.6 Late Infectious Keratitis

Late infection with *M. chelonae* has been reported in a single case 4 weeks after LASEK (see above) [24]. Practitioners should be aware of such late complications so they can be adequately managed and patients informed so that they return promptly with any symptoms of pain, redness, and sudden visual loss occurring in the first few months after surgery.

11.5 Medium Postoperative Complications (Weeks/Months)

11.5.1 Overcorrection/Undercorrection

For LASEK corrections between +4.00 and –8.00 D and up to –5.00 DC, the vast majority of eyes achieve outcomes within ± 0.50 D of that intended [5–8, 10–18], with refractive stability being achieved by 1–3 months in myopic and 3–6 months in hyperopic corrections [16, 17]. Rarely, over- and undercorrection may occur especially in high-order corrections. Reported re-treatment rates vary between 0 and 7% [5–8, 10–15, 18]. In cases of early regression, some practitioners advocate the use of topical corticosteroids, especially in the presence of subepithelial haze [32, 33]. Not all eyes respond, and re-treatment may be indicated.

The optimum timing of re-treatment is unknown, but should not be undertaken before two stable refractive measurements have been obtained at least 3 months apart. It is advisable not to consider re-treatment in cases of myopic surface excimer laser ablation before 6–9 months, and for hyperopic cases before 12 months, due to the risk of precipitating an aggressive healing response. Re-treatment should not occur before any subepithelial haze has been seen to regress. Careful preoperative evaluation is essential to ensure that any regression, especially in myopic cases, is not due to an ectatic process.

11.5.2 Haze

Excimer laser refractive surgery is undertaken on healthy eyes; hence, any deterioration in postoperative corneal trans-

11

parency must be of great concern. In PRK, subepithelial haze develops over the central cornea by the fourth week postoperatively, with maximal disturbances at 3–6 months and is associated with increasing depths of stromal ablation and small optical zone treatments [34–37]. In LASEK, it has been postulated that the creation of an intact epithelial sheet to cover the ablated area might reduce epithelial–stromal cytokine cross-talk during the early phases of postoperative wound healing and induce less haze [1]. Prospective bilateral comparative studies of PRK and LASEK have produced conflicting results. While Hashemi [11] could find no differences, Autrata [6] and Lee [7] demonstrated less haze in LASEK treated eyes. In the author's own series of patients, significant haze formation has been reported as an unusual event even in high myopic and hyperopic corrections, with 89% of eyes being completely clear or showing only the merest trace of haze 6–12 months following surgery [16, 17]. Because of the risks of significant haze development with high-order corrections, small ablation diameters, and increasing depths of stromal ablation, it is the author's protocol to only treat eyes with LASEK between +4 mm and –8.00 D and up to –5 DC, to only use optical zones of greater than 6 mm for myopia and 7 mm for hyperopia and to limit the maximum depth of stromal ablation at 130 μm or less.

Many surgeons advocate the use of topical mitomycin C (MMC) when performing surface excimer laser corrections for high myopia and hyperopia. Carones, in a randomized, controlled study of PRK for high myopia, showed better results with MMC in terms of postoperative haze and refractive and visual outcomes [38]. Camellin, in a non-randomized study of LASEK for myopia, found that although MMC reduced postoperative haze, refractive outcome was less predictable and higher order aberrations increased after LASEK with MMC [39]. At present little is known concerning the long-term effects of MMC usage in refractive surgery. While undoubtedly it is a useful agent in reducing sub-epithelial haze in problematic cases [40], reports of occasional scleral melting associated with MMC usage in pterygium surgery [41] and of postoperative endothelial cell loss in PRK [42] suggest that some caution should be adopted. As acceptable outcomes can be obtained with LASEK for high myopia [17] and hyperopia [16] without MMC usage and until more long-term research in this area has been performed and published, it is recommended to only use MMC in excimer laser re-treatments and complex cases, i.e., post-keratoplasty, post–refractive surgery.

In eyes where haze greater than grade I (easily visible with the slit lamp) develops during the first 3 months, it is recommended to prescribe topical corticosteroid medication (preservative-free Dexamethasone 0.1%) in conjunction with preservative-free topical Timoptol 0.25% twice daily (providing there is no contraindication to its usage) to negate steroid intraocular pressure responses. Although there is evidence to suggest that topical corticosteroids merely delay rather than prevent haze formation [25], the author's experience and that of other practitioners indicate

favorable responses in such eyes [32, 33]. The topical steroid medication should be tapered over a 6- to 8-week period, with careful biweekly monitoring of the intraocular pressure. With time, the haze will clear in the vast majority of eyes with return of any associated loss of BSCVA[(43, 44].

In eyes with persistent and significant haze (>grade 2 beyond 6 months post-surgery) steroid medication will only have a limited effect, and although haze will very gradually clear with time [43, 44], further surgical intervention may be indicated depending on any associated loss of BSCVA, regression of correction and patient preference. Surgical options for persistent post-PRK/-LASEK haze include epithelial debridement with topical application of MMC 0.2 mg/ml applied for 30–45 s [45], phototherapeutic keratectomy (PTK) to remove the haze layer augmented with intraoperative MMC [46], and corneal wavefront topography-assisted excimer laser ablation augmented with intraoperative MMC [47]. The latter procedure is best performed when the refractive status and corneal appearance has been stable for at least 6 months and should not be performed, ideally, until 12 months after the original procedure. The author has found that a transepithelial approach is most beneficial with the laser being used to remove the epithelium, as epithelial hyper/hypoplasia often reduces some of the underlying irregularities caused by the haze formation, and the epithelium is very adherent overlying areas of aggressive haze. When using MMC, it is necessary to reduce the spherical and cylindrical component of the intended refractive correction by about 10%. Very rarely, cases of severe haze cannot be managed with excimer laser re-treatment and may require deep anterior lamellar corneal grafting procedures.

11.5.3 Night Vision Disturbances/Halos

In the early days of excimer laser keratorefractive procedures, night vision disturbances and halo phenomena in mesopic and scotopic conditions were not uncommon with the use of small (4- and 5-mm) diameter optical zone treatments [34, 37, 48], and in some cases have persisted with over 12 years of reported follow-up [45, 48]. With a greater understanding of the need to evaluate the preoperative pupil diameter in mesopic and scotopic conditions, the use of larger optical zone treatments (>6 mm), the advent of wavefront technology the development of aspheric ablation profiles to reduce the induction of fourth-order spherical aberration postoperatively, the incidents of such problems have reduced dramatically [17].

Patients, especially professional drivers, should be counseled preoperatively as to the rare occurrence of night vision disturbances that may preclude driving on unlit roads such as motorways [49]. Careful evaluation of mesopic/scotopic preoperative pupil diameter is mandatory [49]. Matching the optical zone to the pupil diameter should be attempted, and patients in whom matching with 1 mm cannot be achieved, due to the depth of tissue ablation, should not be treated. The use of aspheric ablations profiles, with or without wavefront technology, is important especially in myopic corrections and patients with mesopic/scotopic pupil diameters greater than 6.5 mm [49].

If night vision disturbances should occur, some benefit may be derived from the use of Brimondine tartrate 0.2% or pilocarpine 1% eye drops to induce miosis, taken half an hour before driving on unlit roads [49, 50]. Wavefront-guided re-treatments may be useful in problematic cases [49].

11.5.4 Recurrent Erosion

(See above.) Continuing symptoms 9–12 months after LASEK may be treated with a 360° peripheral anterior stromal puncture procedure. If this does not alleviate the problem, then it may be necessary to perform an epithelial debridement and 20-μm ablation depth, 10-mm-diameter PTK procedure.

11.6 Late Postoperative Complications (Months/Years)

11.6.1 Overcorrection/Undercorrection

See above.
11.6.2 Haze

See above.
11.6.3 Recurrent Corneal Erosion Syndrome

See above.
11.6.4 Ectasia

One of the major contraindications to excimer laser refractive surgery is the presence of overt or even subclinical keratoconus. An association between development/acceleration of corneal ectasia in such eyes and LASIK has been clearly established, with keratoconus both overt and forme fruste being an absolute contraindication to LASIK surgery [51]. While a number of investigators have proposed PTK and PRK as possible treatment modalities for keratoconus [52], recent reports of corneal ectasia after PRK [53–55] strongly suggest that such procedures are not advisable in these eyes, and that keratoconus in all its forms should be regarded as a relative, if not an absolute, contraindication.

Careful preoperative corneal topographic and wavefront evaluation is necessary in all eyes to identify abnormal patterns, and most devices now have statistical packages that identify high-risk cases, which should not be treated. Preoperative corneal pachymetric measurements are essential prior to surface ablative procedures. It is the author's opinion that any eyes with central pachymetric measurements of less than 500 μm should be regarded with great caution. It is also recommended to leave all eyes with a residual minimal stromal thickness of 400 μm as a precaution against problems with long-term corneal biomechanical instability.

In eyes with ectasia after excimer laser corrections (Fig. 11.2a), topical anti-glaucomatous medications may slow/reverse progression and treatment should be initiated [56]. Rigid contact lens fitting is the mainstay of treatment. Riboflavin (vitamin B_2)/UV-A (370 nm) light corneal collagen cross-linkage may perhaps halt progression and should be considered, but only in eyes with residual stromal thicknesses of 400 μm or greater [57]. Intrastromal corneal ring (Intacs) insertion has been show to be of benefit in mild-to-moderate cases, improving both UCVA, BSCVA, and contact lens fitting [58] (Fig. 11.2b). It is the author's preference to generally use single inferior Intacs insertion in such cases (Fig. 11.2b). In eyes with advanced ectasia, deep anterior lamellar keratoplasty may be the only option.

Take-Home Pearls

- Prevention is better than cure.
- Pearls for minimizing complications after LASEK:
  Preoperative
  – Extensive patient counseling concerning potential complications
  – Thorough medical history including:
    – Family history
    – Contact lens problems
  – Thorough ophthalmic examination by appropriately trained ophthalmologist
  – Exclude all unsuitable and at risk patients, including:
    – Form fruste/overt keratoconus
    – Active collagen vascular diseases
    – Overt dry eye
    – Conjunctival cicatrization
    – Corneal limbal stem cell anomalies
    – Preexisting active ocular pathologies
      – Cataract, glaucoma, herpes simplex/zoster
  – Be suspicious in eyes with:
    – Unexplained corneal scars
    – Abnormal corneal topography
    – Central corneal thickness <500 μm
  – Be careful in eyes with:
    – High-order corrections ±8.00 D
    – Central corneal thickness <500 μm
    – Large scotopic pupil diameters (>7 mm)
  – Treat preexisting lid disease, mild dry eye preoperatively
  Operative
  – Meticulous attention to detail
  – Maintain sterile conditions
  Postoperative
  Careful patient monitoring
  – Ensure easy access emergency service is provided.
  – Discuss with patients potential problems and ensure they understand the importance of attending out-patient follow-up visits.
  – Be honest and keep patient informed at every stage.

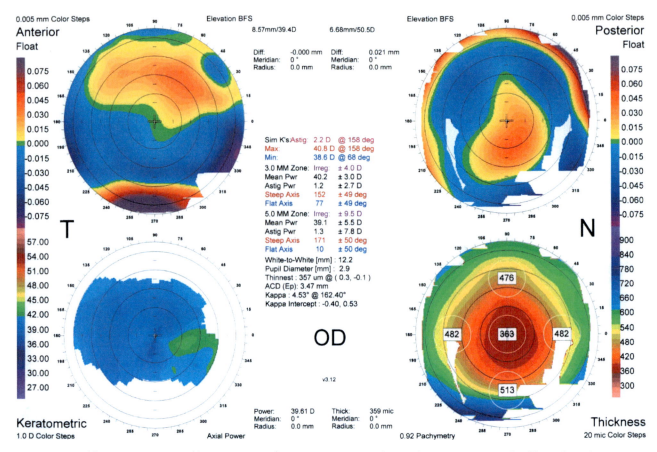

Fig. 11.2 a **a** Mild ectasia in a 42-year-old patient 4 years after LASEK in an eye with some features preoperatively of forme fruste keratoconus. **b** After riboflavin/UV-A corneal collagen cross-linkage and inferior 250-μm Intacs insertion, this eye has an UCVA of 20/20 and BSCVA of 6/5 with +0.25/−0.75 × 50°

References

1. Ciberle M (1999) LASEK may offer the advantages of both LASIK and PRK. Ocular Surgery News, international edn., 28 March
2. Azar DT, Ang RT, Lee JB, Kato T, Chen CC, Jain S, Gabison E, Abad JC (2001) Laser subepithelial keratomileusis: electron microscopy and visual outcomes of flap photorefractive keratectomy. Curr Opin Ophthalmol 12:323–328
3. Shah S, Sebai Sarhan AR, Doyle SJ, Pillia CT, Dua HS (2001) The epithelial flap for photorefractive keratectomy. Br J Ophthalmol 85:393–396
4. Melki SA, Azar DT (2001) LASIK complications: etiology, management and prevention. Surv Ophthalmol 46:95–116
5. Leccisotti A (2003) Laser-assisted subepithelial keratectomy (LASEK) without alcohol versus photorefractive keratectomy (PRK). Eur J Ophthalmol 13:676–680
6. Autrata R, Rehurek J (2003) Laser-assisted subepithelial keratectomy for myopia: two-year follow-up. J Cat Refract Surg 29:661–668
7. Lee JB, Seong GJ, Lee JH, Seo KY, Lee YG, Kim EK (2001) Comparison of laser epithelial keratomileusis and photorefractive keratectomy for low to moderate myopia. J Cataract Refract Surg 27:565–570
8. Litwak S, Zadok D, Garcia-de Quevedo V, Robledo N, Chayet AS (2002) Laser-assisted subepithelial keratectomy versus photorefractive keratectomy for the correction of myopia. A prospective comparative study. J Cataract Refract Surg 28:1330–1333
9. Gabler B, Winkler von Mohrenfels C, Dreiss AK, Marshall J, Lohmann CP (2002) Vitality of epithelial cells after alcohol exposure during laser-assisted subepithelial keratectomy flap preparation. J Cataract Refract Surg 28:1841–1846
10. Autrata R, Rehurek J (2003) Laser-assisted subepithelial keratectomy for the correction of hyperopia: results of a 2-year follow-up. J Cataract Refract Surg 29:2105–2114
11. Hashemi H, Fotouhi A, Foudazi H, Sadeghi N, Payvar S (2004) Prospective, randomized paired comparison of laser epithelial keratomileusis and photorefractive keratectomy for myopia less than −6.50 diopters. J Refract Surg 20:217–222
12. Scerrati E (2001) Laser in situ keratomileusis vs. laser epithelial keratomileusis (LASIK vs. LASEK) J Refract Surg 17:S219–S21
13. Taneri S, Zieske JD, Azar DT (2004) Evolution techniques, clinical outcomes and pathophysiology of LASEK: review of literature. Survey of Ophthalmology 49:576–602
14. Claringbold TV (2001) Laser-assisted subepithelial keratectomy for low to moderate myopia. J Cataract Refract Surg 27:565–570
15. Rouweyha RM, Chuang AZ, Mitra S, Phillips CB, Yee RW (2002) Laser epithelial keratomileusis for myopia with the autonomous laser. J Refract Surg 18:217–224
16. O'Brart DPS, Mellington F, Jones S, Marshall J (2007) Laser epithelial keratomileusis (LASEK) for the correction of hyperopia using a 7.00 mm optical zone with the Schwind ESIRIS flying-spot laser: 12–24 month follow-up. J Ref Surg (in press)
17. O'Brart DPS, Attar M, Hussien B, Marshall J (2006) Laser epithelial keratomileusis (LASEK) for the correction of high myo-

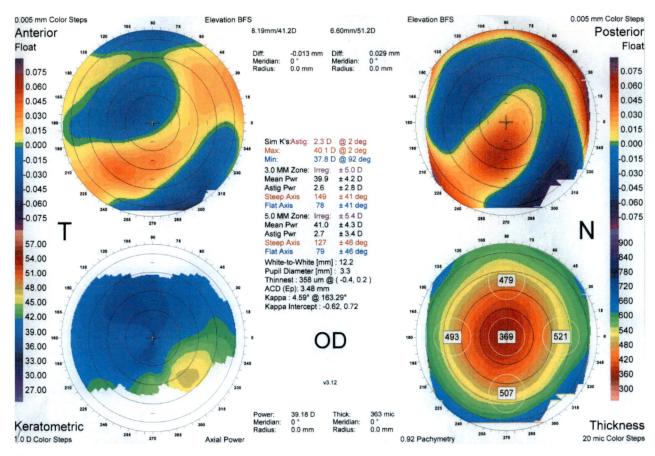

Fig. 11.2 b *(continued)*

pia with the Schwind ESIRIS flying-spot laser. J Refract Surg 22:253–262

18. Camellin M (2003) Laser epithelial keratomileusis for myopia. J Refract Surg 19:666–670
19. Badala F, Fioretto M, Macri A (2004) Effect of topical 0.1% indomethocin solution versus 0.1% fluorometholon acetate on the ocular surface and pain control following laser subepithelial keratomileusis (LASEK). Cornea 23:550–443
20. Verma S, Corbett MC, Heacock G, Patmore A, Marshall J (1997) A comparative study of the duration and efficacy of tetracaine 1% and bupivacaine 0.75% in controlling pain following photorefractive keratectomy (PRK). Eur J Ophthalmol 7:327–333
21. Komilovsky IM (2001) Clinical results after subepithelial photorefractive keratectomy (LASEK). J Refract Surg 17:S222–S223
22. Rouweyha RM, Chuang AZ, Mitra S et al (2002) Laser epithelial keratomileusis for myopia with the autonomous laser. J Refract Surg 18:217–224
23. Laplace O, Bourcier T, Chaumeil C, Cardine S, Nordmann JP (2004) Early bacterial keratitis after laser-assisted subepithelial keratectomy. J Cataract Refract Surg 30:2638–2640
24. Rodriquez B, Holzinger KA, Le LH, Winkle RK, Allen RD (2006) Mycobacterium chelonae keratitis after laser-assisted subepithelial keratectomy. J Cataract Refract Surg 32:1059–1061
25. O'Brart DPS, Lohmann CP, Klonos G, Corbett MC, Pollock WST, Kerr Muir MG, Marshall J (1994) The effects of topical corticosteroids and plasmin inhibitors on refractive outcome, haze and visual performance after excimer laser photorefrac-

tive keratectomy: a prospective, randomised, observer-masked study. Ophthalmology 101:1565–1574
26. Li C, Zhang J, Huang C (1999) The clinical analysis of corticosteroid ocular hypertension and corticosteroid glaucoma after photorefractive keratectomy. Zhonghua Yan Ke Za Zhi 35:179–182
27. Arshinoff SA, Opalinski Y (2003) The pharmacotherapy of photorefractive keratectomy. Comp Ophthalmol Update 4:225–233
28. Hovanesian JA, Shah SS, Maloney RK (2001) Symptoms of dry eye and recurrent erosion syndrome after refractive surgery. J Cataract Refract Surg 27:577–584
29. Dursun D, Kim MC, Solomom A, Pflugfelder SC (2001) Treatment of recalcitrant recurrent erosions with inhibitors of matrix metalloproteinases-9, doxycycline and corticosteriods. Am J Ophthalmol 132:8–13
30. Seiler T, Wollensak J (1992) Complications of laser keratomileusis with the excimer laser. Klin Monatsbl Augenheilkd 200:648–563
31. Fagerholm P, Ohman L, Orndahl M (1004) Phototherapeutic keratectomy in herpes simplex : clinical results in 20 patients. Acta Ophthalmolo 72:457–460
32. Arshinoff SA, Opalinski Y (2003) The pharmacotherapy of photorefractive keratectomy. Comp Ophthalmol Update 4:225–233
33. Lee RW, Lee SB (2004) Update on laser subepithelial keratectomy (LASEK). Curr Opin Ophthalmol 15:333–341

34. Gartry DS, Kerr Muir MG, Marshall J (1991) Photorefractive keratectomy with an argon fluoride excimer laser: a clinical study. Refract Corneal Surg 7:420–435

35. Salz JJ, Maguen E, Nesburn AB et al (1993) A two-year experience with excimer laser photorefractive keratectomy for myopia. Ophthalmology 100:873–882

36. Lohmann CP, Patmore A, O'Brart DPS, Reischl U, Winkler von Mohrenfels C, Marshall J (1997) Regression and wound healing after excimer laser PRK: a histopathological study on human corneas. Eur J Ophthalmol 7:130–138

37. O'Brart DPS, Corbett MC, Lohmann CP, Kerr Muir MG, Marshall J (1995) The effects of the ablation diameter on the outcome of photorefractive keratectomy: a prospective, randomised, double-blind study. Arch Ophthalmol 113:438–443

38. Carones F, Vigo L, Scandola E, Vacchini L (2002) Evaluation of the prophylactic use of mitomycin C to inhibit haze formation after photorefractive keratectomy. J Cataract Refract Surg 28:2088–2095

39. Camellin M (2004) Laser epithelial keratomileusis with mitomycin C: indications and limits. J Refract Surg 20:S693–A698

40. Vigo L, Scandola E, Carones F (2003) Scraping and mitomycin C to treat haze and regression after photorefractive keratectomy for myopia. J Refract Surg 19:449–454

41. Lam DS, Wong AK, Fan DS, Chew S, Kwok PS, Tso MO (1999) Intraoperative mitomycin C to prevent recurrence of pterygium after excision: a 30-month follow-up study. Ophthalmology 106:208–209

42. Morales AJ, Zadok D, Mora-Retana R, Martinez-Gama E, Robledo NE, Chayet AS (2006) Intraoperative mitomycin and corneal endothelium after photorefractive keratectomy. Am J Ophthalmol 142:400–404

43. O'Brart DPS, Patsoura E, Jaycock PD, Rajan MS, Marshall J (2005) Excimer laser photorefractive keratectomy for hyperopia: 7.5 year follow-up. J Cat Ref Surg 31:1104–1113

44. Rajan M, Jaycock P, O'Brart DPS, Marshall J (2004) A long-term study of photorefractive keratectomy: 12 year follow-up. Ophthalmology111:1813–1824

45. Rajan M, O'Brart DPS, Patmore A, Marshall J (2006) Cellular effects of mitomycin-C on human corneas after photorefractive keratectomy. J Cataract Refract Surg 32:1741–1747

46. Proges Y, Ben-Haim O, Hirsh A, Levinger S (2003) Phototherapeutic keratectomy with mitomycin C for corneal haze following photorefractive keratectomy for myopia. J Refract Surg 19:40–43

47. Rajan M, O'Brart DPS, Parel P, Falcon M, Marshall J (2006) Topography-guided customized laser-assisted subepithelial keratectomy for the treatment of postkeratoplasty astigmatism. J Cataract Refract Surg 32:949–957

48. Rajan M, O'Brart DPS, Jaycock P, Marshall J (2006) Effects of ablation diameter on long-term refractive stability and corneal transparency after photorefractive keratectomy. Ophthalmology. 113:1798–1806

49. Salz JJ, Trattler W (2006) Pupil size and corneal laser surgry. Curr Opin Ophthalmol 17:373–379

50. Kesler A, Shemesh G, Rothkoff L, Lazar M (2004) Effect of brimonidine tartrate 0.2% ophthalmic solution on pupil size. J Cataract Refract Surg 30:1707–1710

51. Rabinowitz YS. Ectasia after laser in situ keratomileusis. Curr Opin Ophthalmol 17:421–426

52. Kasparova EA, Kasparov AA (2003) Six-year experience with excimer laser surgery for primary keratoconus in Russia. J Ref Surg 19:S250–S254

53. Randleman JB, Caster AI, Banning CS, Stulting RD (2006) Corneal ectasia after photorefractive keratectomy. J Cataract Refract Surg 32:1395–1398

54. Malecaze F, Coullett J, Calvas P et al (2006) Corneal ectasia after photorefractive keratectomy for low myopia. Ophthalmology 113:742–746

55. Hiatt JA, Wachler BS, Grant C (2005) Reversal of laser in situ keratomileusis-induced ectasia with intraocular pressure reduction. J Cataract Refract Surg 31:1652–1655

56. Wollensak G, Spörl E, Seiler T (2003) Riboflavin/ultraviolet-A-induced collagen cross-linking for the treatment of keratoconus. Am J Ophthalmol 135:620–627

57. Sharma M, Boxer Wachler BS (2006) Comparison of single segment and double segment Intacs for keratoconus and post-LASIK ectasia. Am J Ophthalmol 141:891–895

Chapter 12

Complications of Refractive Keratotomy 12

Carlo F. Lovisolo, Alessandro Mularoni, Antonio Calossi, and Charles Wm. Stewart

Contents

Core Messages

■ Radial keratotomy, initially a Russian technique, was promoted and practiced globally until the availability of the excimer laser.

■ Myriad techniques tried have resulted in a legacy refractive surgeons will continue seeing for decades of very challenging, incision-related, clinical problems.

■ Newer measurement devices and treatment options have provided new options to improve the condition of what would otherwise be a difficult clinical prognosis.

12.1 Introduction

Refractive keratotomy (RK) was the most widely performed refractive surgery in the mid-1980s and early 1990s. Even with its encouraging refractive outcomes, RK resulted in difficult-to-manage or even untreatable complications, and in serious side effects (Table 12.1). Even the most successful RK procedure has irreversibly altered the cornea's natural optical behavior and its life-long corneal stability (biomechanical homeostasis), generating a vulnerability to blunt trauma resultant from the intrinsic and enduring weakness of the wounds [1]. With the appearance of excimer laser technologies, RK has become universally anachronistic. In Italy, we own the record of incisional procedures being intentionally performed on keratoconic eyes [2, 3] (Fig. 12.1). The cessation of RK was a relief; nonetheless, understanding its complications and long-term effects on the eye is important for the practicing surgeon. Therefore, this chapter focuses on management of long-term complications only, without discussion of techniques or patient selection strategies, to prevent and deal with intraoperative and early postoperative complications.

On the other hand, astigmatic–transverse or curvilinear–keratotomies (AKs) continue to be useful, inexpensive, safe, effective, and relatively simple procedures for treating simple astigmatism, as well as more complex cases such as post-keratoplasty eyes [4]. Arcuate incisions, in particular, fully respect the width of the optic pupillary zone, and in most cases improve the physiological corneal profile. Limbal relaxing incisions are a mainstay of lens-based refractive surgery, dealing with even small degrees of astigmatism to optimize the outcome of multifocal, aspheric, accommodative, phakic intraocular lenses (IOLs). With a finite, element analysis-based, biomechanical model of the nonlinear anisotropic hyperelastic behavior of the human cornea [5], empirical nomograms [6] achieve high degrees of predictability and precision.

12.2 Refractive Complications

Contrary to the sequelae of intraoperative complications (e.g., incorrect number, location, depth of incisions, perforation, decentration, intersection of the visual axis and/or the limbus) or postoperative complications, either early or delayed, (e.g., inflammations, infections, healing defects), refractive complications of RK may be approached systematically. It is easy to statistically forecast–the Prospective Evaluation Of Radial Keratotomy (PERK) study estimates that approximately 1.2 million patients were treated with RK only in the United States between 1980 and 1990 [7]–that a large number of patients with either residual refrac-

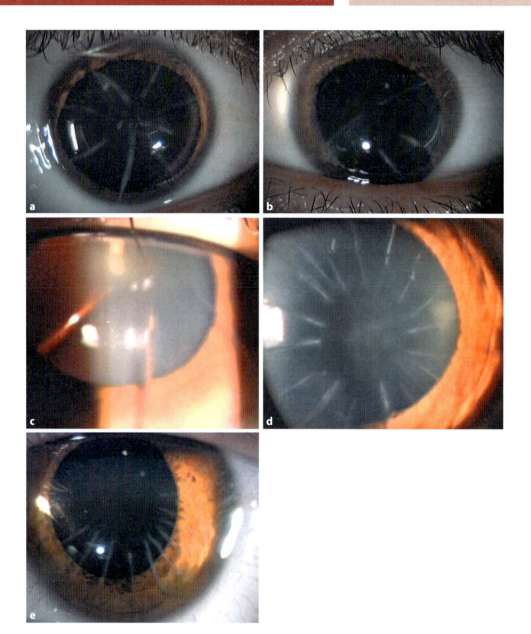

Fig. 12.1 Some typical examples contributing to the bad reputation of RK. Simultaneous "artisan" radial 8-cut (**a**) and asymmetrical 5-cut (**b**) bilaterally performed with non-calibrated steel blades. On-the-visual-axis 8-cut RK (**c**); 18-cut (4 cardinal incisions, 4 in the supra-nasal and 4 in the infra-temporal, 3 in the supra-temporal and 3 in the infra-nasal quadrants), with dense central haze and an iron ring (**d**). 10-Cut asymmetrical RK on the infratemporal cornea for keratoconus (**e**)

tive errors (overcorrection, undercorrection, induced regular, or irregular astigmatism) or more or less disabling visual symptoms are or will be seeking a remedy in the near future. These problematic visual symptoms may be complex and originate from multiple negative attributes of RK. Examples of such symptoms are diurnal or over time instability, starburst, glare, loss of contrast sensitivity, monocular diplopia, diminished night vision, induced anisometropia with imbalance of binocular vision, and meridional aniseikonia (unequal magnification of the retinal image across various meridians from induced asymmetrical astig-

matism). One or more of these problems may distort the patient's spatial perception to levels that are not tolerable by the normal physiological mechanisms of neuroadaptation.

12.3 Reestablishing the Physiological Corneal Shape

After an uneventful RK procedure with an uncomplicated outcome, conventional computerized videokeratography of the anterior corneal surface shows the classic central "blue

Table 12.1 Complicated sequelae of RK (modified from [3])

Secondary to intraoperative complications

Corneal perforations (micro and macro)
Decentered procedures
Incisions intersecting the visual axis
Incisions across the limbus
Incorrect number/meridian of incisions
Incorrect depth of incisions
Incisions intersecting with combined astigmatic cuts

Corneal scars secondary to early or delayed postoperative complications

Bacterial/fungal/viral infections
Healing defects
– Hypertrophic scars
– Haze of the clear optical zone
– Limbal scarring/vascularization
– Inclusion cysts
Recurrent erosions (epithelial basement membrane changes)
Repeated operations
– Multiple, intersecting, abnormal, irregular incisions

Refractive complications

Overcorrection
Undercorrection
Induced regular astigmatism
Induced higher order aberrations
Induced anisometropia
Induced meridional aniseikonia

Biomechanical Complications (iatrogenic keratectasia)

Irregular, asymmetrical astigmatism
Progressive hyperopic drift
RK on unrecognized ectatic corneal disorder (forme fruste KC)

Visual symptoms

Instability
– Diurnal
– Over time
Glare
– Starburst
– Disability glare
Loss of contrast sensitivity
Monocular diplopia
Diminished night vision

Cataract surgery

Intraoperative opening of incisions
Difficulties in calculation of IOL power

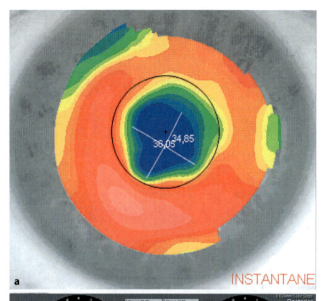

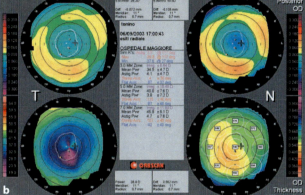

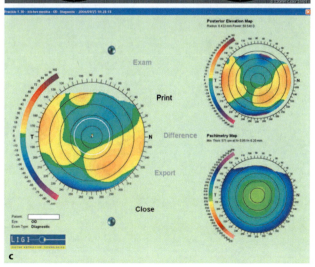

Fig. 12.2 Classic computerized videokeratography pattern (tangential or instantaneous or "true curvature" map) **a** Orbscan elevation maps, **b** after uncomplicated 8-cut RK: similar anterior (*upper left*) and posterior (*upper right*) shape modifications are observed; the pachymetric values (*lower right*) are normal. Precisio elevation and pachymetry maps (**c**) of a decentered 8-cut RK

lake" pattern, with a well-centered 3- to 4.5-mm flattened area. The width of the effective optical zone is inversely correlated to the amount of myopic correction achieved. The central flat area is surrounded by a steepened mid-peripheral red ring (Fig. 12.2a). With Placido disk ring-reflection

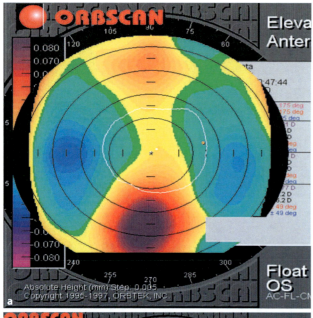

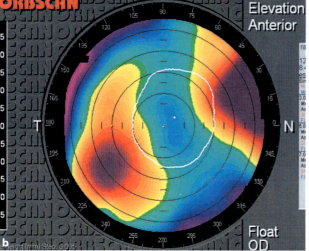

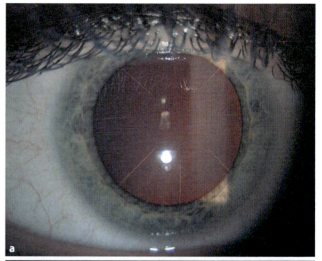

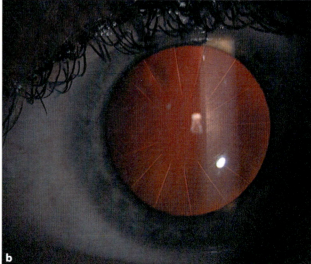

Fig. 12.4 Slit lamp retro-illumination images of 8-cut (**a**) and 16-cut (**b**), well-healed RK treatments with a 3.2-mm clear zone. There is no evidence of wound gape or persistent epithelial plugs

topography, it is not easy to distinguish these maps from those generated after conventional excimer laser myopic photoablations. Sometimes, the slightly irregular, squared or octagonal shape of the mid-peripheral "knee" of the optical zone may help in differentiating RK from the perfectly round and smooth borders of excimer ablations.

In contrast, differential diagnosis becomes very easy when utilizing elevation maps and measuring pachymetry by scanning slit systems such as the Orbscan™ or the various rotating Scheimpflug-based systems now on the market

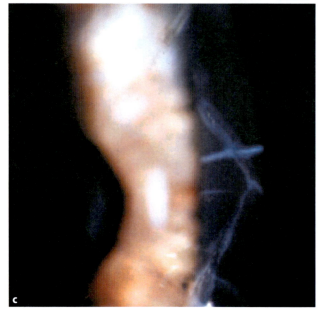

Fig. 12.3 Due to an intraoperative macroperforation of the 6 o'clock incision, an inferior ectasia has occurred (**a**); infranasal and supratemporal ectatic bulgings (**b**) are caused by poor healing that has occurred in the corneal regions where there are crossed radial and arcuate incisions (**c**)

12

(the iVIS Technologies Precisio™, the Oculus Pentacam™, and the Ziemer Galilei™). With elevation or altitudinal tomography, the RK-treated eye's anterior surface pattern is similar to that of the posterior surface, both presenting a central area underlying the best-fit sphere (Fig. 12.2b). The resultant difference between the two similar surfaces, the pachymetric map, displays normal thickness values across the entire cornea. Additionally, even in eyes with the most perfect radial keratotomy, the optical quality of the vision is less than desirable due to the marginal optical performance resulting from a small optical zone, the extremely oblate aspheric shape of the cornea, and the micro- or macro-irregularities at the incisions yielding higher-order aberrations. With small pupils in photopic environments, optical quality is dominantly affected by diffraction, and aberrations have little effect, but the spatial resolution is low. In dim-light conditions with large pupils, the effect of diffraction decreases, and the contribution of optical aberrations becomes significantly larger, increasing with the square of the pupil. More or less irregular patterns, with ectatic bulging of the corneal regions from complicated wounds are frequently observed. Surface irregularities are mainly a function of intraoperative complications or problems arising in the healing phase (see Table 12.1), which induce local bulging of both corneal surfaces. Pachymetry changes are often unremarkable. Topography shows high local dioptric differences in adjacent areas. This localized irregular astigmatism reduces the effective optical zone as well as the resultant optical quality (Fig. 12.3).

As opposed to surgical or healing complications, in many cases, undiagnosed underlying corneal disorders such as forme fruste ectatic corneal disorders (keratoconus or pellucid marginal degeneration) or epithelial basement membrane dystrophy (map-dot-fingerprint disorder), should be considered in determining the main etiology. Widespread awareness and recent improvements in identifying at-risk patients with sophisticated corneal indices [8, 9] will greatly help in properly screening future refractive surgery candidates.

In the excimer laser era, the vast majority of ex-RK patients are looking for a laser-assisted in situ keratomileusis (LASIK) fix. Conventional LASIK can be safely and effectively performed to correct significant amounts of residual ametropia [41–49, 93], provided that: a certain amount of time has passed (at least 2 years), there is a meticulous inspection of the apparently well-healed incisions showing no epithelial cysts or scarring (Fig. 12.4), and the refraction and biomechanics are stable (no irregular astigmatism, no major fluctuations of refraction). Hyperopic ablations for overcorrection may provide good outcomes, by restoring a more physiologically normal corneal asphericity.

The most common secondary surgical strategy consists of using a deeper-than-usual keratome plate (180 or 200 μm) and taking extreme care when manipulating and aligning the flap, taking advantage of the healed wounds as markers. In more than 100 procedures with this type of case, we have been fortunate not to experience any flap fragmentation and only a single buttonholed flap. As opposed to LASIK enhancement for myopic overcorrection, where our nomo-

gram plans for 30% undercorrection, we perform 100% of the hyperopic treatment, as in a virgin eye. This has been consistent across the different laser platforms we have used (Chiron Technolas 217, Alcon Autonomous, Zeiss-Meditec MEL 70 and MEL 80, Wavelight Allegretto, and most recently with the iVIS Technologies iRES). In young patients an expected mean hyperopic shift of 0.15 D per year, we are not concerned with a small overcorrection (110–120% of the treatment) for the same reasons that we would limit the treatment of undercorrected post-RK patients to 80–90%. Patients must be advised of unrealistic expectations. Additionally a number of common problems resultant from RK such as diurnal refractive fluctuations, nighttime visual symptoms, and progressive hyperopic shift with age, will not be addressed, as the underlying cause, the incisions, will not be removed from the eye. However, enlargement of the optical zone and the recovery of a more prolate corneal shape may improve enough of the contributory visual disturbances to make the patient happy.

Preoperatively, significant attention must be paid to the epithelial plugs in the incisions and weighed against the risk of postoperative recurrent and difficult to manage epithelial ingrowths (about 6% in our series).

The use of the laser (femtosecond) keratome may potentially offer minimized flap complications by creating homogeneous flap at a more reproducible depth with less mechanical interaction during flap creation. Our limited experience (three eyes) is in agreement with the only report we could find in the literature [10] on this topic. The RK incisions were made in each of these cases when the flap was lifted, and a LASIK procedure was successfully completed with no occurrences of slipped flaps, microstriae, or epithelial ingrowth. The major complication was an increased postoperative inflammatory response that required extensive steroidal treatment which may explain the loss of best spectacle-corrected visual acuity (BSCVA) in some cases. Efficacy and predictability of the procedure was comparable to that obtained after RK with mechanical keratomes.

12.3.1 Undercorrection

Even perfectly performed, less aggressive, four-incision RK typically achieved only partial improvement of uncorrected visual acuity in patients with non-progressive, low, and moderate amounts of myopia (up to –4.50 D) [50, 52]. Undercorrection occurred more commonly than overcorrection. In the eight-incision-or-more group, the unpredictability of the refractive outcome becomes increasingly evident and stems from significant variability in wound healing responses, surgical "hands" and techniques, difficulty in making all incisions uniformly, and the inability to measure and control the biomechanical properties of the cornea. Improvements or enhancements with re-operation have been described with non-staged techniques [51, 53] (Fig. 12.5), with no evidence of significantly improved safety and efficacy ratios.

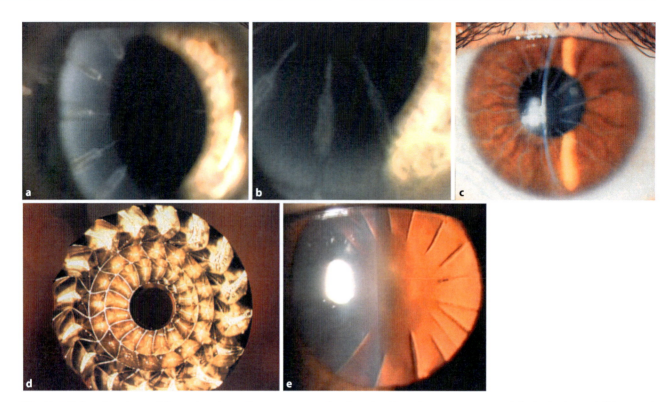

Fig. 12.5 Before the advent of the excimer laser, the management of undercorrected cases was attempted by enhancing the flattening effect on the central cornea with several non-titrated techniques, many of which do not even find citizenship in the medical literature. Examples of these are the intrastromal insertion of polymethylmethacrylate (PMMA) cylinders to keep the incisions open (**a**, **b**); the zigzag, or Kriss's, technique, with its marker (**c**, **d**, courtesy of Fabio and Roberto Dossi, M.D.s); the downhill (American) technique (cut direction from the outer zone toward the limbus) or uphill (Russian) technique (cut direction from the limbus towards the optical zone), single- or double-peripheral (starting from 6 mm) 20-μm re-deepening of cuts; repeated operation (Stan Franks back-cutting technique), and the addition of incisions (**e**). Fancy or creative procedures were frequently combined despite the lack of a true rationale and adequate risk/benefit analysis

The following are cases of surface treatments with modern laser platforms (topography-linked. corneal aberrometry-linked, and wavefront-linked) currently available.

Case 1 (courtesy of Dan Reinstein, M.D., F.A.C.S.): Figure 12.3.5 shows an example of successful reparative treatment for decentration and irregular astigmatism following RK. A 20-year-old male patient underwent RK in the right eye for a –5.75 sphere using eight radial incisions with a 3-mm optical zone. Two further incisions were made as an enhancement at 30° 1 year later. After 2 years, the patient presented to us complaining of severe night vision disturbances (Fig. 12.7a) with no evidence of poor wound healing (Fig. 12.8). On examination, the UCVA in the right eye was 20/40, improving to 20/20 with +1.50 –1.50 × 111°. The contrast sensitivity was below the normal range in the treated right eye and two levels lower than the untreated left eye for 3, 6, and 12 cycles per degree. Topography showed a significant decentration (top left, Fig. 12.6), and the wavefront analysis (WASCA) exam showed that the eye had significantly raised higher-order aberrations, in particular –11.81 μm of Seidel spherical aberration, where a normal eye would typically be approximately –2 μm. Three-dimension-al, layer-by-layer pachymetry maps based on very high frequency echography (Artemis 2, Ultralink) scans (Fig. 12.9) show how the epithelium responds with compensatory behavior. The epithelium thins where the stroma steepens and thickens where the surface curvatures flatten. The patient was treated as photorefractive keratotomy (PRK) with the MEL80 excimer laser (Zeiss Meditec) using a topographically guided treatment generated by the CRS Master II TOSCA system (ablation profile, bottom right, Fig. 12.6). The intended postoperative refraction was plano. Four months postoperatively, the UCVA was 20/20, improving to 20/12.5 with +1.00 –1.00 × 126°; a gain of three lines of UCVA and two lines of BSCVA. The contrast sensitivity was unchanged. The patient reported the haloes had disappeared (Fig. 12.7b), but the starbursts remained. The postoperative topography was well centered with a large optical zone (top middle, Fig. 12.6, plotted on the same scale as the pre-op for direct comparison). The topography difference map (top right, Fig. 12.6) shows an area of inferior flattening that was achieved corresponding to the ablation profile generated by the CRS-Master II TOSCA algorithm. The treatment had also significantly reduced the higher-order aberrations; in particular, the spherical aberration was reduced by 57%

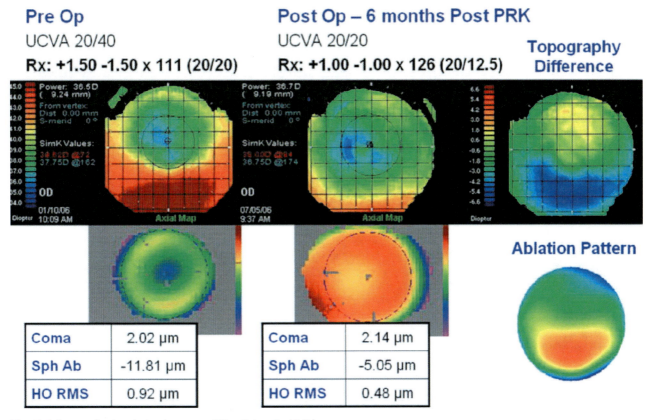

Pre Op
UCVA 20/40
Rx: +1.50 -1.50 x 111 (20/20)

Post Op – 6 months Post PRK
UCVA 20/20
Rx: +1.00 -1.00 x 126 (20/12.5)

Topography Difference

Ablation Pattern

Coma	2.02 µm
Sph Ab	-11.81 µm
HO RMS	0.92 µm

Coma	2.14 µm
Sph Ab	-5.05 µm
HO RMS	0.48 µm

Fig. 12.6 See text for description (courtesy of Dan Reinstein, M.D.)

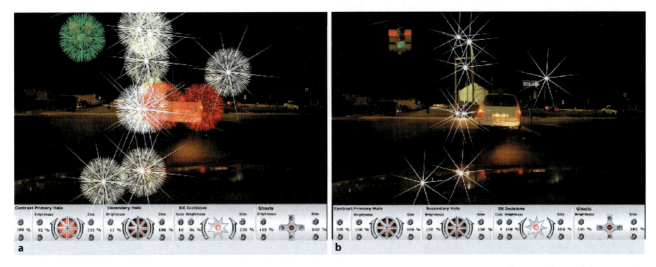

Fig. 12.7 Night-driving quality of vision simulation as based on preoperative (**a**) and postoperative (**b**) wavefront analysis of the case, discussed in text and Fig. 12.6 (courtesy of Dan Reinstein, M.D.)

(bottom middle, plotted on the same scale as the pre-op for direct comparison).

Following the outcomes reported with the original Meditec TOSCA [1] (topography supported custom ablation) system on the MEL70, the new MEL-80 CRS-Master II TOSCA algorithm incorporates both the corneal anterior surface wavefront information (derived from topography) and the intraocular optics to determine the refraction of the front surface and hence the ablation required to remove the irregularities and leave a target toric surface.

Case 2 (courtesy of Massimo Camellin, M.D. and Renzo Mattioli, Ph.D.): In this example, a 26-year-old male patient underwent bilateral RK. Preoperatively OD BSCVA was 20/20 with –3.75 –4.00 × 5°; OS BSCVA was 20/20 with –2.75 –4.00 × 160°. Four radial and four curvilinear incisions were applied (Fig. 12.10). The underlying reasons for the significant variation (intraoperative correction of an incorrect meridian of incision site) from the usual nomogram were not available.

One year after surgery, the patient presented to us complaining of a drop of vision in the left eye and severe night vision disturbances. On examination, BSCVA and manifest refractions were 20/25 with –3.00 –4.00 × 95° OD, 20/30 with –1.00 –7.00 × 170° OS. Contrast sensitivity was well below the normal range in both eyes. Pentacam optical pachymetry (Fig. 12.10b) was considered normal (central OD, 621 μm; OS, 621 μm). Corneal topography (Keratron Scout, Optikon) showed a centered optical zone with a peculiar tetrafoil pattern in the left eye (Fig. 12.11a); corneal wavefront exam (Fig. 12.11b) showed that the eye had significantly increased higher-order aberrations. The left eye of the patient was treated as surface ablation with the ES-IRIS laser (Schwind, Kleinhostein, Germany) using a corneal wavefront link generated by the Keratron Scout videokeratographer (Optikon 2000, Roma, Italy) through the software ORK-w (optimized refractive keratectomy–wavefront) (ablation profile, Fig. 12.11c). Corneal wavefront, the component of the overall aberrometry that is due to the anterior corneal surface alone [18], was obtained by performing a virtual ray tracing on the corneal elevation maps from altitudinal topographies. Mitomycin C 0.02%was applied for 120 s, and the corneal surface carefully washed at the end of the procedure. The intended postoperative refraction was –0.50. Six months postoperatively, the UCVA was 20/25, not improvable with spectacles. No haze could be detected at the slit lamp. Visual symptoms and contrast sensitivity were greatly improved. The postoperative topography showed a well-centered, enlarged optical zone with a regularization of the tetrafoil pattern (Fig. 12.12a). The treatment had also significantly reduced the higher-order aberrations (Fig. 12.12b). The pachymetry differential map (Pentacam, Fig. 12.12c) gave confirmation of the precise execution of the planned ablation profile.

Case 3: Figure 12.3.12 shows an example of an undercorrected post-RK eye treated with a total eye aberrometry wavefront link (Custom Cornea Alcon Autonomous). A 27-year-old male patient underwent RK in the left eye for sphere –10 D, using eight radial incisions in a 2.5-mm clear optical zone. Seven years after surgery, the patient presented to us asking for a laser re-treatment. On examination, the UCVA in OS was count fingers, improving to 20/30 with –5.50 –1.50 × 0°. The contrast sensitivity was far below the normal range. On topography (Fig. 12.13a), the optical zone was irregular and decentered inferiorly. Central pachymetry was 561 μm. Wavefront analysis (Ladar-Wave, Alcon) showed that the eye had significantly raised higher-order aberrations, in particular horizontal and vertical coma, trefoil, and spherical aberration (Fig. 12.13b). A wavefront-linked custom cornea LASIK procedure was performed. The planned depth of the flap was 180 μm. The postoperative topography (Fig. 12.13c) and difference map (Fig. 12.13d) show a nice recentration and a moderate enlargement of the optical zone. The treatment significantly reduced the amount of trefoil and vertical coma, but did not significantly affect the spherical aberration and the horizontal coma. The patient was happy with his UCVA improved to 20/25 (BSCVA was 20/25 with +3.00), but with an unfortunate +4.00 of cycloplegic refraction.

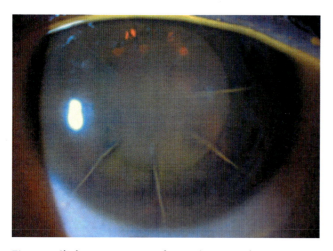

Fig. 12.8 Slit lamp appearance of case 1 (courtesy of Dan Reinstein, M.D.)

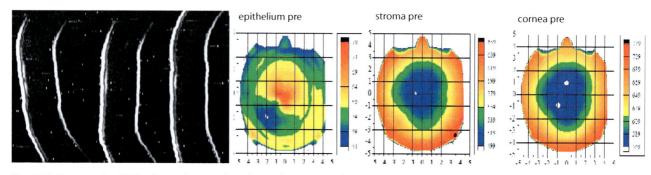

Fig. 12.9 Preoperative VHF echographic meridional scans (Artemis 2, Ultralink) and color-coded, layer-by-layer pachymetry corneal maps (courtesy of Dan Reinstein, M.D.)

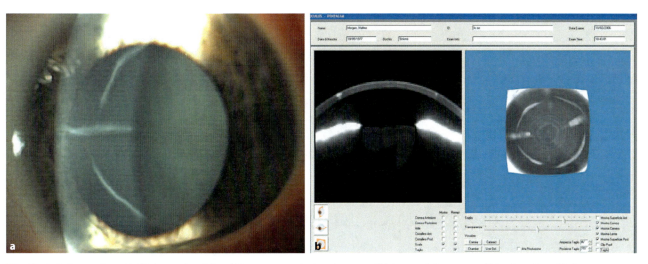

Fig. 12.10 Left eye of case 2. Slit lamp view (**a**) and Pentacam optical pachymetry (**b**) (see text) (courtesy of Massimo Camellin)

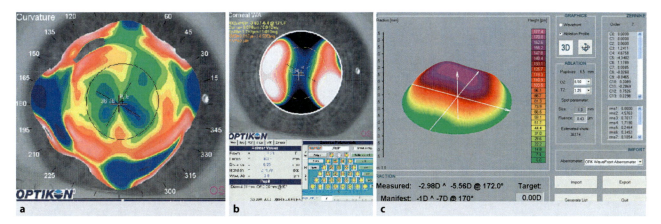

Fig. 12.11 Scout Keratron preoperative topography (**a**) and corneal wavefront (**b**) of case 2; ablation profile using a corneal wavefront link generated through the ORK-w software with the ESIRIS Schwind excimer laser system (**c**) (courtesy of Massimo Camellin and Renzo Mattioli)

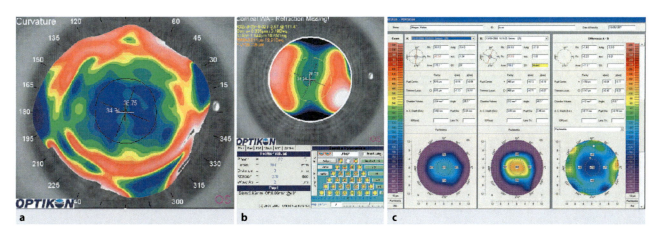

Fig. 12.12 Scout Keratron 6-month postoperative topography (**a**) and corneal wavefront (**b**) of case 2; Pentacam pachymetry differential map (**c**) allows the comparison to the planned ablation profile showed in Fig. 12.11c (courtesy of Massimo Camellin and Renzo Mattioli)

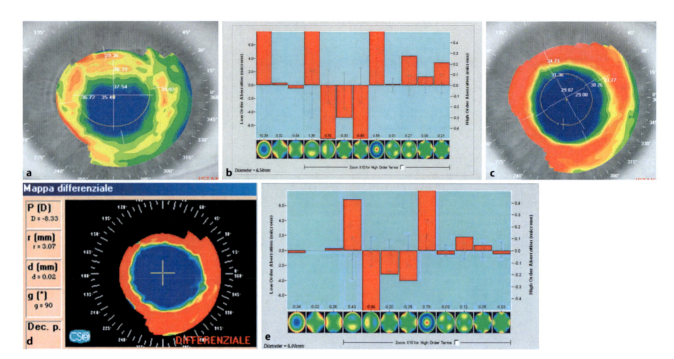

Fig. 12.13 Preoperative CSO topography (**a**), preoperative LadarWave aberrometry (**b**), 2-month postoperative CSO topography (**c**), difference map (**d**), and wavefront analysis of case 3

Case 4: A 39-year-old male patient underwent three consecutive laser procedures (PTK), after a viral keratitis complicated the original AK procedure for a sphere +0.25 cylinder −4.00 × 90° in the right eye. An examination performed 15 years after the first procedure, showed that the UCVA was 20/400, improving to 20/80 with −2.75 −2.00 × 110° and to 20/25 with pinhole. A +2 haze and a slight basement membrane dystrophy were found to be partially responsible for the irregularities in the anterior corneal surface. Corneal topography and corneal wavefront analysis (CSO) showed that the eye had significantly raised higher-order aberrations (Fig. 12.14a, b). The eye was treated using a transepithelial surface ablation procedure, using a topographically guided treatment designed with CIPTA software [12] (ablation profile, Fig. 12.14c) delivered with the iVIS Technologies iRES laser system. Mitomycin C 0.02% was applied for 15 s at the end of the procedure. The intended postoperative refraction was plano. One month postoperatively, the UCVA was 20/20, improving to 20/15 with +0.75 -1.00 × 102! All haloes and starbursts disappeared with impressive subjective and objective improvements. The postoperative topography was well centered with an enlarged optical zone (Fig. 12.15). The iVIS Suite™ integrates high-resolution tomography from Precisio™, a newcomer to the latest-generation topography systems (Fig. 12.16) and detailed pupil function analysis using the pMetrics™ dynamic pupillometer. pMetrics provides a full understanding of the patient's dynamic range of pupil sizes, relative reactivities from scotopic to photopic, and a unique statistical analysis with lifestyle weighting. This "ideal pupil" dimension represents the diameter which will cover two standard deviations (95%) of all pupil sizes encountered with the individual's lifestyle re-

lated conditions and activities. The iVIS Suite uses the new iRES laser, which is controlled by a proprietary technology that produces two separate beams, each with a very regular Gaussian profile of micrometric size, 0.65 mm. Combining the dual-beam technology with the laser head repetition rate, iRES delivers a frequency of 1,000 Hz (approximately 10 times faster the conventional systems) on the corneal plane leaving a very smooth surface without inducing any acoustic shock effect. Moreover, the iRES's high repetition rate is leveraged to use a new technique in which a variable pulse rate is delivered to the cornea achieving a Constant Frequency per Area™ (CF/A) (Fig. 12.17).

12.3.1.1 Considerations about Laser Treatments on Post-RK Eyes

1. Adopting topography [13], elevation maps or the Zernike polynomial coefficients of the corneal wavefront for a laser link in post-RK eyes, in which the internal components of the total amount of ocular aberrations can be considered of little relevance, seems more convenient and potentially more accurate than using total eye wavefront analysis. First, the data from total eye aberrometry is more artifactual and less reliable [19] in cases of distorted corneas; second, the measurements obtained by elevation topography for large pupil diameters are not influenced by additional factors, such as accommodative or cycloplegic state [20] and environmental light conditions.

2. As with other custom treatments, post-RK topography planned surgeries include higher-order aberrations and are unforgiving for any misalignment between ablation

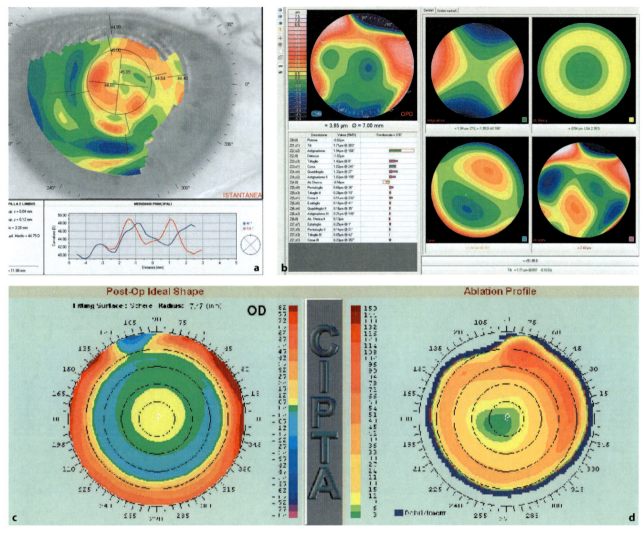

Fig. 12.14 Illustrative example of application of CIPTA software in a patient wih corneal irregularities. In this patient the preoperative corneal topography is shown in figure (**a**). The corneal derived aberrations are shown in **b**. The ablation profile planned to achieve the postoperativeideal shape (**c**) with CIPTA software is shown in **d**.

plan and the proper position on the cornea. Perfect registration (calibration of the topographer, elimination of artifacts, good repeatability of consecutive maps, and proper placement of the planned ablation on the corresponding corneal tissue) and proper tracking of the entrance pupil are requirements. The laser eye tracker centers the ablation pattern on the pupil or the geometric center of the cornea and relies on the patient's cooperation to maintain fixation, since it cannot distinguish between a lateral movement of the head and a fixation loss that would unavoidably introduce a parallax error.

3. The correct choice of the corneal asphericity is crucial. The correction of the topographic peripheral knee from RK that causes high degrees of spherical aberration is critical to restore a more prolate physiological profile, to influence the lower orders (spherocylinder), and is often responsible for the overcorrection (such as reported above in case 3). The exact amount of change in corneal asphericity (Q or e) is open to debate [21–23]. It

is uniquely dependant on the diameter referenced, and several other factors:
(a) Preoperative asphericity
(b) Sign (positive or negative) and dioptric amount of lower-order aberrations to be corrected
(c) Patient's age, taking into account the internal aberrations
(d) Corneal biomechanics

4. A typical postoperative finding in eyes in which a secondary, standard PRK was performed over prior RK without the application of mitomycin C, was haze associated with a lack of predictability [34]. Anecdotally, we have also observed two cases of moderate haze with difficult explanation. With the first case, +2 haze spontaneously appeared bilaterally 7 years after an eight-cut procedure. Subjective and objective vision was OD UCVA, 20/40; BSCVA, –0.50 –1.25 × 90° 20/20– and OS UCVA, 20/25; BSCVA, plano –1.00 × 90° 20/20 (Fig. 12.18). In the second case, haze showed up 3 months after RK was

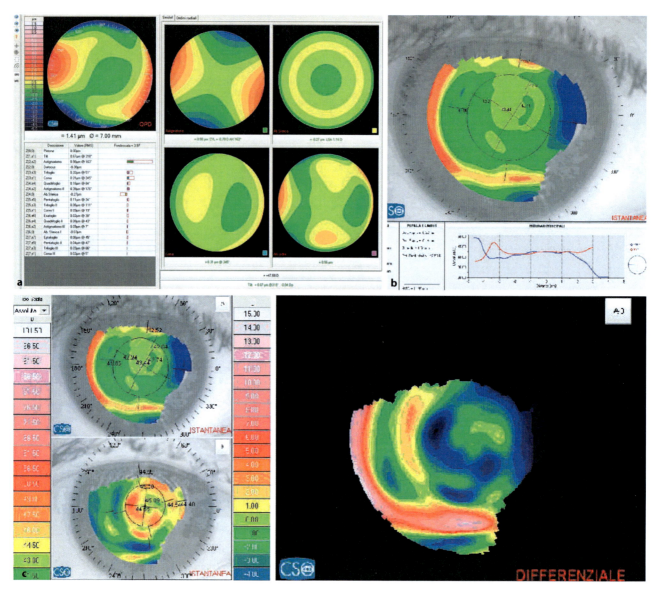

Fig. 12.15 Post-operative topography (**a**), corneal wavefront (**b**), and differential map (**c**) of case 4

performed as an enhancement on an undercorrected PRK performed 12 months prior [35]. The lack of predictability of cutting flaps in post-RK eyes [36] (no post-RK eye is similar to another from the biomechanical standpoint) and, above all, the great outcomes obtained with modern topography [11–14] or wavefront-linked [17] surface ablations plus mitomycin C (MMC) applications [16, 17, 92] have recently converted our practices to the exclusive use of surface ablations [87]. At present, all post-RK eyes in our practice that are enrolled for excimer laser surgery receive a customized surface ablation plus 15 s' application of a sponge imbibed with 0.02% MMC, with protection of the limbal stem cells by means of a specifically cut, ring-shaped standard soft contact lens.

5. When RK incisions are found gaped, they are usually filled with pearl-like, persistent clusters of keratin plugs

[96] (Fig. 12.19). Despite a moderate number of adjacent activated keratocytes observed in confocal microscopy [24], these epithelial inclusions prevent formation, remodeling and cross-linking of new collagen fibers. The continuity of anterior stromal lamellae is never repaired completely, thus causing an intrinsic weakness of the wound integrity (Fig. 12.20). Significant vulnerability of the incised cornea to blunt trauma [25], intraocular surgery–like phacoemulsification [26, 94] or penetrating keratoplasty [91], or even external treatment like conductive keratoplasty [37], has been reported even decades after surgery [39]. The wounds are also prone to develop delayed or recurrent eye-surface erosion defects and infections [27, 38]. In our experience, epithelial plugs do not ablate at the same rate as the adjacent stroma and thus cause irregular postoperative surfaces when treated with surface ablation procedures if not dealt with

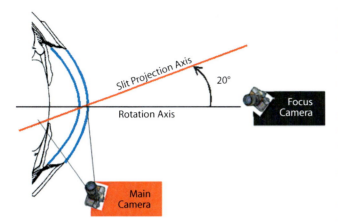

Fig. 12.16 Based on triangulation combined with the rotation of a white light slit that is detected using a Scheimpflug optical system, the Precisio™ provides high-resolution measurements across a wide viewing angle, which includes both the anterior and posterior surfaces' morphology of the cornea, while calculating point-by-point pachymetry. Its slit is projected onto the cornea with an incidence angle of 20° with respect to the axis of rotation of the system (**a**). A dedicated fixation target allows the patient to align his visual axis with the rotation axis of the system (**b**). During the acquisition, the slit is imaged serially and recorded through an integrated system composed of two different CCD cameras (MAIN and FOCUS) working in harmony. An intelligent eye-tracker system, whose references are the corneal reflections of four infrared LEDs, allows the correct location of acquired points in three-dimensional spaces. All points collected by the MAIN and FOCUS cameras are stored in conjunction with the position of the limbus vessels, which are visible through the proprietary illumination system

12.3.2 Overcorrection

12.3.2.1 Consecutive Hyperopia after RK

Twenty to 30% of the eyes previously operated with RK are now hyperopic with a strong probability that this percentage will grow with time [1]. The pace of the hyperopic shift can be roughly estimated to be 1.00 D every 6–8 years. The blurring of vision at both distance and near is referred to as being "relentless progressive." Early techniques focused on steepening the central cornea by compressing the mid-periphery with placement of a variety of circumferential and interrupted intrastromal purse-string sutures. Our limited experience (three cases) with the "lasso" 10-0 nylon compression suture (Fig. 12.21) did not confirm the good outcomes reported in the literature [31–33]. We found all the approaches of intrastromal suturing for overcorrected RK (purse-string, interrupted radial, or combined stitches) to be unacceptable in predictability, complicated by a significant regression of the effect during the early postoperative period, and a challenging technique even for the meticulous, expert corneal surgeon. A stable result was not expected to be achieved for at least 6–12 months postoperatively. The depth of suturing must be at least 50% of the stromal thickness; otherwise, the unpleasant "gift" of irregular astigmatism, recurrent corneal erosions, and extrusion through a melted superficial stroma may be experienced. As progressive hyperopization with corneal instability may be interpreted as an ongoing peripheral keratoectatic process, a riboflavin-mediated stromal collagen cross-link procedure (i.e., a 30-min application of UV-A light–5.4 J/cm^2 at 370 nm of wavelength–after topical application on the debrided corneal surface of a solution of 0.1% riboflavin-5-phosphate and dextran, every 3–5 min) may be a treatment option. Preliminary, although anecdotal, results suggesting stabilization have been already reported (Brian S. Boxer Wachler, M.D., free paper presented at the American

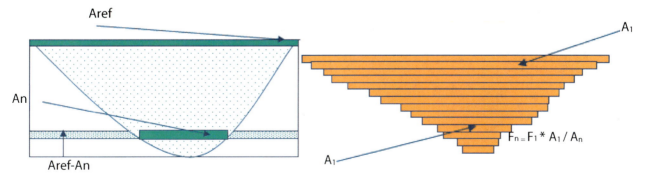

Fig. 12.17 An ablation volume is composed of a fixed number of layers. In the standard method's randomization, the repetition rate varies per area in each ablation layer based upon the layer's total area; spot delivery is specifically designed to avoid firing subsequent shots in the same or adjacent areas. This is effective only for large areas, in which a sufficient time passes between adjacent shots, but as the layer area becomes smaller, randomization does not allow enough time to pass to avoid firing through plume. This can significantly affect various aspects of the ablation: the amount of energy delivered due to the plume's absorption, thermal effects, predict-ability of the resultant treatment, and the completeness of the total desired surface affecting smoothness of the pattern. Surgeons or manufacturers attempt to partially mitigate these issues by using nomograms or algorithms, which cannot be specific to the nature of these unknown variables. By varying the frequency layer by layer and planning equal ablation time for each reference area (*Aref*), the iRES technology delivers a constant frequency per square millimeter for all layers. *A1* first layer area, *An* last layer area, *F1* frequency per square millimeter at first layer, *Fn* frequency per square millimeter at last layer

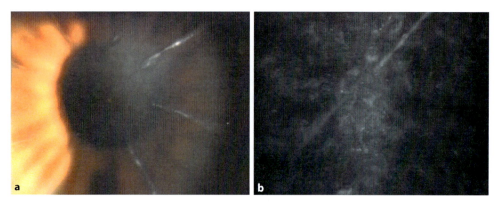

Fig. 12.18 Central haze +2 and iron line (hemosiderin deposition) (**a**) developed seven years after uneventful RK surgery and unremarkable course. Confocal microscopy (**b**) showed the typical pattern of haze after excimer laser ablation, i.e., high reflectivity of subepithelial dense matrix and activated keratocytes around the healed RK wound

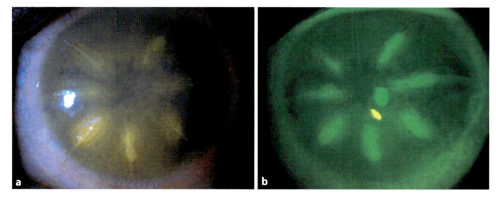

Fig. 12.19 Slit lamp evidence of epithelial plugs in seven out of eight radial keratotomies after fluorescein staining (**a**) and under cobalt-blue filter (**b**) (courtesy of Dan Reinstein, M.D.)

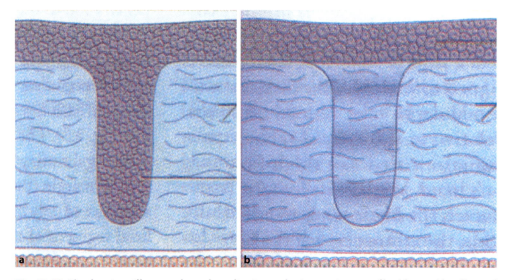

Fig. 12.20 The drawings illustrate the early replication and migration of epithelium into the wound, followed by the formation of a plug (days 1–2 postoperatively) (**a**); the successive stromal phase of wound healing (months 1–2 postoperatively) activates keratocytes into myofibroblasts with collagen deposition and plug displacement; late phase or stromal healing (months 3-12 postoperatively) includes collagen formation and cross-linking (**b**) (modified from Probst LE [2000] Complex cases with LASIK, Slack, Thorofare, N.J.)

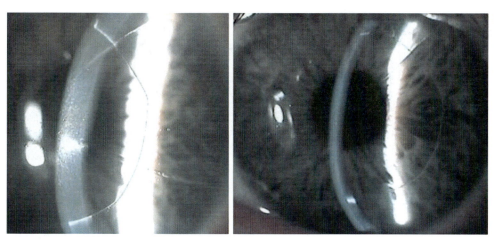

Fig. 12.21 Lasso circumferential 10-0 nylon compression suture after overcorrected RK (courtesy of Gianni Alessio, M.D.)

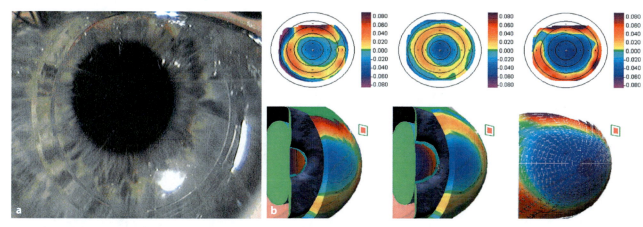

Fig. 12.22 Slit lamp image (**a**) and postoperative versus preoperative Orbscan anterior elevation difference maps (**b**) of an undercorrected RK treated with Intacs insertion

Academy of Ophthalmology, Las Vegas, November 2006), but longer follow-up data is obviously needed.

12.3.2.2 Intrastromal Corneal Ring Segments Option

The same concepts of corneal bioptics validated for excimer laser surgery [28, 29] are applicable to undercorrected or complicated sequelae of radial and astigmatic keratotomy. Intrastromal corneal ring segment implantation finely tunes the refractive outcome, enlarges the functional optical zone, reduces higher-order aberrations (irregular astigmatism), and improves the physiological corneal shape toward being more prolate (Fig. 12.22). This sometimes translates into a gain of four or five lines of UCVA and BCVA and always in a significant improvement of contrast sensitivity and quality of vision in general.

When a post-RK true iatrogenic keratectasia shows progression, photoablative surgery is forbidden and lamellar or penetrating keratoplasty becomes an option. However, before proceeding with a transplant surgery, we believe it is worth treating these cases with a couple of symmetrical (same thickness), asymmetrical (different thickness) (Fig.

12.2.22), or a single Intacs or Ferrara ring segment. The rationale of segment's choice is still controversial and mainly left to surgeon's experience.

Despite these apparent ideal features, we must remain aware of the following safety issues:

- The risk of incision dehiscence during channel dissections or segment positioning. Similar to what has been described during penetrating keratoplasty [30],when the dissector passes through the cuts, even though no particular resistance is encountered, it always creates torque that separates, and potentially opens the old wounds. This separation would require watertight closure with placement of extra sutures in the keratotomies and discouraging any placement of the implants.
- Delayed postoperative opening and wound melt. Due to the fact that these elements are space occupying, strain enhancing, and place the wound under constant tension over time. (Fig. 12.2.23).
- Neovascularization (Fig. 12.2.24)

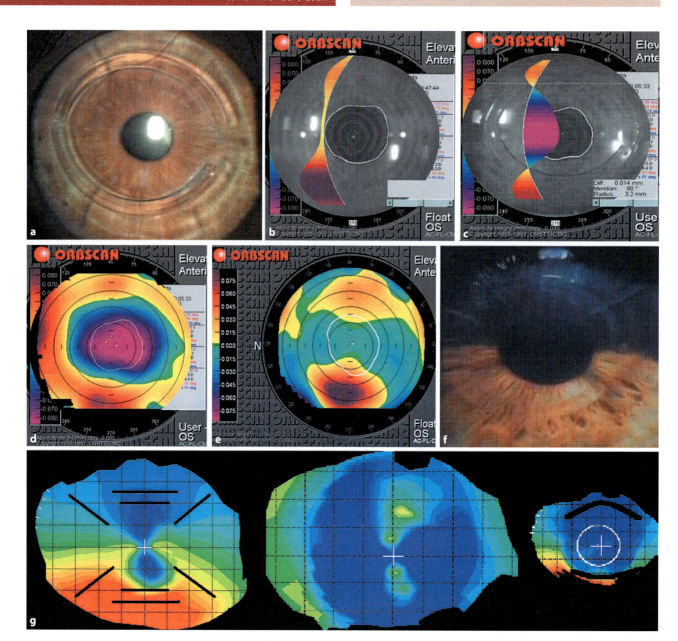

Fig. 12.23 Case 5. A superior 0.25-mm and an inferior 0.45-mm Intacs (**a**) were implanted at 70% of stromal depth, with incision site positioned temporally, to treat the high–against-the-rule (ATR) astigmatism (BSCVA, 20/100 with +2.75 –6.00 × 85°) caused by the inferior ectasia (preoperative elevation map is shown in Fig. 12.4a, the anterior corneal surface profile in **b**). Early postoperative outcome was improved (BSCVA, 20/25 with +1.25); Orbscan profile (**c**) and topography (**d**) show the central flattening and wide optical zone created by the rings. At the 6-year postoperative follow-up exam, a moderate instability can be observed (**e**); BSCVA is still acceptable (20/30 with +0.75 +1.50 × 20°). Case 6 was managed similarly, with insertion of a pair of symmetrical Ferrara ring segments (**f**), and gave an even better outcome (postoperative UCVA, 20/25). Orbscan anterior elevation map difference (**g**, *middle*) shows the coupling effect (steepening of the flattest meridian and flattening of the steepest one) induced by the segments

12.3.2.3 Phakic IOL Option

Case 10: A 25-year old lady submitted to 16-cut RK for high myopia (–8.00) and one unsuccessful circumferential intrastromal suturing for extreme overcorrection (2 years after surgery BSCVA was 20/25 with + 8.00 +2.50 × 0°). Significant (minimum keratometric [K] reading was 28.76 D) but regular, symmetrical flattening of the central cornea was observed on examination (Fig. 12.26a). A custom-made hyperopic toric phakic IOL (Visian ICL, STAAR) was implanted horizontally through a temporal incision in the posterior chamber. Since a wide anterior segment was available for the implant, despite the very flat cornea, the white-to-white rule of thumb was considered unreliable for this case, and the choice of the overall length of the implant was made on the basis of the horizontal sulcus diameter, as measured with very high frequency (VHF) echography (Arte-

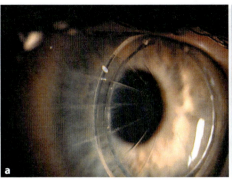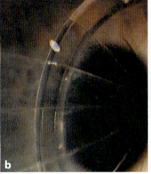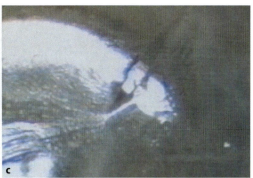

Fig. 12.24 During the dissection pass of case 7–undercorrected, decentered RK–we experienced the external dehiscence of the cuts at 8:30 and 10 o'clock. We decide to position two symmetrical Intacs implants and not to place sutures. Three days postoperatively the eye was unremarkably tranquil, vision was 20/20 uncorrected (!), the oblate shape of the cornea partially restored, and the depth of implantation was 70% of the corneal thickness. After 3 months, we noticed a slightly grayish opacity of epithelium and superficial stroma above the segments in the two opened wound (**a, b**). After 6 months at those sites, significant epithelial erosions and stromal melt occurred, and we were compelled to remove the segments. A similar case (8) happened 3 months after insertion of one single Ferrara ring in a post-RK severe iatrogenic corneal ectasia, probably an unrecognized forme fruste keratoconus (**c**)

mis 2, Ultralink) and by using the Lovisolo Phakic IOL Sizer software [40] (Fig. 12.26b). A slight overcorrection was planned, taking into account the age of the patient and the relentless progression of the hyperopic shift. On day 1 after surgery, UCVA was 20/25. Three years after implantation, BSCVA is 20/20 with –0.50, UCVA is 20/30+.

12.3.2.4 Wavefront-Based Glasses Option

Beyond the clear transparency and the uneven, smooth regularity of its surface, the ideal optical qualities of the cornea, from a purely theoretical standpoint, should have an ellipsoidal geometry with an adequate shape factor (asphericity) and with its apex perfectly centered on the visual axis. Inadequate shape factor (as in oblate geometries) results in spherical aberration, while a decentered apex generates coma, and oblique incidence astigmatism. Higher-order aberrations (HOA) are mainly caused by surface irregularities. After a successful RK procedure, the lower-order aberrations (spherical defocus and cylinder, regular astigmatism) generally find a significant improvement. However, the most frequent visual complaints reported by RK patients are a loss of best-corrected vision, or a loss of quality of vision such as with ghost images, double vision, glare, halos, comets, starburst radiating lines or other light distortions, essentially at night. These disturbances are essentially due to iatrogenically induced higher-order aberrations (HOA) that are not correctable by conventional means like standard glasses and soft contact lenses that are designed to correct only the lower orders (spherocylinder). Recently, wavefront-guided spectacle lenses (iZon, Ophthonix) have become available on the market (Fig. 12.27). The iZon optics are programmed on a point-for-point basis to address beyond the lower orders up to the sixth order of Zernike polynomials, they have the potential to reduce the unique aberrations of the keratotomized eye, thus improving symptoms, and may correct the lack of crisp-

ness and clarity of vision (visual acuity, low-contrast visual acuity, and contrast sensitivity). Requisite for any aspheric lens introduced in the eye's optical system, these lenses require meticulous mounting and alignment with the visual axis to be optimally efficient. The distance between lens and ocular surface should be minimized, as well as the eye movements, in favor of the movements of the head. Since they are expensive, the real utility of these glasses is still debatable. Wavefront-guided contact lenses are expected to be launched by the same company soon.

12.3.2.5 Contact Lenses Option

Case 11: Five years after a 16-cut RK procedure, the right eye of a 29 year-old lady showed a BSCVA of 20/20 with +1.25 +5.00 × 5° (Fig. 12.28). Disabling visual symptoms, mainly glare, were described under mesopic light conditions, which did not improve with glasses. Videokeratoscopy (Fig. 12.28c) and corneal topographies (Fig. 12.28e) showed the ectatic changes of the inferior incisions, which were responsible for the nighttime complaints of the patient. While with a photopic pupil size of 3 mm, the optical quality of the central corneal zone remained good, as soon as the pupil dilated, the patient suffered increasing amounts of coma (due to the vertical asymmetry), spherical aberration (due to the hyperoblate profile) and HOA (due to surface irregularities) (Fig. 12.28d). Given its lack of flexibility, a rigid gas-permeable (RGP) contact lens may perfectly compensate for the aberrations caused by the altered shape and profile of the anterior corneal surface. The tear meniscus that centrally fills the space behind the posterior surface of the contact lens compensates for more than 90% of the anterior corneal surface aberrations, thus reducing the aberrations to less than 10% of their manifest values. Therefore, when the front surface is designed with the optimized curvature, the RGP lens compensates for both lower and higher orders of aberration, providing the best

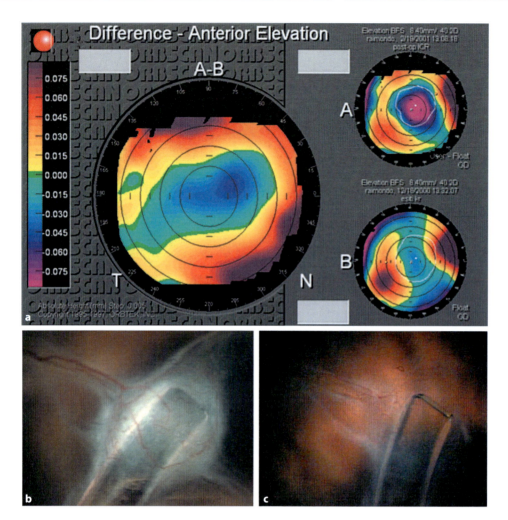

Fig. 12.25 In case 9, a combination of radial and curvilinear cuts caused an irregular corneal shape with high asymmetric astigmatism (BSCVA, 20/90 with –6.00 cylinder × 40°). Intraoperatively, immediately after activating the suction, the old radial wound adjacent to the new incision site (positioned at 105°) opened. Surgery was completed with insertion of two 0.45-mm Intacs segments, and the opened cut was sutured with one 10-0 nylon stitch. Suture was removed after 3 months. The outcome can be observed in the Orbscan anterior elevation difference map (**a**). Five months after surgery, a new vessel developed from the limbus, in correspondence with the opened wound, and invaded the superficial corneal around the edge of the ring (**b**). Steroid topical therapy plus argon laser applications induced a significant regression. Four years postoperatively, the ring segments are still in situ and the cornea looks clinically quiet (**c**). BSCVA is 20/50 with +1.25 +1.75 × 125°

visual performance achievable with any means. The rigid, inflexible nature of the lens collaterally creates positioning and stability problems especially when conventional RGP geometries are used. Standard RGP contact lenses have been designed for physiologically prolate corneas and are too mobile and, in general, poorly tolerated. When the RGP optical zone is optimally aligned to the center of the cornea, the lens will have excessive edge lift. Conversely, if the back optical zone radius (BOZR) is reduced to minimize the peripheral edge lift, then the optical zone excessively vaults at the center of the cornea. Instead, the oblate elliptical shape of post-RK corneas requires a reverse geometry RGP contact lens [88, 89, 97, 98]. This non-standard design utilizes a peripheral zone curve that is steeper than the optical zone, thus allowing a proper alignment of

both critical areas. Figure 12.3.28 shows the reverse geometry RGP CL used in case 10.

12.3.3 IOL Power Calculation after RK

When keratotomized eyes undergo cataract surgery, overestimation of the corneal power made by conventional keratometers is the main factor responsible for the choice of an IOL power that is too low, with an undesired hyperopic refractive surprise using conventional calculation formulas [90, 95]. The origin of the error lies in the inaccuracy of the approximations made in the measurement of corneal power. Conventional keratometers measure the sagittal curvature of the anterior surface in a small paracentral area [53].

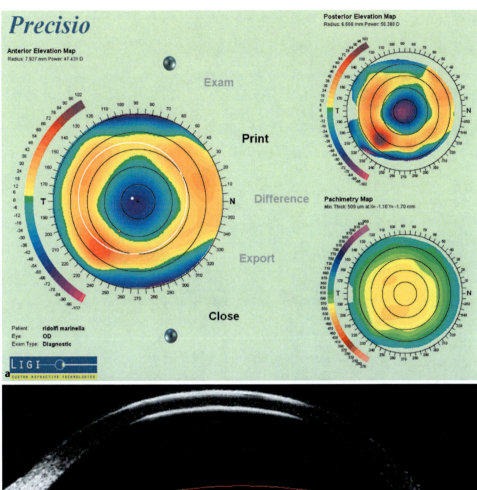

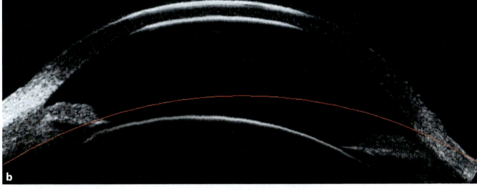

Fig. 12.26 Precisio corneal maps (**a**) and VHF echography image with hyperopic ICL simulation (**b**) obtained with the Lovisolo ICL Sizer Software [42] of case 10

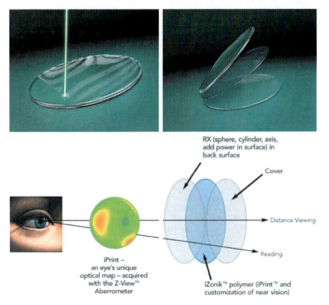

Fig. 12.27 In the iZon™ (Ophthonix) wavefront glasses, a programmable polymer undergoes a point-by-point process on the basis of the digital aberrometry data; then it is sandwiched between front and back surface blanks to create a multiple composition layer of the lens, a 1.6 index with anti-reflective, UV-blocking, scratch-resistant, and hydrophobic coat

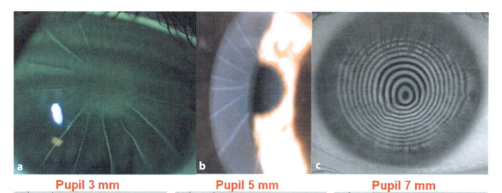

Fig. 12.28 Slit lamp images with and without fluorescein staining (**a**, **b**), keratoscopy (**c**), corneal aberrometry (**d**), and tangential, axial, altitudinal, and refractive corneal maps, where the *circles* represent the photopic pupil diameter (**e**) of the case 11 (see text for description)

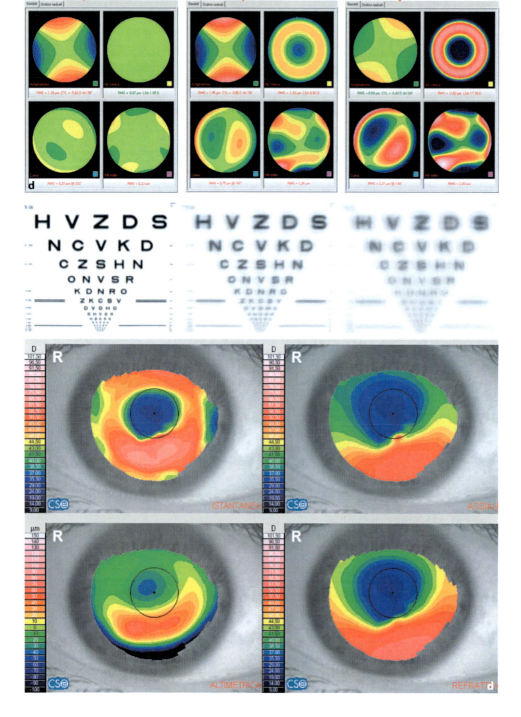

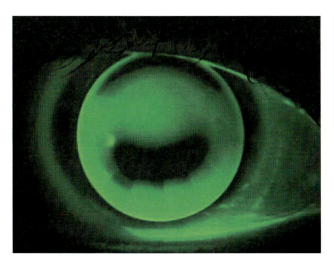

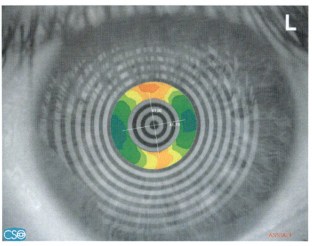

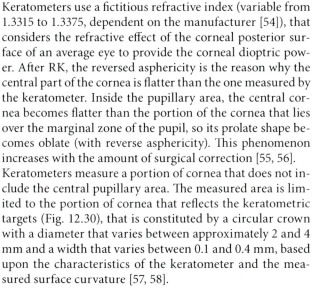

Fig. 12.29 Reverse geometry RGP contact lens fit in the case 11 (see text for description). Fluorescein staining under cobalt-blue filter illustrates the significant vertical asymmetry. The steeper peripheral zone allows the lens to stay stable and centered

Fig. 12.30 The circular crown *colored area* represents the zone of the cornea utilized for keratometry measurements and for computerized videokeratography SimK index. The central pupillary area is not measured

Keratometers use a fictitious refractive index (variable from 1.3315 to 1.3375, dependent on the manufacturer [54]), that considers the refractive effect of the corneal posterior surface of an average eye to provide the corneal dioptric power. After RK, the reversed asphericity is the reason why the central part of the cornea is flatter than the one measured by the keratometer. Inside the pupillary area, the central cornea becomes flatter than the portion of the cornea that lies over the marginal zone of the pupil, so its prolate shape becomes oblate (with reverse asphericity). This phenomenon increases with the amount of surgical correction [55, 56]. Keratometers measure a portion of cornea that does not include the central pupillary area. The measured area is limited to the portion of cornea that reflects the keratometric targets (Fig. 12.30), that is constituted by a circular crown with a diameter that varies between approximately 2 and 4 mm and a width that varies between 0.1 and 0.4 mm, based upon the characteristics of the keratometer and the measured surface curvature [57, 58].

With the same keratometer on a steeper cornea, a portion of cornea closer to the center is measured, whereas on a flatter cornea a more peripheral zone is measured. Due to the Stiles-Crawford effect (SCE) of the first type [59, 60], the area of the cornea that covers the central pupillary zone provides a brighter image than the one formed by the portion of the cornea that covers the marginal zone of the entrance pupil. It follows that the central cornea, which is not measured, has a more dominant role in the formation of the foveal image than the portion of the cornea that is usually measured by keratometers. In a normal cornea with an average asphericity, this phenomenon is of little impact because the sagittal curvature varies slightly from the center to the keratometer measuring area, but when asphericity has high absolute values, differences between central and paracentral curvature cannot be neglected (Fig. 12.31). It is for these reasons that the

measurement of the corneal curvature for optical purposes should provide the average value, weighted by the SCE (i.e., a Gaussian weighing) of the whole corneal area covering the entrance pupil (mean pupil power). For the reasons we have described, this measurement cannot be performed by conventional keratometers, but can be obtained by computerized videokeratographers.

In a conventional IOL power formula, K readings are also used to calculate the effective lens position (ELP), which is the estimated postoperative distance between the anterior corneal surface and the principal optical plane of the IOL. The assumption is that flat cornea curvatures generally mean shallow anterior chamber depths and more anterior positioning of the IOL; this principle is obviously not applicable to post-RK eyes, whose anterior corneal surface has been flattened but the unaltered anterior chamber is usually deep and wide [61, 62].

To correct this artifact, which is subject to the error produced by the corneal power overestimation, Aramberri proposed a modification to the SRK/T formula, by using the presurgical K value, obtained by preoperative keratometry or topography for the ELP calculation and the postsurgical K value by the clinical history method for IOL power calculation by the vergence formula [61]. Double-K modification of the SRK/T formula greatly improves the accuracy of IOL power calculation after RK, but it is sometimes impossible to adopt because the preoperative corneal curvatures are not always available.

Several methods have been proposed for optimizing the the IOL power calculation in RK patients. An oversimplified, empirical method proposed by Lyle and Jin 63], proposed a fixed subtraction of 1.00 D from the average K reading (adjusted K), which is inserted in a formula that averaged the result between the Binkhorst and the Holladay formulas, and unfortunately showed no significant accuracy [64].

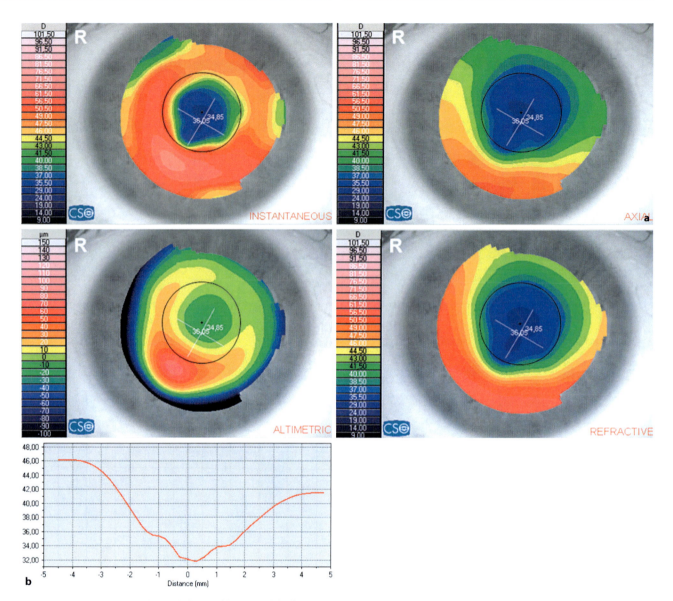

12

Fig. 12.31 a Instantaneous (*upper left*), Axial (*upper right*), Elevation (*lower left*), and Refractive (*lower right*) corneal maps and the corresponding sagittal curvature profile (**b**) of a typical post-RK cornea. The average simulated keratometry (SimK) is 35.74 D, while the mean pupil power is 32.75 D

The clinical history method [65, 66] and its variants [67–69] substantially considered the changes in refraction induced by the procedure from the preoperative keratometric readings.

The contact lens method [65, 66, 70] subtracts the difference between the manifest refraction with and without a hard contact lens of known base curve from that base curve plus the power of the lens. The drawbacks of this method lie in the high variability of refractive measurements with and without contact lenses. Accuracy varies because of the rigid contact lens fit and significantly decreases with decreasing visual acuity and with increasing media opacity [71].

The intraoperative aphakic refraction technique has many variants proposed by different authors. Mackool et al. [80, 81] first described a technique in which the cataract is removed, the aphakic eye is refracted 30 min later, the IOL power is calculated by using a nomogram developed by the same authors, and the IOL is eventually implanted. Ianchulev et al. [82] used intraoperative automated refraction, while Ahmed and Toufeeq [84] performed intraoperative retinoscopy after the fit of +10-D disposable soft contact lens to minimize retinoscopic error. The latter authors concluded that intraoperative retinoscopy after phacoemulsification is useful but not accurate in estimating corneal power or axial length of the eye. The obvious disadvantage of this approach is the need to return to the operating room for IOL implantation. It also uses oversimplified formulas (Mackool and Ianchulev multi-

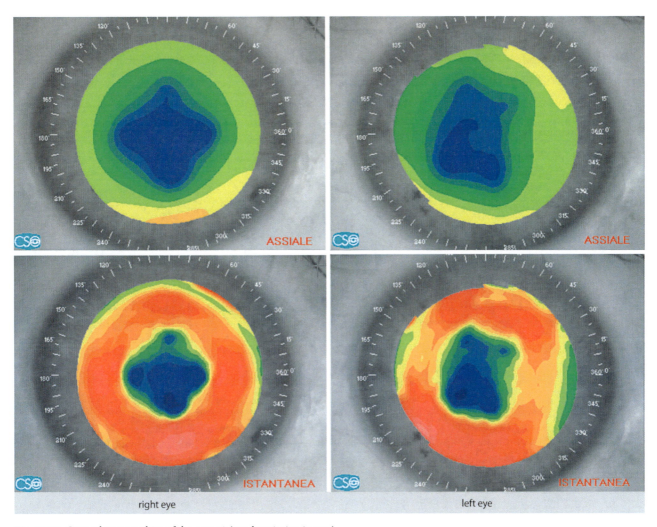

right eye   left eye

Fig. 12.32 Corneal topographies of the case 12 (see description in text)

plied the measured refractive error by a fixed, albeit different, value: 1.75 and 2.01, respectively) and is prone to the errors secondary to the vertex distance dependence of the aphakic refraction and the biomechanical instability of the keratotomized cornea immediately after cataract surgery [85], which commonly show variable amounts of transient hyperopia in the early postoperative period. This is felt to be due to the stromal edema around the radial incisions, producing a temporary enhancement of central corneal flattening.

The use of topographic data has been advocated by several authors and is actually considered the more precise alternative to standard keratometry [72–77]. Modern computerized videokeratographers allow us to measure thousands of points in a wide area of the anterior corneal surface and provide us plenty of keratometric indices: simulated keratometry (SimK), minimum K reading (K_{min}), curvatures at 3, 5 and 7 mm, central keratometry (K_c), ACP (average corneal power) etc. However, the crucial question remains "Which one is the most adequate for calculating IOL power?" Han and Lee [77] recently re-

ported that in highly myopic eyes with previous RK, the flatter keratometric value between SimK and the 3-mm zone mean keratometric value from Orbscan II was the closest to the true postoperative RK keratometric value of the central cornea. However, Chen et al. [64] reported a large variability of results.

In our opinion, the use of topographic data (we strongly suggest the use of the average curvature of the corneal area that covers the entrance pupil weighted on the Style-Crawford effect [78]) offers the greatest precision of IOL power calculation as compared with keratometric data. Importantly however, clinical experience teaches us that repeatability of measurements is lower with computerized videokeratographs than with keratometers, and that the possibilities of error increase in short distance videokeratographer [79]. For this reason, we suggest an accurate verification of the instrument calibration and taking more measurements of the same eye with elimination of the extremes and calculating the average of the central values. If the conventional keratometric targets have a regular appearance, then it is useful to compare keratometric read-

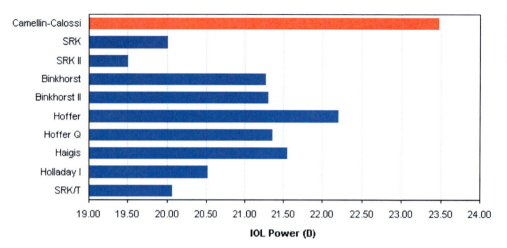

Fig. 12.33 Comparison of IOL power obtained in the case 12, *left eye*, with different formulae

ings with SimK, and if these values greatly differ, new measurements should be obtained.

In post-RK eyes, we have been using the Camellin-Calossi formula [78] for more than 6 years, and 100% of our postoperative refractions lie in the ±1.00-D range (predicted versus achieved refraction), 95% are in the ±0.75-D range. The formula originates from a theoretical one that was empirically adjusted in two parameters (1) the corneal power (D_c) and (2) and the prediction of effective lens position (ELP).

Different from other third-generation formulas that often use keratometry as the main predictor, and similar to Haigis [85], Camellin and Calossi have chosen a K-independent method to estimate ELP. The variable ACD_{post} is a function of the anterior chamber depth previous to cataract surgery (ACD_{pre}), of the lens thickness (CT), of the axial length (L), and of the ACD constant (ACD_{const}). To estimate the real corneal power, they use the average curvature, weighted according to the SCE, of the corneal area that covers the entrance pupil. The real corneal power is calculated considering a relative keratometric refractive index, which is a function of the actual corneal curvature (r), the type of keratorefractive surgery performed, and the surgically induced refractive change (SIRC). In the case of laser ablative surgery, the prime cause of error is the conversion from curvature radius to dioptric power of the cornea [86] since photokeratectomy modifies the ratio between anterior and posterior corneal surfaces. The real corneal power is calculated using a relative keratometric refractive index that is a function of the SIRC. When incisional surgery has been performed (the ratio between anterior and posterior corneal surfaces has not been modified), the average central curvature is considered as the radius (r), weighted according to SCE, of the corneal area that covers the entrance pupil. This value can be measured with a corneal topographer with these capabilities, e.g., CSO (CSO Ophthalmic, Florence, Italy), EyeSys (EyeSys Technologies, Houston, TX), Keratron (Optikon 2000, Rome, Italy), and TMS (Tomey, Japan). Then, the real corneal power is calculated using Gaussian optics equation

adopting a keratometric refractive index (n) of 1.332. After RK, conventional K readings should only be used when reliable topographic measurements are not available (for instance, when huge variations of corneal asphericity or reflections of the Placido disk mires out of the optical zone are found).

Case 12: A 58-year-old man was referred for IOL power calculation, as a corticonuclear cataract had developed in his left eye, 16 years after bilateral RK for compound myopic astigmatism (pre-RK refraction was OD, –4.00 –1.50 × 20°; OS –4.75 –2.00 × 150°). As shown by corneal topographies (Fig. 12.32), the excessive flattening of central cornea led to significant overcorrection (BSCVA was OD, 20/20 with +5.00; OS, 20/200 with +3.00 +0.50 × 180°). A-scan ultrasound biometry data of the left eye was axial length, 25.9 mm; lens thickness, 4.45 mm; anterior chamber depth, 3.87 mm. Mean keratometry was 37.50 D. Asphericity of the optical zone was strongly oblate (Q = 2.14). To calculate the actual corneal power, we utilized the averaged power in the pupillary area, as obtained from the CSO topographer, that with the Camellin-Calossi formula gave us a power of 35.86 D (very close to the corrected keratometric value given by the same formula for an achieved correction of –8.00 D, 36.02 D). For an A-constant equal to 118.5, the Camellin-Calossi formula calculated a power of +23.66 D for emmetropia. Figure 12.3.32 summarizes the IOL powers obtained with different formulae with standard keratometry values. An IOL of +24 D was implanted; 1 month after surgery, uncorrected visual acuity was 20/20, improving to 20/20+ with –0.50 × 90°. The great outcome and the anisometropic difficulties in binocular vision (the right eye was the dominant one) motivated to consider the option of a clear lens extraction surgery in the right eye.

Considering the good visual acuity of the right eye, we have tried to compare the data obtained from different methods to get the effective corneal power. OD mean K reading was 36 D, the contact lens method gave us a value of 33.75 D, while the mean pupillary power obtained from videokeratography (CSO) was 34.5 D. By using the Camellin-Calossi formula, the corrected keratometric val-

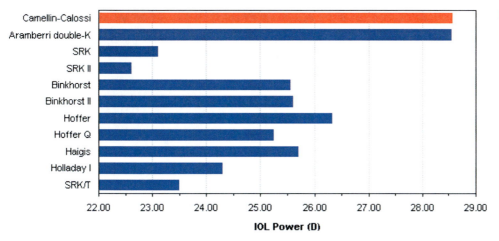

Fig. 12.34 Comparison of IOL power calculated for the right eye of the case 12, with different formulae and methods

ue for a myopic corneal correction of –9.00 D was 34.49. The Q value of the optical zone was 4.5. A-scan US axial length was 25.2 mm; lens thickness, 4.45 mm; and ACD, 3.64 mm. For an A-constant of 118.5, the Camellin-Calossi gave us a power of +28.56 D for emmetropia. A similar value (+28.54 D) was obtained by using the double-K Aramberri formula as combined with the value of effective corneal power obtained with the contact lens method. Figure 12.3.33 makes the comparison of IOL power obtained with different formulae with standard keratometry values.

Take-Home Pearls

- Following the marketing hype of RL in the 1980s and 1990s, refractive surgeons will be faced with several decades of iatrogenic challenges.
- RK patients are likely to increase progressively toward hyperopia at a mean rate of 1.00 D per 6–8 years.
- RK patients may have multiple contributory factors to visual disturbances such as too-small optical zones, prolate asphericity, irregular astigmatism, and decentrations beyond the lower order progressive aberrations.
- Elevation topography may be beneficial in the differential diagnosis of RK sequelae.
- LASIK for correction of stable RK refractive errors should be considered with a thicker-than-normal flap to minimize possibility of flap fragmentation.
- A number of common RK problems will not be resolved by LASIK, but correction of some of the causes of visual disturbances may improve the patient's condition.
- Larger numbers of RK incisions typically means that the predictability suffers.
- Whole-eye wavefront may not be accurate for complex RK corneas; whereas repeatable corneal elevation–based custom refractive surgery may be more accurate.

- Restoring physiologically normal asphericity is an important aspect of decreasing visual disturbances.
- Gaped incisions with plugs should have plugs removed, sutured, and allowed to heal for 1 year or more before any further refractive treatment.
- Intrastromal rings may improve asphericity, but as space-occupying elements, may contribute to wound strain and delayed wound opening sequelae.
- Relentless progressive hyperopia is difficult to manage even with suturing techniques.
- Keratometer readings on RK eyes are unreliable for use with IOL calculations.
- The Camellin-Calossi formula currently produces the highest IOL predictability for post-RK eyes.

References

1. Waring GO III (1992) Refractive keratotomy for myopia and astigmatism. Mosby–Year Book, St. Louis
2. Lombardi M, Abbondanza M (1997) Asymmetric radial keratotomy for the correction of keratoconus. J Refract Surg 13:302–307
3. Utine CA, Bayraktar S, Kaya V et al (2006) Radial keratotomy for the optical rehabilitation of mild to moderate keratoconus: more than 5 years' experience. Eur J Ophthalmol 16:376–384
4. Poole TR, Ficker LA (2006) Astigmatic keratotomy for postkeratoplasty astigmatism. J Cataract Refract Surg 32:1175–1179
5. Alastrue V, Calvo B, Pena E et al (2006) Biomechanical modeling of refractive corneal surgery. J Biomech Eng 128:150–160
6. Kaufmann C, Peter J, Ooi K et al (2005) Limbal relaxing incisions versus on-axis incisions to reduce corneal astigmatism at the time of cataract surgery. J Cataract Refract Surg 31:2261–2265
7. Waring GO III, Lynn MJ, McDonnell PJ (1994) Results of the Prospective Evaluation Of Radial Keratotomy (PERK) study 10 years after surgery. Arch Ophthalmol 112:1298–1308
8. Ambrosio R Jr, Alonso RS, Luz A, Coca Velarde LG (2006) Corneal-thickness spatial profile and corneal-volume distribution: tomographic indices to detect keratoconus. J Cataract Refract Surg 32:1851–1859

9. Lovisolo CF, Calossi A, Cybo AO (2002) Intrastromal inserts in keratoconus and ectatic corneal disorders. In: Lovisolo CF, Fleming JF, Pesando PM (eds) Intrastromal corneal ring segments. Fabiano, Canelli, Italy, pp 95–163

10. Munoz G, Albarran-Diego C, Sakla HF et al (2006) Femtosecond laser in situ keratomileusis after radial keratotomy. J Cataract Refract Surg 32:1270–1275

11. Wygledowska-Promienska D, Zawojska I, Gierek-Ciaciura S, et al (2000) Correction of irregular astigmatism using excimer laser MEL 70 G-Scan with the TOSCA program--introductory report. Klin Oczna 102:443–447

12. Alessio G, Boscia F, La Tegola MG, Sborgia C (2001) Corneal interactive programmed topographic ablation customized photorefractive keratectomy for correction of postkeratoplasty astigmatism. Ophthalmology 108:2029–2037

13. Jankov MR II, Panagopoulou SI, Tsiklis NS et al (2006) Topography-guided treatment of irregular astigmatism with the wavelight excimer laser. J Refract Surg 22:335–344

14. Rajan MS, O'Brart DP, Patel P et al (2006) Topography-guided customized laser-assisted subepithelial keratectomy for the treatment of postkeratoplasty astigmatism. J Cataract Refract Surg 32:949–957

15. Carones F, Vigo L, Scandola E (2006) Wavefront-guided treatment of symptomatic eyes using the LADAR6000 excimer laser. J Refract Surg 22:S983–S989

16. Abraham LM, Selva D, Casson Rr, Leibovitch I (2006) Mitomycin: clinical applications in ophthalmic practice. Drugs 66:321–340

17. Lacayo GO III, Majmudar PA (2005) How and when to use mitomycin-C in refractive surgery. Curr Opin Ophthalmol. 16:256–259

18. Mattioli R, Tripoli NK (1997) Corneal geometry reconstruction with the Keratron videokeratographer. Optom Vis Sci 74:881–894

19. Mattioli R, Camellin M (2004) La aberrometria corneale ed il link "topo-aberrometrico." In: Camellin M (ed) LASEK & ASA. Fabiano, Canelli, Italy, pp 232–253

20. He JC, Burns SA, Marcos S (2000) Monochromatic aberrations in the accommodated human eye. Vision Res 40:41–48

21. Gatinel D, Hoang-Xuan T, Azar DT (2001) Determination of corneal asphericity after myopia surgery with the excimer laser: a mathematical model. Invest Ophthalmol & Vis Sci 42:1736

22. Eghbali F, Yeung K, Maloney R (1995) Topographic determination of corneal asphericity and its lack of effect on the refractive outcome of radial keratotomy. Am J Ophthalmol 119:275–280

23. Marcos S, Cano D, Barbero (2003) Increase in corneal asphericity after standard laser in situ keratomileusis for myopia is not inherent to the Munnerlyn algorithm. J Refract Surgery 19: S592–S596

24. Leung DY, Yeung EF, Law RW et al (2004) In vivo confocal microscopy of epithelial inclusions from aberrant wound healing after astigmatic keratotomy. Cornea 23:299–301

25. Lee BL, Manche EE, Glasgow BJ (1995) Rupture of radial and arcuate keratotomy scars by blunt trauma 91 months after incisional keratotomy. Am J Ophthalmol 120:108–110

26. Behl S, Kothari K (2001) Rupture of a radial keratotomy incision after 11 years during clear corneal phacoemulsification. J Cataract Refract Surg 27:1132–1134

27. Bergmanson J, Farmer E, Goosey J (2004) Epithelial plugs in radial keratotomy: the origin of incisional keratitis? Cornea 20:866–872

28. Fleming JF, Lovisolo CF (2000) Intrastromal corneal ring segments in a patient with previous laser in situ keratomileusis. J Refract Surg 16:365–367

29. Lovisolo CF, Calossi A, Fleming JF (1989) Corneal bioptics. Improving success and managing complications of refractive surgery. In: Lovisolo CF, Fleming JF, Pesando PM (eds) Intrastromal corneal ring segments. Fabiano (Canelli, Italy, pp 171–204

30. Rashid ER, Waring GO III (2002) Complications of radial and transverse keratotomy. Surv Ophthalmol 34:73–10

31. Lyle WA, Jin GJ (1995) Long-term stability of refraction after intrastromal suture correction of hyperopia following radial keratotomy. J Refract Surg 11:485–489

32. Damiano RE, Forstot SL, Frank CJ et al (1998) Purse-string sutures for hyperopia following radial keratotomy. J Refract Surg 14:408–413

33. Alió J, Ismail M (1993) Management of radial keratotomy overcorrections by corneal sutures. J Cataract Refract Surg 19:595–599

34. Ribeiro JC, McDonald MB, Lemos MM et al (1995) Excimer laser photorefractive keratectomy after radial keratotomy. J Refract Surg 11:165–169

35. Shoji N, Hayashi E, Shimizu K et al (2003) Central corneal haze increased by radial keratotomy following photorefractive keratectomy. J Refract Surg 19:560–565

36. Sinha R, Sharma N, Vajpayee RB (2004) Microkeratome-induced reduction of astigmatism after RK. J Refract Surg 20:89–90

37. Kymionis GD, Titze P, Markomanolakis MM et al (2003) Corneal perforation after conductive keratoplasty with previous refractive surgery. J Cataract Refract Surg 29:2452–2454

38. Levy J, Hirsh A, Klemperer I et al (2005) Late-onset *Pseudomonas* keratitis after radial keratotomy and subsequent laser in situ keratomileusis: case and literature review. Can J Ophthalmol 40:217–221

39. Sony P, Panda A, Pushker N (2004) Traumatic corneal rupture 18 years after radial keratotomy. J Refract Surg 20:283–284

40. Lovisolo CF, Reintein DZR (2005) Phakic intraocular lenses. Surv Ophthalmol 50:549–587

41. Attia WH, Alió JL, Artola A et al (2001) Laser in situ keratomileusis for undercorrection and overcorrection after radial keratotomy. J Cataract Refract Surg 27:267–272

42. Lyle WA, Jin GJ (2003) Laser in situ keratomileusis for consecutive hyperopia after myopic LASIK and radial keratotomy (2000) J Cataract Refract Surg 29:879–888

43. Yong L, Chen G, Li W et al (2000) Laser in situ keratomileusis enhancement after radial keratotomy. J Refract Surg 16:187–190

44. Oral D, Awwad ST, Seward MS et al (2005) Hyperopic laser in situ keratomileusis in eyes with previous radial keratotomy. J Cataract Refract Surg 31:1561–1568

45. Shah SB, Lingua RW, Kim CH et al (2000) Laser in situ keratomileusis to correct residual myopia and astigmatism after radial keratotomy. J Cataract Refract Surg 26:1152–1157

46. Lipshitz I, Man O, Shemesh G et al (2001) Laser in situ keratomileusis to correct hyperopic shift after radial keratotomy. J Cataract Refract Surg 27:273–276

47. Clausse MA, Boutros G, Khanjian G et al (2001) A retrospective study of laser in situ keratomileusis after radial keratotomy. J Refract Surg 17:S200–S201

48. Francesconi CM, Nose RA, Nose W (2002) Hyperopic laser-assisted in situ keratomileusis for radial keratotomy induced hyperopia. Ophthalmology 109:602–605

49. Agarwal A, Agarwal A, Agarwal T et al (2001) Laser in situ keratomileusis for residual myopia after radial keratotomy and photorefractive keratectomy. J Cataract Refract Surg 27:901–906

50. Leroux les Jardins S, Frisch E, Bertrand I et al (1990) Current limitations of radial keratotomy. Ophtalmologie 4:346–349

51. American Academy of Ophthalmology (1993) Radial keratotomy for myopia. Ophthalmology 100:979–980

12

52. Durand L, Monnot JP, Burillon C (1991) Radial keratotomy: analysis of undercorrected patients, based on 200 successive operations. J Fr Ophtalmol 14:211–217

53. Bennett AG, Rabbetts RB (1991) What radius does the conventional keratometer measure? Ophthalmic Physiol Opt 11:239–247

54. Bennett AG, Rabbetts RB (1989) Clinical visual optics, 2nd edn. Butterworths, London ,p 468

55. Fleming JF (1993) Corneal asphericity and visual function after radial keratotomy. Cornea 12:233–240

56. Schwiegerling J, Greivenkamp JE, Miller JM et al (1996) Optical modeling of radial keratotomy incision patterns. Am J Ophthalmol 122:808–817

57. Layman PR (1987) Measuring corneal area utilizing keratometry. Optician 154:261

58. Holladay JT, Waring III GO (1992) Optics and topography of radial keratotomy. In: Waring III GO (ed) Refractive keratotomy for myopia and astigmatism. Mosby–Year Book, St. Louis

59. Applegate RA, Lakshminarayanan V (1993) Parametric representation of Stiles-Crawford functions: normal variation of peak location and directionality. J Opt Soc Am A 10:1611–1623

60. Stiles WS, Crawford BH (1933) Luminous efficiency of rays entering the eye pupil at different points. Proc Roy Soc Lond 112:428–450

61. Aramberri J (2003) Intraocular lens power calculation after corneal refractive surgery: double-K method. J Cataract Refract Surg 29:2063–2068

62. Holladay JT (1998) Intraocular lens power calculation for the refractive surgeon. Oper Tech Cataract Refract Surg 1:105–117

63. Lyle WA, Jin GJ (1997) Intraocular lens power prediction in patients who undergo cataract surgery following previous radial keratotomy. Arch Ophthalmol 115:457–461

64. Chen L, Mannis MJ, Salz JJ et al (2003) Analysis of intraocular lens power calculation in post-radial keratotomy eyes. J Cataract Refract Surg 29:65–70

65. Holladay JT (1989) Consultations in refractive surgery. Refract Corneal Surg 5:203

66. Hoffer KJ (1995) Intraocular lens power calculation for eyes after refractive keratotomy. J Refract Surg 11:490–493

67. Ladas JG, Stark WJ (2004) Calculating IOL power after refractive surgery. J Cataract Refract Surg 30:2458; author reply 2458–2459

68. Walter KA, Gagnon MR, Hoopes PC Jr et al (2006) Accurate intraocular lens power calculation after myopic laser in situ keratomileusis, bypassing corneal power. J Cataract Refract Surg 32:425–429

69. Sambare C, Naroo S, Shah S et al (2006) The AS biometry technique–a novel technique to aid accurate intraocular lens power calculation after corneal laser refractive surgery. Cont Lens Anterior Eye 29:81–83

70. Haigis W (2003) Corneal power after refractive surgery for myopia: contact lens method. J Cataract Refract Surg 29:1397–1411

71. Joslin CE, Koster J, Tu EY (2005) Contact lens overrefraction variability in corneal power estimation after refractive surgery. J Cataract Refract Surg 31:2287–2292

72. Celikkol L, Pavlopoulos G, Weinstein et al (1995) Calculation of intraocular lens power after radial keratotomy with computerized videokeratography. Am J Ophthalmol 120:739–750

73. Husain SE, Kohnen T, Maturi R et al (1996) Computerized videokeratography and keratometry in determining intraocular lens calculations. J Cataract Refract Surg 22:362–366

74. Holladay JT (1997) Corneal topography using the Holladay Diagnostic Summary. J Cataract Refract Surg 13:209–221

75. Maeda N, Klyce SD, Smolek MK at al (1997) Disparity between keratometry-style readings and corneal power within the pupil after refractive surgery for myopia. Cornea 16:517–524

76. Muraine M, Siahmed K, Retout A et al (2000) Phacoemulsification following radial keratotomy. Topographic and refractive analysis concerning an 18-month period (apropos of a case). J Fr Ophtalmol 23:265–269

77. Han ES, Lee JH (2006) Intraocular lens power calculation in high myopic eyes with previous radial keratotomy. J Refract Surg 22:713–716

78. Camellin M, Calossi A (2006) A new formula for intraocular lens power calculation after refractive corneal surgery. J Refract Surg 22:187–199

79. Mandell RB (1992) Everett Kinsey lecture. The enigma of the corneal contour. Clao J 18:267–273

80. Mackool RJ (1998) The cataract extraction-refraction-implantation technique for IOL power calculation in difficult cases [letter]. J Cataract Refract Surg 24:434–435

81. Mackool RJ, Ko W, Mackool R (2006) Intraocular lens power calculation after laser in situ keratomileusis: Aphakic refraction technique. J Cataract Refract Surg 32:435–437

82. Ianchulev T, Salz J, Hoffer K et al (2005) Intraoperative optical refractive biometry for intraocular lens power estimation without axial length and keratometry measurements. J Cataract Refract Surg 31:1530–1536

83. Bardocci A, Lofoco G (1999) Corneal topography and postoperative refraction after cataract phacoemulsification following radial keratotomy. Ophthalmic Surg Lasers 30:155–159

84. Ahmed I, Toufeeq A (2005) Accuracy of intraoperative retinoscopy in corneal power and axial length estimation using a high plus soft contact lens. Ophthalmic Physiol Opt 25:52–56

85. Haigis W (2004) The Haigis formula. In: Shammas HJ (ed). Intraocular lens power calculations. Slack, Thorofare, N.J., pp 41–57

86. Seitz B, Langenbucher A (2000) Intraocular lens power calculation in eyes after corneal refractive surgery. J Refract Surg 16:349–361

87. Joyal H, Gregoire J, Faucher A (2003) Photorefractive keratectomy to correct hyperopic shift after radial keratotomy. J Cataract Refract Surg 29:1502–1506

88. Hau SC, Ehrlich DP (2003) Contact lens fitting following unsuccessful refractive surgery. Ophthalmic Physiol Opt 23:329–340

89. Titiyal JS, Dutta R, Sinha R et al (2003) Contact lens fitting for post-radial-keratotomy residual myopia. Clin Experiment Ophthalmol 31:48–51

90. Stakheev AA (2002) Intraocular lens calculation for cataract after previous radial keratotomy. Ophthalmic Physiol Opt 22:289–295

91. McNeil JI (1993) Corneal incision dehiscence during penetrating keratoplasty nine years after radial keratotomy. J Cataract Refract Surg 19:542–53

92. Majmudar PA, Forstot SL, Dennis RF et al (2000) Topical mitomycin-C for subepithelial fibrosis after refractive corneal surgery. Ophthalmology 107:89–94

93. Afshari NA, Schirra F, Rapoza PA et al (2005) Laser in situ keratomileusis outcomes following radial keratotomy, astigmatic keratotomy, photorefractive keratectomy, and penetrating keratoplasty. J Cataract Refract Surg 31:2093–2100

94. Freeman M, Kumar V, Ramanathan US et al (2004) Dehiscence of radial keratotomy incision during phacoemulsification. Eye 18:101–13

95. Packer M, Brown LK, Hoffman RS et al (2004) Intraocular lens power calculation after incisional and thermal keratorefractive surgery. J Cataract Refract Surg 30:1430–1434

96. Patel SM, Tesser RA, Albert DM et al (2005) Histopathology of radial keratotomy. Arch Ophthalmol 123:104–105

97. Martin R, Rodriguez G (2005) Reverse geometry contact lens fitting after corneal refractive surgery. J Refract Surg 21:753–756

98. Bufidis T, Konstas AG, Pallikaris IG et al (2000) Contact lens fitting difficulties following refractive surgery for high myopia. CLAO J 26:106–110

12

Contents

Core Messages

■ Intraoperative complications
  and their management

■ Early postoperative complications
  and their management

■ The complications of different types of AS-PIOLs

■ Complications that may lead to explantation
  of the AS-PIOLs

■ Explantation techniques of AS-PIOLs

■ Prevention of complications
  – Surgical technique
  – AS-PIOL design
  – Anterior imaging and appropriate
    AS-PIOL sizing

13

13.1 Anterior Chamber Angle-Supported Complications: Prevention and Treatment

Orkun Muftuoglu and Jorge L. Alió

13.1.1 Introduction

Anterior chamber angle-supported phakic intraocular lenses (AS-PIOLs) are attractive for the practical surgeon, as the anterior chamber (AC), especially in myopic eyes, is the largest space in the anterior segment of the eye, and its anatomy can be studied easily both preoperatively and postoperatively. The iridocorneal angle was chosen by Dannheim [1], Baron [2], and Strampelli [3] in the early 1950s as the first, easy-to-maneuver anatomical space reached by the surgeon for inserting a lens into a phakic eye. In the 1950s, Strampelli and Barraquer were the first surgeons to use angle-supported AC lenses for the correction of high myopia [3, 4]. Unfortunately, the initial designs of these lenses were plagued by major complications, such as corneal decompensation and chronic iritis. This was due to manufacturing imperfections as well as to inherent biological defects in the principle of angle fixation [5]. Angle-supported lenses were solid and extremely thick at their edges. Therefore, the first generation of these lenses eventu-

ally was abandoned [4, 5]. Other factors contributing to the termination of the procedure were inferior surgical techniques [2].

Because of the disastrous experiences with myopia correction, it took about 30 years before the correction of high myopia with intraocular lenses was reconsidered. New surgical techniques with lens glides, the use of viscoelastics, and improved manufacturing technique allowed the development of new types of phakic AC lenses [6, 7]. In the late 1980s, a second generation of AS-PIOLs was introduced by Baikoff, which were followed by several others [8]. Studies emphasized good visual and refractive outcomes of these second-generation phakic lenses [9–15]. As the related complications were not as severe or frequent as those seen with the first generation, and because they are easy to implant with basic surgical tools, in most cases AS-PIOLs became more popular [16].

Despite the effectiveness of second-generation lenses, problems and complications related with cataract, endothelial decompensation, and pupil ovalization remained. Besides, the incision sizes of most of the phakic IOL models were large enough to create at least some astigmatism [16]. The latest-generation of angle-fixated phakic lenses with a foldable optic to be inserted through a self-sealing small incision (less than 3.5 mm), was introduced in the late 1990s. Preliminary studies with these newest AS-PIOLs showed promising results in terms of safety ratio and accuracy of the refractive outcomes [16–18].

Implanting a phakic AC IOL in highly myopic eyes has generated renewed interest recent years because it achieves better optical results than do other procedures for the correction of high myopia [9, 19, 20]. However, this procedure raises many questions concerning the long-term potential risks to corneal endothelium, lens, anterior uvea, and other eye structures [21–23]. Therefore, treatment and prevention of complications are essential for ophthalmologists who use these types of PIOLs [22–25].

13.1.2 Intraoperative Complications

Intraoperative complications include ocular hypotony (iris prolapse, choroidal hemorrhage), damage to the natural lens, and endothelium or iris. These are usually due to inappropriate surgical technique or IOL size and design.

13.1.3 Early Postoperative Complications

13.1.3.1 Ocular Hypertension

When viscoelastic substance removal has been incomplete, intraocular pressure (IOP) rises because of transient trabecular blockage by the residual viscous molecules (the chamber is deep and the angle is open). If viscoelastic in the AC is visible, then the anterior lip of the incision should be depressed in order to allow the viscoelastic to leave the AC. Treatment includes the use of antihypertensive and hyperosmotic agents.

Intraocular hypertension also can be seen between the second and the fourth week after the surgery, likely related to the corticosteroid eye drops prescribed postoperatively. Intraocular hypertension typically resolves after the steroid treatment is discontinued. Although its rate is low with the recent designs of PIOLs, pupillary block should be always be considered as a possible reason of IOP increase after PIOL implantation. The AC depth (ACD) and the competency of iridotomy or iridectomy should be evaluated. Rapid intervention is necessary as endothelial decompensation can occur due to decreased ACD [9, 12–16].

13.1.3.2 Acute Uveitis

In the first examination a few hours after the surgery, there may be a mild inflammation in the AC due to the remnants of additives introduced into the AC or from breaking the blood–aqueous barrier through surgery. This can be induced by a traumatic operation, and it requires treatment with anti-inflammatory and mydriatic drugs. Due to the surgical trauma, contact with the trabecular meshwork, and iris root some degree of erosion, vessel disturbance, pigment dispersion, and synechiae formation is inevitable after phakic IOL implantation, hence the concern about glaucoma, iridocyclitis, and breakdown of the blood–aqueous barrier [12–16].

13.1.3.3 Decentration, Displacement, or Rotation of the IOL

Decentration, displacement, or rotation of the PIOL is usually due to inappropriate surgical technique or IOL sizing. This requires repositioning or replacement with another lens of appropriate size.

13.1.3.4 Endophthalmitis

Endophthalmitis can complicate any open-eye procedure. However, the literature offers only anecdotal reports of septic intraocular inflammation after phakic IOL implantation, with an exceedingly low incidence [16]. Compared with cataract surgery, the severity of the complication seems to be limited by the maintenance of the crystalline lens barrier, which may delay the catastrophic spread of the infection to the vitreous chamber. It is hope that this is a rare complication, which requires the retrieval of the implant and antibiotic treatment as for any postoperative endophthalmitis. It would be gratifying to think that the antibacterial property of the heparin coating was a factor, but there are no definitive data available to substantiate that premise [16].

13.1.3.5 Corneal Edema

Corneal edema is usually secondary to excessive manipulation during surgery, inflammation, or to ocular hypertension.

13.1.3.6 Residual Refractive Error

Requires replacing the lens or correction by means of a corneal procedure (photorefractive keratectomy [PRK], laser in situ keratomileusis [LASIK], laser epithelial keratomileusis [LASEK] or intracorneal rings)

13.1.4 Complications after Implantation of Different Types of ASP-IOLS and Their Management

13.1.4.1 ZB, ZB5M, and NuVITA

ZB (Domilens, Lyon, France) is a monoblock lens made of polymethylmethacrylate (PMMA) obtained by modifying an AC lens for correcting aphakia, the Kelman Multiflex lens. This lens had four angle-support points, an anterior haptics of angle of 25°, and an optical zone of 4.5 mm. This lens was soon found to induce endothelial damage [7]. The ZB model was replaced by the ZB5M model, whose haptics were angled at 20° and had a considerably reduced peripheral thickness of the optic zone. This model was available in three diameters (12.5, 13, and 13.5 mm) and had a biconcave optic zone of overall diameter 5 mm and effective diameter of 4 mm. Lens power ranged from –7.00 to –20 D in 1.00-D increments. Surface treatment of the lens with "fluorine plasma" to improve biocompatibility gave rise to the ZB5MF model. Successive modifications of the ZB5MF lens generated a third-generation lens, the NuVita MA20 (Chiron Vision, Claremont, California), only available in minus powers. This design attempted to reduce the incidence of night vision problems described by patients by increasing the real optical zone to 4.5 mm (total optical zone, 5 mm) thinning its rim by 20%, changing the biconcave shape of the lens to a meniscus shape, and subjecting it to "peripheral detail technology" to reduce glare. Its haptic support zones were enlarged to achieve better support at the angle and thus reduce the incidence of pupil ovalization. However, the NuVita MA20 lens was taken off the market probably because of the continued problems such as glare and monocular diplopia [26].

13.1.4.1.1 Complications

The 12-year data showed severe pupil ovalization in 12.3% of ZB5M implants, while low or moderate pupil ovalization has been found in 24.6% cases. Pupil ovalization is produced because of ischemia due to compression of the haptics at the iris root. The difficulty of adapting the three lens sizes available to all possible diameters of the AC, added to the imperfect measurement methods, makes this complication one of the most difficult to avoid. In many cases, ovalization is discrete and does not affect the patient, but in others, the lens needs to be removed due to severe atrophy of the iris.

The ZB lens was associated with several cases of endothelial decompensation through lens endothelium contact [27]. Subsequent models have been designed to reduce this contact. Despite this, in one series, the ZB5M model has been related to an average cell loss of 22.4% after 12 years. Other long-term studies involving the ZB5M lens have shown low or moderate endothelial cell loss [28].

In a series, a statistically significant increase in flare values was found in every patient 12 years after surgery. However, the inflammation in the AC was usually mild without severe complications.

Given that the "effective optical zone" size is always smaller than the "intended" optical zone size, the percentage of patients complaining about halos and night glare were found to be always higher than desired.

The prevalence of nuclear cataracts 12 years after surgery was 10% [9].

13.1.4.2 ZSAL-4 and ZSAL-4/Plus Phakic Refractive IOLS

The ZSAL-4 angle-supported AC IOL (Morcher, Stuttgart, Germany) is a plano-concave lens made of a single-piece PMMA, with Z-shaped haptics. The total optical zone is 5.5 mm, with an effective optical zone of 5 mm to reduce night-vision problems. The optic has a three-side edge to reduce refracted glare. The haptics are angulated 19° anteriorly [7, 8]. The overall length of the lens is 12.5 of 13 mm, and the lens power ranges from −6.00 D to −20 D in 1.00-D steps. The ZSAL-4 lens was replaced by the ZSAL-4/Plus lens, which is a plano-concave, one-piece PMMA lens. This lens has an effective optical diameter enlarged from 5 to 5.3 mm (total optical zone. 5.8 mm), keeping the transitional edge of the optic to reduce night halos. This lens is available in 12-, 12.5-, and 13-mm overall lengths, and the lens power ranges from −6.00 D to −20 D in 0.50-D steps. The haptic geometry was modified to increase haptic flexibility and disperse compression forces against angle structures (Fig. 13.1.1) [29].

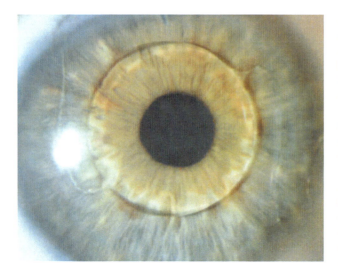

Fig. 13.1.1 ZSAL-4/Plus phakic lens 6 months after surgery. Note the large optic and the thin haptics

13.1.4.2.1 Complications (according to the series of Perez-Santonja and coauthors [29], which included 23 eyes)

Although mild AC inflammation was frequently observed, it disappeared by 1 month after surgery in all eyes. However, in two eyes (8.7%), a slight inflammatory response was observed in the AC up to 6 months after surgery, which improved with corticosteroid therapy.

Inflammatory deposits on the IOL surface were seen in 5 eyes (21%) up to 6 months postoperatively, but disappeared over time [30].

Postoperative elevated IOP greater than 22 mmHg complicated the postoperative course in three eyes (12%) during the first month after surgery. However, the elevated IOP resolved after the corticosteroids were discontinued. In none of the operated eyes did the rise of IOP persist more than 8 weeks after surgery.

Decentration was calculated as the distance between the center of the pupil and that of the IOL, using slit lamp beams of 0.2, 0.5, and 1 mm. With this method, 65.2% of eyes showed a decentration between 0 and 0.25 mm, 30.4% of eyes between 0.26 and 0.5 mm, and 4.3% between 0.51 and 0.75 mm. When decentration was present, the center of the pupil was always nasal in relation to the center of the IOL.

In 26.1% of eyes, night halos were present at 12 and 24 months after surgery. There was no significant relationship between decentration and halos at 12 and 24 months.

Pupillary ovalization was observed in 2 of 23 eyes (8.7%) at 1, 3, and 6 months after surgery, and in 4 of 23 eyes (17.4%) at 12 and 24 months. Pupil ovalization was always discrete and non-progressive. Pupil ovalization occurred along the axis of the first haptic footplate in three eyes, and in one eye along the main axis of the IOL. Although all pupil ovalization appeared in eyes with long IOLs (overall length, 13 mm), no significant relationship was found between pupil ovalization and IOL length.

Twenty-four months after surgery, the IOL axis remained in the horizontal meridian in 13 of 23 eyes (56.5%), rotated counter-clockwise between +25 and +50° in 26% of eyes, between +70 and +90° in 13%, and rotated clockwise between −70 and −90° in 4.3%. These data show that some IOLs rotate early after surgery and, after 1 month, the IOLs tend to become stable.

No contact was noted between the IOL and the natural lens, with either a narrow or a wide pupil. Lens opacities, retinal detachment, or pupillary block was not observed in this series.

In a prospective clinical study with 20 eyes and 1-year follow-up, the clinical results with the ZSAL-4/Plus phakic lens regarding effectiveness, predictability, and stability were similar to those found after ZSAL-4 lens implantation. The endothelial cell loss was 3.8% at 12 months, which is similar to that found after ZSAL-4 implantation. However, the ZSAL-4/Plus phakic lens reduced the rate of night halos (none) and pupil ovalization (10%) found with the previous ZSAL-4 model [31].

13.1.4.3 Phakic 6, 6H, and 6H2 Lenses

The Phakic 6 and 6H IOLs (Ophthalmic Innovations International, Ontario, Calif.) are made of PMMA and follow the ideas of M. Galin and H Gould. The 6 and 6H ("H" for heparin coating) have a 1-mm vault, optic of 6 mm up to –10 D, and then 5.5 mm up to –25 D. The haptic sizes ranged from 11.5 to 14 mm in increments of 0.5 mm. In addition, the patented IOL heparin coatings are believed to impart anti-inflammatory and antibacterial properties. A more recent modification of the footplates and a reduction of the optic edge from 0.77 to 0.56 mm in the higher dioptric powers is designated as Phakic 6H2 [31, 32].

13.1.4.3.1 Complications

In the early series using the early versions of these lenses, a number of cases ultimately required IOL explantation, cataract removal, and keratoplasty. In this early series of prior IOL models, all experienced full vision recovery. All of the complications could be explained primarily by inadequate ACD or angle openness and, in one case, IOL mobility with an undersized IOL.

According to the main investigators, the mean endothelial cell loss from preoperative baseline for the Phakic 6 myopic implants was 2.5% at the 6-month interval and 1.9% at 18 months. In another series, the annualized rate of endothelial cell loss was 1.2% in the treated eyes and 1.3% in the fellow (control) eyes. It was concluded that the cell loss for eyes implanted with these AC IOLs is within the normal range of annual cell loss in untreated eyes. The most significant influencing factor for both untreated and treated eyes was found to be postoperative time [31, 32]. On the other hand, recently in a series of AS-PIOL explantation, the time interval of implantation and endothelial cell loss was found to be much shorter with Phakic 6 than with the ZB5M lens [33].

The small series of Phakic 6 implants done in the United States prior to 1999 showed minimal ovalization. None of the ovalization went beyond the optic or produced any visual symptoms; nevertheless, they were mildly objectionable cosmetically. To date, the Phakic 6H2 with its "ski-edge" haptic foot has not produced significant iris ovalization.

According the series of main investigators, in one case, a slight overcorrection made the patient mildly hyperopic and warranted maintenance on daily pilocarpine drops. One-year postoperatively, pupillary block occurred, with iris deformation and visual compromise. The patient had some endothelial loss and required keratoplasty.

Glare was a significant problem with a smaller optic in the early models. The design of the Phakic 6 configurations with a 6-mm optic was implemented to address this problem. The downside of increased optic diameter was a deeper ACD requirement and increased possibility of endothelial damage. However, even with a scotopic/mesopic pupil of greater than 6 mm, subjective complaints of glare was found to be rare.

13.1.4.4 GBR/Vivarte Angle-Supported Foldable Phakic IOL

The Vivarte IOL and the GBR are very similar but distributed by two different companies. This is a one-piece, AC, three-point angle-supported lens (tripod support), and was the first foldable phakic lens on the market with angle support. This one-piece and three-point angle-supported IOL has a soft hydrophilic acrylic optic with rigid PMMA haptics that finish with soft acrylic footplates. Iridocorneal angle irritation is low because the footplates are very flexible. The 5.5-mm biconcave optic is tangentially fixed in the middle of the large haptic bow, which permits insertion of the haptic through a less than 3-mm incision. The Vivarte IOL is available in overall diameters of 12, 12.5, and 13 mm, and only for myopic correction from 7.00 to –25 diopters. Using the specific forceps, the lens can be folded into an N shape and implanted under topical anesthesia through a 3.2-mm clear-corneal incision [34].

13.1.4.4.1 Complications

The most frequent and important complications are related to sudden unfolding of the lens into the AC. Another is selection of the wrong lens length in relation to the actual size of the AC.

The Vivarte IOL is a phakic lens simple to implant, and its self-centration has been excellent when the previous measurement of the AC is well planned. However, the IOL geometric center does not always correspond with the pupillary center, especially in some high ametropic patients. The relatively large optic diameter of the Vivarte IOL, make small decentrations more tolerable and less symptomatic than other phakic IOLs.

Transient incisional edema can be induced when hydrating that resolves spontaneously during the first 24 f. Significant corneal edema due to endothelial damage is unusual and is mainly seen at the beginning of the learning curve, as the surgeon may damage the corneal endothelium when the lens unfolds or with the instruments used to put the lens in place.

In the first examination a few hours after the surgery, there may be a mild inflammation in the AC due to the remnants of additives introduced into the AC or from breaking the blood–aqueous barrier through surgery.

About 40% of our patients had a significant increase (>2 mmHg) of the IOP in the first 24 f, although it was over 25 mmHg in only two cases (20%). These cases responded well to topical treatment, as well as oral acetazolamide in cases of IOP above 30 mmHg. This rise in the IOP is due to the remaining viscoelastic that was not removed during the surgery. Another group of patients (30%) developed intraocular hypertension between the second and the fourth week after the surgery, likely related to the corticosteroid eye drops. All of them resolved after the steroid treatment was discontinued.

Endothelial cell loss 1 week after surgery was 2.5% and was probably secondary to surgical stress, since the endothelial cells did not decrease significantly in the 2-year follow-up.

It is important to check lens position in the postoperative examinations. Although rare, significant dislocations (>2 mm), which require replacement with a larger diameter lens due to monocular diplopia, are possible.

The most common late complication was the rotation of the lens. In one case, the lens was well centered, but it rotated until the simple haptic found an iridotomy and did not rotate anymore [34].

Halos and glare symptoms after surgery are possible. These symptoms are related to pupil diameter and the effective optical zone of the IOL [16]. Mild pupil ovalization was observed in one case that started to develop at 1-year follow-up. Other complications (different from those described above) were not observed [34].

13.1.4.5 Kelman Duet Phakic AC Lens

This lens was designed by Kelman, is manufactured by Tekia (Irvine, Calif.), and was implanted for the first time by Jorge L. Alió. This innovative, foldable AC IOL has two independent parts, a tripod haptic made of PMMA and a silicone optic of 5.5 mm in diameter (Fig. 13.1.2). The haptic overall length ranges from 12 to 13 mm, in 0.5-mm steps, and the lens power from –8.00 to –20 D. The IOL is implanted in two steps. First, the haptic is implanted into the AC and positioned, within the AC, and second, the optic is fixated to the haptic by means of small haptic tabs. A glare-preventing shield has been added to the periphery of the 6.3-mm (effective diameter: 5.5 mm) optic [35].

The preliminary pillow study was published in 2003 and proved the feasibility of the concept, which reduces the incision size for implantation down to 2.75 mm, the smallest incision available for an AC-PIOL. A potential concern, common to the GBR/Vivarte, is the tendency to move around the angle when a patient blinks or rubs his eye, as it was found with previous tripod lenses [16, 25].

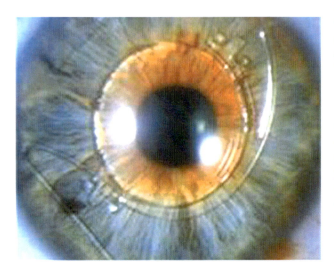

Fig. 13.1.2 Kelman-Duet angle-supported phakic IOL

In a recent study [36], 169 consecutive eyes of 110 patients (range, 18–45 years of age) were implanted with the Kelman-Duet PIOL, with a minimum of 12 months of follow-up. Surgery was completely successfully in all eyes with no intraoperative complications. Postoperatively, no lens opacification, chronic increased IOP, or pupillary block occurred, and none of the lens had to be explanted during the follow-up period. Only one eye experienced synechiae (0.59%) between the iris and the optic of the lens in the early postoperative period, which was solved by widening the iridotomy. This eye suffered endothelial cell density loss of more than 20%.

Pupil ovalization, considering mild and severe levels of ovalling, was present in 17 eyes (10.06%). Haptic exchange was performed in 9 eyes (5.33%) and haptic repositioning in 3 eyes (1.78%). Mild decentration of the lens could be appreciated by slit lamp biomicroscopy in 9 eyes (5.33%). Night-vision disturbances such as halos or glare were a significant complaint in 11.24% of eyes at 1 month, but this frequency decreased to 4.73% at 3 months.

At 12 months, no severe complications were present. Halos and glare were a disturbing phenomenon in only 1.18% of cases. No retinal complication was reported. No statistically significant differences were found between preoperative endothelial cell density and the postoperative value at 3 months. However, the preoperative endothelial density was higher than the 1-year postoperative measurement. Therefore, a significant decrease in endothelial cell density occurred.

13.1.4.6 Alcon AcrySof

AcrySof (Alcon, Forth Worth, Tex.) is a single-piece foldable lens in acrylic material with 5.5-mm meniscus optic and peculiar T-shaped haptic design. It is manufactured with the standard AcrySof material and implanted with an injector. This lens is facing the last stage of its clinical investigation in a multicenter trial with a 6-mm optic, implantable through a mean incision of 3 mm. First results with the AcrySof phakic implant have been very encouraging, with excellent tolerance and stability and minimal induction of pupil ovalling. Upside-down implantation of the IOL is reported; therefore, recent designs will have a mark in order to prevent this complication [16].

13.1.4.7 ICARE

ICARE (Corneal, Pringy, France) is a hydrophilic acrylic monobloc lens, with 5.75-mm optic size and four independent feet to provide a wider contact surface in the angle support. The forces developed under compression are therefore supposed to be smaller, to maximally preserve iridocorneal angle and iris structures. It was designed to provide a longer mid-peripheral distance from the endothelium to the optic's edge. The ICARE lens requires an incision of 3.5 mm; it also reports good tolerance and adequate visual and refractive outcomes. Foldable PIOLs have the potential of vaulting due to the intrinsic characteristics of the biomaterial, a fact that can be enhanced by the temperature of the aqueous humor due to their thermosensitivity. Intermittent endothelial touch might be the consequence of such intrinsic instability. For this reason, long-term follow-up data concerning corneal endothelial cell stability are necessary for these foldable designs [16].

13.1.5 Treatment of Late Complications That Require Explantation of Phakic IOLS

Recently Alió and coauthors evaluated 100 eyes that have undergone explantation of angle supported PIOLs [33]. The models of lenses included in this study were ZB, ZB5M, ZSAL-4, and Phakic 6.

Cataract was the main cause of explantation (64%) of angle supported AC PIOLs (Fig. 13.1.3). The mean time interval between AS-PIOL implantation and explantation surgery was 10.04±3.66 (range, 2–14) years. In all of these cases, cataracts were nuclear according to the LOCS III. Some cases had areas of pigmentary dispersion on the anterior capsule, typically at the midperiphery of the anterior lens surface. Cataract development is four times more frequent in patients with high myopia than in the general population [23]. Previous reports have not demonstrated a relationship between AS-PIOL implantation and cataract development, but instead have shown that the probability of cataract development increases when an eye with an axial length of over 30 mm is implanted in patients older than 40 years, leading to nuclear cataract development in the following 2 years [23]. Surgery also might increase the speed of nuclear cataract development because of surgical trauma, postoperative inflammation, and the postoperative use of topical steroids [10, 12]. Phakic IOL implantation in eyes with early changes of the nucleus might promote the progression of these changes into the development of a clinically significant nuclear cataract [23]. Hence, the physician should pay careful attention to recent changes in refraction and densi-

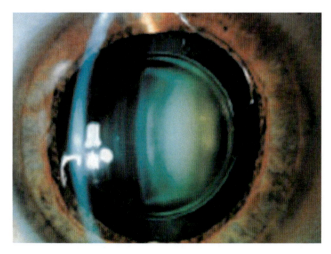

Fig. 13.1.3 Nuclear cataract in a patient implanted with the Baikoff ZB5M angle-supported AC phakic IOL

ty of the lenses of highly myopic eyes before this surgery is recommended [33].

Although chronic inflammation may contribute to the development of cataract [10, 12], none of the cases that developed cataract in this series suffered from clinical inflammatory reactions, such as acute postoperative iritis or chronic inflammation, after AS-PIOL implantation [33].

No adhesions between the phakic lens and the iris or the angle were observed in any patient. However, iris prolapse occurred frequently during surgery and was the most common intraoperative inconvenience. This complication was never observed in cases operated using the microincisional cataract surgery (MICS) technique. Alió and coauthors have found in this study that the use of the MICS technique in bilensectomy surgery enhanced intraocular fluid control [33, 37]. They observed that the AC was more stable, with less liability to iris prolapse, when MICS was used. The final refractive correction achieved with a posterior chamber (PC) IOL as well as best spectacle-corrected visual acuity (BSCVA) were mildly reduced from those obtained 3 months after PC-IOL implantation. This may be due to a relatively large interval between the two procedures and the natural history of high myopia. The presence of an AS-PIOL had minimal influence on axial length measurement [33].

Endothelial cell loss was the second most frequent cause of AS-PIOL explantation (24%). The mean interval between implantation and secondary intervention due to progressive endothelial cell loss was 8.97±2.21 years (range, 2–14) years. In most of the cases, the PIOL was the Baikoff ZB, ZB5M or Phakic 6 (Fig. 13.1.4). The mean interval between implantation and explantation of Phakic 6 cases (3.22±1.07 years) was much shorter than that for the Baikoff ZB5M cases (12.33±1.15 years) (p < 0.02) [33, 36]. Reasons for endothelial cell loss are related to AS-PIOL design and inadequate anatomy of the AC. The findings of both ultrasound biomicroscopy and Artemis suggested that the excessive vault of the Phakic 6 model, together with the relatively large optic diameter, might contribute to endothelial cell damage (Fig. 13.1.5). In all these cases, explantation was performed without complications. No synechia or iris adhesions were observed [33].

Pupil ovalization has been reported as a common finding in patients implanted with AS PIOLs (Fig. 13.1.6) [15]. Ten eyes (10%) in this series with the Baikoff ZB5M AS PIOL had marked pupillary ovalization extending beyond the edge of the PIOL and atrophic findings at the iris, and bilensectomy surgery was indicated. However, the explantation of the lens in these cases was difficult due to the frequent presence of iris synechia and angle adhesions. AC bleeding occurred in four cases and was severe in two. Pupil recentration was attempted in all cases by sectorial iris stretching or purse string suturing with variable success [33, 37].

In one case (1%), after the implantation of the largest available overall size of the ZSAL-4 AS-PIOL, the lens appeared to be undersized, and rotation of the lens threatened the endothelium and angle. This lens was exchanged for a

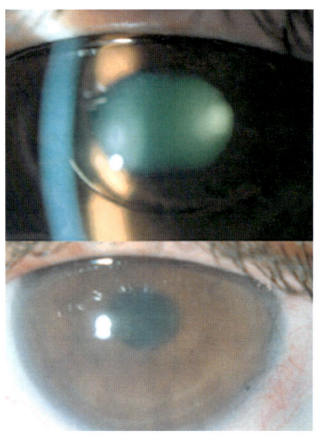

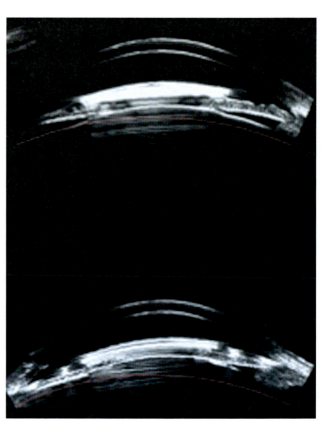

Fig. 13.1.5 Artemis pictures of two cases that developed severe endothelial cell loss because of Phakic 6 IOL implantation

Fig. 13.1.4 Corneal decompensation in a patient implanted with the Phakic 6 IOL. *Bottom*, the same case 1 week after phakic IOL explantation

13

custom-made Kelman Duet implant of 13.5-mm overall diameter, which remained stable [33].

In one case (1%), implanted with the Baikoff ZB5M, the patient developed RD, and the PIOL had to be removed 2.5 years later to enhance fundus visualization for retinal reattachment surgery [33].

In none of the cases in this series was the AS PIOL explanted due to glaucoma, postoperative inflammation, or uveitis [33].

13.1.6 Techniques Used for Phakic IOL Explantation

13.1.6.1 Bilensectomy

Bilensectomy surgery is recommended when BSCVA decreased by at least 2 lines from the BSCVA documented after AS-PIOL implantation and related to evident lens sclerosis or cataract. Bilensectomy is also recommended, even without development of cataract, when the endothelial cell count decreased markedly to approach 1,500 cells/mm² or when severe pupillary ovalization developed in patients older than 45 years.

Posterior chamber IOLs are used to correct aphakia after PIOL removal. Lens power can be calculated using the

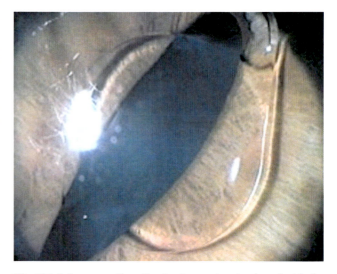

Fig. 13.1.6 Severe pupil ovalization in a patient implanted with the Baikoff ZB5M angle-supported AC phakic IOL

SRK/T formula. Bilensectomy can be performed using coaxial phacoemulsification or MICS in order to increase surgical control during the phacoemulsification procedure [43]. The AS-PIOL can be explanted through a 6-mm incision and then can be sutured after PIOL removal. Afterward, MICS surgery can be performed through two 90°-apart, 1.5-mm incisions, as previously reported [38]. After phacoemulsification of the nucleus and cortex removal, the initial 6-mm incision is reopened, and a PC IOL can be placed in the capsular bag.

In the series of Alió et al., synechiae seldom were found in the explanted cases, except those with extreme pupil ovalization. The endothelial cell count was 2,271±403 cells/mm^2 just before bilensectomy, and it was 2,137±401 cells/mm^2 3 months after bilensectomy. Also, corneal endothelial cell loss after bilensectomy was similar to that in another study of cell loss after conventional phacoemulsification with PC IOL implantation. No complications were observed during follow-up. Mean cylindrical power was not significantly changed by the PIOL explantation surgery [33, 38].

13.1.6.2 Phakic Intraocular Lens Exchange

This procedure can be performed when the PIOL is improperly sized or when significant endothelial cell loss occurred related to the PIOL. To exchange the PIOL, peribulbar anesthesia is usually preferred. Then, using steps similar to those previously described for bilensectomy but with only one side port, the PIOL can be explanted and the new PIOL can be implanted [33].

13.1.6.3 Phakic Intraocular Lens Explantation and Penetrating Keratoplasty

This procedure can be performed when there is severe corneal endothelial decompensation. In the series of Alió et al., four cases that developed corneal endothelial decompensation as a result of Baikoff ZB AS PIOL implantation underwent lens explantation and penetrating keratoplasty with good results [33].

13.1.6.4 Simple Phakic Intraocular Lens Removal

This procedure can be performed when significant endothelial cell loss occurred related to the PIOL or to enhance posterior segment visualization when retinal surgery is indicated. Simple PIOL explantation is usually eventless [33].

13.1.7 How to Prevent Complications

In all the intraoperative complications, possible endothelial or lens damage when introducing, unfolding, or placing the lens in the angle should be noted.

Potential complications, such as lens material deterioration, endothelial cell loss higher than the physiological rate, glaucoma, iris atrophy, and/or severe pupil ovalization could appear in these patients in the future, and a careful and exhaustive informed consent is highly recommended for implanting any type of phakic lens [16].

13.1.7.1 Surgical Technique

For the successful implantation of angle supported PIOLs, surgeons should avoid ocular hypotony because of the consequences of excessive vitreous pressure (iris prolapse, choroidal hemorrhage). It is also important to have a sufficient AC depth to avoid damaging the natural lens, endothelium, or iris. In addition, it is necessary to have a self-sealing incision of suitable width to aid the maneuvers needed to introduce the lens and prevent intraoperative athalamia. Finally, good miosis is essential to avoid introducing the optic of the IOL or any haptic through the pupil [16].

13.1.7.2 IOL Design

Until recently, the incision sizes of most of the phakic IOL models were large enough to create at least some astigmatism. In addition, insertions of phakic IOLs were sometimes traumatic to the endothelium and the iris. The danger of inducing opacities in the natural lens are not only theoretical, but have been documented. The long-term effects of the redirection of aqueous flow and its clinical significance have yet to be determined. If the implant has to be removed, the surgery becomes quite extensive, and the damage to endothelium and natural lens is more likely

Successful PIOLs should have some properties (defined by Charles Kelman [35]) that should:

- Not put pressure on the angle
- Not move in the AC
- Not flex against the peripheral endothelium
- Not rub against the iris
- Not cause damage to the natural lens on insertion
- Not require an incision of more than 1.5–2 mm
- Not be difficult to insert
- Not be difficult to remove
- Not be difficult to exchange

13.1.7.3 Anterior Segment Imaging and PIOL Sizing

AC is in the middle of delicate structures such as the cornea, endothelium, iris, iridocorneal angle, and crystalline lens. Therefore, the eye's tolerance of PIOLs depends on accurate measurements of the internal biometry of the AC. Recently, devices to image anterior segment, based on the optical principles of the Scheimpflug method, high- and very high–ultrasound frequency scanning and optical coherence tomography, are introduced.

Although the Scheimpflug technique provides good images, it is impossible to define the tip of the iridocorneal angle precisely and the real internal diameter of the AC since the cornea–sclera junction zone is overexposed because of the extremely whiteness of scleral tissue. This may lead to a difference up to 1.5 mm in angle-to-angle measurements between the Scheimpflug technique and other techniques (Fig. 13.1.7). In addition, the optical cuts are oblique and require fairly complex reconstruction software as the dis-

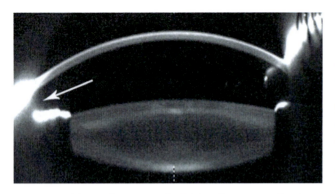

Fig. 13.1.7 Scheimpflug image of AC. Note the cornea–sclera junction zone is overexposed because of the extreme whiteness of scleral tissue

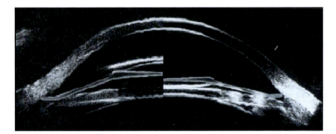

Fig. 13.1.8 Four superimposed VHF echographic images (Artemis 2) showing the evolution of the "safety distance," that is, the clearance from mid-peripheral endothelium and edge of the myopic optic of different generations of angle-fixated phakic IOLs. Compared to the old ZB (*top left*) and ZB5MF (*bottom left*), the Nuvita (*top right*) and the foldable GBR/ Vivarte (*bottom right*) show the modern trend for a significantly lower vault to respect the corneal endothelial cell layer

tances observed on the images vary depending on the position in the anterior segment [39–46].

The ultrasound biomicroscopy allows good imaging of iridocorneal angle. However, it explores a very small zone that needs to be reconstructed by juxtaposing images to evaluate anterior segment. The Artemis very high–frequency digital ultrasound arc scanner (Ultralink) can provide measurement of intraocular dimensions such as the angle-to-angle width and AC depth (Fig. 13.1.8) [38–42]. Recently, the Artemis system is demonstrated to have accurate, repeatable, and reproducible measurements of the anterior segment [39–47]. It is possible to evaluate the posterior chamber behind the iris pigments with the ultrasound scanning. On the other hand, there are disadvantages of the ultrasound imaging: a water or gel bath should placed between the tip of the ultrasound device, the examined eye and the operator has to identify the axis under study on the control screen, effects of accommodation should be evaluated by inducing the fellow eye or with pilocarpine eye drops, and the variation in ultrasound acoustic transmissions can produce shadowing behind the prosthesis or iris showing notches and repetition echoes [39–47].

The AC optical coherence tomography (AC-OCT; Visante OCT, Carl Zeiss, Meditec) enables all the required AC measurements (AC diameter, AC depth, corneal pachymetry, crystalline lens thickness, and iridocorneal angle opening). It is shown to have accurate, repeatable, and reproducible measurements of the anterior segment. Since the infrared light beam is stopped by the pigments, a satisfactory view of the structures situated behind the iris is not possible. The advantages of the AC-OCT are no contact is needed for examination, easy examination, accommodation can be induced, and calculations in the AC are simple. With these advantages, AC-OCT seems to be the most convenient device to scan the AC for AS-PIOLs [39–47].

Angle-supported AC IOLs must respect three parameters: perfect adjustment to the internal diameter of the AC, minimum distance from the endothelium, and no contact with the iris and the crystalline lens [39].

13.1.7.3.1 Internal Diameter of the AC

To date, the internal diameter of the AC has only been estimated form the horizontal corneal diameter (white-to-white measurements). However, no anatomical correlation was found between white-to-white measurements and internal diameter of AC.

Using the Artemis in a series of 14 eyes, Rondeau et al. [48] found that the internal shape of the iridocorneal angle is a circle. On the other hand, Werner et al., found that the vertical diameter of the AC (iridocorneal angle or sulcus) was generally larger than the horizontal diameter in 20 cadaver eyes, using the same Artemis device. Using AC-OCT in 107 eyes, Baikoff et al. found that the internal vertical diameter of the AC was larger than the internal horizontal diameter, with a mean difference of 310 mm. This differs from the white-to-white evaluation, which generally assumes that the horizontal diameter is larger than the vertical diameter.

Oversized IOLs are the main reason of pupil ovalization seen after AS-PIOL implantations. Also, careful placement of the footplates is another factor that should be considered. Adapting AS-PIOLs to the largest internal diameter of the AC may avoid the propeller effect. When the IOL is perfectly adapted to the largest axis, it will usually rest in the angle without any displacement or rotation [39–48].

13.1.7.3.2 AC Depth

The clearance between the endothelium and AS-PIOL is critical. Therefore, determination of ACD is very important. Measurement of the internal depth of the AC (crystalline lens to endothelium) should be preferred over the measurement of the ACD between the crystalline lens and the epithelium. The clearance between the IOL and the endothelium is not the distance from the center of the optic to the posterior face of the endothelium along the eye's axis, but the shortest distance from the optic to the endothelium. It was clearly demonstrated that there should be a minimum of 1.5 mm distance between the edge of the optic and the

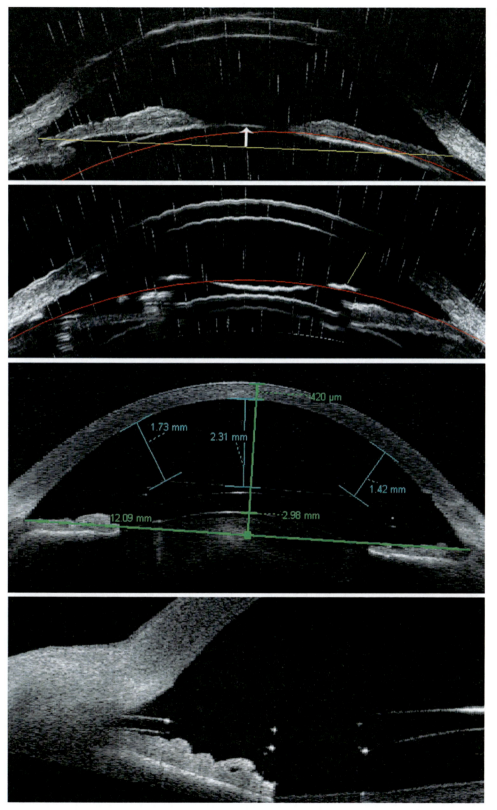

Fig. 13.1.9 Safety distances from the endothelium and the crystalline lens for angle supported phakic IOL implantation demonstrated in the anterior segment optical coherence tomography image

endothelium to prevent the risk for corneal damage. If the edge of the optic is less than 1.5 mm from the endothelium, then corneal distortions that occur during eye rubbing can give rise to endothelial alterations by contact with the edge of the IOL. If the IOL is closer than 1 mm from the endothelium, then explantation should be considered [39–48].

13.1.7.3.3 Implant Vaulting

The vault of AS-IOLs enables them to remain in front of and at a distance from the iris surface and the anterior pole of the crystalline lens when they move. The modifications of the shape of the natural lens should be considered during determination of the vault distance. The shape of the iris dome is conditioned by the forward protrusion of the anterior pole onto which the iris molds itself. All AS-PIOLs rest in the iridocorneal angle, which is the only zone of the anterior uvea that remains fixed throughout a person's life and during accommodation. To determine the forward protrusion of the crystalline lens dome, the line joining the two iridocorneal angles along the horizontal corneal diameter is used as a fixed reference. The distance between the anterior pole of the crystalline lens and the median of this base line is considered the crystalline lens rise. In addition, with every diopter of accommodation, the anterior pole of the crystalline lens moves forward 30 µm, and the natural lens thickens with age with a mean of 18–20 µm forward movement of its anterior pole every year. This means that after 20 years, the anterior pole of the crystalline lens has moved forward by 400 µm.

An AS-PIOL should have a sufficient clearance relative to the endothelium (minimum of 1.5 mm from the optic edge) and sufficient vault to be able to remain in front of the crystalline lens dome with the consideration effects of accommodation and aging to the natural lens. The IOL must therefore be placed within a safety zone delimited at the front by a 1.5-mm distance from the endothelium, and at the back by the theoretical 400-mm protrusion of the anterior pole of the crystalline lens or 700 µm from the base line joining the two iridocorneal sinuses (considering the mean crystalline lens height in a young subject is approximately 300 mm, Fig. 13.1.9) [39–48].

Take-Home Pearls

- Intraoperative and early postoperative complications can easily be prevented or treated with appropriate surgical techniques.
- Each AS-PIOL has its own specific complications. Therefore, PIOLs should be chosen and patients should be followed regarding the specific properties of each AS-PIOL.
- The results of explantation of AS-PIOLs are usually excellent with the appropriate techniques such as bilensectomy and PIOL explantation.
- Cataract incidence is much lower with the new generation IOLs.
- AS-PIOLs that require smaller incision for implantation and easily explantable should be preferred.
- Anatomical imaging, preferably with AC-OCT, is important for correct PIOL sizing:
  - Correct measurement of angle-to-angle distance for IOL diameter
  - Sufficient clearance with the endothelium (more than 1.5 mm)
  - Sufficient clearance with the crystalline lens (more than 700 µm)

As long as the meticulous care is given to the prevention or treatment of the complications reviewed above, the implantation of the AS-PIOLs will give good results with the least damage to the patient.

References

1. Dannheim H (1962) Types of AC lenses with elastic loops. Ann Inst Barraquer 3:570–2, 1962
2. Baron A (1953) Tolérance de l'oeil a`la matière plastique: prothéses optiques cornéennes, prothéses optique cristalliniennes. Bull Soc Ophthalmol Fr 9:982–988
3. Strampelli B (1958) Lentilles camerulaires apres 6 annees d'experience. Acta Conc Ophthalmol Belgica 11:1692–1698
4. Barraquer J (1959) AC plastic lenses. Results and conclusions from five years experience. Trans Ophthalmol Soc UK 79:242–393
5. Drews RC (1982) The Barraquer experience with intraocular lenses: 20 years later. Ophthalmology 89:386–393
6. Waring GO III (1998) Comparison of refractive corneal surgery and phakic IOLs. J Refract Surg 14:277–279
7. Hosny M, Alió JL, Claramonte P et al (2000) Relationship between AC depth, refractive state, corneal diameter, and axial length. J Refract Surg 16:336–340
8. Baikoff G, Arne JL, Bokobza Y et al (1998) Angle-fixated AC phakic intraocular lens for myopia of –7 to –19 diopters. J Refract Surg 14:282–293
9. Pérez-Santonja JJ, Alió JL, Jiménez-Alfaro I, Zato MA (2000) Surgical correction of severe myopia with an angle-supported phakic intraocular lens. J Cataract Refract Surg 26:1288–1302
10. Perez-Santonja JJ, Iradier MT, Sanz-Iglesias L et al (1996) Endothelial changes in phakic eyes with AC intraocular lenses to correct high myopia. J Cataract Refract Surg 22:1017–122
11. Perez-Santonja JJ, Hernandez JL, Benitez del Castillo JM et al (1994) Fluorophotometry in myopic phakic eyes with AC intraocular lenses to correct severe myopia. Am J Ophthalmol 118:316–21
12. Alió JL, de la Hoz F, Ismail M (1993) Subclinical inflammatory reactions induced by phakic AC lens for the correction of high myopia. Ocul Immunol Inflamm 1:219–223
13. Alió JL, Ruiz-Moreno JM, Artola A (1993) Retinal detachment as a potential hazard in surgical correction of severe myopia with phakic AC lenses. Am J Ophthalmol 115:145–148
14. Pérez-Santonja JJ, Ruíz-Moreno JM, de la Hoz F et al (1999) Endophthalmitis after phakic intraocular lens implantation to correct high myopia. J Cataract Refract Surg 25:1295–1298
15. Alió JL, de la Hoz F, Perez-Santonja JJ et al (1999) Phakic AC lenses for the correction of myopia: a 7-year cumulative analysis of complications in 263 cases. Ophthalmology 106:458–466
16. Levisolo CF, Reinstein DZ (2005) Phakic intraocular lenses. Surv Ophthalmol 50:549–587
17. Kaufman HE, Kaufman SC (2004) Phakic intraocular lenses–where are we now? In: Alió JL, Perez-Santonja JJ (eds) Refractive surgery with phakic IOLs: fundamentals and practice. Highlights of Ophthalmology International, El Dorado, Republic of Panama, pp 5–12
18. Elies D, Coret A (2004) GBR/Vivarte Angle-supported foldable phakic IOL. In: Alió JL, Perez-Santonja JJ (eds) Refractive surgery with phakic IOLs: fundamentals and practice. Highlights of Ophthalmology International, El Dorado, Republic of Panama, pp 121–127
19. Ferreira de Souza R, Allemann N, Forseto A et al (2003) Ultrasound biomicroscopy and Scheimpflug photography of angle-supported phakic intraocular lens for high myopia. J Cataract Refract Surg 29:1159–1166

13

20. Garcia-Feijoó J, Hernández-Matamoros JL, Castillo-Gómez A et al (2003) High-frequency ultrasound biomicroscopy of silicone posterior chamber phakic intraocular lens for hyperopia. J Cataract Refract Surg 29:1940–1946

21. Jiménez-Alfaro I, García-Feijoó J, Pérez-Santonja JJ, Cuiña R (2001) Ultrasound biomicroscopy of ZSAL-4 AC phakic intraocular lens for high myopia. J Cataract Refract Surg 27:1567–1573

22. Colin J (2000) Bilensectomy: the implications of removing phakic intraocular lenses at the time of cataract extraction. J Cataract Refract Surg 26:2–3

23. Alió JL, de la Hoz F, Ruiz-Moreno JM, Salem TF (2000) Cataract surgery in highly myopic eyes corrected by phakic AC angle-supported lenses. J Cataract Refract Surg 26:1303–1311

24. Mamalis N, Davis B, Nilson CD et al (2004) Complications of foldable intraocular lenses requiring explantation or secondary intervention–2003 survey update. J Cataract Refract Surg 30:2209–2218

25. Schmidbauer JM, Peng Q, Apple DJ et al (2002) Rates and causes of intraoperative removal of foldable and rigid intraocular lenses: clinicopathological analysis of 100 cases. J Cataract Refract Surg 28:1223– 1228

26. Iradier MT, Moreno E, Hoyos-Chacon J. Baikoff (2004) (ZB, ZB5M, NuVita) angle-supported phakic IOLs. In: Alió JL, Perez-Santonja JJ (eds) Refractive surgery with phakic IOLs: fundamentals and clinical practice. Highlights of Ophthalmology International, El Dorado, Republic of Panama, pp 83–93

27. Baikoff G, Arne JL, Bokobza Y et al (1998) Angle-fixated AC phakic intraocular lens for myopia of -7 to -19 diopters. J Refract Surg 14:282–293

28. Saragoussi JJ, Cotinat J, Renard G et al (1991) Damage to the corneal endothelium by minus power AC intraocular lenses. Refract Corneal Surg 7:277–285

29. Perez-Santonja JJ, Ruiz-Moreno JM, Alió JL (2004) ZSAL-4 and ZSAL-4/PLUS angle supported phakic IOLs. In: Alió JL, Perez-Santonja JJ (eds) Refractive surgery with phakic IOLs: fundamentals and clinical practice. Highlights of Ophthalmology International, El Dorado, Republic of Panama, pp 95–107

30. Perez-Santonja JJ, Iradier MT, Benitez del Castillo JM et al (1996) Chronic subclinical inflammation in phakic eyes with intraocular lenses to correct myopia. J Cataract Refract Surg 22:183–187

31. Gould HL, Galin M (2004) Phakic 6H angle-supported phakic IOL. In: Alió JL, Perez-Santonja JJ (eds) Refractive surgery with phakic IOLs: fundamentals and clinical practice. Highlights of Ophthalmology International, El Dorado, Republic of Panama, pp 109–120

32. Galin MA, Gould HL (2000) Angle supported phakic AC lenses. Operative techniques. Cataract Refractive Surgery 3:43

33. Alió JL, Abdelrahman AM, Javaloy J et al (2006) Angle-supported AC phakic intraocular lens explantation. Ophthalmology 113:2213–2220

34. Elies D, Coret A (2004) GBR/Vivarte angle-supported foldable phakic IOL. In: Alió JL, Perez-Santonja JJ (eds) Refractive surgery with phakic IOLs: fundamentals and clinical practice. Highlights of Ophthalmology International, El Dorado, Republic of Panama, pp 121–127

35. Kelman CD (2004) The Kelman DUET angle-supported phakic IOL. In: Alió JL, Perez-Santonja JJ (eds) Refractive surgery with phakic IOLs: fundamentals and clinical practice. Highlights of Ophthalmology International, El Dorado, Republic of Panama, pp 128–133

36. Alió JL, Piñhero D (2007) Long-term complications of Kelman-Duet phakic intraocular lens. J Refractive Surgery (in press)

37. Werblin TP (1993) Long-term endothelial cell loss following phacoemulsification: model for evaluating endothelial damage after intraocular surgery. Refract Corneal Surg 9:29–35

38. Alió JL, Rodríguez-Prats JL, Galal A, Ramzy M (2005) Outcomes of microincision cataract surgery versus coaxial phacoemulsification. Ophthalmology 112:1997–2003

39. Baikoff G (2006) Anterior segment OCT and phakic intraocular lenses: a perspective. J Cataract Refract Surg 32:1827–1835

40. Kim DY, Reinstein DZ, Silverman RH et al (1998) Very high frequency ultrasound analysis of a new phakic posterior chamber intraocular lens in situ. Am J Ophthalmol 125:725–729

41. Ferreira de Souza R, Allemann N, Forseto A et al (2003) Ultrasound biomicroscopy and Scheimpflug photography of angle-supported phakic intraocular lens for high myopia. J Cataract Refract Surg 29:1159–1166

42. Boker T, Sheqem J, Rauwolf M, Wegener A (1995) AC angle biometry: a comparison of Scheimpflug photography and ultrasound biomicroscopy. Ophthalmic Res 27(Suppl):104–109

43. Werner L, Izak AM, Pandey SK et al (2004) Correlation between different measurements within the eye relative to phakic intraocular lens implantation. J Cataract Refract Surg 30:1982–1988

44. Reinstein DZ, Archer TJ, Silverman RH, Coleman DJ (2006) Accuracy, repeatability, and reproducibility of Artemis very high-frequency digital ultrasound arc-scan lateral dimension measurements. J Cataract Refract Surg 23:1799–1802

45. Garcia-Feijoó J, Hernández-Matamoros JL, Castillo-Gomez A et al (2003) High-frequency ultrasound biomicroscopy of silicone posterior chamber phakic intraocular lens for hyperopia. J Cataract Refract Surg 29:1940–1946

46. Garcia-Feijoó J, Hernández-Matamoros JL, Mendez-Hernandez C et al (2003) Ultrasound biomicroscopy of silicone posterior chamber phakic intraocular lens for myopia. J Cataract Refract Surg 29:1932–1939

47. Izatt JA, Hee MR, Swanson EA et al (1994) Micrometer-scale resolution imaging of the anterior eye in vivo with optical coherence tomography. Arch Ophthalmol 112:1584–1589

48. Rondeau MJ, Barcsay G, Silverman RH et al (2004) Very high frequency ultrasound biometry of the anterior and posterior chamber diameter. J Refract Surg 20:454–464

Core Messages

■ Iris-supported phakic IOLs are available internationally from –23 to +12, and Toric lenses are available from –2.00 to –7.50 and from +2.00 to +7.50.

■ ARTISAN/ARTIFLEX is independent of the internal dimensions of the eye ("one size fits all").

■ Good selection of patients and good surgical techniques are the keys to avoid complications.

■ Complications include iris prolaps, bleeding, decentration, high intraocular pressure, postoperative inflammation, and endothelial cell loss. However, the complication rates of iris-supported phakic IOLs remain low.

13.2 Complications of Iris-Supported Phakic IOLs

Antonio A P. Marinho

13.2.1 Introduction

In this chapter, we try to show the possible complications associated with implantation of iris-supported phakic IOLs. As many of the complications found are related not to the lenses themselves, but to poor selection of the candidates for implantation or to somewhat rough surgery, we cover briefly both of these aspects after presenting the available models of iris-supported phakic IOLs.

13.2.2 Iris-Supported Phakic IOLs

The concept of implantation of an IOL supported by the mid-periphery of the iris was developed by Jan Worst for aphakia in 1979.The great success and safety of this implant led Jan Worst and Paul Fechner [15, 16] to implant the first iris-supported phakic IOL for myopia in1986. It was originally a biconcave lens, which was sometimes too close to the corneal endothelium, possibly causing damage. In 1991, the phakic IOL was redesigned to a safer planoconcave shape. This IOL was renamed ARTISAN in 1997. We describe summarily the different available iris-supported phakic IOLs, pointing to their material, optic diameter, and powers. All these lenses have in common the following characteristics [1, 5, 7, 8, 10, 12, 14, 23]:

■ Anterior chamber lenses consisting of an optic and two haptics
■ The haptics are in the form of a lobster claw to receive the enclavation of iris tissue.
■ The overall size of these lenses is 8.5 mm for all eyes

(except for a very rarely used pediatric model), so it is independent of the size of the anterior chamber. This is what we call "one size fits all."
■ All these lens are manufactured by OPHTEC (The Netherlands) and distributed worldwide by OPHTEC (ARTISAN/ARTIFLEX) and Advanced Medical Optics ([AMO] United States) under the brand names of Verisyse/Veryflex.

13.2.2.1 Characteristics of Different Models of Iris-Supported Phakic IOLs

■ Model 206, ARTISAN Myopia 5/8.5 mm
 – Material: PMMA
 – Optic: 5 mm
 – Power: –3.00 to –23.50 (Fig. 13.2.1)

■ Model 204, ARTISAN Myopia 6/8.5 mm
 – Material: PMMA
 – Optic: 6 mm
 – Power: –3.00 to –15.50 (Fig. 13.2.2)

■ Model 203, ARTISAN Hyperopia 5/8.5 mm
 Material: PMMA
 Optic: 5 mm
 Power: +1.00 to +12 (Fig. 13.2.3)

■ ARTISAN Toric 5/8.5 mm
 – Material: PMMA
 – Optic: 5 mm
 – Power: cylinder from –2.00 to –7.50, and +2.00 to +7.50. Both negative and positive cylinders are available at 0° (type A) and 90° (type B) (Figs. 13.2.4, 13.2.5).

■ ARTIFLEX Myopia 6/8.5 mm
 – Material: Polysiloxane (silicone) optic/PMMA haptics
 – Optic: 6 mm
 – Power: –3.00 to –14.5 (Fig. 13.2.6)

13.2.3 Patient Selection

The selection of candidates for implantation of ARTISAN/ARTIFLEX follows the general rules of refractive surgery, such as 1–21 years minimum age (an exception is pediatric anisometropia), with a stable refraction. Absence of intraocular vascular (diabetes) or inflammatory (uveitis) dis-

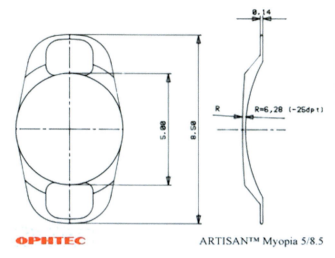

Fig 13.2.1 ARTISAN Model 206 (Myopia PMMA 5 mm)

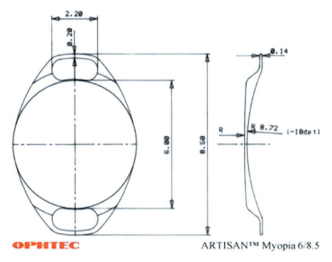

Fig 13.2.2 ARTISAN Model 204 (Myopia PMMA 6 mm)

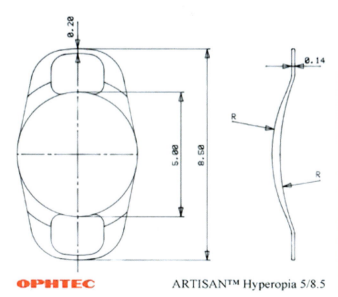

Fig 13.2.3 ARTISAN Model 203 (Hyperopia PMMA 5 mm)

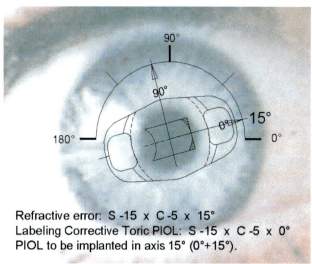

Refractive error: S -15 x C -5 x 15°
Labeling Corrective Toric PIOL: S -15 x C -5 x 0°
PIOL to be implanted in axis 15° (0°+15°).

Fig 13.2.4 Toric ARTISAN (type A)

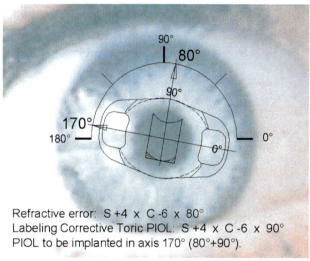

Refractive error: S +4 x C -6 x 80°
Labeling Corrective Toric PIOL: S +4 x C -6 x 90°
PIOL to be implanted in axis 170° (80°+90°).

Fig 13.2.5 Toric ARTISAN (type B)

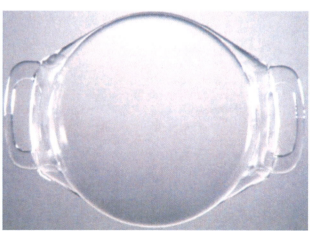

Fig 13.2.6 ARTIFLEX (foldable)

eases is also mandatory. As the IOL will be implanted in the anterior chamber, it is very important to be sure that no damage is inflicted to the corneal endothelium. The anterior chamber depth must be carefully measured. Classically, it was stated that an anterior chamber depth (from endothelium to natural lens) should be at least 2.8 mm. However, the central anterior chamber depth is not the main issue; because of the shape of the cornea (dome-shaped) and the great thickness of the lens in periphery (myopia lens), the critical distance between the IOL and the endothelium must be 1.5 mm [1] (Fig. 13.2.7). This measurement is not available by ultrasound biometry or Orbscan (Bausch & Lomb). Although there are data that provide parameters for this distance from the central anterior chamber depth and the power of the IOL, it is much safer to simulate the implantation and actually measure the distances with devices such as the anterior chamber OCT (Visante, Zeiss, Germany). Devices like this will certainly be clinical routine in the near future.

Despite the safety of these lenses to the corneal endothelium, we must not implant ARTISAN/ARTIFLEX in eyes with endothelial disease. Endothelial cell count of at least 2,400 cells/mm^2 and absence of significant polymegathism and polymorphism are criteria for implantation (except in eyes after penetrating keratoplasty, in which lower counts can be accepted).

One last very important point concerning the inclusion/exclusion criteria for implantation of ARTISAN/ ARTIFLEX deals with the shape of the iris. Eyes with a convex iris (mostly hyperopes) should not be implanted with this kind of phakic IOL [6, 17].

13.2.4 Surgery

It is very important to review in detail the surgical technique of implantation of ARTISAN/ARTIFLEX, because many of the complications associated with these IOLs are caused by an imperfect surgery, and so complications can be avoided if the rules are strictly followed for each step [4].

13.2.4.1 Preoperative Preparation
Before surgery, we must constrict the pupil. In most patients, two or three drops of 2% pilocarpine are enough. Alternatively, you may achieve the same goal by using intracameral acetylcholine. If you are planning a peribulbar/retrobulbar anesthesia, then a perfusion of intravenous Mannitol may be useful to reduce vitreous pressure (see next section).

13.2.4.2 Anesthesia
ARTISAN/ARTIFLEX can be implanted with different types of anesthesia. Generally, we think general anesthesia is the most adequate for the procedure, and it is mandatory for the inexperienced surgeon. Retrobulbar/peribulbar

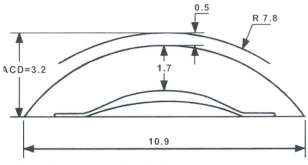

ARTISAN® Hyperopia 5/8.5 (Ref. 203)

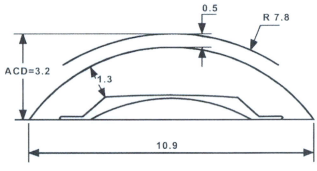

ARTISAN® Myopia 5/8.5 (Ref. 206)

Fig 13.2.7 Critical distances to the endothelium in myopia (bottom) and hyperopia (top)

block is not recommended, because it is usually associated with increased vitreous pressure and consequent shallowing of the anterior chamber, increasing surgical difficulty. Topical anesthesia is possible with ARTIFLEX (small incision), especially when the surgery is performed by an experienced surgeon.

13.2.4.3 Surgical Steps
The first surgical step (common to all these lenses) is to implement two side ports. These side ports are classically done at the 10 and 2 o'clock positions (assuming the main incision is at 12 o'clock), but their location can change according to the desired position of the IOL. These side ports must be 1.5-mm wide. After completing the side ports, the anterior chamber is filled with cohesive, viscoelastic material. Dispersive viscoelastics should never be employed. The next step is the main incision. When using PMMA IOLs the incision is 5.2 or 6.2 mm, according to the model. The incision can be clear corneal, sclerocorneal, or scleral, with or without a tunnel. The importance of the location of the incision relates to the possible induction of astigmatism with these large incisions. In most hands, slightly posterior incisions give better results. When implanting ARTIFLEX, a clear-cornea 3.2-mm incision is the rule [7, 8]. The IOL is then introduced in the anterior chamber and rotated to the desired position. This position is critical when implanting Toric ARTISAN [4, 10, 12, 14]. In this case, we must de-

fine the axis of implantation by marking the limbus with a surgical pen (preferably sitting to avoid cyclotorsion). In all the other models, the axis of implantation is irrelevant. Once the ARTISAN/ARTIFLEX is in the proper position, we proceed to the most critical point of the surgery–the enclavation. In this step, the ARTISAN/ARTIFLEX is fixated to the midperiphery of the iris. We achieve this fixation with a bimanual technique (Fig. 13.2.8). One hand holds the IOL with a forceps–with ARTISAN, the forceps holds the optic of the lens [4], while with ARTIFLEX, as the optic is soft, special forceps were designed to hold the haptics [7, 8]. With the other hand, a blunt "needle" is introduced through the side port and a sufficient amount of iris tissue is introduced (enclavate) in the claw of the haptic. This is repeated in both haptics. It is very important at this stage to check the correct and the perfect centration of the ARTISAN/ARTIFLEX with the pupil. In this type of phakic IOL, the centering of the IOL is the exclusive responsibility of the surgeon. The next step consists of performing a small iridotomy or iridectomy (this can also be done with YAG laser capsulotomy preoperatively). After completing the iridotomy/iridectomy, the viscoelastic material must be completely removed. We usually use passive irrigation to achieve this goal. The last step of the surgery is the suture of the incision for ARTISAN and simple hydration of the wound for ARTIFLEX (sutureless surgery).

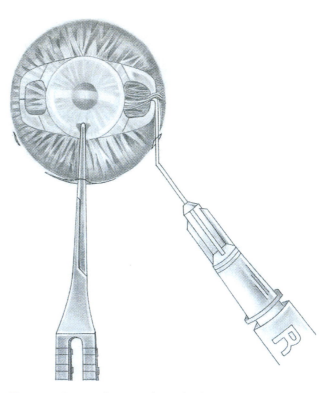

Fig 13.2.8 Fixating the IOL to the iris (enclavation using the needle)

13.2.4.4 Postoperative Care

At the end of the surgery, a subconjunctival injection of antibiotic and steroids is recommended. The postoperative regimen consists of topical Ofloxacin and topical prednisone acetate four times daily for 2 weeks. Oral prednisone for a week is recommended in patients with heavily pigmented eyes.

13.2.5 Complications

The complications related to the implantation of iris-supported phakic IOLs can be divided into three groups. Short-term complications are those found during surgery or in the first postoperative days. Medium-term complications occur during the first 3 weeks postoperatively and long-term complications are those beyond that period of time [3,9,18].

13.2.5.1 Short-Term Complications

The most common complications found during implantation of ARTISAN are iris prolapse and loss of anterior chamber depth [3]. These problems are related to the large incision (5.2 or 6.2 mm) and mostly to high vitreous pressure. This high vitreous pressure is related mostly to patient anxiety and high volume of retrobulbar/peribulbar anesthetic. This loss of anterior chamber makes the surgery very difficult and usually leads to other complications. The best way to avoid it is to use general anesthesia, and if peribulbar is needed, association of preoperative Mannitol can help. In the presence of iris prolapse, an iridectomy/iridotomy should be performed immediately; usually the eye calms down, and the surgery may continue. These two complications are very rarely observed with ARTIFLEX, as the small incision (3.2 mm) allows us to work in a closed system [7, 8, 23].

Bleeding can occur during surgery. If the iris is pulled too vigorously during the enclavation process, we can observe some bleeding from the root of the iris. In addition, when performing iridectomy, bleeding is possible. Generally, this complication is avoided with gentle surgery, and if bleeding does occur, it is usually stopped easily by putting some viscoelastic in the bleeding site. Postoperative hyphema is exceptional.

Centration of the IOL and sufficient amount of iris tissue enclavated in the haptic (grasp) are very important, and failure to achieve these will lead to later complications. The suture, when needed (ARTISAN) must be astigmatic free.

Corneal edema may be present in the first day after surgery. It usually caused by a traumatic surgery with excessive manipulation. It is a more common complication during the learning curve of the procedure, or if the surgical conditions of the eye are not perfect (loss of anterior chamber). This edema generally goes away in a matter of days, but later damage to the endothelium is possible. It is easily avoidable with good surgery and adequate surgical conditions.

Another complication seldom seen but possible in the first days postop is a flat anterior chamber with the possible touch of the IOL to the cornea. This flat anterior chamber can occur in two different settings. We can observe a flat anterior chamber with low ocular pressure or with high ocular pressure. In the former case, it is due to inadequate closure of the surgical incision. In this condition, the suture must be fixed. More serious is the latter situation of a flat anterior chamber with high ocular pressure. This can be related to retained viscoelastic, but more often to not patent iridectomy. In this situation, we must immediately to avoid the risk of a permanent dilated pupil (Urrets-Zavalia syndrome). YAG laser iridotomy usually solves the problem.

The most feared complication in the first days postoperatively is the infectious endophthalmitis. In this exceptional event (common to every intraocular surgery) routine endophthalmitis treatment (systemic and intravitreal) must be used.

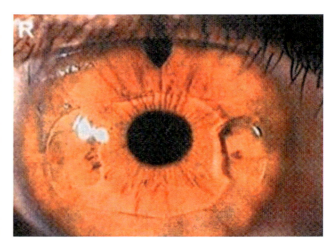

Fig 13.2.9 Decentered ARTISAN

13.2.5.2 Medium-Term Complications

In the first 3 months after the surgery, some complications may occur. As we shall see, they are mostly related to poor surgery or failure to follow the guidelines for patient selection.

During the first 2 weeks postoperatively, high ocular pressure is sometimes present. This is due to the topical steroids. Suspension of the steroids brings the pressure to normal levels, and no further treatment is needed. However, the most important complications in this period are optical and inflammatory in nature. The most common optical complication is the complaint of halos and glare. This is more frequent if the optic is small (5 mm) or the pupil is large. Decentration of the IOL (even slight) (Fig. 13.2.9) may cause a lot of halos and glare, especially if the lens is decentered superiorly. To avoid (or to minimize) this problem, centration of the IOL must be carefully done, and we should not implant patients with mesopic pupil larger than the optic of the ARTISAN/ARTIFLEX [3, 9]. If we find a decentered IOL with symptoms in the postoperative period surgical recentering of the lens is advised. Although halos and glare may be present in patients with perfect surgeries and normal pupils, these symptoms tend to wane over time, and it is exceptional (we never done it personally) to have to explant the lens.

Another optical problem we may find is the induction of astigmatism. This can occur with Toric ARTISAN if the IOL is not implanted in the right axis, or in ARTISAN if the suture is poorly constructed. Doing slightly posterior incisions (avoiding clear cornea) reduces the risk. It also very important in Toric ARTISAN to mark carefully (sitting position) the axis of implantation. To manage this complication, we may try to do a new suture, but most often more reliably, we manage the residual astigmatism with laser corneal surgery (if corneal conditions allow). With ARTIFLEX, we never observed any significant change in astigmatism [7, 8, 23].

However, the most feared complications in the first 3 months after surgery are inflammatory complications [6,17]. Acute uveitis immediately after surgery is a rare event and is usually associated with a very traumatic surgery. Standard uveitis treatment solves the problem. Pigment deposits on the surface of the lens are commonly observed between 2 weeks and 3 months. These pigment deposits are asymptomatic, tend to disappear with time, and do not require treatment. These pigment deposits are seen in both ARTISAN and ARTIFLEX lenses. Giant cell deposits have also been observed in some eyes implanted with ARTIFLEX (Fig. 13.2.10). In these cases, there is normally decrease of visual acuity, with only very mild inflammatory signs. In our personal series of 120 eyes implanted with ARTIFLEX, these giant cell deposits have been observed in 4 eyes [7, 8, 23]. To avoid this complication, we suggest the subconjunctival injection of steroids at the end of the surgery. If these deposits occur, then topical and oral steroid treatments lead to full recovery.

Late-onset uveitis (after 3 weeks of surgery) associated with cyclitic membranes and posterior synechiae have been described mostly in hyperopic eyes. This is due to special anatomic conditions of the iris (convex iris) [6, 17]. As was stated above (in Sect. 13.2.3), this form of the iris is a contraindication for the implantation of these lenses. In the presence of such a situation, aggressive therapy with oral and topical steroids should be implemented. If the treatment does not succeed or the situation recurs, then explantation is recommended.

13.2.5.3 Long-Term Complications

One possible complication observed later than 3 months after surgery (may also be seen sooner) is the luxation of the IOL [3, 9]. This means that one (Fig. 13.2.11) (exceptionally both) haptic of the IOL became free from the iris tissue, leading to the luxation of the IOL. This is always due to insufficient amount of iris tissue enclavated in the claw of the lens (weak grasp). A good grasp definitively avoids this problem. In the event of a luxation of an iris-supported phakic IOL, surgical reposition must be done immediately, as the loose lens may damage the corneal endothelium.

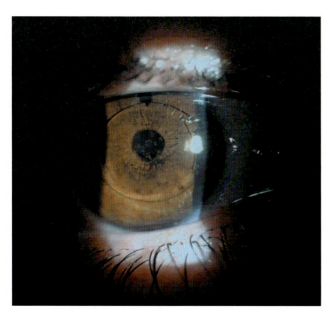

Fig 13.2.10 ARTIFLEX with pigment deposits

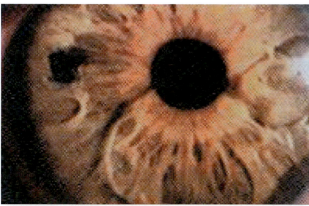

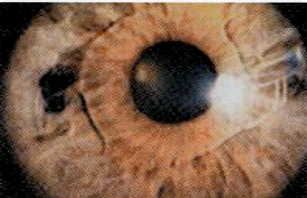

Fig 13.2.11 Luxation of ARTISAN (top) and after management (bottom)

The relationship between phakic IOLs (mostly anterior chamber) and corneal endothelium has been widely discussed. Several studies concerning the affect of ARTISAN

implantation and endothelial cell loss have been done. The most complete study is the European Multicenter Study published in 2000 [13], where 518 eyes implanted with AR-TISAN showed a loss of endothelial cell count of 4.8% at 3 months (surgically induced), but only a further loss of 1.7% at 2 years and a 0.4% at 3 years. Most other published studies (however much smaller) show similar results [2, 14, 19, 20, 23]. A classic paper by Perez Santonja et al. [22] in 1996 stated important losses of endothelial cells in eyes implanted with ARTISAN. In this paper however, there is no relationship of these losses with power of the implanted IOLs and the anterior chamber depths. Of course, if the anterior chamber is not deep enough, then endothelial cell loss will occur. Personal data show that ARTISAN/ARTIFLEX are safe for the corneal endothelium as long as the selection criteria for implantation are met [7–9]. Nevertheless, it is advised to check the corneal endothelium yearly after surgery and to explant if endothelial cell count or shape (polymorphism, polymegathism) degrades significantly.

Being at a safe distance from the natural lens, the iris-supported phakic IOLs do not induce anterior subcapsular cataract, as do the posterior chamber phakic IOLs. However, some nuclear cataracts have been observed in eyes implanted with ARTISAN. These nuclear cataracts are age related, but in implanted eyes tend to be present at younger age (late forties, early fifties). The reason for this is not clear, but it has been suggested that the opening of the eye during surgery or the misdirection of the aqueous humor (due to the iridectomy) may account for the earlier development of nuclear cataracts [11, 18, 21] .

13.2.6 Conclusion

Like any surgery, the implantation of iris-supported phakic IOLs can be associated with many complications. What is important at this point is to differentiate the complications related to the IOL itself from those arising from other factors such as the selection of candidates for implantation or the surgical technique. The most frequent complications are:

- Complications due to incorrect surgery (or anesthesia)
  Iris prolapse
  Hyphema
  Endothelial touch (corneal edema; endothelial cell loss);
  IOL decentration (glare)
  Induced astigmatism (ARTISAN)
  IOL luxation (weak grasp)
  Acute uveitis
- Complications due to poor selection of candidates for implantation
  Late-onset uveitis with posterior synechia (convex iris);
  Endothelial cell loss (shallow anterior chamber)
  Glare and halos (large pupils)

Take-Home Pearls

■ Most of the complications associated with the implantation of ARTISAN/ARTIFLEX Phakic IOLs are surgeon related, and so easily avoidable with a good selection of candidates and a perfect surgery.

■ In the selection of candidates, special attention should be paid to the depth of the anterior chamber and to the shape of the iris. Patients with shallow anterior chambers and convex iris must be excluded.

■ During surgery, the key points to avoid problems are non-traumatic surgery and a sufficient amount of iris tissue enclavated in the haptics.

■ Following these guidelines, the implantation of these IOLs is virtually complication free.

References

1. Ophtec (2004) Lens power calculation and critical distance. ARTISAN phakic IOL training manual. Ophtec BV, The Netherlands

2. Budo C (2004) Clinical results. In: Budo C (ed) The ARTISAN Lens. Highlights of Ophthalmology International, El Dorado, Republic of Panama

3. Budo C (2004) Complications. In: Budo C (ed) The ARTISAN lens. Highlights of Ophthalmology International, El Dorado, Republic of Panama

4. Budo C (2004) Surgical procedures. In: Budo C (2004) The ARTISAN Lens. In: Budo C (ed) The ARTISAN lens. Highlights of Ophthalmology International, El Dorado, Republic of Panama

5 Budo C (2004) Types of lenses and applications. In: Budo C (ed) The ARTISAN lens. Highlights of Ophthalmology International, El Dorado, Republic of Panama

6. Izak M, Izak A (2004) Inflammatory reaction associated with ARTISAN phakic refractive IOL implantation. In: Budo C (ed) The ARTISAN lens. Highlights of Ophthalmology International, El Dorado, Republic of Panama

7. Marinho A (2005) ARTIFLEX: a new phakic IOL. In: Garg A, Pandey S, Chang D et al (eds) Advances in ophthalmology 2. Jaypee Brothers, New Delhi

8. Marinho A, ARTIFLEX: a new phakic IOL. In: Garg A, Pandey S, Chang D et al (eds) Advances in ophthalmology 2. Jaypee Brothers, New Delhi

9. Marinho A, Salgado R (2005) Complications of phakic IOLs. In: Garg A, Alió J, Marinho A et al (eds) Lens-based refractive surgery (phakic IOLs). Jaypee Brothers, New Delhi

10. Marinho A, Salgado R (2005) Toric Phakic IOLs. In: Garg A, Alió J, Marinho A et al (eds) Lens-based refractive surgery (phakic IOLs). Jaypee Brothers, New Delhi

11. Alió J et al (1999) Phakic anterior chamber lenses for the correction of myopia: a 7 year cumulative analysis of complications in 263 cases. Ophthalmology 106:458–466

12. Bartels M, Santana N, Budo C et al (2006) Toric phakic intraocular lens for the correction of hyperopia and astigmatism. J Cataract Refract Surg 32:243–249

13. Budo C, Hessloehl J, Izak M (2000) Multicenter study of the ARTISAN phakic intraocular lens. J Cataract Refract Surg 26:1163–1171

14. Dick H, Alió J, Bianchetti M et al (2003) Toric phakic intraocular lens: European multicenter study. Ophthalmology 110:150–162

15. Fechner P, van der Hejde G, Worst J (1989) The correction of myopia by lens implantation into phakic eyes. Am J Ophthalmol 107:659–663

16. Fechner P, Wichman W (1993) Correction of myopia by implantation of minus optic (worst iris claw) lenses in the anterior chamber of phakic eyes. Eur J Imp Ref Surg 5:55–59

17. Izak M (1998) Surgical trauma not lens design is responsible for myopia claw IOL irritation. Ocular Surgery News 9:38

18. Marinho A (2006) Phakic IOLs: what could go wrong? Ophthalmol Times 2:29–33

19. Menezo JL, Cisneros A, Cervera M et al (1994) Iris claw phakic lens immediate and long-term corneal endothelial changes. Eur J Implant Refract Surg 6:195–199

20. Menezo JL, Cisneros A, Rodriguez-Salvador V (1998) Endothelial study of iris claw phakic lens. Four-year follow-up. J Cataract Refract Surg 24:1039–1049

21. Menezo JL, Peris-Martinez C, Cisneros A et al (2004) Rate of cataract formation in 343 highly myopic eyes after implantation of three types of phakic intraocular lenses. J Refract Surg 20:317–324

22. Perez-Santonja J, Iradier M,Sanz-Iglesias L et al (1996) Endothelial changes in phakic eyes with anterior chamber intraocular lenses to correct high myopia. J Cataract Refract Surg 22:1017–1022

23. Tehrani M, Dick H (2005) Short-term follow-up after implantation of a foldable iris-fixated intraocular lens in phakic eyes. Ophthalmology 112:2189–2195

13

Core Messages

■ Collamer® posterior chamber phakic IOL (Visian ICL™) implantation is a predictable and effective method to correct high myopia and hyperopia. Toric phakic IOLs (TICL™) are currently available to correct combined high astigmatisms, including stable keratoconus and post-keratoplasty eyes.

■ Current ICL models show better clinical outcomes and a decrease in the incidence of cataracts postoperatively.

■ To guarantee their long term safety, these lenses require a thorough preoperative anatomical evaluation of the anterior segment with specialized high-resolution biometry technologies, such as VHF ultrasonography and dedicated software to size their overall length.

■ Most of the complications related to the use of modern ICL models may be avoided by adequate preoperative implant sizing and a proper surgical technique.

13.3 Complications of Posterior Chamber Phakic Intraocular Lenses

Carlo F. Lovisolo and Fabio Mazzolani

13.3.1 Introduction

Posterior chamber intraocular lenses (IOLs), also called sulcus or lens-supported phakic IOLs, are widely used today. Their implantation through minimally invasive procedures is likely to produce excellent results in terms of precision, predictability, and stability of the refractive outcome [34, 45, 49, 54, 56, 57, 65]. When compared with eyes that receive a myopic conventional laser-assisted in situ keratomileusis (LASIK) procedure, the postoperative quality of vision has been shown to be better in the implanted eyes, yielding significantly less higher-order aberrations [55, 59]. The outstanding outcomes reported after implantation of toric optics [58] have allowed authors to expand indications to highly astigmatic patients, including stable keratoconus [10] and post-keratoplasty eyes. Refractive inaccuracies may be easily adjusted with complementary fine-tuning excimer laser corneal surgeries [7, 51, 70]. In the event of implanting a lens with an inadequate size, or with reported visual symptoms, the implants can be removed or exchanged with an anastigmatic small incision, permitting potential reversibility to the preoperative condition [34, 63].

However, as a consequence of the anatomic site of fixation–posterior chamber phakic IOLs are vaulted between the iris posterior pigmented layers and the anterior crystalline lens with the anterior zonules–these implants may possibly cause acute angle closure and/or malignant glau-

coma, ischemic "blown" pupil (Urretz-Zavalia syndrome), pigmentary dispersion syndrome, anterior subcapsular cataract, damage to the zonules with dislocation, and chronic uveal inflammation [12, 14, 37, 21, 28, 29, 51, 52, 66, 67].

13.3.2 Posterior Chamber Phakic IOLs

Since the original "collar button" silicone lens introduced by Fyodorov in the early 1980s [23], some different models have been proposed through the years, but only one has reached a successful, widespread use, the Visian ICL™ (STAAR Surgical, Monrovia, Calif.) [34]. The "top hat" elastomer lenses provided by Adatomed (Munich, Germany) in the mid-1990s [35, 40] have been abandoned due to significant inflammatory complications and to the fibrotic changes induced to the anterior crystalline lens, though no convincing evidence has been published as to whether these complications were due to hydrophobic properties of the low refractive index silicone material or to the design contour.

Although thousands of new-generation silicone models (PRL™, Zeiss-Meditec, Jena, Germany) were implanted in Europe with satisfactory refractive outcomes [18, 19], a significant decentration rate (about 10% in our experience, versus 0% of the ICL) [37] and the concerns about some design-related severe complications anecdotally reported at meetings, mainly zonular damage and dislocation into the vitreous chamber, are the reasons why the PRL is now slowly falling into disuse worldwide.

At the time of writing, newcomer acrylic material models, like the Sticklens™ (IOLTECH, La Rochelle, France), the Epi.Lens™ (AcriTec, Henningsdorf, Germany), and the ThinOpt-X™ (Medford Lakes, N.J.) are in the very early phases of experimental trial application and only preliminary reports have been heard.

This chapter summarizes the use of ICL and its most relevant complications. Particular attention is paid to lens implant sizing and the new safety guidelines based on internal anatomy provided by specialized biometry techniques, such as very high frequency (VHF) ultrasonography and a dedicated software [37].

13.3.2.1 The Visian ICL

The ICL is made of Collamer®, a so-called collagen–copolymer material where the addition of a 0.2% collagen to the silicone (60% poly-HEMA) makes the implant more hydrophilic (36% water) and more permeable to gas and nutrients. ICL by attracting the deposition on its surface of a monolayer of fibronectin, which inhibits aqueous protein binding, is more biocompatible with the nearby structures [61].

After the first prototypes were implanted in Italy and Austria in the fall of 1993 [1, 8], several clone models followed, with variations of the built-in vault height (Fig. 13.3.1a). Current ICL models (V4 or Version Four for myopia, V3 or Version Three for hyperopia) marketed in Europe are measured in a bath of NaCl solution. The ICL is a rectangular, 7-mm wide lens implant, available in four

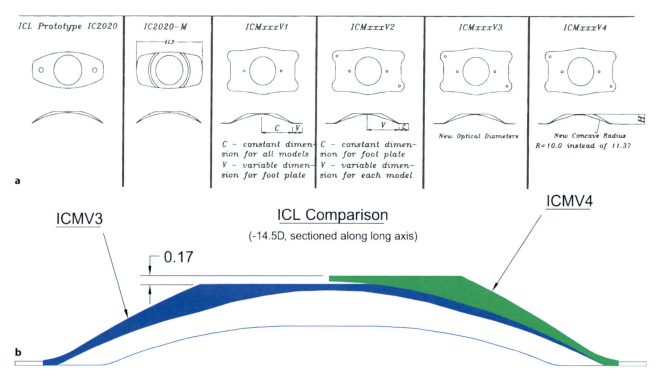

Fig. 13.3.1 Technical drawings of successive generations of myopic ICL (**a**) and direct comparison of the last model (V4) versus the previous one (V3) (**b**)

overall lengths (11.5, 12, 12.5 and 13 mm for the myopic lenses, called ICM; 11, 11.5, 12 and 12.5 mm for the hyperopic ones, called ICH). The optic diameter ranges from 4.65 to 5.5 mm in the ICMs, depending on the dioptric power, and is always 5.5 mm for ICHs. The basic design change of the most used V4 ICM is in the vaulting. In an attempt to increase the clearance from the anterior crystalline lens surface, and therefore to minimize the risk of iatrogenic subcapsular anterior opacities, the V4 has an additional 0.13–0.21 mm of anterior vault height, due to the steeper radius of curvature of the base curve and depending on the dioptric power (Fig. 13.3.1b) [34]. When implanted into the intraocular environment or immersed into balanced salt solution (BSS), the ICL swells, thus increasing its dimensions to about 5.2%. So the lens implant width becomes 7.37 mm, an optic of 5 mm corresponds to 5.26 mm and an overall length of 13 to13.6 mm. In the US market, the lenses are labeled based on measurements taken in BSS rather than NaCl.

For comparative reasons, the overall ICL patient population was divided into three groups based on the lens model implanted and the method utilized for choosing its overall length.

1. Group A: 139 myopic eyes implanted with first- to third-generation ICLs (41 ICLs implanted with the forceps, 98 lenses injected), from September 1993 until April 1998, with a mean follow-up of 39 months (maximum:14 years).

2. Group B: 401 myopic eyes implanted with the last-generation (V4, Version Four) ICL sized according to the "white-to-white, +0.5-mm rule of thumb" (from April 1998 until December 2003). The mean follow-up was 37 months (maximum: 9 years).

3. Group C: 287 myopic eyes implanted from January 2002 to June 2007, with the last model (V4), including toric correction (V4 TICL), whose sizing was made with a software based on the ciliary sulcus dimensions (sulcus to sulcus) obtained with the Artemis 2 (Ultralink, St. Petersburg, Fla.) VHF echographer and the Lovisolo Custom ICL Sizer [37, 48]. The mean follow-up was 29 months (maximum: 65 months).

Table 13.3.1 shows a comparison of complication rates among the three groups and group D, including the data provided by the STAAR International Vigilance Office on the eyes implanted with the pre-V4 generation of ICL, September 1993 to January 1998 [34, 36], and group E, presenting the results of the post-V4 ICL eyes enrolled in the long-term, multicenter STAAR Myopic Implantable Contact Lens trial, which led to US Food and Drug Administration (FDA) approval in late 2005 [57].

13.3.3 Intraoperative Complications

Intraoperative complications are extremely rare and almost exclusively connected to human error in the surgical tech-

Table 13.3.1 Synopsis of complication rates (percentages) in different populations of ICL-implanted myopic eyes

Complication	Group A (n = 139)	Group B (n = 401)	Group C (n = 287)	Group D (n = 1,285)	Group E (n = 526)
Safety index	91.7	108.9	127.4	NR	105
Eyes in the ±1.00-D range at 6 month	73.1	91.4	100	78.4	99
Disabling visual symptoms	0.8	0	0	0.2	0.6
Intraoperative ICL tear	2.6	0.5	0	NR	NR
Inverted implantation	1.7	1	0	NR	NR
Explantation–replacement	2.6	0.5	0	0.4	1.7
Corneal haze/edema after 1 week postoperatively (endothelial cell loss >30%)	0.8	0.25	0	NR	0
3-year cumulative endothelial cell loss	11.6	5.8	2.8	7.7	8.4–9.7
Non-disabling halos	7.9	4.75	5.8	NR	NR
Decentration >0.5 mm	7.9	0	0	1.2	0
Late anterior chamber dislocation	0.8	0	0	0	0
Late vitreous dislocation	0	0	0	0	0
Maculopathy	1.6	1.5	0.9	0.2	NR
Retinal detachment	0.8	0.25	0.3	0.2	0.6
Atonic pupil (Urretz-Zavalia syndrome)	3.2	0.25	0	0.4	NR
Pupil ovalization–iridopathy	1.6	0.75	0	NR	NR
Endophthalmitis	0	0.25	0	0	0
Malignant glaucoma	0.8	0	0	0.1	0
Angle closure glaucoma	6.4	3	0.6	0.9	NR
Open angle/pigmentary glaucoma (IOP >25 mmHg or >10-mmHg increase)	0.8	0	0	0.6	0.2
Increased IOP on medications	16.9	2.5	0	NR	0.4
Anterior subcapsular lens opacities	8.2	1.75	0	1	2.7a
Clinically significant cataract	5.6	0.75	0	0.4	1.4b

NR not reported

[a] Most of these opacities are early, presumably surgically induced

[b] All the cataract are found in the subgroup of myopia >10 D

nique (Fig. 13.3.2). Given their reduced thickness (less than 100 μm in the footplate and the thinnest part of the optic), ICLs are extremely delicate and should be handled with great care to avoid splits and tears. The most frequent cause of a torn lens is an incorrect loading technique (Fig. 13.3.3). In our learning curve (our first 30 cases when we used a metal head injector designed for aphakic top hat silicone lenses), we registered an incidence of one out of ten damaged ICLs, from minor (allowing safe implantation) to major damages (requiring postponement of intervention). In our last 500 cases, the incidence of that complication was 0%. In certain cases, we must deal with sticky, upbent haptics–tricky to detach inside the eye and always requiring the patience of an expert "butterfly surgeon" for additional manipulations (Fig. 13.3.4) [34]. The injection of an upside-down lens may also happen. With the first ICL models, whose footplates had no landmarks, the inverted implantation was more frequent and difficult to recognize. Thus, many surgeons preferred using the forceps technique to achieve maximum control of the intraocular opening of

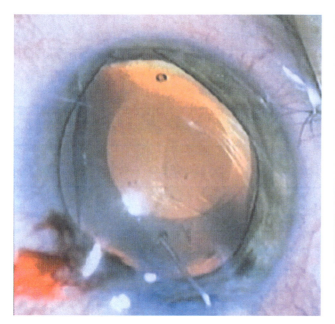

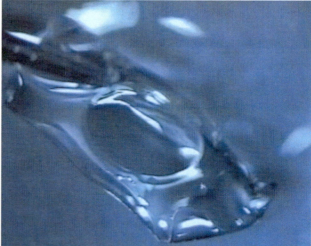

Fig. 13.3.4 Upbent haptics

Fig. 13.3.2 Iatrogenic intra-operative Y-shaped lens opacity that appeared immediately after unwanted contact between the tip of the spatula and the anterior lens capsule

13

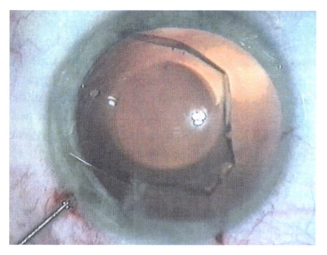

Fig. 13.3.3 Total fracture of the proximal haptic. The ICL must be removed and replaced

the lens. With the latest models, the surgeon can easily intervene by pronosupinating the hand, keeping monomanual shooter before the optic has completely unfolded and overturn the implant. If, however, an inverted implantation does occur, then the surgeon should never try to turn the lens around inside the anterior segment, because of the high risk of damaging the crystalline lens or the corneal endothelium. The recommended solution is to enlarge the incision to 3.5–4 mm, to remove the lens with specially textured forceps (Lovisolo ICL Removal Forceps, American Surgical Instruments Corporation, Westmont, Ill.) under the protection of a viscoelastic substance, and to reim-

plant it with appropriate forceps. Then, a suture could be required to ensure incision tightness and astigmatic neutrality. The same technique should be used in the event of an ICL exchange [34], when replacing is needed because of inadequate optical performance or sizing, or alternatively, if the surgeon has to perform a cataract extraction procedure (bilensectomy) (Fig. 13.3.5).

Intra-operative pupillary block can occur if the surgeon does not perform completely patent yttrium aluminum garnet (YAG) peripheral iridotomies in the preliminary workup, or alternately, if he/she overfills the globe with an excessive amount of viscoelastic or the irrigation bottle is placed too high. It may be useful to avoid the pressure thrust linked to fluids (viscoelastic and balanced saline solution), lower the height of the irrigation bottle, and relax the patient. If this does not help, the surgeon must perform a surgical iridectomy.

13.3.4 Postoperative Complications

13.3.4.1 Visual Outcomes

13.3.4.1.1 Loss of Best Corrected Visual Acuity

We evaluated the safety of the ICL procedure by comparing the postoperative best-spectacle corrected visual acuity (BSCVA) in Snellen lines with the preoperative values of BSCVA. A safety index ≥100 would indicate that BSCVA lines are not lost as a result of surgery–in contrast with a value of <100, which indicates BSCVA was better prior to surgery–and that the procedure can be reasonably considered safe. Respectively, the mean safety indexes were 91.7±21.6, 108.9 ±17.1, and 127.4±26.3 in groups A, B, and C, respectively. In group C, the index was ≥100 for all patients. The differences between groups A and B, B and C, and A and C were statistically significant (p < 0.001).

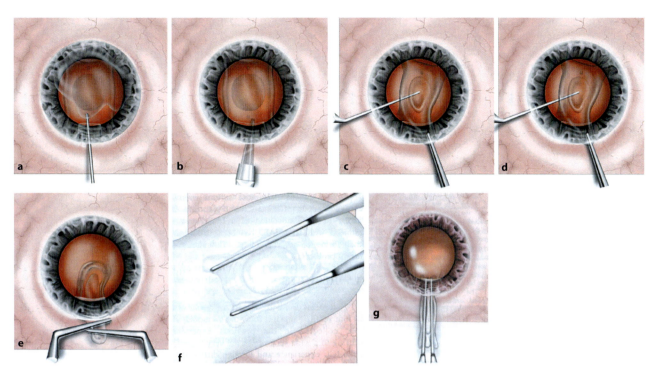

Fig. 13.3.5 Suggested ICL-removal technique. **a** Inject Healon above and below the ICL. **b** Enlarge the incision to 4 mm, with a calibrated knife. **c** Catch the right proximal footplate with Lovisolo ICL Removal Forceps and pull it toward the incision. The finely sandblasted tips firmly grasp the lens without damaging it. **d** As soon as the haptic starts to appear from the incision, using a second forceps catch the footplate perpendicular to the first (tangentially to the limbus) and continue pulling outward. **e** Release the first hold and catch with the other hand in a direction parallel to the second, repeating the maneuver two to three times, until the most part of the lens is outside the eye. Never go below the ICL with the forceps arms in the central zone to avoid damaging the anterior crystalline lens. **f** Extract the lens and wash it with BSS. **g** Fold it using Lovisolo ICL Loading Forceps and reinsert it with the forceps technique

13.3.4.1.2 Overcorrection and Undercorrection

Toric ICLs (TICLs) require an astigmatically neutral surgical incision and robust fixation site to provide rotational stability over time, as the cylinder correction decreases with increasing deviation of the lens implant from the target axis by following a non-linear relationship. To prevent rotation of a small implant, again, precise sizing is essential.

As shown in a study where the position of 30 TICLs sized with VHF echography was documented by superimposable slit lamp photographs [37], the mean lens deviation from the original meridian over time (3 years) was less than 5°, i.e., compatible with a maximum of 10% loss of astigmatic correction in all cases.

If we consider the threshold range of ±1.00 D as a significant level of over or undercorrection, the predictability of the ICL refractive outcome showed a great improvement, 26.9% in group A, to 9.6% of group B, and to 2.6% in group C, where 88.1% of eyes were within the ±0.50 D range.

As for refractive stability of the ICL, at 6 months almost 97% of the myopic eyes were within the ±0.50-D range, significantly better than the average 82% obtainable with excimer laser surgery [53]. However, when evaluated at the 2-year gate, most of the eyes showed a limited regression, such that the ratio decreased to 68% (as a comparison, ±0.50-D range stability with LASIK is 77%), possibly due to a reduction of vault height that we observed over time in all implanted eyes (unpublished data) or a progression of the myopia. We now therefore aim at a slight overcorrection (+0.50 sphere) in all patients younger than 38 years.

13.3.4.1.3 Quality of Vision Disturbances

Different degrees of nighttime visual disturbances when driving vehicles [39] are spontaneously reported by 5–8% of our ICL patients, although only one patient (one eye in group A) requested the removal of the ICL for these complaints. No significant differences were noticed among the three groups (p = 0.852, p = 0.196, p = 0.087). Visual symptoms under dim light conditions are caused by mesopic entrance pupil diameters that do not match small optic sizes, whose edges consequently cause higher-order aberrations, mainly spherical aberration, of the retinal image. The deeper the chamber and the steeper the corneal curvature, the greater the effect. Binocular infrared pupillometry, a helpful tool to predict these side effects, has shown that scotopic pupil diameter in young myopic patients–the average candidates to ICL surgery–is significantly larger than in the emmetropic group. Our observations on Caucasians myopic eyes, ranging from 21 to 39 years of age, showed a mean scotopic pupil diameter of 6.87±0.72 mm, the range of minimum-maximum values going from 5.6 to 8.9 mm. For surgeons used to judge the pupil size on the corneal plane, an approximate mean conversion rate of 1.26 for the ICL-equivalent optical zone versus the LASIK one should be applied (Table 13.3.2).

The combination of an additional excimer laser corneal procedure (BIOPTICS) [70] has highlighted the need for a wide functional optical zone. For a –16-D correction in a patient with a 6-mm mesopic pupillary diameter, for instance, postoperative quality of vision is unquestionably better if we select a wide-optic implant (a –12 ICL has a 5.5-mm diameter and corrects approximately –9.50), and combine it with a –6.50, 6-mm optical zone excimer laser ablation, instead of implanting a –20, 4.65-mm optic ICL, fully correcting the ammetropia. As a trend, taking advantage of new designs and higher index materials, it is easy to foresee that the average effective optical zone of future lenses will

Table 13.3.2 Corneal vs. retropupillary plane equivalent optical zones (in millimeters)

ICL (retropupillary plane)	LASIK (corneal plane)
4.65	5.86
5	6.3
5.2	6.55
5.5	6.9

soon be made larger with an aspherical shape factor to respect physiology.

13.3.4.2 Clinical Complications

13.3.4.2.1 Ocular Hypertension and Iridopathy
An early acute intraocular pressure (IOP) rise is relatively frequent (7–8%). When hypertension occurs within the first 24 h and without chamber shallowing, it is almost always moderate (less than 30 mmHg), asymptomatic, and rapidly transient in 24–48 hours. Since it is mainly caused by trabecular blockage by retained ophthalmic viscosurgical devices (OVD) (Fig. 13.3.6a), it should be prevented with thorough intraoperative removal of the viscoelastic gel and carbonic anhydrase inhibitor administration (acetazolamide tablets, orally, twice a day). ICL surgery should be planned in the morning to allow a comfortable check after 5–6 hours. Very rarely, painful IOP spikes require decompression from the side port at the slit lamp with a blunt spatula.

When peripheral iridotomies (PIs) were not performed or they were not patent, or occluded (by the lens footplate or by dense viscoelastic gel), physiological aqueous flow through the pupil is blocked; the iris root is pushed forward leading to angle closure glaucoma. The anterior chamber is flat and the ICL overvaulted (Fig. 13.3.6b). The surgeon can try to take time, dilating the pupil with isonephrine 30% or phenylephrine 10%, and lowering the IOP by dehydrating the vitreous with mannitol or acetazolamide intravenous infusion, while the OVD is fully reabsorbed. Additionally,

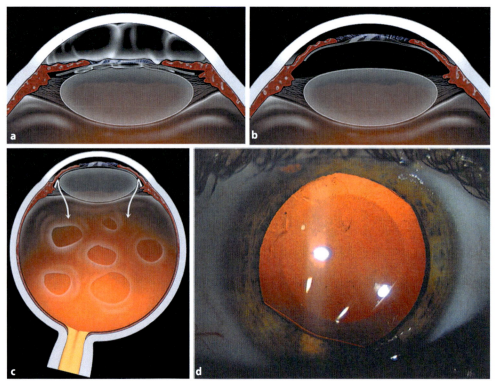

Fig. 13.3.6 Viscoelastic-related IOP rise with deep chamber and normal expected vaulting (a). Pupillary block in an ICL-implanted eye. The chamber is shallow and the lens vaulting exaggerated (b). Malignant glaucoma: flat chamber with both crystalline lens and ICL pushing forward (c). Urretz-Zavalia syndrome 20 days after hyperopic ICL surgery (d)

13

the surgeon can re-YAG the eye at the existing sites of PIs, eventually performing a new one at 6 o'clock, doing a Y-shape or a surgical iridectomy. An urgent ICL removal, theoretically necessary in case the previous steps are ineffective, has never been required in our series.

If the acute IOP rise is associated with a markedly flat anterior chamber with the entire iridolenticular block (iris–ICL–crystalline lens) pushed forward (Fig. 13.3.6c), then the block of the aqueous flow is posterior and typically refractory to the iridectomy. The aqueous inverts its physiological direction, moving toward the vitreous, where it accumulates forming pools of fluid (malignant glaucoma). The surgeon must intervene by urgently dehydrating the vitreous with osmotic agents (intravenous mannitol) and atropinization. If no results are observed after a few hours, then the patient must return to the operating room for implant removal. In extreme cases, via pars plana vitreous decompression through a 25-ga needle or phacoemulsification combined with posterior vitrectomy (the so-called Chandler's procedure) may be necessary.

Urrets-Zavalia syndrome refers to intermittent pupillary block with sudden IOP rise, causing iris sphincter muscle ischemia and atonic (blown) pupil (Fig. 13.3.6d). The syndrome, described after other intraocular procedures [26, 64], usually occurs at night with no apparent symptoms. The non-reactive pupil, around 7 mm in diameter, is often irreversible and will not respond to pharmacological treatment. In some cases, the pupil diameter shows a slight tendency to contract under the effect of non-steroidal anti-inflammatory (NSAID) eye-drops. The most important disturbances are the visual symptoms resulting from optical aberrations induced by the edge of the optic. If the patient does not complain about these problems, then the surgeon should leave the lens inside the eye and possibly widen (repeat YAG) the iridotomies. One of our patients benefited from this conservative behavior; after 4 years, although the pupil is still atonic, her pupil diameter improved from 7 to 5.5 mm and does not interfere with night driving. It stands to reason that the removal of the ICL will not change the situation to any great degree; given the fragility of the atrophic iris stroma, a pupilloplasty with Prolene purse-string suture should not be advisable. One alternative solution could be to exchange the ICL with a new wide optic implant or to perform a clear lens extraction and implant a low-power, wide-optic IOL in the capsular bag.

In a recognized steroid responder population like high myopia, it is no surprise that aggressive postoperative cortisone treatment often created considerable IOP rises, which always regressed to preoperative values with the suspension of the therapy (by 2–4 weeks after surgery), but sometimes required the prolonged use of an hypotonizing regimen, topical beta-blocker twice daily in general. At present, steroid-induced hypertension is no longer a problem, given that the postsurgical anti-inflammatory therapy has been greatly reduced. After routine, uneventful surgery, we do not use dexamethazone eye drops for more than 3 days any longer, tapering it soon in favor of NSAID eye drops.

Pigment movement successive to posterior chamber phakic IOL surgery is an undesired but inevitable event due to the chosen site of implantation. In slit-lamp retroillumination, small windows defects, trace deposition in the trabecular meshwork–gonioscopically, a sort of moderate, inferior Sampaolesi line–and pigment spots on the lens surfaces (Fig. 13.3.7) are frequently seen, but in our experience, the mechanical chafing of the posterior layer of the iris has always been moderate and self-limiting, never reaching a level of clinical importance. The increased pigmentation of the trabecular meshwork observed at the early postoperative period, in particular, returns to the preoperative level after 12–18 months.

Not all experts fully accept our position of reassurance, but the concerns voiced some years ago relative to a long-term risk of chronic glaucoma secondary to the pigmentary dispersion syndrome [6, 69] have not been confirmed by the recent literature. Prevention of post-ICL glaucoma includes the general rule to always perform at least one, well-patent, minimum 500-µm-wide preliminary YAG peripheral iridotomy or an intraoperative surgical iridectomy located perpendicularly at ICL position. The potential for avoiding PIs is being investigated with ICL centrally or peripherally holed ICL implants. Our preliminary results, 3 years after surgery, suggest ensuring a uniform physiological perfusion flow of the aqueous on both sides of the implant (Fig. 13.3.8).

Following guidelines supplied by the manufacturer (choosing the ICL overall length based on the external white-to-white distance and excluding from surgery the eyes with ACD–central distance between the endothelium and the anterior surface of the crystalline lens–of less than 2.8 mm) is questioned, since it has been artificially derived from old studies [1, 15, 17, 30, 38] in eyes with naturally occurring angle closure glaucoma (Fig. 13.3.9).

Although an obvious medicolegal reference point, a single measurement of the central anterior chamber depth, done by a conventional A-scan ultrasound biometry or by more or less sophisticated optical devices (slit lamp, IOL-Master*, Scheimpflug camera-based of slit scanning tomog-

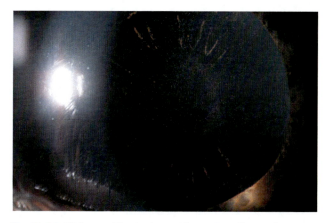

Fig. 13.3.7 High magnification image of non-clinically significant pigmentary deposition on the anterior and posterior surfaces of the ICL

raphers) is not a reliable predictor of the risk of developing angle closure glaucoma, as it shows no precise correlation with the shape of the anterior segment and to the width and the occludability of the iridocorneal angle [32, 37] Similar ACDs often show very different, individual, anterior segment shape [68], angle aperture, iris configuration, and original asymmetries. Angle-to-angle and sulcus-to-sulcus measurements obtained with VHF ultrasound or anterior segment optical coherence tomography showed significant differences among four meridians analyzed, suggesting that the human eye is not geometrically round [68]. The longest meridian may be located horizontally, vertically, or obliquely (Fig. 13.3.10). For surgical anatomy, the only rule is that there is no rule. In spite of ACD, only the clinical judgment based on a thorough high-precision examination of the anatomy, provided by very high frequency ultrasonography and a software showing the statistical risk carried out by certain linear and angular measurements, may help the surgeon to perform safe implantations [32, 34, 37] (Fig. 13.3.11).

Because of the biometric changes occurring over time, age is a fundamental factor to be considered in the ICL-safety preliminary evaluation. Due to the life-long mitotic activity of the subcapsular epithelial cells at the lens equator, the thickness of the human lens increases as it gradually grows, with an anterior change in displacement by 0.4 mm during the lifetime of a 90-year-old [41]. As a consequence, the anterior chamber depth drops by 0.75 mm over a 50-year span [22, 25, 41], particularly in the periphery. It is thus essential to bear these points in mind when dealing with very young patients. Nobody knows how much the anterior chamber volume available to the aqueous circulation of a normal eye (average 157 µl) can be reduced by the physical presence of the ICL implant, without risking angle closure or crowded anterior segment glaucoma. The limit of the angle opening to risk pupillary block in pristine eyes has been set to around 15° [62]. According to the Orbscan and echographic data, properly sized myopic ICL ideally vaulted 500 µm, reduce the post-ICL iridocorneal angle by an average of 25% (from about 42 to 29°) [34]. Long-term

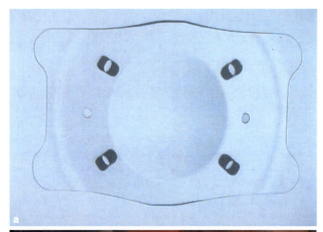

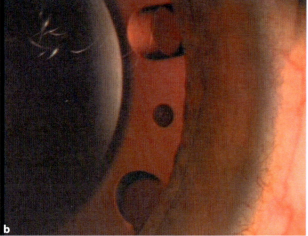

Fig. 13.3.8 ICL with four oblique through holes in the haptics, 0.6 mm in diameter, outside (**a**) and inside (**b**) the eye

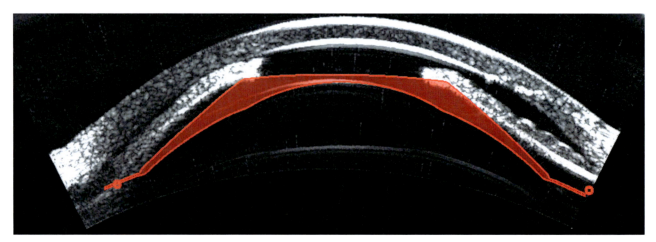

Fig. 13.3.9 Artemis 2 VHF echography image of an angle closure glaucoma caused by exaggerated ICL vault height. Preoperative ACD was 3.09 mm. Since the white-to-white was 12.5 mm, the overall length was correctly (?) chosen to 13 mm. Instead, the sulcus-to-sulcus distance was 10.9 mm

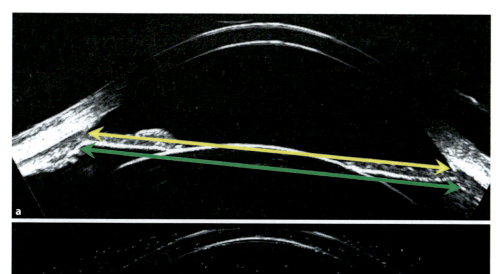

Fig. 13.3.10 In a sample of 288 eyes scanned with VHF Echography (Artemis 2), the largest cross-sectional internal sulcus diameter was found to be horizontal in 27%, oblique in 15%, vertical in 58%. The horizontal external diameter (white-to-white) was found to be the largest in all eyes. White-to-white was found to be smaller than sulcus-to-sulcus (a) in 41%, larger (b) in 59% of eyes

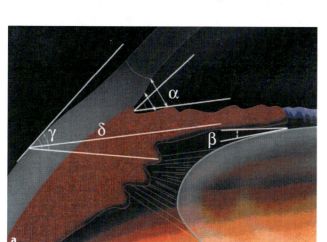

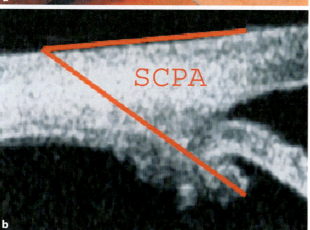

effects of potential redirection of aqueous flow have yet to be determined in ICL-implanted eyes.

Moreover, information on the degree of anatomical variability of the hidden ciliary body and the nearby structures is necessary to understand the dynamics after positioning an ICL (intermittent touch during accommodation, chafing of posterior structures, cysts or abnormalities of the ciliary body, forward rotation of ciliary processes after scleral buckling, etc.). All candidates should have a complete, in-depth examination of the size and morphology of the anterior segment. This is part of the overall procedure that is often omitted for reasons of cost and substituted with unacceptable, empirical approaches.

13.3.4.2.2 Inflammation

Considering the inflammatory response within the eye or the long-term integrity of the anterior uveal barrier mechanisms, evidence to date supports the safety of ICL implantation. Clinical assessments of anterior chamber flare and cellular reaction for up to 3 years after surgery were reported as absent in 99.6–100% of the cases [53]. The inhibition of protein binding provided by the interaction between collagen and fibronectin seems to be the main reason for the superior biocompatibility of the Collamer® material [61]. One

Fig. 13.3.11 Angle biometric parameters. α: Irido-corneal angle; β: iris-lens angle, γ: sclera-ciliary processes angle (SCPA); δ: sclera-iris angle (a). SCPA defined in a UBM image (b)

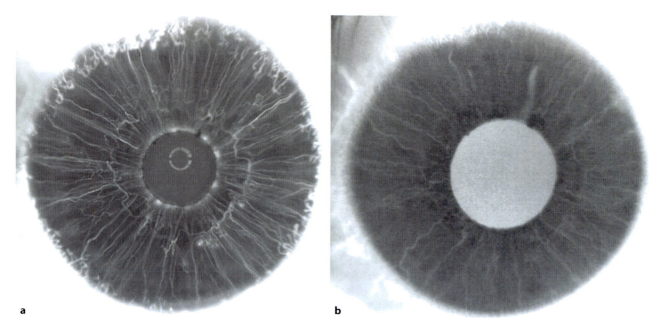

Fig. 13.3.12 Late-phases iris angiography, 1 month after ICL surgery, after the injection of fluorescein (**a**) and indocyanine green (**b**). The dye leakage appears to be moderate to absent

13

week after surgery, the photometric levels measuring the aqueous flare appeared to have increased by twofold, but by the third month, the values had returned to baseline levels in all implanted eyes [34]. The early leakage of the dye observed with fluorangiographic examination of the permeability of iris vessels [34] (Fig. 13.3.12), and the laser flare and cell meter measurements taken between 3 months and 3 years after surgery were within the normal range [53]. In the light of this evidence, we no longer consider the preoperative presence of posterior syncline, secondary to low-grade uveal inflammation after previous operations (such as penetrating keratoplasty, for instance), as a contraindication to ICL surgery.

On the side of anterior chamber phakic IOL implantation (both angle fixated and iris supported), however, transient low-grade acute postoperative iritis was observed in 3.4–10.7% of cases [3–5]. Although fluorophotometric evaluations were controversial, some of them indicated a prolonged breakdown of the blood–aqueous barrier and a reduction in the transmittance of the crystalline lens [11, 42, 43].

Endophthalmitis
Septic contamination, which may happen in every intraocular procedure, can complicate phakic IOL implantation. Endophthalmitis can occur as an early acute (within 5 days of surgery), subacute (up to 6 weeks after surgery) or late chronic low-grade uveitis of septic origin. Very few cases have been fully described in the peer-reviewed phakic IOL literature [1, 15], and even considering the see-no-evil attitude of ophthalmologists, a very rare incidence (1/8,000) of post-ICL surgery endophthalmitis may be roughly estimated. Though endophthalmitis is a potentially blinding complication, it may be prevented with maximum care by using

a sterile technique, and with early diagnosis and prompt treatment. As compared with what happens in the average after cataract surgery endophthalmitis case, we observed a peculiar clinical outcome (anatomic restitutio ad integrum and 20/20 uncorrected 2 weeks after surgery and intraocular antibiotic administration) in the only case we had [34], thus suggesting a sort of "barrier" effect provided by the ICL and/or by the crystalline lens to prevent diffusion to the vitreous chamber, therefore determining the better final prognosis.

13.3.4.2.3 Crystalline Lens Opacity (Anterior Subcapsular Cataract)

Early crystalline lens opacities caused by excessive surgical trauma (highly powered YAG PIs and rough intraocular maneuvers) may complicate the early course of the ICL procedure. These iatrogenic opacities are easy to identify, as they appear at an early stage (up to a maximum of 60 days postoperatively). They are focal and densely white, as they directly involve the anterior capsule. These opacities usually do not progress when visual interference is limited, but require follow-up on yearly basis (Fig. 13.3.13). Other factors classically recognized as interfering with the lens metabolism, like excessive intraoperative and postoperative IOP rise, air and OVD residuals, and prolonged steroid therapy, do not seem to play a role in determining the formation of a cataract.

Apart from these conditions, the close position of the material to the anterior lens surface is the main criticism against posterior chamber phakic IOLs and is likely to be the main issue of future scientific investigations. Researchers are far from completely understanding the mecha-

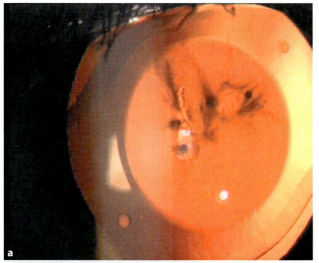

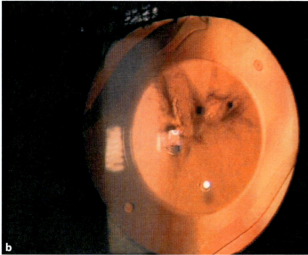

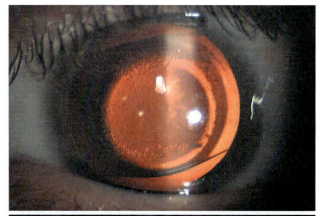

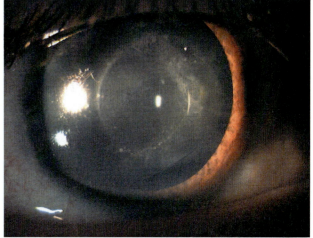

Fig. 13.3.14 Mid-peripheral anterior capsular and subcapsular opacities 4 years after Adatomed silicone posterior chamber phakic IOL implantation

Fig. 13.3.13 Non-evolutive, iatrogenic, anterior capsular opacities provoked by intraoperative inadvertent touch 2 months (a) and 6 years (b) after surgery. The uncorrected vision was 20/20−, and only minor interference with the quality of vision was noticed by the patient, who decided to keep the ICL in situ

nisms of cataract formation. However a few years ago, it was believed that the hydrophilic nature of the Collamer* were crucial in avoiding cataract formation, in contrast with what happens with hydrophobic silicone lenses (Fig. 13.3.14). Now, more attention is given to perfect sizing of the lens, to achieve adequate vaulting, or space separation between the IOL and the crystalline lens that allows aqueous exchange essential to the metabolism of the subcapsular epithelium of the lens. Given the oblate aspherical shape of the anterior crystalline lens surface, the vaulting of myopic lenses is reduced peripherally, especially when higher powers and thicknesses are involved. If the ICL is poorly sized, its short overall length sizing causes circular contact of the edges, with the semi-peripheral regions of the crystalline lens trapping a pool of aqueous. The metabolic stagnation leads to hyperplasia and fibrometaplasia by the

subcapsular epithelial cells of the lens. This theory is confirmed by the fact that in our practice, no hyperopic ICL induced opacities have been documented to date, even if the implant is closer to the crystalline lens in these short eyes. Due to the geometrical shape of the hyperopic optic, aqueous circulation is not impaired. The design of the lens is also critical. In our series, we saw no cataracts with the earlier, more vaulted models, but we reported a significant incidence of cataract–8.2%, with a 5.8% of surgical extraction (bilensectomy), with the flatter base curve of V2 and V3 ICL designs (Fig. 13.3.15).

Since the introduction of the V4 (April 1998), seven (1.75%) ICL-induced subcapsular opacities, and three (0.75%) cataract procedures have been recorded in the group were the lenses were sized following the white-to-white rule; no (0%) opacities have been observed in the group where the overall length was chosen with the Lovisolo Custom ICL Sizer, based on VHF echography measurements of the sulcus dimension.

The issue of potential intermittent touching during accommodation [24] when the crystalline lens moves forward, was recently addressed with partial coherence interferometry studies [46]. As the sulcus retracts with accommodation, no significant changes in distance between the ICL and the crystalline lens were found; the ICL vaulting increases as necessary, compensating the 200- to 600-μm forward movement of the anterior lens surface. On the other hand, under photopic environmental conditions or after application of pilocarpine, pupil constriction reduces the vault height by forcing the ICL against the crystalline lens [46].

Although inconclusive, the evidence provided by more than 14 years of experience in human beings should reassure about the potential threat of decay of the material, that is deterioration of transparency, permeability to nutrients,

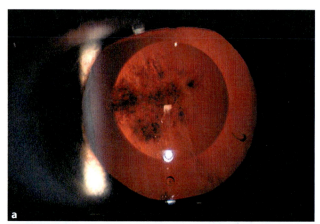
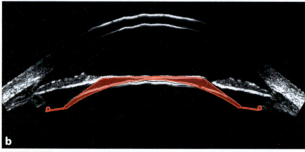
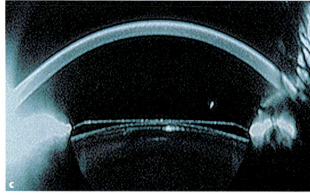

Fig. 13.3.15 Typical ICL-related iatrogenic subcapsular anterior opacities (**a**) 26 months after surgery; the VHF echography (**b**) and the Scheimpflug camera (EAS 1000, Nidek, Japan) images show the lack of vault between the ICL (V2) and the crystalline lens. The 12-mm V2 myopic ICL, selected based on the 11.6-mm external corneal diameter, turned out to be too small for a sulcus diameter of 12.3 mm

and biocompatibility of the Collamer® that could occur in the long-term.

13.3.4.2.4 Corneal Decompensation

Maximum long-term preservation of the corneal endothelium has always been an important issue for the entire area of phakic IOL implantation, in view of the high rates of corneal decompensation reported after the first implantations [9]. Our data allow us to state that currently refined ICL surgical techniques can minimize [33] the sacrifice of endothelial cells. Almost 40% of the postoperative cell counts and morphologies of group C actually improved at the month-3 follow-up gate. Beyond the actual bias of the instruments measuring the endothelium, the apparent paradox can be explained by cell centripetal migration and enhanced metabolism after stopping wearing contact lenses.

In the long run, the protective role of the iris barrier to prevent ongoing endothelial cell loss through mechanical chafing has been almost unanimously recognized by different authors [20, 34]. Although metabolic interference was hypothesized by Dejaco-Ruhswurm and coauthors [16], their report is the only one in the literature with worrying rates of progressive loss (5.5% at 1 year, 12.3% at 4 years) during a 4-year follow-up of ICL-implanted eyes. In their study, however, only the first-year data were statistically significant, and the cell morphological indices (polymorphism and polymegathism) remained stable during the follow-up period.

In our long-term (≥6 years of follow-up), the mean annual loss is very similar to the 14 cells/mm^2 (0.5–0.6%) a year that is considered physiological in non-implanted healthy eyes. Therefore, we believe that the current cell density limits proposed for ICL implantation should not be shared with anterior chamber (angle fixated or iris enclaved) phakic IOLs, that have proven to be less safe for the corneal endothelium [4, 13, 44, 47].

Moreover, beyond the usual recommendations of taking into consideration the patient's age to assess the minimum cell density, asking the patients not to rub their eyes and checking yearly the endothelial images with specular or confocal microscopy, we feel comfortable to safely implant eyes that are presently excluded from surgery, such as post-penetrating keratoplasty, keratoconus, chronic contact lens wearers with poor endothelial cell count.

13.3.4.2.5 Vitreoretinal Complications

The overall incidence of vitreoretinal complications in ICL-implanted eyes is approximately 1–2% and seems generally caused by predisposition more than by surgery or by the presence of the implant itself [1]. By the way, it is well known that the high myopic population suitable for phakic IOL implantation is at high risk for:

1. Progressive posterior retinal atrophy, secondary to mechanical and vascular stress from congenital scleral

weakness and deterioration of choriocapillary and retinal pigmented epithelium.

2. Spontaneous or neovascular macular hemorrhage (the risk is 6%, compared with 0.002% in normal young persons).

3. Rhegmatogenous retinal detachment secondary to vitreous liquefaction, asymptomatic peripheral retinal breaks, or degenerations and posterior vitreous detachment (the risk is 2.4% in the first 60 years of life, compared with 0.06% in the normal population).

To minimize the risk of coincident pathologies, the role of the vitreoretinal expert should be emphasized, as he or she is the person who will be entrusted with providing documentation, treatment, and prophylaxis of any pathology that may complicate the natural history of such vulnerable eyes. Potential negative influences during surgery (iridotomy and shallowing of the anterior chamber) may stimulate the vitreous to contract, potentially generating avulsion of the base and giant retinal tears [3]. For that reason, we feel more comfortable operating on an eye with an already detached posterior vitreous [27].

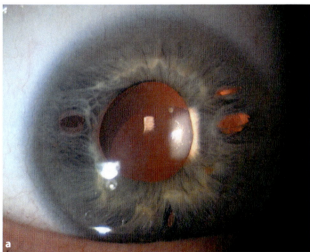

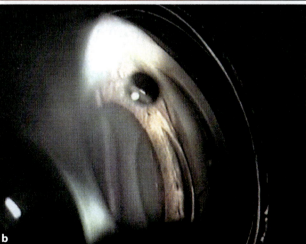

ICLs seem to be well tolerated by the myopic retina. They do not disturb fluorangiography or the observation of the retinal periphery since the pupil dilates normally and the haptics do not interfere with the display of the image. In eyes operated with episcleral procedures, great care must be taken. Scleral buckles generate an anterior displacement of the ciliary body and crystalline lens, and reduce the depth of the anterior chamber and the width of the iridocorneal angle [60]. The indentation devices may interfere with peripheral choroidal venous drainage through compression of the vorticose veins, resulting in edema of the ciliary body, in such a way that the surgeon should consider better to remove the buckle before ICL positioning, particularly if the chorioretinal scars are old and no vitreal traction is visible.

13.3.4.2.6 Zonular Damage, Decentration, Anterior and Posterior Dislocation

Although further studies are necessary to definitely prove this statement in the long run, well-sized, recent design and carefully implanted (no dialing maneuvers for retro-iris positioning!) ICLs can be safely implanted even in eyes with a limited (less than 60°) encoche of the Zinn apparatus. We have implanted six highly myopic eyes with moderate zonular disruption, taking care to put the haptics in the healthy areas; after more than 3 years of follow up, we did not observe even a minimal decentration.

Although we saw decentration, and spontaneous dislocation into the anterior chamber years after unremarkable clinical course [34] (Fig. 13.3.16) with the old generation of lenses, with the latest models of ICL, decentration larger than 1 mm has never been an issue even when the sizing has been patently inaccurate.

For another posterior chamber phakic implant (the PRL), instead, the commonly used one-size-fits-all 11.3-mm overall length, claimed as "floating inside the posterior chamber with no anatomical fixation sites," frequently (about 10%) decenters more than 1 mm. Moreover, our experience confirms the concerns of significant (design-related?) risk of cataract, damage to the zonules and dislocation into the vitreous chamber (Fig. 13.3.17).

Fig. 13.3.16 Inferior decentration of the first ICL prototype (IC2020) implanted in the western world in September 1993 (courtesy of Paolo Pesando, M.D.) (**a**). Gonioscopic view of a V2 ICL spontaneously dislocated in the anterior chamber (**b**)

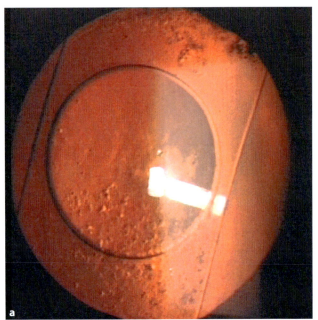

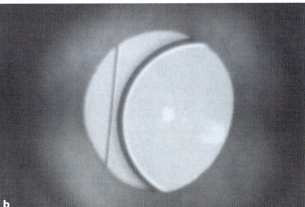

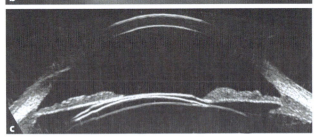

Fig. 13.3.17 PRL-induced iatrogenic anterior subcapsular opacities 2 years after surgery (**a**); Scheimpflug retroillumination (**b**) and Artemis 2 (**c**) images of a decentered PRL

13.3.5 The Lovisolo Custom Phakic IOL Sizer. How to Get Rid of Implant-Related Complications

Since 1999 [31], we have been using proprietary software–the Lovisolo Custom Phakic IOL Sizer–(Fig. 13.3.18) to predict postoperative vault height and the expected clearances between corneal endothelium, iris, and crystalline lens before implanting phakic IOLs, based on high-resolution

images of the anterior segment. Accurate measurements of these parameters may be obtained with instruments that use VHF ultrasound waves in the 35- to 50-MHz range, like the Artemis 2 and the Vu-Max (Sonomed, New York, N.Y.) (Fig. 13.3.19a,b). Optical devices like slit scanning systems with or without rotating Scheimpflug camera (like the Precisio, Ligi, Taranto, Italy [Fig. 13.3.19c,d], the Pentacam, Oculus, Germany, and the Galilei, Ziemer, Germany), or infrared light optical coherence tomographers (Visante OCT*, Zeiss-Meditec) (Fig. 13.3.19e) permit high-definition cross-sectional anterior segment imaging with excellent reproducibility of measurements by using the interference profile of the reflections from the cornea, the iris, and the crystalline lens. However, these methods are not interesting for sizing the ICL, since the retro-irideal space cannot be perfectly visualized by optical devices and the statistical correlation between angle and sulcus diameters is as poor as between external white-to-white and internal dimensions [68].

For the ICL, the latest version of the software takes into account:

- The position (the sclerociliary processes angle) (Fig. 13.3.10) and the whole dimension of the ciliary sulcus, as measured under cycloplegic conditions
- The crystalline lens rise on the iris plane or the sclera-iris angle (Fig. 13.3.20)
- The iridocorneal angle
- The specific features of the chosen lens implant (overall length, vault at rest, central and peripheral optic thickness, flexibility)
- A corrective factor for BSS ICL, as those marketed in the United States (the European ICL are labeled as measured in NaCl). Intraocularly, for instance, a European 125V4 ICL enlarges from 12.5 to 13.2 mm
- The implant behavior under compression, as predicted by finite element analysis, given the elasticity of the material (Fig. 13.3.21)
    - The age (life expectancy) of the patient. An average reduction of the anterior chamber depth of 0.015 mm per year is calculated to predict the anatomic relationships even after 50 years.
    - A warning signal is automatically given if one parameter shows a difference higher than 20% from normal values.

In our most recent personal series (group C) on 287 eyes implanted with the ICL V4, with a mean follow-up of 29 months, we have not yet observed any cases of iatrogenic cataract, pigmentary dispersion, or angle closure glaucoma. The mean central vault height was 386 μm, with a standard deviation of ±113 μm. The minimum vault obtained was 189 μm. An expected-versus-achieved vault height in the ±150-μm range was obtained in the 95% confidence interval. In comparison with the group control (group B), where the ICL was implanted based on the white-to-white, the mean central vault height was 406 μm (the difference

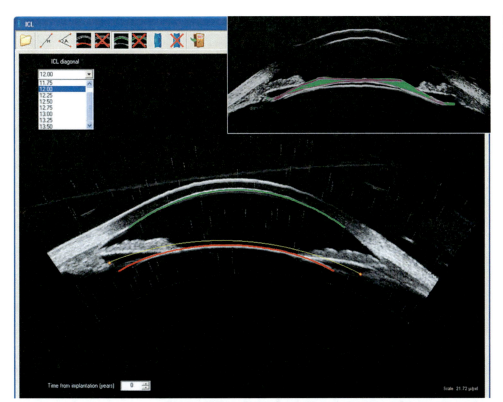

Fig. 13.3.18 Snapshot of the last version of the Lovisolo Custom Phakic IOL Sizer

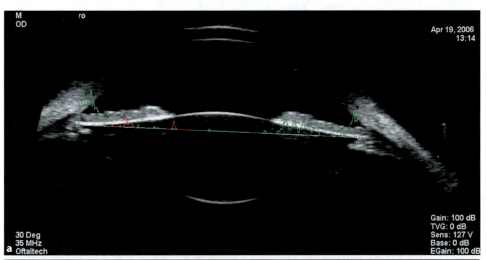

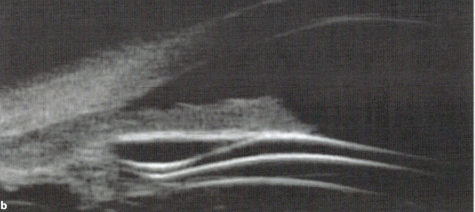

Fig. 13.3.19 Thirty-five–MHz VHF echography images (Vu-Max II): overall image of the anterior segment (**a**) and detail of the site of fixation of the ICL haptics (**b**). Precisio anterior chamber map and Scheimp-flug scan (**c, d**); Visante OCT scan of the same eye (**e**)

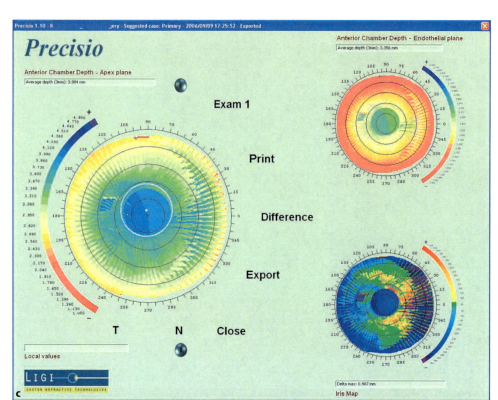

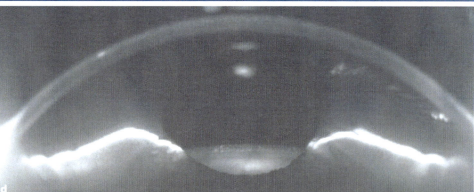

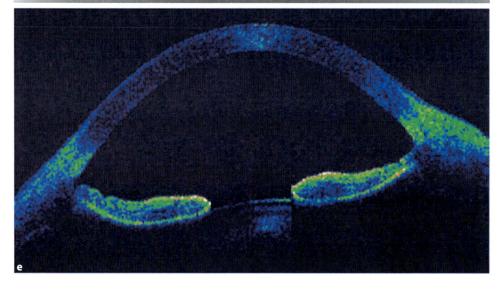

Fig. 13.3.19 c–e *(continued)*

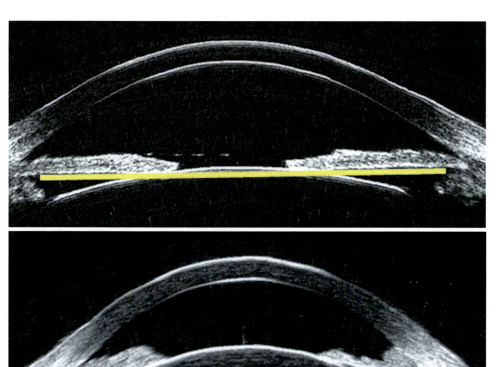

Fig. 13.3.20 Flat or steep shapes of the anterior segment as imaged by the crystalline lens rise on the iris plane (yellow line)

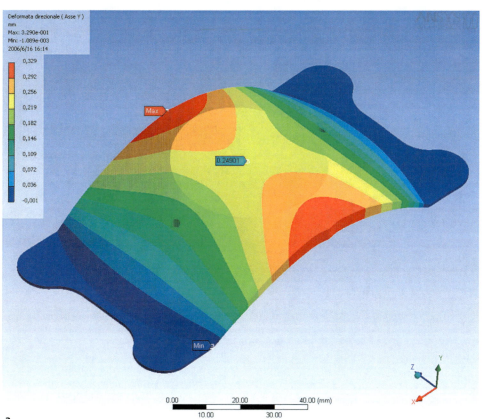

a

Fig. 13.3.21 a, b Finite element analysis computer simulation representing a three-dimensional geometrical model of an ICL by multiple, linked representations of discrete regions. Equations of equilibrium are applied to each element, and a system of simultaneous equations is constructed. A set of compressions in order to simulate the intraocular ICL behavior for different powers, lens implant and sulcus sizes is performed and ICL deformation recorded in every point

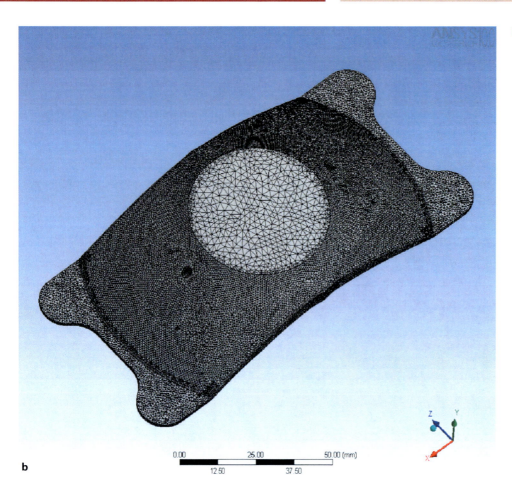

Fig. 13.3.21 b *(continued)*

b

0.00   25.00   50.00 (mm)
      12.50   37.50

13

was not statistically significant), but the standard deviation was highly significant (±667 μm). The minimum vault achieved was 0 μm, and the incidence of size-related complications (angle-closure glaucoma, cataract, and clinically significant pigmentary dispersion) was around 8%. The reference point of the 95% confidence interval as referred to the expected-versus-achieved vault height was reached for the range of ±730 μm [59]. Similar values are obtained from multivariate regression analysis by sizing the ICL on the basis of anterior chamber depth, corneal pachymetry, opening of the iridocorneal angle, angle-to-angle distance, and axial length–also shoe, hat, or glove size!

Take-Home Pearls

■ Posterior chamber phakic lenses (ICLs) are safe for the corneal endothelium, most probably safer than other models of phakic lenses.

■ Adequate and specific surgeon training is mandatory prior to using ICLs, as this may prevent most of the intraoperative and early postoperative complications.

■ Most late-postoperative ICL complications (including iatrogenic anterior subcapsular cataract) are size related. Sizing cannot be based on external anatomy (the horizontal corneal diameter or white-to-white distance), because it has shown to correlate poorly with the internal dimensions.

■ To accurately predict the postoperative intraocular implant-to-tissue clearances, the project of an ICL must be customized to the individual, internal biometric measurements of the anterior segment, obtained with very high frequency echography and calculated by accomplished software.

■ After surgery, the implanted eyes should be monitored at least yearly with very high frequency echography.

References

1. Albirsk PH (1976) Primary angle-closure glaucoma. Oculometry, epidemiology and genetics in a high-risk population. Acta Ophthalmol 54:127–135
2. Aliò J L, de la Hoz F, Ismail MM (1993) Subclinical inflammatory reaction induced by phakic anterior chamber lenses for the correction of high myopia. Ocular Immun Inflamm 1:219–223
3. Aliò JL, Ruiz-Moreno JM, Artola A (1993) Retinal detachment as a potential hazard in surgical correction of severe myopia with phakic anterior chamber lenses. Am J Ophthalmol 115:143–148

4. Aliò JL, de la Hoz F, Pérez-Santonja JJ (1999) Phakic anterior chamber lenses for the correction of myopia: a seven years cumulative analysis of complications in 263 cases. Ophthalmology 106:448–456

5. Aliò JL, Mulet ME, Shalaby AM (2002) Artisan phakic iris claw intraocular lens for high primary and secondary hyperopia. J Refract Surg 18:697–707

6. Arne JL, Lesueur LC (2000) Phakic posterior chamber lenses for high myopia: functional and anatomical outcomes. J Cataract Refract Surg 26:369–374

7. Arne JL, Lesueur LC, Hulin HH (2003) Photorefractive keratectomy or laser in situ keratomileusis for residual refractive error after phakic intraocular lens implantation. J Cataract Refract Surg 29:1167–1173

8. Assetto V, Benedetti S, Pesando PM (1996) Collamer intraocular contact lens to correct high myopia. J Cataract Refract Surg 22:551–556

9. Barraquer J (1959) Anterior chamber plastic lenses. Results and conclusions from five years experience. Trans Ophthalmol Soc UK 79:393–424

10. Battle J (2004) Toric phakic IOL may be alternative for treating keratoconus. Ophthalmology Times Meeting E-News. Available via http://www.ophthalmologytimes.com/ophthalmologytimes

11. Benitez del Castillo JM, Hernandez JL, Iradier MT et al (1993) Fluorophotometry in phakic eyes with anterior chamber intraocular lens implantation to correct myopia. J Cataract Refract Surg 16:607–609

12. Brandt JD, Mockovak ME, Chayet A (2001) Pigmentary dispersion syndrome induced by a posterior chamber phakic refractive lens. Am J Ophthalmol 131:260–263

13. Budo C, Hessloehl JC, Izak M et al (2000) Multicenter study of the Artisan phakic intraocular lens. J Cataract Refract Surg 26:1163–1171

14. Bylsma SS, Zalta AH, Foley E et al (2002) Phakic posterior chamber intraocular lens pupillary block. J Cataract Refract Surg 28:2222–2228

15. Coakes RL, Lloyd-Jones D, Hitchings RA (1979) Anterior chamber volume. Its measurement and clinical application. Trans Ophthalmol Soc UK 99:78

16. Dejaco-Ruhswurm I, Scholz U, Pieh S et al (2002) Long-term endothelial changes in phakic eyes with posterior chamber intraocular lenses. J Cataract Refract Surg 28:1589–1593

17. Delmarcelle Y, Francois J (1976) Biometrie oculaire clinique (oculometrie). Bull Soc Belge Ophthalmol pp 172–181

18. Dementiev DD, Hoffer KJ, Sborgia G et al (1999) Phakic refractive lenses (PRLs). In: Lovisolo CF, Pesando PM (eds) The implantable contact lens (ICL) and other phakic IOLs. Fabiano, Canelli, Italy

19. Dementiev DD, Hoffer KJ, Sonecka A (2004) PRL-Medennium posterior chamber phakic intraocular lens. In: Aliò JL, Perez-Santonja JJ (eds) Refractive surgery with phakic IOLs. Fundamentals and practice. Highlights of Ophthalmology International, El Dorado, Republic of Panama

20. Edelhauser HF, Sanders DR, Azar R et al (2004) Corneal endothelial assessment after ICL implantation. J Cataract Refract Surg 30:576–583

21. El-Sheikh HF, Tabbara KF (2003) Cataract following posterior chamber phakic intraocular lens. J Refract Surg 19:72–73

22. Fontana ST, Brubaker RF (1973) Volume and depth of the anterior chamber in the normal aging human eye. Arch Ophthalmol 98:1803

23. Fyodorov SN, Zuev VK, Tumanyan ER (1987) Modern approach to the stagewise complex surgical therapy of high myopia. Transactions of International symposium of IOL. Moscow, RS-FSP Ministry of Health, pp 27427–27429

24. Garcia-Feijoo J, Alfaro IJ, Cuina-Sardina R et al (2003) Ultrasound biomicroscopy examination of posterior chamber phakic intraocular lens position. Ophthalmology 110:163–172

25. Glasser A, Campbell MC (1998) Presbyopia and the optical changes in the human crystalline lens with age. Vision Res 38:209–229

26. Halpern BL, Pavilack MA, Gallagher SP (1995) The incidence of atonic pupil following cataract surgery. Arch Ophthalmol 113:448–450

27. Hikichi T, Trempe CL, Schepens CL (1995) Posterior vitreous detachment as a risk factor for retinal detachment. Ophthalmology 102:527–528

28. Keuch RJ, Bleckmann H (2002) Pupil diameter changes and reaction after posterior chamber phakic intraocular lens implantation. J Cataract Refract Surg 28:2170–2172

29. Kodjikian L, Gain P, Donate D et al (2002) Malignant glaucoma induced by a phakic posterior chamber intraocular lens for myopia. J Cataract Refract Surg 28:2217–2221

30. Lee DA, Brubaker RF, Ilstrup DM (1984) Anterior chamber dimensions in patients with narrow angles and angle-closure glaucoma. Arch Ophthalmol 102:46

31. Lovisolo CF (1999) Methods of sizing ICLs should be improved, surgeon says. Ocular Surg News 10:34–35

32. Lovisolo CF (2003) Posterior chamber phakic IOLs. ISRS/AAO 2003 Refractive Surgery comes of age. Subspecialty Day Syllabus, pp 33–41

33. Lovisolo CF, Giacomotti E (2004) Implantation of phakic intraocular lenses for hyperopia correction. In: Aliò JL, Perez-Santonja JJ (eds) Refractive surgery with phakic IOLs. Fundamentals and practice. Highlights of Ophthalmology International, El Dorado, Republic of Panama

34. Lovisolo CF, Pesando PM (2000) The Implantable Contact Lens (ICL⁻) and other phakic IOLs. Fabiano, Canelli, Italy

35. Lovisolo CF, Pesando PM (2004) Posterior chamber phakic intraocular lenses. In: Aliò JL, Perez-Santonja JJ (eds) Refractive surgery with phakic IOLs. Fundamentals and practice. Highlights of Ophthalmology International, El Dorado, Republic of Panama

36. Lovisolo CF, Pesando PM (2004) ICL posterior chamber phakic IOL. In: Aliò JL, Perez-Santonja JJ (eds) Refractive surgery with phakic IOLs. Fundamentals and practice. Highlights of Ophthalmology International, El Dorado, Republic of Panama

37. Lovisolo CF, Reinstein DZ (2005) Phakic intraocular lenses. Surv Ophthalmol 50:549–587

38. Lowe RF (1970) Aetiology of the anatomical basis for primary angle-closure glaucoma. Biometrical comparisons between normal eyes and eyes with primary angle-closure glaucoma. Br J Ophthalmol 54:161

39. Maroccos R, Vaz F, Marinho A et al (2001) Glare and halos after phakic IOL surgery for the correction of high myopia. Ophthalmologe 98:1055–1059

40. Menezo JL, Peris-Martínez C, Cisneros AL et al (2004) Phakic intraocular lenses to correct high myopia: Adatomed, Staar, and Artisan. J Catar Refract Surg 30:40–51

41. Okabe I, Taniguchi T (1992) Age related changes of the anterior chamber width. J Glaucoma 1:100

42. Pérez-Santonja JJ, Hernandez JL, Benitez del Castillo M et al (1994) Fluorophotometry in myopic phakic eyes with anterior chamber intraocular lenses to correct severe myopia. Am J Ophthalmol 118:316–321

43. Pérez-Santonja JJ, Iradier MT, Benitez del Castillo JM et al (1996) Chronic subclinical inflammation in phakic eyes with intraocular lenses to correct myopia. J Cataract Refract Surg 22:183–187

44. Pérez-Santonja JJ, Bueno JL, Zato MA (1997) Surgical correction of high myopia in phakic eyes with Worst-Fechner myopia intraocular lenses. J Refract Surg 13:268–284

13

45. Pesando PM, Ghiringhello MP, Tagliavacche P (1999) Posterior chamber collamer phakic intraocular lens for myopia and hyperopia. J Refract Surg 15:415–423

46. Petternel V, Koppl CM, Dejaco-Ruhswurm et al (2004) Effect of accommodation and pupil size on the movement of a posterior chamber lens in the phakic eye. Ophthalmology 111:325–331

47. Pop M, Payette Y (2004) Initial results of endothelial cell counts after Artisan Lens for Phakic Eyes. Ophthalmology 111:309–317

48. Reinstein DZ, Silverman RH, Raevsky T et al (2000) A new arc-scanning very high-frequency ultrasound system for 3D pachymetric mapping of corneal epithelium, lamellar flap and residual stromal layer in laser in situ keratomileusis. J Refract Surg 16:414–430

49. Rosen E, Gore C (1998) STAAR collamer posterior chamber phakic intraocular lens to correct myopia and hyperopia. J Cataract Refract Surg 24:596–606

50. Sanchez-Galeana CA, Smith RJ, Rodriguez X et al (2001) Laser in situ keratomileusis and photorefractive keratectomy for residual refractive error after phakic intraocular lens implantation. J Refract Surg 17:299–304

51. Sanchez-Galeana CA, Zadok D, Montes M et al (2002) Refractory intraocular pressure increase after phakic posterior chamber intraocular lens implantation. Am J Ophthalmol 134:121–123

52. Sanchez-Galeana CA, Smith RJ, Sanders DR et al (2003) Lens opacities after posterior chamber phakic intraocular lens implantation. Ophthalmology 110:781–785

53. Sanders DR (2003) ICL in Treatment of Myopia Study Group. Postoperative inflammation after implantation of the implantable contact lens. Ophthalmology 110:2335–2341

54. Sanders DR (2007) Matched population comparison of the Visian Implantable Collamer Lens and standard LASIK for myopia of –3.00 to –7.88 Diopters. J Refract Surg 23:537–553

55. Sanders D, Vukich JA (2006) Comparison of implantable collamer lens (ICL) and laser-assisted in situ keratomileusis (LASIK) for low myopia. Cornea 25:1139–1146

56. Sanders DR, Vukich JA, Doney K et al (2003) Implantable Contact Lens in Treatment of Myopia Study Group. U.S. Food and Drug Administration clinical trial of the Implantable Contact Lens for moderate to high myopia. Ophthalmology 110:255–266

57. Sanders DR, Doney K, Poco M (2004) ICL in Treatment of Myopia Study Group. US FDA clinical trial of the Implantable Collamer Lens (ICL) for moderate to high myopia: three-year follow-up. Ophthalmology 111:1683–1692

58. Sanders DR, Schneider D, Martin R et al (2007) Toric Implantable Collamer Lens for moderate to high myopic astigmatism. Ophthalmology 114:54–61

59. Sarver EJ, Sanders DR, Vukich JA (2003) Image quality in myopic eyes corrected with laser in situ keratomileusis and phakic intraocular lens. J Refract Surg 19:397–404

60. Schepens CL (1994) Increased intraocular pressure during scleral buckling Ophthalmology 101:417–421

61. Sechler JL, Corbett SA, Wenk MB et al (1998) Modulation of cell-extracellular matrix interactions. Ann N Y Acad Sci 857:143–154

62. Shaffer RN (1960) Gonioscopy, ophthalmoscopy and perimetry. Trans Am Acad Ophthalmol Otorlaryngol 64:112

63. Trindade F, Pereira F (2000) Exchange of a posterior chamber phakic intraocular lens in a highly myopic eye. J Cataract Refract Surg 26:773–776

64. Urrets-Zavalía A Jr (1963) Fixed, dilated pupil, iris atrophy and secondary glaucoma; a distinct clinical entity following penetrating keratoplasty in keratoconus. Am J Ophthalmol 56:257–265

65. Uusitalo RJ, Aine E, Sen NH et al (2002) Implantable contact lens for high myopia. J Cataract Refract Surg 28:29–36

66. Visessook N, Peng Q, Apple DJ et al (1999) Pathological examination of an explanted phakic posterior chamber intraocular lens. J Cataract Refract Surg 25:216–222

67. Werner L, Apple DJ, Pandey SK et al (2001) Phakic posterior chamber intraocular lenses. Int Ophthalmol Clin 41:153–174

68. Werner L, Lovisolo CF, Chew J et al (2007) Meridional differences of internal dimensions of the anterior segment of human eyes evaluated with two imaging systems. Ophthalmology (submitted)

69. Zaldivar R, Davidorf JM, Oscherow SA (1999) Posterior chamber phakic intraocular lens. In: Lovisolo CF, Pesando PM (eds) The Implantable Contact Lens (ICL⁻) and other phakic IOLs. Fabiano, Canelli, Italy

70. Zaldivar R, Oscherow S, Piezzi V (2002) Bioptics in phakic and pseudophakic intraocular lens with the Nidek EC-5000 excimer laser. J Refract Surg 18:336–339

Contents

Core Messages

■ This chapter approaches retinal complications, in particular retinal detachment after lens surgery in high-myopic patients.

■ The incidence of retinal detachment in high-myopic patients corrected by intraocular surgery is reported based on the experience of the authors and on a review of published reports.

■ The cumulative risk of retinal detachment development in high-myopic patients after intraocular refractive surgical procedures (whether lens exchange or phakic intraocular lenses) is reported.

■ Various options for the treatment of retinal detachment in high-myopic patients after ocular refractive surgery is outlined.

14.1 Retinal Detachment

José Mª Ruiz-Moreno, Jorge L. Alió,
and Mohamed H. Shabayek

14.1.1 Introduction

There is some controversy regarding the risk of retinal complications after refractive surgical procedures. Before approaching retinal complications after refractive surgery, an important issue is to determine whether refractive surgery leads to an increase in the development of retinal complications. Retinal complications especially in myopic patients after refractive surgery is mainly due to two possible causes: higher incidence of predisposing retinal lesions in myopic eyes compared with general population and the hypothesis that refractive surgery might induce several iatrogenic factors that will increase the incidence of such pathology.

Several factors may contribute to induce iatrogenic retinal detachment after refractive surgery. They depend mainly on the type of refractive surgical procedure: corneal (as in photorefractive keratectomy [PRK] or laser in situ keratomileusis [LASIK]) or intraocular (as in phakic intraocular lens implantation [PIOL] or clear lens extraction [CLE]). Such procedures might influence the retina, especially in high-myopic patients, due to the pressure induced by the microkeratome suction ring, the impact of laser pulses during PRK or LASIK, the hypotension or other intraoperative factors that can be induced during PIOL/CLE, and the postoperative inflammatory reaction.

The main point addressed in this chapter is whether the incidence of retinal detachment in high-myopic patients increases after keratorefractive surgery, PIOL implantation, CLE, or uneventful cataract surgery. An understanding of the preexisting risk factors in high myopia is necessary before we can attribute an increase of the rate of retinal detachment (RD) by ocular refractive surgery.

14.1.2 Retinal Detachment in Highly Myopic Eyes

Previous studies reported a higher incidence of RD in unoperated-on highly myopic eyes compared with non-myopic eyes (whether emmetropic or hypermetropic) [31, 48]. These studies reported risk that ranged between 0.71 and 3.2% [31, 48]. These previous published reports studied high myopic eyes with spherical equivalent (SE) greater than –6.00 D and included 1,000 eyes [48]. The annual incidence was 0.015% in eyes with myopia ≤ 4.75D, 0.07% in myopic eyes ranging between –5.00 D and –9.75 D, and 0.075% in eyes with myopia greater than 10 D [34]. While in high-myopic patients more than –15 D, the risk of developing RD increases from 15-fold up to 110-fold when compared with general population. Burton [13] reported that high-myopic patients greater than –5.00 D with degeneration are prone to extraordinary risk of developing RD, especially with long-life expectancy, and in such patients the risk of developing RD during the second, third, or fourth decade of life is very high, which is mainly due to trophic retinal holes. However, in this report he did not provide results on severe myopia with high axial length.

Also, in low-to-moderate myopia, early posterior vitreous detachment in patients with peripheral retinal degeneration can be a predisposing factor for retinal detachment development between the fourth and sixth decade.

14.1.3 Incidence of Retinal Detachment in High-Myopic Patients Corrected by Refractive Surgery

Surgical correction of high myopia, on intraocular basis, can be achieved by PIOL by anterior or posterior chamber, or by lens surgery (clear or cataractous) and implantation of a posterior chamber pseudophakic IOL.

RD after PIOL implantation has been reported by several authors [2, 46, 38, 23, 39, 58]. In 1993, Alió et al. [2] were the first to report retinal detachment after PIOL implantation for correcting high myopia. Fechner [23] reported RD in one case out of 125 myopic patients corrected with PIOLs. The incidence rate reported by other studies varied from 0.8 to 5.26% (Pesando [39], Zaldivar [58], and Panozzo [38]). We reported eight cases of RD in a series of 168 eyes (4.8%) [46]. An analysis of 12 eyes that developed RD out of 294 (4.08%) consecutive high myopic eyes after PIOL implantation followed [45]. Due to the variation in incidence rates, the survival rate was studied to avoid errors in the estimated real incidence. Kaplan-Maier analysis showed a cumulative risk of RD after PIOL implantation of 1.36% at 5 months, 2.6% at 17 months, 3.61% at 27 months, and 5.63% at 52 months [45].

We conducted a retrospective study to evaluate RD development in 522 consecutive highly myopic eyes after PIOL implantation [47]. In this case series, we reported on 15 eyes that developed RD with an incidence of 2.87%. We further estimated the cumulative risk of RD with time using Kaplan-Maier analysis. A cumulative risk of 0.57% at 3 months, 1.64% at 12 months, 2.73% at 36 months, and 4.06% at 92–145 months was observed [47].

However, both studies [45, 47] included highly, if not severe, myopic eyes (with mean SE of –18.5 D in the first study [45], and –18.1 D in the second [47]). Therefore, comparing the risk of RD in these studies to unoperated myopic eyes, with different degrees of myopia, would not be clinically valid.

The time interval (laps time) between PIOL implantation and the development of RD ranged between 1 and 52 months in the first study [45], (four eyes with laps time less than 6 months) compared to a range of 1–92 months in the second study [47]. Therefore, the relationship between PIOL implantation and RD development is not clear. A large case-control study with the same degree of myopia and with longer follow-up is needed to validate such a relationship.

Comparing the annual incidence of RD of unoperated high myopia –10 D (0.075%) [34] to our results after PIOL implantation, we observe a higher incidence after PIOL (2.87%) and almost similar to those of severe myopic patients (3.2%), but with higher annual risk; therefore, it is considered that the development RD is higher in our study of myopic eyes corrected with PIOL than in unoperated-on high-myopic population, and that further follow-up for these patients with a longer period might even reveal a greater incidence of RD. However, and keeping in consideration that the SE of our study, –18 D is significantly higher than –10 D is (higher degree of myopia), which can be a factor contributing to this higher incidence of RD in addition to the surgical intervention, therefore the comparison is not valid.

14.1.4 Incidence of Retinal Detachment in High-Myopic Patients Corrected by Lens Exchange

During lens surgery, whether clear lens extraction or cataract surgery, a transient decrease of the intraocular pressure (decompression effect) is induced that can cause changes in the vitreous, especially if it is degenerative as in high myopic eyes [2]. In addition to this fact, another possible "theoretical" pathogenic mechanism of such a refractive surgical procedure that may be added is the changes induced on the vitreous cavity during lens surgery [4, 7–9, 26, 32, 35, 37, 49, 50, 53].

The presence of cortical material in the anterior vitreous is an established fact after cataract surgery, but the effect of such material is not exactly established. The presence of lens proteins (cristalinase αA, αB, βA4, βB2, and γS) have been detected in the anterior vitreous of pseudophakic eyes, without a trace in the posterior vitreous of pseudophakic nor in the vitreous of phakic eyes (unoperated-on eyes). Also, in pseudophakic eyes changes have been detected in transitrretin concentration, alpha-antitrypsin "retinoic acid binding protein," and a decrease in the concentration proteins (antioxidants proteins, carbonic anhydrase and isomerase tri-phosphate) in posterior vitreous [4, 7–9, 26, 32, 35, 37, 49, 50, 53].

In addition, an inversion in the anteroposterior viscosity gradient has been detected in the vitreous of pseudophakic eyes. When added together, this sustains the hypothesis that the changes induced in the protein of pseudophakic eyes, coincides with the alterations in the structure of the vitreous humor and that these alteration in the retinal environment can contribute to the appearance of retinal complications after lens surgery [4, 7–9, 26, 32, 35, 37, 49, 50, 53].

Another surgical alternative for correcting high myopia is through lens (clear or cataractous) extraction and pseudophakic posterior lens implantation. Analyzing the reported incidence of RD in high myopic eyes corrected by lens extraction, we observe that the incidence of RD is higher than in high myopia corrected with PIOL.

Analyzing previous reports studying the incidence of RD after lens surgery in high-myopic patients is difficult. Some previous studies compared different surgical techniques, extracapsular cataract extraction (ECCE) and phacoemulsification; others compared the incidence of RD after clear and cataractous lens extraction. The mean follow-up, SE, and age group highly varied in various published reports.

Fernandez-Vega reported an incidence of 2.10% in 190 myopic eyes after CLE "phacoemulsification" after a mean follow-up of 4.78 years [24]. Pucci reported an incidence of 4.0% in 25 high myopic eyes (>12 D) [40]. Whereas Fan, in a study with mean axial length of 20.13 mm, reported a 1.69% incidence of RD [22]. Han reported a 3.2% incidence of RD in 62 eyes [29]. In a report that included 930 high myopic eyes with SE ranging from –30 D to –15 D, Ripandelli reported an incidence of 8% with mean age of 62.5% years and mean follow-up of 36 months [42]. Tosi, on the other hand, with a mean follow-up of 62.3 months and mean axial length of 30.22mm reported a 1.3% incidence of RD in 73 eyes [52]. Ravalico reported RD incidence of 0.26% in 388 cases after cataract surgery after a mean follow-up of 47 months [41]. Gabric in 72 eyes with a mean follow-up of 48 months reported only 1 case of RD 1.38% [25]. Other authors reported incidence rates of Cahstang [15] 6.1%, Barraquer [5] 7.3%, and Colin [18] 8.1% of RD.

Colin [18] suggests that the risk of RD after CLE in high-myopic patients may increase with time, and that studies with less than 4 years of follow-up demonstrate excellent results. Surprisingly, he reported a 0% incidence rate of RD [16] after 12 months, 1.9% [17] after 48 months, and 8.1% after 84 months [18].

The incidence rates of RD after CLE and cataract extraction cannot be compared in high myopia (as the incidence is lower after the latter), especially in young patients where CLE can induce vitreous changes and increase the traction on the retina over time, this is not expected to occur in elderly patients "after cataract extraction" [41].

We conducted a retrospective study [3] in which the incidence rate of RD in 439 high-myopic eyes of 274 patients after lens surgery (CLE and cataract) was determined. Pseudophakic posterior chamber IOLs were implanted by different surgeons after coaxial phacoemulsification between January 1996 and December 2000 at Vissum-Instituto Oftalmológico de Alicante, Spain. The mean age of patients was 62.2±11.7 years (ranging from 21 to 90 years); 32.4% were males and 67.6% were females. The mean follow-up was 61.5±29.6 months (ranging from 2 to 147 months). Highly myopic eyes with an axial length of over 26 mm and spherical equivalent ±6.00 D were included in the study. Eyes previously operated for RD or other intraocular surgeries (three eyes) were excluded.

The retrospective review of the patients' charts included preoperative examination: uncorrected visual acuity (UCVA), refraction, best spectacle-corrected visual acuity (BSCVA), slit lamp biomicroscopy, intraocular pressure, fundus examination, and ultrasonic biometry to determine the axial length and calculate the intraocular lens power. Data regarding the surgical complications such as posterior capsular tears and vitreous loss were also compiled. Postoperative data such as UCVA, BSCVA, and the visual outcome before and after retinal surgery in eyes with RD were gathered (postoperative examination was performed at 1 day, 1 week, 1, 3, 6, and 12 months after surgery and then annually).

Mean outcome measures included, in addition to postoperative BSCVA and spherical equivalent, occurrence of RD, age, axial length, operative complications (vitreous loss), posterior capsular opacification, and Nd:YAG.

Patients were divided into two groups according to age at the time of surgery, group 1 patients of 50 years or less (82 eyes) and group 2 patients over 50 years of age (357 eyes). Eyes were also stratified according to axial length (≤28-mm 274 eyes and >28-mm 165 eyes) for analyzing the risk of RD with time (Kaplan-Meier analysis).

RD occurred in 12 eyes of 12 patients out of 439 eyes, an incidence of 2.7%. The mean age of the patients affected by RD was 56.16±9.96 years (range, from 38 to 70 years). Mean axial length in retinal detached eyes was 27.85±1.83 mm (range, from 26.00 to 31.34), and mean spherical equivalent was –13.4±5.8 (range, from –28 D to –6.50 D). The incidence rate per age group was the following: group 1, 3.65% (3 out of 82 eyes) and group 2, 2.52% (9 out of 357 eyes). The incidence rate was 2.18% (6 out of 274 eyes) in eyes with axial length ≤ 28 mm and 3.36% in eyes with axial length >28 mm (6 out of 165 eyes).

Kaplan-Meier analysis was performed in order to establish the risk of RD in high-myopic eyes after coaxial phacoemulsification. The cumulative risk of RD onset among all 439 eyes was 0.47% at 3 months, 0.71% at 6 months, 1.71% at 15 months, 2.59% at 48 months, and 3.28% at 63 until 105 months. In group 1, the risk increased to 1.23% at 3 months and 4.46 at 63 until 147 months. In group 2, the incidence rate was 0.58% at 6 months, 1.83% at 15 months, 2.56% at 48 months, and 2.96% at 52 until 118 months. The cumulative risk of RD onset in eyes with axial length ≤28 mm was 0.40, 1.64, 2.12, and 2.62% for 6, 15, 48, and 52 until 147 months respectively. In eyes with axial length >28 mm, the cumulative risk was 1.22, 1.87, 3.35, and 4.42% for 4, 14, 42 and 63 until 117 months, respectively [3].

A trend was found indicating an association between age, axial length, and risk of RD, in which younger age groups and eyes with axial length >28 had increased risks of developing RD. A larger sample size study is necessary to obtain significant correlations; assuming that the risk of RD for group 1 (<50 years) was 4.46% at 146 months compared with 2.96% at 118 months for group 2 (>50 years), it would be necessary to include 1,066 eyes in each group, making a total of 2,132 eyes. Similarly, assuming that the cumulative risk of RD was 2.62% at 147 months for eyes with axial length ≤28 mm and 4.42% at 117 months for eyes with axial length >28 mm, it would be necessary to include 680 eyes in each group, ending up with 1,360 eyes in the study to obtain a significant difference [3].

Two factors are important when analyzing RD development after lens surgery, intraoperative capsular tear with vitreous loss and Nd:YAG laser capsulotomy after posterior capsular opacification (PCO).

Previous studies demonstrated an important difference in the incidence rates of PCO after lens surgery. Fernandez-Vega reported an incidence of 77.89% [24], Horgan 61% [29], our study 34.6% [3], Gabric 30.5% [25], Tosi 16.4% [52], and Colin 61.2% with 7 years follow-up [18]. However, it is difficult to make a reliable conclusion regarding the influence of Nd:YAG capsulotomy on RD development out of this data due to variations in follow-up periods, different age groups (the younger the age the greater the incidence of posterior capsular opacification), and different types of IOLs.

In summary and after an extensive analysis of the literature and our case series (439 eyes), we could not pinpoint any particular risk factor related to the development of retinal detachment, even though a trend, albeit not statistically significant, toward a higher incidence in patients with high axial length (>28 mm) and aged younger than 50 years was observed. A large multicenter collaborative study is recommended to gather a large number of cases to ascertain conclusively risk factors associated with the occurrence of retinal detachment in high myopic eyes and assess the real risk of this complication on patients' lifestyle. This will help in future indications for lens removal and medicolegal implications.

14.1.5 Treatment of Retinal Detachment in High-Myopic Patients after Ocular Refractive Surgery

Before treating RD after high-myopia correction with ocular refractive surgery, a serious and sight threatening complication, we should search for a therapeutic alternative that can offer the best results. The challenge is to treat RD and maintain the achieved emmetropia obtained by the previous ocular refractive surgical procedure.

The placement of a scleral buckling as a treatment for RD as a primary procedure vs. vitrectomy is an old dilemma [21], existing prospective comparative multicenter studies till the present time try to figure out the best procedure [1]. Both procedures offer reattachment data in cases of pseudophakic RD with multiple surgeries around 90% [6, 10, 12, 14, 20, 51, 55, 57]. However, by means of scleral buckling as a primary procedure, the incidence of initial failure to reattach the retina varies between 20 and 38.5% [20, 28, 57].

In cases of pseudophakic RD, vitrectomy seems to offer better results, with a rate of almost 90% retinal reattachment from the first procedure [10, 20, 56]. The development of new instruments and techniques, such as the usage of liquid perfluorocarbon, and present better visualization systems allow identification of small breaks, as in pseudophakic RD, with a prevalence of missed break of 20% [43, 57]. In addition to difficulties in exploring the retinal periphery, due either to capsular opacification or to aberrations induced by IOL during primary scleral buckling, all these factors rendered vitrectomy as the preferable primary procedure for pseudophakic RD [6, 10, 14, 51]. In addition, scleral buckling induces an average of 1.50 D of myopia [44].

Although the rate of retinal reattachment is similar with both procedures with multiple interventions and the final visual outcome is similar after one year, pars plana vitrectomy is considered an effective procedure, as it provides better localization and identification of the breaks responsible for pseudophakic RD, in addition to the success rate in achieving retinal reattachment by a single procedure [11].

Combining both procedures does not offer any difference in the final outcome. In such patients, vitrectomy as an initial treatment without the encircling band is indicated by many retinal surgeons [54].

14.1.6 Conclusion

The surgeon should keep in mind two facts of RD in high-myopic patients after lens surgery: (1) capsular integrity, whether inevitable, tear during lens surgery (cataract or CLE) or (2) as-indicated Nd:YAG capsulotomy after PCO will increase the incidence of retinal disease [19, 27, 30, 33, 36]. In addition, the IOL and anterior or posterior capsular fibrosis increases the difficulty in exploring the retina.

Take-Home Pearls

■ Avoid intraoperative posterior capsular tears with vitreous loss, as they increase the incidence of retinal complications.

■ Remove all cortical matter with meticulous elimination of the epithelial cells of the anterior capsule to decrease the incidence and delay of PCO as much as possible and to provide better and proper future fundus examination.

■ Perform large capsulorhexis to avoid the risk of capsular phimosis that will render fundus examination difficult and to decrease the number of anterior capsule epithelial cells.

■ Pars plana vitrectomy should be considered as the best therapeutic alternative especially for high myopic pseudophakic RD.

References

1. Ahmadied H, Moradian S, Faghihi et al (2005) Anatomic and visual outcomes of scleral buckling versus primary vitrectomy in pseudophakic and aphakic retinal detachment. Report no. 1. Ophthalmology 112:1421–1429

2. Alió JL, Ruiz-Moreno JM, Artola A (1993) Retinal detachment as a potential hazard in surgical correction of severe myopia with phakic anterior chamber lenses. Am J Ophthalmol. 115:145–148

3. Alió JL, Ruiz-Moreno JM, Shabayek MH et al (2007) The risk of retinal detachment in high myopia after small incision coaxial phacoemulsification. Am J Ophthalmol 144:93–98

4. Balazs EA, Denlinger JL (1984) The vitreous. In: Davson J (ed) The Eye, vol. 1A, 3rd edn. Academic, New York, pp 535–589

5. Barraquer C, Cavelier C, Mejía LF (1994) Incidence of retinal detachment following clear-lens extraction in myopic patient; retrospective analysis. Arch Ophthalmol 112:336–339

6. Bartz-Schmidt KU, Kirchof B, Heimann K (1996) Primary vitrectomy for pseudophakic retinal detachment. Br J Ophthalmol 80:346–349

7. Bertelmann E, Kojetinsky C (2001) Posterior capsule opacification and anterior capsule opacification. Curr Opinion Ophthalmol 12:35–40

8. Bettelheim FA, Popdimitrova N (1992) Hyaluronic acid-syneretic glycosaminoglycan. Curr Eye Res 11:411–419

9. Bishop PN, Takanosu M, Le Goff M et al (2002) The role of the posterior ciliary body in the biosynthesis of vitreous humour. Eye 16:454–460

10. Bovey EH, Gonvers M, Sahli O (1998) Surgical treatment of retinal detachment in pseudophakia: comparison between vitrectomy and scleral buckling. Klin Monatsbl Augenheilkd 212:314–317

11. Brazitiko PD, Androudi S, Christen WG et al (2005) Primary pars plana vitrectomy versus scleral buckle surgery or the treatment of pseudophakic retinal detachment. Retina 25:957–964

12. Brazitikos PD, D'Amico DJ, Tsinopoulos IT et al (1999) Primary vitrectomy with perfluoro-n-octane use in the treatment of pseudophakic retinal detachment with undetected retinal breaks. Retina 19:103–109

13. Burton TC (1990) The influence of refractive errors and lattice degeneration on the incidence of retinal detachment. Trans Am Ophthalmol Soc 87:143–155

14. Campo RV, Sipperley JO, Sneed SR et al (1999) Pars plana vitrectomy without scleral buckle for pseudophakic retinal detachments. Ophthalmology 106:1811–1815

15. Chastang P, Ruellan YM, Rozembaum JP et al (1998) Phakoémulsification à visée réfractive sur cristallin clair; a propos de 33 yeux myopes fortes. J Fr Ophtalmol 21:560–566

16. Colin J, Robinet A (1994) Clear lensectomy and implantation of a low-power posterior chamber intraocular lens for the correction of high myopia. Ophthalmology 101:107–112

17. Colin J, Robinet A (1997) Clear lensectomy and implantation of a low-power posterior chamber intraocular lens for the correction of high myopia: four-year follow-up. Ophthalmology 104:73–77

18. Colin J, Robinet A, Cochener B (1999) Retinal detachment after clear lens extraction for high myopia: seven-year follow-up. Ophthalmology 106:2281–2285

19. Coonan P, Fung WE, Webster RG Jr et al (1985) The incidence of retinal detachment following extracapsular cataract extraction. A ten-year study. Ophthalmology 92:1096–1101

20. Cousins S, Boniuk I, Okun E et al (1986) Pseudophakic retinal detachment in the presence of various IOL types. Ophthalmology 93:1198–1208

21. Escoffery RF, Olk RJ, Grand MG, et al (1985) Vitrectomy without scleral buckling for primary rhegmatogenous retinal detachment. Am J Ophthalmol 99:275–281

22. Fan DS, Lam DS, Li KK (1999) Retinal complications after cataract extraction in patients with high myopia. Ophthalmology 106:688–691

23. Fechner PU, Strobel J, Wicchmann W (1991) Correction of myopia by implantation of a concave Worst-iris claw lens into phakic eyes. Refract Corneal Surg 7:286–298

24. Fernandez-Vega L, Alfonso JF, Villacampa T (2003) Clear lens extraction for the correction of high myopia. Ophthalmology 110:2349–2354

25. Gabric N, Dekaris I, Karaman Z (2002) Refractive lens exchange for correction of high myopia. Eur J Ophthalmol 12:384–387

26. Garland DL, Duglas-Tabor Y, Jimenez-Asensio J et al (1996) The nucleus of the human lens: demonstration of a highly characteristic protein pattern by two-dimensional electrophoresis and introduction of a new method of lens dissection. Exp Eye Res 62:285–291

27. Glacet-Bernard A, Brahim R, Mokhtari O et al (1993) Retinal detachment following posterior capsulotomy using Nd:YAG laser. Retrospective study of 144 capsulotomies. J Fr Ophtalmol 16:87–94

28. Ho PC, Tolentino FI (1984) Pseudophakic retinal detachment. Surgical success rate with various types of IOLs. Ophthalmology 91:847–852

29. Horgan N, Condon PI, Beatty S (2005) Refractive lens exchange in high myopia: long term follow-up. Br J Ophthalmol 89:670–672

30. Javitt JC, Tielsch JM, Canner JK et al (1992) National outcomes of cataract extraction. Increased risk of retinal complications associated with Nd:YAG laser capsulotomy. The Cataract Patient Outcomes Research Team. Ophthalmology 99:1487–1497

31. Kaluzny J (1970) Myopia and retinal detachment. Polish Medical Journal 9:1544–1549

32. Kim KI, Miller JW (2002) Management of dislocated lens material. Seminar in Ophthalmology 17:162–166

33. Lois N, Wong D (2003) Pseudophakic retinal detachment. Surv Ophthalmol 48:467–487

34. Michels RG, Wilkinson CD, Rice TA (1990) Retinal detachment. Mosby, St Louis, pp 83–84

35. Neal RE, Bettelheim FA, Lim C et al (2005) Alterations in human vitreous humor following cataract extraction. Exp Eye Res 80:337–347

36. Olsen G, Olson RJ (2000) Update on a long-term, prospective study of capsulotomy and retinal detachment rates after cataract surgery. J Cataract Refract Surg 26:1017–1021

37. Osterlin S (1977) Preludes to retinal detachment in the aphakic eye. Mod Probl Ophthalmol 18:464–467

38. Panozzo G, Parolini B (2001) Relationships between vitreoretinal and refractive surgery. Ophthalmology 108:1663–1670

39. Pesando PM, Ghiringhello MP, Tagliavacche P (1999) Posterior chamber Collamer phakic intraocular lens for myopia and hyperopia. J Refract Surg 5:415–423

40. Pucci V, Morselli S, Romanelli F et al (2001) Clear lens phacoemulsification for correction of high myopia. J Cataract Refract Surg 27:896–900

41. Ravalico G, Michieli C, Vattovani O et al (2003) Retinal detachment after cataract extraction and refractive lens exchange in highly myopic patients. J Cataract Refract Surg 29:39–44

42. Ripandelli G, Scassa C, Parisi V et al (2003) Cataract surgery as a risk factor for retinal detachment in very highly myopic eyes. Ophthalmology 110:2355–61

43. Rosen PH, Wong HC, McLeod D (1989) Indentation microsurgery: internal searching for retinal breaks. Eye 3:277–281

44. Rubin ML (1975) The induction of refractive errors by retinal detachment surgery. Trans Am Ophthalmol 73:452–490

45. Ruiz-Moreno JM, Alió JL (2003) Incidence of retinal diseases following refractive surgery in 9,239 eyes. J Refract Surg 19:534–547

46. Ruiz-Moreno JM, Alió JL, Pérez-Santonja JJ et al (1999) Retinal detachment in phakic eyes with anterior chamber intraocular lenses to correct severe myopia. Am J Ophthalmol 127:270–275

47. Ruiz-Moreno JM, Montero J, de la Vega C et al (2006) Retinal detachment in myopic eyes after phakic intraocular lens implantation. J Refract Surg 22:247–252

48. Schepens CL, Marden D (1966) Data on the natural history of retinal detachment: further characterization of certain unilateral non traumatic cases. Am J Ophthalmol 61:213–226

49. Sebag J (1987) Age-related changes in human vitreous structure. Graefes Archive for Clin Exp Ophthalmol 225:89–93

50. Sebag J (1998) Macromolecular structure of vitreous. Prog Polymer Science 23:415–446

51. Senn P, Schmid MK, Job O et al (2002) Pars plana vitrectomy for pseudophakic retinal detachment. Klin Monatsbl Augenheilkd 219:226–230

52. Tosi GM, Casprini F, Malandrini A et al (2003) Phacoemulsification without intraocular lens implantation in patients with high myopia: long-term results. J Cataract Refract Surg 29:1127–1131
53. Watanabe H, Komoto M, David LL et al (1990) Changes in crystallin concentration in rat aqueous and vitreous humors after selenium-induced reversible cortical cataract. Jpn J Ophthalmol 34:472–478

54. Weichel ED, Martidis A, Fineman MS et al (2006) Pars plana vitrectomy versus combined pars plana vitrectomy-scleral buckle for primary repair of pseudophakic retinal detachment. Ophthalmology 113:2033–2040

55. Wilkinson CP (1985) Pseudophakic retinal detachment. Retina 5:1–4

56. Wu WC, Chen MT, Hsu SY et al (2002) Management of pseudophakic retinal detachment with undetectable retinal breaks. Ophthalmic Surg Lasers 33:314–318

57. Yoshida A, Ogasawara H, Jalkh AE et al (1992) Retinal detachment after cataract surgery. Surgical results. Ophthalmology 99:460–465

58. Zaldivar R, Davidorf JM, Oscherow S (1998) Posterior chamber phakic intraocular lenses for myopia of –8 to –1:467–487

14

Core Messages

- The natural history of high-myopic eyes is associated with a small incidence of choroidal submacular neovascularization

- RLE is applicable to younger patients than generally undergo cataract surgery.

- There is a clearer distinction between RLE in myopic eyes than in hyperopic eyes, which are not subject to the effects of the retinal stretching that can lead to premature macular subretinal neovascularization and macular degeneration.

- Light toxicity as a potential cause of premature macular degeneration has to be considered in relation to the light blocking characteristics of replacement lens implants.

- UV light– and blue light–blocking pigments in IOLS have to be balanced against their potential to degrade dim light vision quality.

- Clinical signs associated with premature onset of AMD and family history of AMD are important counseling points for patients considering undergoing RLE.

14.2 Refractive Lens Exchange and Choroidal Neovascularization

Emanuel Rosen

14.2.1 Introduction

Refractive lens exchange (RLE) comprises exchange of the clear or relatively clear crystalline lens for a lens implant for the purpose of refractive relief, i.e., adjustment of the refraction of the eye to any desired end. As its name implies, this is a process applicable to a younger cohort of patients than those patients undergoing lens exchange for removal of a visually disabling cataract. The surgical process is the same, but the age range is different. In the older group of cataract patients (with geographic and racial variants) age-related central retinal (macular) pathology is prevalent as its name implies. On the other hand, RLE is applicable to highly myopic eyes, whose natural history embraces macular pathology in particular the effects of retinal stretching an aspect of the larger eye globe of the high myopic eye as well as posterior staphyloma, local hyper-stretching phenomena.

Cataract surgery is much more prevalent than RLE is and though it embraces a different age related cohort, lessons can be learned from the data provided in relation to the risks to macular function through subretinal pathology, which is the subject of this chapter. We are also able to derive conclusions from study of pathological specimens allowing the relationship between clinical ophthalmoscopic signs and subretinal pathology to be better understood. The role of light in the causation of macular pathology is also relevant, for RLE involves the exchange of a yellowing (but optically well functioning) lens for a intraocular lens implant (IOL), which in general do not have the light filtration qualities of the natural lens.

There is a clearer distinction between RLE in myopic eyes than in hyperopic eyes, which are not subject to the effects of the retinal stretching that can lead to premature macular subretinal neovascularization and macular degeneration.

14.2.2 Pathology

Age-related macular degeneration (AMD) is clinically less common in Indian compared with Caucasian eyes, whereas cataract surgery is applicable in general to a younger age group. Therefore, potential lessons may be learned from postmortem eyes, which can be related to clinical signs in eyes of patients being considered for RLE [1]; 48% had some form of age-related macular change. These included basal laminar deposits, hard drusen, soft drusen, extensive retinal pigment epithelium atrophy of the macula, and disciform degeneration of macula with a combination of changes often seen. Illustrations of clinical aspects of these pathological changes can be seen in Figs. 14.2.1–14.2.10.

Spraul et al. [2] performed a histopathologic study to compare eyes with different stages of AMD with age-matched eyes to identify characteristics associated with exudative vs. nonexudative AMD. They showed that in the macular area, a statistically significant difference was observed for the degree of calcification ($p = 0.02$) and fragmentation ($p = 0.03$) of Bruch's membrane in eyes with exudative AMD (1.6 and 5 per eye, respectively) compared with eyes with nonexudative AMD (0.8 and 1 per eye, respectively) and control eyes (0.8 and 0 per eye, respectively). Eyes with AMD

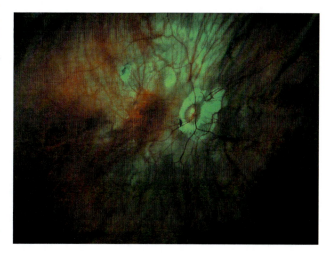

Fig. 14.2.1 Myopic RLE myopic retinal thinning and central RPE atrophy precursor of choroidal neovascularization

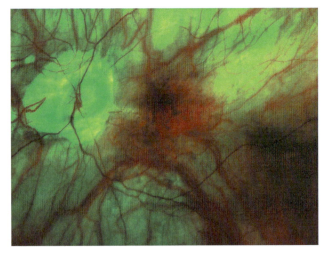

Fig. 14.2.2 Myopic RLE myopic retinal thinning and central RPE atrophy precursor of choroidal neovascularization

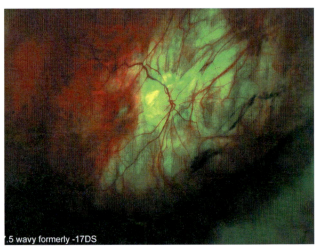

Fig. 14.2.5 Myopic RLE myopic retinal thinning and central RPE atrophy with early choroidal neovascularization and distorted vision

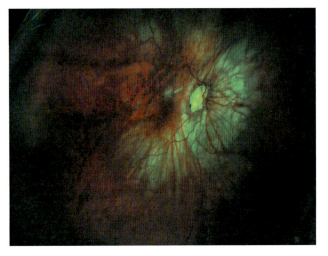

Fig. 14.2.3 Myopic RLE myopic retinal thinning and central RPE atrophy precursor of choroidal neovascularization

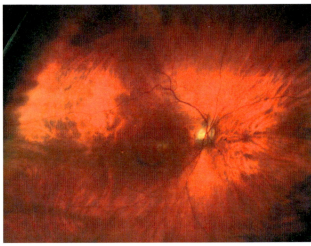

Fig. 14.2.6 Hyperopic RLE subretinal neovascular membrane (SRN-VM) with retinal pigment epithelium detachment

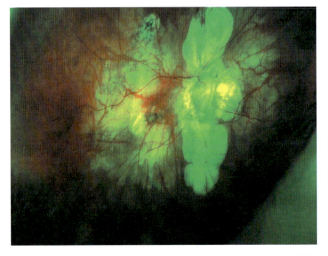

Fig. 14.2.4 Myopic RLE myopic retinal thinning and central RPE atrophy plus early choroidal neovascularization

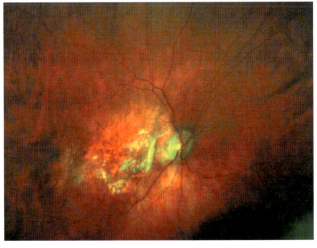

Fig. 14.2.7 Hyperopic RLE SRNVM with lipid exudate

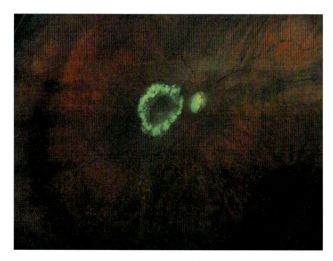

Fig. 14.2.8 Pseudophakia SRNVM with lipid circinate exudate

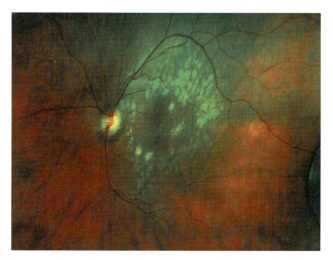

Fig. 14.2.9 Pseudophakia soft drusen and good vision (6/6)

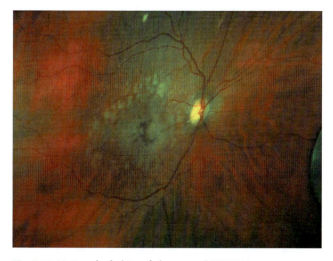

Fig. 14.2.10 Pseudophakia soft drusen and SRNVM

displayed notably softer, more confluent, and larger drusen and basal laminar (linear) deposit in the macular area compared with control eyes. Calcification and fragmentation of Bruch's membrane, soft, confluent, and large drusen, and basal laminar (linear) deposit but not hard drusen correlate with the histological presence of AMD. The degree of calcification and fragmentation of Bruch's membrane is greater in eyes with exudative compared with non-exudative AMD.

14.2.2.1 Retina in High Myopia

Pruett [3] notes that macular choroidal neovascularization occurs more often in those with moderate staphyloma than in those with advanced atrophy in the posterior pole. Indocyanine green angiography has improved our knowledge of this complication, which has been correlated with an increased number of posterior choroidal drainage systems. Clinically, RLE while offering refractive relief to the severely myopic, patients must be aware that natural progression of retinal stretching can result in loss of the anticipated longer-term benefit of this surgery.

14.2.2.2 Prevalence

Choroidal neovascularization (CNV) is an uncommon cause of vision loss in patients <50 years of age. In these patients, CNV is often the result of pathologic myopia, but other pathologies such as angioid streaks may be coexistent in myopic eyes being considered for refractive relief through RLE. Of course, untreated CNV may cause rapid deterioration of central vision and with a poor prognosis [4].

Lessons related to RLE may be derived from studies of characteristics of choroidal neovascularization in highly myopic patients corrected by the implantation of phakic intraocular lenses (PIOLs) Ruiz-Moreno et al. [5] determined CNV occurred in five eyes (1.7%); three eyes were in women, and two were in men. The interval between phakic anterior chamber lens implant (PACL) implantation and CNV was 63.2 ± 27.3 months (range, 18–87 months). The CNV was subfoveal in four eyes and juxtafoveal in one case. The mean BSCVA after PACL implantation and before the appearance of CNV was 0.53 ± 0.18 (range 0.4 [20/50] to 0.8 [20/25]); after CNV appeared, it was 0.26 ± 0.18 (range 0.05 [20/400] to 0.5 [20/40]), a statistically significant difference ($p = 0.001$, paired Student t test). The cumulative risk for CNV (Kaplan-Meier survival analysis) in highly myopic patients corrected by PACL implantation was 0.43% at 18 months and 5.4% at 87 months.

Ruiz- Moreno et al. [6] studied 522 consecutive highly myopic eyes (spherical equivalent refraction ±6.00 D and/or axial length >26 mm) (323 patients) corrected by the implantation of PIOLs, before and after treatment of CNV, and the interval between refractive surgery and the development of choroidal neovascularization. CNV developed after PIOL implantation at a mean interval time of 33.7 ± 29.6 months (range, 1 to 87 months). Using Kaplan-Meier analysis, the risk of choroidal neovascularization in patients with high myopia corrected by PIOL implantation was 0.57% at 5 months, 0.81% at 18 months, 1.31% at 24 months, and 3.72% at 87–145 months While phakic intraocular lens implantation for the correction of high myopia does seemingly not play a role in the development of CNV, the study reflects the potential natural incidence of CNV in a population similar to one which would undergo RLE, albeit for higher degrees of myopia than in this study cohort.

On the other hand, Fernandez-Vega et al. [7] evaluated the postoperative outcomes and intra- and postoperative complications of RLE with PACL implantation in highly myopic eyes in a retrospective case series of 107 patients (190 eyes) who had been observed for at least 3 years after surgery. Highly myopic eyes (axial length >26 mm) over 7 years (January 1990 to December 1996) were reviewed. Subfoveal CNV developed in 4 eyes (2.10%) of 3 patients; all of these eyes presented with a macular lacquer crack. Hayashi K et al. [8] considered the incidence and characteristics of (CNV) in patients with high myopia more than 8.00 D who underwent cataract surgery between September 1991 and March 2000. CNV was found in 6 eyes (12.5%) of 6 patients. The mean interval between cataract surgery and the development of CNV was 34±17 months (range, 12–48 months). The CNV was subfoveal in all cases. Subfoveal CNV developed more frequently in eyes when the fellow eye showed evidence of CNV preoperatively (40.0%) than in eyes when the fellow eye exhibited no evidence of CNV (9.3%). Implantation of a PACL to correct high myopia was followed by a small incidence of CNV (cumulative risk of 5.4% at 87 months). The appearance of CNV was followed by a significant decrease in BSCVA.

Cataract surgery is undertaken in an older age group than RLE patients, and the underlying age related phenomena in cataractous eyes are undoubtedly different from the younger eyes undergoing RLE. Early clinical case series reports suggested a link between cataract surgery and late AMD [9–11]. A report on postmortem eyes also suggested that neovascular AMD was more frequently observed in pseudophakic than phakic eyes. Pollack et al. [10, 11] in a small number of cases, carefully documented that the risk of AMD increased within 6 to 12 months after surgery in patients with bilateral, symmetric, early AMD. In contrast, Armbrecht et al. [12] could not confirm such an observation between surgical and nonsurgical patients.

On the other hand, myopic eyes undergoing RLE already have degenerative elements specific to myopia. Therefore, as the relationship between pseudophakia and AMD remains unclear but positive in the sense that there does appear to be a relationship, we can only speculate on the potential mechanisms that may cause RLE eyes to be more susceptible to earlier onset AMD with or without choroidal neovascularization. This could be mediated via inflammatory reactions associated with the surgery postoperative biochemical environmental changes within the eye (increased free radicals or growth factors) [14, 15] or increased light exposure either during or after surgery [16, 17]. The question of whether or not blue light–filtering IOLs are helpful in this regard remains unresolved [18, 19].

14.2.2.3 Light Toxicity and Potential Macular Effects

RLE patients may be in their sixth or seventh decade, and those younger patients are going to get older, so retinal health if not an immediate issue may be compromised by retinal light exposure at least according to some theories. Therefore, there is at least a hypothetical risk that RLE could lead to premature AMD. Photoxicity is one possible mechanism that could disturb central retinal balance.

There are at least two forms of retinal phototoxicity: blue–green and UV–blue. Blue–green phototoxicity is mediated by rhodopsin, the same photopigment involved in scotopic vision. The second type of retinal phototoxicity, UV–blue, increases with decreasing wavelength. In other words, UV radiation (100–400 nm) is more hazardous than is violet light (400–440 nm), which in turn is more hazardous than blue light (440–500 nm). UV radiation is responsible for 67% of acute UV–blue phototoxicity in the part of the spectrum that can reach the retina through an IOL, while violet light accounts for 18% and blue light for 14%.

The potentially harmful effects of UV radiation eventually led to the inclusion of UV-blocking chromophores in nearly all IOLs on the market today. It has been suggested that violet- and blue-blocking lenses (AcrySof Natural, Alcon Laboratories; AF-1, Hoya Corporation) may help prevent AMD as they to some degree mimic the color degradation of the ageing crystalline lens.

Blue light is much more important for mesopic and scotopic vision than it is for photopic vision because of rod as opposed to cone photoreceptor sensitivities. This is due to the photopigment rhodopsin, which has peak sensitivity near 500 nm, the border between blue and green light.

Age-related pupillary miosis and crystalline lens yellowing conspire to reduce older adults' effective blue light exposure to a tenth that of younger people.

The pathogenesis of AMD, the most common cause of visual loss after the age of 60 years, is indeed a complicated scenario that involves a variety of hereditary and environmental factors. For many years there has been concern, yet unfounded, that light exposure might play a role, but this relationship remains unproven. The availability of visible light-blocking intraocular lenses emphasizes the importance of continuing research in this area. There may be a tradeoff between blocking blue light and maintaining optimum mesopic vision [20, 21].

Cumulative sunlight exposure and cataract surgery are reported risk factors for AMD [21]. Laboratory studies suggest that accumulation and photochemical reactions of A2E (*N*-retinylidene-*N*-retinylethanolamine) and its epoxides, components of lipofuscin, are important in AMD. To relate this data to the clinical setting, Meyers et al. [22] modeled the effects of macular irradiance and spectral filtering on production of A2E and reactive oxygen intermediates (ROIs) in pseudophakic eyes with a clear or yellow IOL and in phakic eyes. They calculated the relative changes in macular irradiance as a function of light (390–700 nm) intensity, pupil size, age, and lens status, and modeled resulting all-transretinal concentration and rates of production of A2E-related photochemicals and photon-induced ROIs in rods and retinal pigment epithelium (RPE). They compared these photoproducts after cataract surgery and IOL implantation with and without spectral sunglasses to normal age-related nuclear sclerotic lens changes. Following cataract and IOL surgery, all-transretinal and lipofuscin photochemistry would theoretically increase average generation of (1) A2E-related photochemicals, (2) ROI in rods, and (3) ROI in RPE, respectively, 2.6-fold, 15-fold, and 6.6-fold, with a clear IOL, and 2.1-fold, 4.1-fold, and 2.6-fold with a yellow IOL, but decrease approximately 30-fold, approximately 20-fold, and 4-fold with a vermillion filter sunglass and clear IOL compared with an average 70-year-old phakic eye.

Sunglasses that strongly decrease both deep blue light and rod photobleaching, while preserving photopic sensitivity and color perception, could provide upstream protection from potential photochemical damage in subjects at risk for AMD progression after cataract (and RLE) surgery. If this is relevant for cataract surgery then it should be more so for RLE where life expectancy after RLE may be up to 60 years!

Take-Home Pearls

■ RLE is applicable to younger patients than generally undergo cataract surgery.
■ There is a clearer distinction between RLE in myopic eyes than in hyperopic eyes, which are not subject to the effects of the retinal stretching that can lead to premature macular subretinal neovascularization and macular degeneration.

References

1. Biswas J, Raman R (2002) Age-related changes in the macula. A histopathological study of fifty Indian donor eyes. Indian J Ophthalmol 50:201–204
2. Spraul CW, Grossniklaus HE (1997) Characteristics of Drusen and Bruch's membrane in postmortem eyes with age-related macular degeneration. Arch Ophthalmol 115:267–273
3. Pruett RC (1998) Complications associated with posterior staphyloma. Curr Opin Ophthalmol 9:16–22
4. Miller DG, Singerman LJ (2006) Vision loss in younger patients: a review of choroidal neovascularization. Optom Vis Sci 83:316–325
5. Ruiz-Moreno JM, de la Vega C, Ruiz-Moreno O, Aliò JL (2003) Choroidal neovascularization in phakic eyes with anterior chamber intraocular lenses to correct high myopia. J Cataract Refract Surg 29:270–274
6. Ruiz-Moreno JM, Montero JA, de la Vega C, Alió JL, Zapater P (2006) Macular choroidal neovascularization in myopic eyes after phakic intraocular lens implantation. J Refract Surg 22:689–694
7. Fernandez-Vega L, Alfonso JF, Villacampa T (2003) Clear lens extraction for the correction of high myopia. Ophthalmology 110:2349–2354
8. Hayashi K, Ohno-Matsui K, Futagami S, Ohno S, Tokoro T, Mochizuki M (2006) Choroidal neovascularization in highly myopic eyes after cataract surgery. Jpn J Ophthalmol 50:345–348
9. Schaft TL van der, Mooy CM, de Bruijn WC, Mulder PG, Pameyer JH, de Jong PT (1994) Increased prevalence of disciform macular degeneration after cataract extraction with implantation of an intraocular lens. Br J Ophthalmol 78:441–445
10. Pollack A, Marcovich A, Bukelman A, Oliver M (1996) Age-related macular degeneration after extracapsular cataract extraction with intraocular lens implantation. Ophthalmology 103:1546–1554
11. Pollack A, Marcovich A, Bukelman A et al (1999) Development of exudative age-related macular degeneration after cataract surgery. Eye 11:523–530
12. Seward HC (1998) Do patients with age related maculopathy and cataract benefit from cataract surgery? Br J Ophthalmol 83:253–254
13. Cugati S, Mitchell P, Franzco ER et al (2006) Cataract surgery and the 10-year incidence of age-related maculopathy: the Blue Mountains Eye Study. Ophthalmology 113:2020–2025
14. Algvere PV, Marshall J, Seregard S (2006) Age-related maculopathy and the impact of blue light hazard. Acta Ophthalmol Scand 84:4–11
15. Oliver M (1966) Posterior pole changes after cataract extraction in elderly subjects. Am J Ophthalmol 62:1145–1148
16. Anderson DH, Mullins RF, Hageman OS, Johnson LV (2002) A role for local inflammation in the formation of drusen in the aging eye. Am J Ophthalmol 134:411–431
17. Mainster MA, Ham WT Jr, Delori PC (1983) Potential retinal hazards: instrument and environmental light sources. Ophthalmology 90:927–932
18. Libre PE (2003) Intraoperative light toxicity: a possible explanation for the association between cataract surgery and age-related macular degeneration [letter]. Am J Ophthalmol 136:961
19. Braunstein RE, Sparrow JR (2005) A blue-blocking intraocular lens should be used in cataract surgery. Arch Ophthalmol 123:547–549
20. Mainster MA (2005) Intraocular lenses should block UV radiation and violet but not blue light. Arch Ophthalmol 123:550–555
21. Mainster MA (2005) Spectral trasmittance of intraocular lenses and retinal damage from intense light sources. Am J Ophthalmol 85:167–175
22. Meyers SM, Ostrovsky MA (2004) Bonner RFA model of spectral filtering to reduce photochemical damage in age-related macular degeneration. Trans Am Ophthalmol Soc. 2004;102:83

Core Messages

- Refractive surprises after cataract post–corneal surgeries are mostly related to curvature changes induced by corneal refractive surgeries.

- Refractive surprises after cataract post–corneal surgeries are in hyperopic shifts (<3.00 D may be resolved in 1 to 3 months; >3.00 D suggest an IOL calculation error–exchange).

- Progressive myopia or astigmatism can announce a secondary ectasia.

- The quality of vision can be altered by an increase in spherical aberrations (addition of asphericity loss after photoablation + spherical lens implantation).

14.3 Refractive Surprises after Cataract Post–Corneal Refractive Surgery

Béatrice Cochener and Jean Louis Arne

14.3.1 Introduction

Population aging and increase in visual needs leads to increased surgical cataracts. This evolution will undoubtedly be observed in patients who have undergone refractive surgery in the past. Indeed, those patients used to emmetropia and satisfied by the removal of glasses could very early detect visual changes induced by the beginning of lenticular opacification. Furthermore, they will require cataract surgery to avoid a return to glasses.

However, difficulties in IOL power calculations represent one major limitation of cataract surgery after previous corneal refractive surgery, essentially related to corneal curvature and asphericity changes. This could lead to postoperative refractive and visual surprises and require delicate enhancement procedures for inadequate outcomes [1–4].

These complications justify an adjustment of calculation formulas, integrating keratometry, and refractive changes induced by the initial corneal surgery [5–8]. This chapter focuses on photoablative surgeries.

A review of these unexpected results after pseudophakic IOL implantation after corneal refractive surgery are described as well as the therapeutic solutions that have been proposed for their correction. Various modified methods for IOL calculations, their principles, interests, and limitations are discussed.

Surprises after cataract post–corneal refractive surgeries can be essentially summarized as inadequate calculations of the IOL, especially if these were based on keratometry data secondary to photoablation. Note that after phakic implantation, measurements such axial length can be modified by the intraocular lens, suggesting the recommendation of archiving preoperative information of virgin eyes in order to facilitate IOL calculation.

14.3.2 Hyperopic Shift

A hyperopic shift commonly complicates incisional corneal surgery (cf. Chap. 12 on radial keratotomy) and photoablation for myopia. Concerning RK, surgery causes edema surrounding the incisions that regularly induces a transitory hyperopia (around +3.00 D) spontaneously resolved in 1–3 months. This potential favorable evolution suggests not surgically correcting this secondary ametropia.

Adversely, when hyperopia is superior to a +3.00-D level, an IOL calculation error can be suspected that could be associated with this corneal response. The same assumption of an inadequate implant calculation can be made when a hyperopic shift is noted after a cataract surgery after excimer surface photoablation or LASIK.

This ametropia is particularly difficult to tolerate in an initially myopic patient who became hyperopic, with discomfort in far and near vision. Therefore, this patient will ask for an improvement and will be reluctant to glasses, especially multifocal, which he/she was not used to before the surgery.

14.3.3 Myopic Shift

Its occurrence is rare, but it is easier to manage myopia than hyperopia. Theoretically, it could appear after a surgery for hyperopia with an overestimation of keratometry.

A secondary ectasia should be eliminated in case of progressive myopia that would be often associated to a loss in BCVA and irregular induced astigmatism.

14.3.4 Induced Astigmatism

This complication can be reported after any cataract surgery and can result from the incision procedure. The risk of postoperative astigmatism was considerably reduced by the advent of mini- and micro-incisions. Nevertheless, it may potentially increase the size of the preoperative cylinder if the size and the site of incision had not been correctly adapted.

However, because mechanical integrity is better preserved in photoablation compared to corneal incisions, the occurrence of irregular astigmatism is very uncommon.

In long-term corneal surgery, the occurrence of a progressive astigmatism should be suspected to announce a secondary ectasia, even more specifically than a progressive postoperative myopia.

14.3.5 Decentration

Photoablation, whatever the profile (including the use of scanning beam and wavefront custom treatment) is responsible for edging effects. However, this effect has been decreased by the creation of progressive transitional edges, enlargement in the optical zone, and introduction of the transition zone.

The crucial role of good laser centration on visual results is perfectly demonstrated and has justified the development of options such as cyclotorsion and pupil shift compensation. At the intraocular implantation stage, the adequate positioning of the lens in terms of centration and tilt admittedly plays a major role in the quality of vision. If positioning/centration are not perfect, then a conflict appears between the ablation area and the IOL, inducing degradation in qualitative vision with halos, glare, diplopia, and an increase in high order aberrations.

14.3.6 Alteration of Vision Quality

Alteration of the quality of vision can be induced by all the complications previously described. The addition of an IOL behind a cornea whose physiologic curvatures have been surgically modified systematically causes changes in optical properties. These degradations are sources of functional symptoms and increases in high-order aberrations.

Before the advent of wavefront sensors, many inadequate outcomes were unexplained because of limitations of available measurement concepts. First, geometrical optics provides only the pure spherocylindrical refraction and is based on the Gaussian assumption that the eye can be simplified to a convergent diopter. This concept appears too approximative in cases of an imperfect optical system, such in an eye modified by surgery. Furthermore, the measurement is paraxial, centrated, and static (does not integrate the effects of pupil dilation). Videotopography is considered (whichever, Placido or elevation system), if it can assess toricity, symmetry and more recently quantify asphericity; none of the available devices can access the periphery of the cornea for a true three-dimensional evaluation and a real-time measurement.

Elaboration of aspherical ablation profiles would help to preserve natural characteristics of the cornea. These adjustments should contribute to minimize the impact on the quality of vision. The new design of aspherical IOLs has the same goal and is based on two concepts, a lens with negative spherical aberrations (in order to compensate positive spherical aberrations of the cornea), and a lens-free of aberration. The good choice of an aspherical IOL after corneal refractive surgery would be, at that date, the second model, since the photoablation has changed the corneal profile resulting in an increase in positive spherical aberration in case of hyperopic correction and in the adverse for myopic treatment. Therefore, we would first try not to increase high order aberrations in using an implant with neutral effects on spherical aberrations.

14.3.7 Management of Refractive Complications after Cataract Surgery Post-Corneal Surgery

14.3.7.1 Optical Equipment
Adaptation of glasses represents the most common and the safest solution to correct imperfect visual results after cataract extraction. When we consider that visual recovery in

that specific surgical condition takes time (1–3 months), the option of glasses offers the advantages of safety and adjustability. However, if the residual ametropia is responsible for anisometropia, then glasses may not be tolerated by the patient. In the case of irregular astigmatism, an adjustment of contact lenses could be recommended in order to optimize visual performances. This contact lens adaptation is easier to conduct after photoablation than after radial keratectomy, but requires specific experience from the physician.

14.3.7.2 Lens Exchange
This option is the most commonly discussed since the most frequent complication is the hyperopic shift resulting from an IOL calculation error. Patience is required from the patient for at least 2 weeks in order to control the stability of induced ametropia, despite an unusual regression compared to radial keratectomy. Over 3.00 D can be discussed for a high-power lens exchange (based on the addition of the residual hyperopic value to the initial IOL power).

The need of an IOL exchange was estimated to one case per four surgeries, until a better approach of IOL calculation was issued from refined formulas, and an increase in surgical experience was observed. Therefore, it appears crucial to inform the patient of this eventuality. Furthermore, preoperative keratometry and refractive data should be provided to patients who underwent corneal refractive surgery in order to facilitate IOL calculations and to decrease the occurrence of this complication.

Care and caution are required for the selection of the IOL that has to be easy to manipulate and remove. Moreover, when an exchange is required, it should be performed early for safer mobilization in the capsular bag.

14.3.7.3 Photoablation
A complementary photoablation can be justified in the case of low spherical and/or cylindrical refractive error. That could consist of excimer correction by PRK or under a LASIK flap (newly created or re-lifted). The choice of the technique will depend on the initial method, on the type of ametropia, and on surgeon conviction.

A particular vigilance is required for the eye-tracker connection because it may be disturbed by the lens reflect. The presence of an intraocular lens may also make the aberrometry measurement difficult (even impossible in cases of high irregular astigmatism after radial keratectomy). However, when this one is accessible, it is interesting to perform a custom ablation to improve quality of vision.

In all cases, especially secondary hyperopia, it is necessary to maintain an optical zone as large as possible in order to minimize functional symptoms resulting from the superposition of different successive surgeries.

14.3.7.4 Incisions
For surgeons experienced in incisional surgical techniques, it is common to perform incisions at the same stage of

phacoemulsification; arcuate incisions on the axis of the meridian flatten it for the correction of preoperative astigmatism.

The efficacy of this single-step technique depends on the surgical expertise and is limited by the unpredictability of the postoperative refraction, as has already been underlined. It could appear logical to discuss a two-step correction, with the adjustment of incisions according to the refraction after cataract surgery. But, as we know that persistent refractive errors are mostly hyperopic, incisions will be rarely indicated.

14.3.7.5 Piggyback Multifocal IOL

This method corresponds to a secondary implantation of an IOL in the sulcus in front of an IOL previously placed in the bag. The initial lens provides an incomplete correction, resulting in residual ametropia that defines the value of the secondary IOL (with an addition of around 20%) [9, 10].

The second lens will be chosen with the same biomaterial as the first one. Its design has to be compatible with positioning in the sulcus, which means associating rigid haptics in a three-piece model will allow correct centration and stability. Particular care will be brought to the interface cleaning between the two intraocular lenses in order to prevent cell ingrowth that would be the source of transparency and vision alteration.

A promising concept is under development, based on the concept of a piggyback, multifocal IOL, designed for the correction of the residual sphere after cataract surgery combined with an addition for near vision. The first model was created by Ioltech (Zeiss) laboratory under the name of Acor, which is made of a one-piece acrylic hydrophilic material. One of the current limitations to this piggyback implantation is represented by the difficulty to measure the sulcus diameter and thus to adapt the precise overall diameter of the lens. Different sizes should be available. In current accurate conditions, a decentration is difficult to avoid, inducing a loss of the expected multifocal effect. New designs are currently under evaluation.

14.3.7.6 Perspectives: Multifocal IOLs? Toric?

High difficulties in IOL calculation in cataract extraction after corneal refractive surgery make the use of multifocal lenses very delicate. Despite convincing results achieved with the new generation of diffractive IOLs, they could result, in that specific context, in under- or overcorrection, or difficulty in tolerating them, leading to a major alteration in the quality of vision untenable for the operated patient.

Among currently available concepts, the elective choice would move to an aberration-free aspherical profile in order not to add to these multioperated-on eyes high-order aberrations, which are difficult to quantify and neutralize. It has been demonstrated that corneas that had a photoablation have increased (in case of myopic correction) or reversed (in case of hyperopic correction) preoperative positive spherical aberrations. Whatever the ablation profile, these induced changes presume that aspherical IOLs with negative spherical aberrations would partially compensate or in the adverse increase initial corneal spherical aberrations.

It might not be difficult to imagine that the ideal IOL could one day be customized to the eye, like a mirror of the wavefront map coming from the eye candidate to a cataract surgery. This would be an interesting method to achieve the exact compensation of corneal aberrations, especially for those corneas that have received refractive surgery in the past [11–21].

14.3.8 Prevention of Surprises: Adjusted Implant Calculation

In an eye that has had refractive surgery, miscalculation of IOL power frequently occurs, leading to hyperopia after myopic surgery and to myopia after hyperopic surgery [22, 23], for which patients had expectations of perfect vision without correction after cataract surgery.

A significant hyperopic result after cataract surgery in eyes that had previous RK has been reported when the IOL power was calculated using corneal power obtained by manual keratometry [24, 25].

IOL lens power calculation depends on the axial lens (AL), ACD, and keratometry readings. Studies of axial length changes after corneal refractive surgeries have shown no significant changes [26]; with few exceptions (corneal rings), ACD is not changed after corneal refractive surgery. Factors leading to errors are inaccurate estimation of corneal power, and use of an inappropriate IOL power-calculation formula [27].

Corneal refractive surgery produces an abnormally shaped cornea: The center of the cornea becomes flatter than the peripheral cornea after refractive surgery for myopia. Manual keratometry measures two points approximately 3 mm apart. If these points are measured outside the flatter central area, then the manual keratometer reads steeper values [28, 29].

Current instruments measure the anterior corneal radius of curvature (Ra) by measuring the reflected images of the projected mires; the posterior radius of curvature is not assessed but is compensated for by the use of a modified (effective) index of refraction. The keratometric diopters are derived from the anterior radius of curvature using an effective refractive index (n) in the paraxial formula: keratometric power (D) = $(n - 1)/Ra$.

However, this effective refractive index is valid only if the proportion between the radius of the anterior and posterior surfaces of the cornea resembles that of a model eye.

Following RK, both the anterior and posterior corneal surfaces undergo a relatively proportional flattening, and the relationship between them is not changed. The central cornea flattens more than the Para central transition (knee) zone, which leads to an overestimate of the curvature of the central flat optical zone.

Following PRK or LASIK, if the treatment zone is large, then the anterior radius of curvature measurement can be still accurate because the transition area is far outside the 2.6- to 3-mm measured zone. In this instance, the lack of accuracy in the K reading results from the fact that the normal relationship between the anterior and posterior corneal surface curvature is disrupted as a result of anterior corneal surface flattening, while the posterior surface curvature remains unchanged. Therefore, the use of an effective index of refraction, which was generated in normal corneas, does not compensate correctly for the posterior corneal surface power which results in an inaccurate K readings [23, 30].

Another problem is that it is impossible to quantify accurately the discrepancy between measured corneal power change and refractive change to determine a correction factor that could derive true evaluations from the measured corneal power.

14.3.8.1 Correcting the Variance

There are two ways of correcting the variance when calculating the IOL power. The first involves the development of a method that accurately estimates corneal power and the second the development of a more appropriate formula.

14.3.8.1.1 Estimation of Corneal Power after Corneal Refractive Surgery [31]

Standard office keratometers estimate central corneal power. The problem is that the reflected ring of the keratometer measures the cornea at approximately the 3-mm diameter zone, which is often a steeper area after myopic surgery than the flatter optical centre (vice versa after hyperopic surgery).

Another method is measuring the corneal power within 3 mm of the center of the cornea using a videokeratometer. Corneal topography measures more than 1,000 points in the central 3- mm zone, while conventional keratometry only measures 2 points located 3.2 and 2.6 mm from the corneal centre. Simulated keratotopographic readings (SimK) values seem the most accurate among measured keratometric power [32]. However, it is often admitted that the central corneal power should be used with topography, as it gives a more reliable central power measurement than the stimulated keratometry value after refractive surgery.

However, it has often been noted that videokeratography-derived K values are inaccurate in eyes with abnormal or surgically altered corneal surfaces.

Sonego-Krone et al. (33) think that OrbscanII total mean and total optical power maps accurately assess the corneal power after myopic LASIK independent of preoperative data or correcting factors and should improve IOL calculation.

Generally, with all the techniques, it is safer to use a smaller value to prevent a hyperopic shift after surgery for myopia and a larger value after hyperopic surgery. To avoid underestimation of intraocular lens power after surgery for myopia, the measured corneal power must be corrected. There are no universal and absolutely reliable methods but many surgeons subtract 1.00 D from the measured value.

After surgery for hyperopia, the measured value must be increased.

The hard contact lens method, introduced by Holladay [34] is based on determining the difference between the manifest refraction with and without a rigid "plane" contact trial lens of a known base curve. An unchanged refraction indicates the tear lens between the cornea and contact lens has zero power, and that the effective anterior corneal radius is equal to the posterior radius (base curve) of the trial lens. If a myopic shift in refraction occurs with the contact lens, the base curve is steeper (i.e., the tear lens forms a plus lens) and vice versa. The idea is to determine the corneal radius by finding the trial lens that does not change the refraction with and without contact lenses and then read the power from the contact lens.

This method takes a relatively long time. It cannot be used if visual acuity is too low because of the lens opacity. It is widely used after RK but has not been validated for use after PRK or LASIK. Dense cataracts may give rise to a false refraction.

Case example: hard contact lens method

- Plane hard contact lens curvature: 40.5 D
- SE (corneal plane vertex 12.5 mm) without contact lens: 0.50 D
- SE with contact lens: → unchanged refraction
  - **Mean corneal power** = [40.5 + 0 (−0.50) − (0.50)] = 40.5 →S.E. = −1.00 D
  - **Mean corneal power** = [40.5 + 0 + (−1.00) − (0.5)] = 40 → S.E. = +1.00 D
  - **Mean corneal power** = [40.5 + 0 + (+1.00) − (−0.5)] = 42

Clinical history method [34, 35]:
Postoperative corneal power is obtained by subtracting the refractive change (calculated at the corneal plane using a standard vertex distance of 12 mm) induced by surgery from the preoperative keratometry readings in myopic eyes. The refractive change must be determined once refraction has been stabilized after corneal surgery by subtracting the postoperative from the preoperative spherical equivalent refraction, but both must be corrected by the vertex distance to the plane of the cornea. These values can be calculated with the following formula: $R_c = R_s + (1 − vR_s)$, where R_c = power (D) at the corneal plane, R_s = power (D) at vertex (v) distance, and V = vertex distance (meters); a vertex distance of 0.012 m is often assumed. However, myopia induced by the opacification of the crystalline lens is an important factor of error.

Case example: clinical history method

- Preoperative keratotomy: 44 D
- Preoperative refraction: –7.00 D
- Postoperative refraction: –2.00 D
- Change in SE: (–7.00) – (–2.00) = –5.00 D
  - Calculated keratometry for determination of IOL power: 44 – 5.00 = 39 D

Refraction-derived corrected keratometric value (K_c.rd): According to this method, which Shammas [15] derived from the clinical history method, the corneal power is the result of the formula $K_c \times rd = K_{post} (-0.25 \times CR_c)$, where K_{post} is the actual keratometry reading, and CR_c is the amount of myopia corrected at the corneal plane.

Clinically derived corrected keratometric value (K_c.cd): This method (also developed by Shammas from the historical method) calculates the corneal power by means of the following equation: $Kc \times cd = 1.14 Kpost - 6.8$, where $Kpost$ is the actual keratometry reading [36].

Correction factor method by ROSA et al. [37]: The postoperative radius, as measured by videokeratography, is multiplied by a correcting factor that varies between 1.01 and 1.22 according to the axial length of the eye.

Theoretical variable refractive index (TRI) as proposed by FERRARA et al. [38]: The change in the corneal refractive index after excimer laser surgery is correlated to the axial length. Such correlation is expressed by the formula: $TRI = -0.0006 \times (AL \times AL) + 0.0213 \times AL + 1.1572$, where AL is axial length. Corneal power (P) can be calculated using the formula: $P = (TRI - 1)/r$, where r is the corneal curvature in meters.

Separate consideration of anterior and posterior corneal curvature: This method is based on the assumption that the total corneal refractive power of the cornea (P) can be calculated by adding the power of the anterior (P_a) and posterior (P_p) corneal surfaces [39]: $P = P_a + P_p = (n_2 - n_1)/r_1 + (n_3 - n_2)/r_2$, where n_1 is the refractive index of air (–1), n_2 is the refractive index of the cornea (1.376), and n_3 is the refractive index of the aqueous humor (1.336).

Both preoperatively and postoperatively, the P_a can be obtained by multiplying the videokeratographic corneal power by 1.114 (corresponding to 376/337.5) [40]. Hence, $P_p = P_a - P = (SimK \times 1.114) - SimK$.

To measure the total corneal power after excimer laser surgery, there are two options:

1. If the preoperative videokeratographic power is available and thus the posterior corneal surface can be calculated, then the postoperative P_a may be added to P_p (which is assumed not to be significantly altered by surgery) as expressed by the formula: $P = $ postop $P_a + P_p = $ postop $SimK \times 1.114 + $ (preop $SimK \times 1.114 - $ preop $SimK$).
2. If the preoperative videokeratographic power is not available, thus precluding calculation of P_p, then the latter is substituted by a mean value 4.98. The resulting formula is $P = $ postop $P_a + P_p = $ postop $SimK \times 1.114 - 4.98$ [41].

14.3.8.1.2 Methods to Calculate IOL Power

The list of methods for IOL calculations after refractive surgery is long and growing (Table 14.3.1). As it is always the case when there are several solutions to a problem, none is perfect.

The Feiz-Mannis vertex IOL power method [42]: The IOL power for emmetropia is based on pre-LASIK keratometry values. The SE change resulting from LASIK is then used to modify the IOL power, assuming 1.00 D of change in IOL produces only 0.70 D of change in refraction at the spectacle plane. This is based on the IOL position behind the iris and a vertex distance of 12–13 mm. This method produces higher IOL powers after myopic LASIK and lower IOL powers after hyperopic LASIK. Furthermore, the higher the amount of treatment, the more inaccurate the traditional keratometry readings. Based on these results, the authors created a nomogram using linear regression analysis as a basis.

Errors often advise when calculating IOL powers the using SRK/T formula.

The reason for the residual hyperopia is incorrect effective lens position (ELP) estimation calculated by third-generation theoretical formulas in which the post refractive surgery K value is used. This usually short value underestimates the ELP and IOL power after surgery for myopia resulting in a hyperopia.

Aramberri [43] modified the SRK/T formula to use the pre–refractive surgery K value (K_{pre}) for the ELP calculation and the post–refractive surgery K value for IOL power calculation by the vergence formula.

The K_{pre} value is obtained by keratometry or topography and the K_{post} by the clinical history method, once the refraction stabilized. This value is converted to the corneal plane and subtracted from K_{pre}.

Rosa [44] et al. tried to calculate IOL power in cases where pre–refractive surgery data are not available by adjusting the corneal radius based on the axial eye length.

Latkany et al. [45] described regression formulas based on both the average and flattest post–refractive surgery keratometric readings when pre–refractive surgery data are not available.

They describe two methods:

1. Calculation of IOL power using mean keratometry readings obtained using the Javal keratometer and modifying it by $-0.46x + 0.21$, where x equals the surgically induced change in refraction.
2. Calculation of IOL power using the flat K modified by $-0.47x + 0.85$.

Presented at the ASCRS convention of March 2006, the BEESt formula developed by Borasio and Stevens is based on an improved version of the Gaussian optics formula for para-axial imagery. This method requires measurement of the anterior and posterior corneal radii and central corneal thickness; these values are taken from the Oculus Pentacam [46].

Methods were described to calculate IOL power after refractive surgery without using the inaccuracies of the post LASIK corneal power.

Walter et al. [47] assumed the patient never had myopic LASIK to calculate IOL power and then targeted the IOL at the pre-LASIK amount of myopia. The pre-LASIK keratometry values, pre-LASIK manifest refraction, and the current axial length are placed in the Holladay formula by passing the post-LASIK corneal power.

With Masket's formula [48], one calculates IOL power in a standard fashion and simply modifies the final value of the IOL as a function of the LASIK-induced refractive change. An advantage of this method is that there is less reliance on historical data, as the LASIK-induced change is multiplied by 0.323. Therefore, if there is a 1.00-D error in the historical data regarding the refractive change, then this translates to only a 0.32-D error in IOL selection.

Ianchulev et al. [49] used an intraoperative autorefractive retinoscopy to obtain aphakic autorefraction and measured the aphakic spherical equivalent before lens implantation.

Mackool et al. [50] described a technique in which the cataract is removed without IOL implantation. Approximately 30 min later, manifest aphakic refraction is performed. The calculation of the IOL power is obtained using a specific algorithm. The patient then returns to the operating room for lens implantation.

14.3.9 Specific Problems

In the case of cataract surgery after RK, all eyes experience an initial hyperopic shift caused by early postoperative corneal flattening due to a stromal edema [51].

Corneal edema normally resolves within a few weeks after cataract surgery. A significant amount of hyperopic error will also regress, and it is suggested to wait at least 3 months before performing IOL exchange. However, a larger hyperopic error does not totally regress, and the IOL exchange must be done earlier. The benefit of performing secondary surgery earlier is that the same incision can be used and lens replacement is easier. The disadvantage is that accurate IOL power selection is difficult because the corneal curvature and power are still unstable [52].

The newly approved techniques for the treatment of low-to-moderate hyperopia, conductive keratoplasty (CK) and laser thermokeratoplasty (LTK), have postulated effect similar to the RK procedure, where both surfaces of the cornea are shifted together in the same direction. The anterior–posterior corneal surface relationship is not disrupted, the effective optical zone is relatively large, and the transition zone is far outside the measured area. Thus, accurate K readings with the current instruments might be anticipated after CK and LTK.

What should the clinician do when faced with the daunting problem of post–refractive surgery IOL power calculation after excimer corneal refractive surgery [53]?

Table 14.3.1 Methods for lens power calculation

Methods requiring pre–refractive surgery data:
– Double-K VKG
– Double-K clinical history
– Single-K refraction–derived method
– Feitz-Mannis formula
– Double-K based on separate consideration of anterior and posterior corneal curvatures (with preoperative data)
– Latkany's regression formula
– Feitz-Mannis monogram
– Walter method
– Masket formula

Methods not requiring pre–refractive surgery data:
– Single-K clinically derived method
– Rosa's single-K method
– Ferrara's single-K method
– Double-K based on separate consideration of anterior and posterior corneal curvatures (without preoperative data)
– Mackool method
– Ianchulev method

To evaluate the corneal power, it is recommended to choose the lowest value after myopic surgery and the highest after hyperopic surgery.

For the IOL power calculation, the surgeon must use several approaches and look for values that are consistent with at least one other reading.

Patients should be informed that the accuracy of these methods to calculate the IOL power after refractive surgery has not yet be validated, and that an exchange of the IOL or other interventions may be necessary.

To minimize this problem, all candidates for refractive surgery should be given a wallet card containing their preoperative data (pretreatment average keratometric power, proposed treatment, preoperative refraction, and refraction at a suitable postoperative time when the cornea has stabilized and before the development of lens opacity).

Take-Home Pearls

■ Management of refractive surprises after cataract post–corneal surgeries
  – Optical equipment: the safest method but partial and /or transitory solution
  – Lens exchange: preoperative patient information ++ (not too early , >3.00 D)
  – Photoablation (surface or LASIK): for low-residual refractive error post-cataract
  – Incision: rarely indicated at the day of surgery for residual cylinder
  – Piggyback implantation: in sulcus or in the bag, 2° IOL brings residual error
  – (New designs under evaluation)

■ Perspectives of cataract surgery after corneal surgeries
  – Prevention of surprises: archiving keratometry
    + axial lens pre–refractive surgery
  – Ideal implantation?
  – Multifocal IOLs (pseudophakic, piggy back)
  – Aspherical profile (aberration free…customized
    as a mirror of the operated cornea)?

References

1. Sridhar MS, Rao SK, Vajpayee RB, Aasuri MK, Hannush S, Sinha R (2002) Complication of laser in situ keratomileusis. Indian J Ophthalmol 50:265–282
2. Hamilton DR, Hardten DR (2003) Cataract surgery in patients with prior refractive surgery. Curr Opin Ophthalmol 14:44–53
3. Seitz B, Langenbucher A, Haigis W (2002) Pitfalls of IOL power prediction after photorefractive keratectomy for high myopia – case report, practical recommendations and litterature review. Klin Monatsbl Augenheilkd 219:840–850
4. Kushner BJ, Kowal L (2003) Diplopia after refractive surgery: occurrence and prevention. Arch Ophthalmol 121:315–321
5. Feiz V, Mannis MJ (2004) Intraocular lens power calculation after corneal refractive surgery. Corr Opin Ophthalmol 15:342–349
6. Randleman JB, Loupe DN, Song CD, Waring GO III (2002) Stulting RD. Intraocular lens power calculations after laser in situ keratomileusis. Cornea 21:751–755
7. Langenbucher A, Haigis W, Seitz B (2004) Difficult lens power calculations. Curr Opin Ophthalmol 15:1–9
8. Wang L, Booth MA, Koch DD (2004) Comparison of intraocular lens power calculation methods in eyes that have undergone laser assisted in situ keratomileusis. Trans Am Ophthalmol Soc 102:189–196; discussion 196–197
9. Gills JP, Van der Karr MA (2002) Correcting high astigmatism with piggiback toric intraocular lens implantation. J Cataract refract Surg 28:547–549
10. Odenthal MT, Eggink CA, Melles G, Pameyer JH, Geerards AI, Beekhuis WF (2003) Clinical and theoretical results of intraocular lens power calculation for cataract surgery after photorefractive keratectomy for myopia. Arch Ophthalmol 120:500–1/Arch Ophthalmol 121:584
11. Aizawa D, Shimizu K, Komatsu M, Ito M, Suzuki M, Ohno K, Uozato H (2003) Clinical outcomes of wavefront-guided laser in situ keratomileusis: 6 month follow-up. J Cataract Refract Surg 29:1507–1513
12. Preussner PR, Wahl J, Weitzel D (2006) Topography-based intraocular lens power selection. J Cataract Refract Surg 32:1591; discussion 1591–1592
13. Mesa JC, Marti T, Arruga J (2005) Intraocular lens (IOL) power calculation after keratorefractive procedures. Arch Soc Esp Oftalmol 80:699–703
14. Feiz V, Moshirfar M, Mannis MJ, Reilley CD, Garcia-Ferrer F, Caspar JJ, Lim MC (2005) Nomogram-based intraocular lens power adjustment after myopic refractive keratectomy and lasik: a new approach. Ophthalmology 112:1381–137
15. Rosa N, Capasso L, Lanza M, Iaccarino G, Romano A (2005) Reliability of a new correcting factor in calculating intraocular lens power after refractive corneal surgery. J Cataract Refract Surg 31:1020–1024
16. Liberek I, Kolodziajezyk W, Szaflik JP, Szaflik J (2006) Intraocular lens power calculation in patients after keratorefractive surgery – personal experience. Klin Oczna 108:214–219
17. Masket S, Masket SE (2006) Simple regression formula for intraocular lens power adjustment in eyes requiring cataract surgery after excimer laser photoablation. J Cataract Refract Surg 32:430–434
18. Camellin M, Calosis A (2006) A new formula for intraocular lens power calculation after refractive corneal surgery. J refract Surg 22:735 ; author reply 735–736
19. Sambara C, Naroo S, Shah S, Sharma A (2006) The AS biometry technique—a novel technique to aid accurate intraocular lens power calculation after corneal laser refractive surgery. Cont lens Anterior Eye 29:81–83
20. Taberno J, Piers P. Benito A, Renondo M, Artal P (2006) Predicting the optical performance of eyes implanted with IOLs to correct spherical aberrations. Invest Ophthtalmol Vis Sci 47:4651–4658
21. Wang L, Booth MA, Koch DD (2004) Comparison of intraocular lens power calculation methods in eyes that undergone LASIK. Ophthalmology 111:1825–1831
22. Seitz B, Langenbucher A, Nguyen NX et al (1999) Underestimation of intraocular lens power for cataract surgery after myopic photorefractive keratectomy. Ophthalmology 106:693–702
23. Holladay JT (1997) Cataract surgery in patients with previous keratorefractive surgery (RK, PRK, and LASIK). Ophthalmic Pac 15:238–244
24. Celikkol L, Pavlopoulos G, Weinstein B (1995) Calculation of intraocular lens power after radial keratotomy with computerized videokeratography. Am J Ophthalmol 120:739–770
25. Lyle WA, Jin GCC (1997) Intraocular lens power prediction in patients who undergo cataract surgery following previous radial keratotomy. Arch Ophthalmol 115:457–461
26. Hoffer KJ, Darin JJ, Pettit TH et al (1981) UCLA clinical trial of radial keratotomy: preliminary report. Ophthalmology 88:729–736
27. Olsen T (1992) Sources of error in intraocular lens power calculation. J Cataract Refract Surg 18:125–129
28. Kalski RS, Danjoux JP, Fraenkel GE et al (1997) Intraocular lens power calculation for cataract surgery after photorefractive keratectomy for high myopia. J Refract Surg 13:362–366
29. Koch DD, Wakil JS, Samuelson SW et al (1992) Comparison of the accuracy and reproducibility of the keratometer and the EyeSys Corneal Analysis System Model I. J Cataract Refract Surg 18:342–347
30. Olsen T (1986) On the calculation of power from curvature of the cornea. Br J Ophthalmol 70:152–154
31. Kim JH, Lee H, Joo FK (2002) Measuring corneal power for intraocular lens power calculation after refractive surgery. J Cataract Refract Surg 88:1932–1938
32. Stakheev AA, Balashevich LJ (2003) Corneal power determination after previous refractive surgery for intraocular lens calculation. Cornea 22:214–220
33. Sonego-Krone S, Lopez-Moreno G, Beaujon-Balbi G et al (2004) A direct method to measure the power of the central cornea after myopic laser in situ keratomileusis. Arch Ophthalmol 122:159–166
34. Holladay JT (1989) Consultations in refractive surgery. Refract Corneal Surg 5:20
35. Hoffer KJ (1995) intraocular lens power calculation for eyes after refractive keratotomy J Refract Surg 11:490–493
36. Shammas HJ, Shammas MC, Garabet A et al (2003) Correcting the corneal power measurements for intraocular lens power calculations after myopic laser in situ keratomileusis. Am J Ophthalmol 136:426–432
37. Rosa N, Capasso L, Romano A (2002) A new method of calculating intraocular lens power after photorefractive keratoectomy. J Refract Surg 18:720–724

14

38. Ferrara G, Cennamo G, Marotta G et al (2004) New formula to calculate corneal power after refractive surgery. J Refract Surg 20:465–471

39. Speicher L (2001) Intraocular lens calculation status after corneal refractive surgery, Curr Opin Ophthalmol 12:17–29

40. Mandell RB (1994(Corneal power correction factor for photorefractive keratectomy. J Refract Corneal Surg 10:125–128

41. Savini G, Barboni P, Zanini M (2006) Intraocular lens power calculation after myopic refractive surgery. Theoretical comparison of different methods. Ophthalmology 113:1271–1282

42. Feitz V, Mannis MJ, Garcia-Ferrer F et al (2001) Intraocular lens power calculation after laser in situ keratomileusis for myopia and hyperopia a standardized approach, Cornea 20:792–797

43. Aramberri J (2003) Intraocular lens power calculation after corneal refractive surgery double-K method. J Cataract Refract Surg 29:2063–2068

44. Rosa N, Capasso L, Romano A (20020 A new method of calculating intraocular lens power after photorefralctive keratectomie. J Refract Surg 18:720–724

45. Latkany RA, Chokshi AR, Speaker MG et al (2005) Intraocular lens calculations after refractive surgery. J Cataract Refract Surg 31:562–570

46. Borasio E, Stevens J, Smith GT (2006) Estimation of true corneal power after keratorefractive surgery in eyes requiring cataract surgery: BESSt formula. J Cataract Refract Surg 32:2004–2014

47. Walter KA, Gagnon MR, Hoopes PC Jr et al (2006) Accurate intraocular lens power calculation after myopic laser in situ keratomileusis bypassing corneal power. J Cataract Refract Surg 32:425–429

48. Masket S (2006) Simple regression formula for intraocular lens power adjustement in eyes requiring cataract surgery after excimer laser potoablation, J Cataract Refract Surg 32:430–434

49. Ianchulev T, Salz J, Hoffer K et al (2005) Intraoperative optical refractive biometry for intraocular lens power estimation without axial length and keratometry measurements. J Catarac Refract Surg 31:1530–1536

50. Mackool RJ, Ko W, Mackool R (2006) Intraocular lens power calculation after laser in situ keratomileu:the aphakic refraction technique. J Cataract Refract Surg 32:435–437

51. Koch DD, Lin JF, Hyde LL et al (1989) Refractive complications of cataract surgery after radial keratotomy. Am J Ophthalmol 108:676–682

52. Gimbel H, Sun R, Kaye GB (2000) Refractive error in cataract surgery after previous refractive surgery. J Cataract Refract Surg 26:142–144

53. Koch DD (2006) New options for IOL calculation after refractive surgery. J Cataract Refract Surg 32:371–372

Chapter 15

Complications of Radial Keratotomy and Conductive Keratoplasty

15

Contents

Core Messages

■ Post-RK patients present unique challenges for cataract surgeons and must be counseled regarding possible complications and a hyperopic result in the early postoperative period.

■ Accurate IOL power calculations are more difficult in post-RK patients and require unique measurements of corneal power.

■ RK incision rupture is a potential complication, especially if it is necessary to have the phaco hand piece directly under an RK incision.

■ Zonular weakness and subsequent lens movement are also possible complications for post-RK patients.

■ You may want to consider not using multifocal IOLs to reduce unwanted retinal images.

■ Do not make any alterations or changes until several months have passed.

■ Piggyback IOLs are the best method for enhancing refractive results in post-RK patients.

15.1 Cataract Surgery Complications of Radial Keratotomy

*Howard Fine, Richard S. Hoffman,
Mark Packer, and Laurie Brown*

A patient post–radial keratotomy (RK) presents several challenges for cataract surgery. It is very important that people who have had radial keratotomy and are confronting cataract surgery, or refractive lens exchange, be counseled extensively about the difficulties of lens power calculation, the increased potential for complication including zonular dialysis or rupture, loss of a lens into the vitreous, and the high potential for hyperopia in the early postoperative weeks and months.

The first, and most commonly encountered, challenge is intraocular lens (IOL) power calculations. We have studied this and have recently published a paper on our technique for lens power calculations after radial keratotomy [1]. The primary challenge to calculating appropriate IOL power in post-RK patients is to determine accurately the corneal refractive power [2, 3]. Due to the methods by which their measurements are obtained, standard keratometry and computerized corneal topography are not as accurate in their K readings for patients post-RK as they are for patients who have not undergone keratorefractive surgery. Similar to previous research [4], we found that when we used K readings taken only from the central portion of the cornea, we were better able to accurately predict postoperative refractive results [1]. We currently use the effective refractive power (EffRP, Holladay Diagnostic Summary, EyeSys, Topographer), a corneal power value representing the central 3-mm pupil zone, taking into account the Stiles-Crawford effect, as part of the Holladay 2 IOL Consultant to calculate IOL power. In addition to proper K readings, accurate biometry, in the form of partial coherence interferometry (IOL Master) for axial length, provides further improvement to postoperative refractions.

An additional complication is the potential for rupturing radial incisions during the course of phacoemulsification surgery. One technique for avoiding this is to make scleral tunnel incisions and to avoid, as best possible, going directly under a radial incision. Obviously, this is impossible if one is performing coaxial phacoemulsification in corneas in which there are more than eight incisions. Our preferred technique for surgery is to utilize bimanual micro-incision phacoemulsification and go between the radial incisions, which is always possible for 8 incisions or less (Fig. 15.1.1) and sometimes even in the presence of 16-incision post-RK patients.

The surgical technique has been described in detail [5]. The procedure is performed under topical anesthesia after informed consent is obtained, preoperative measurements for an IOL are made, and preoperative dilation and antibiotics are administered. A Paratrap diamond keratome (Mastel Precision Surgical Instruments, Rapid City,

S.D.), or a 1.1- to 1.3-mm 3D diamond knife (Rhein Medical, Tampa) is utilized to create two trapezoidal 1.1-mm clear corneal incisions, 30–45° from the temporal limbus and 60–90° from each other (Fig. 15.1.2). In post-RK patients it is very important to limit the length of the micro-incisions so as not to approach to converging radial incisions. After 0.5 ml of non-preserved lidocaine 1% is instilled into the anterior chamber, complete exchange of the anterior chamber aqueous humor by sodium hyaluronate 3.0%–chondroitin sulfate 4.0% (Viscoat*) is performed. A capsulorhexis forceps, designed to fit and function through a 1mm incision (Fine-Hoffman Micro-incision Capsulorhexis forceps, MicroSurgical Technology, Redmond, Wash.) is then inserted through one of the same incisions and used to complete a 5- to 6-mm capsulorhexis (Fig. 15.1.3).

Cortical cleaving hydrodissection [6] with decompression is then performed in two distal quadrants followed by

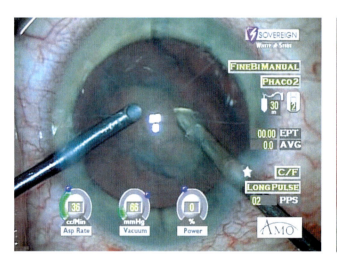

Fig. 15.1.1 The bimanual micro-incision incision hand pieces are positioned between the RK incisions, allowing for phacoemulsification without trauma to the RK incisions

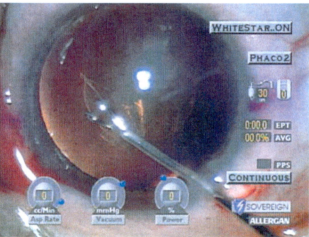

Fig. 15.1.3 A capsulorhexis is formed with a micro-incision capsulorhexis forceps

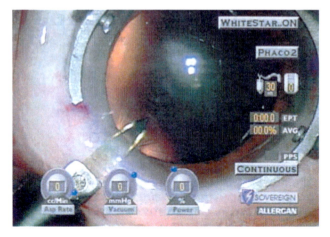

Fig. 15.1.2 A left-handed 1.2-mm clear corneal incision is placed 45° from the temporal limbus with a diamond knife

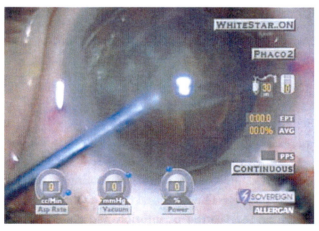

Fig. 15.1.4 The beveled irrigating hand piece is placed in the left-handed micro-incision

15

a third round of hydrodissection to prolapse the entire lens, or at least half of the lens, out of the capsular bag. The Duet System micro-incision irrigating hand piece (MicroSurgical Technology) (Fig. 15.1.4) is placed in the left-hand incision and the sleeveless phaco needle is inserted through the right-hand incision. Lens extraction is then performed, without phaco power in most cases, involving clear or soft lenses, using high levels of vacuum while carouselling the relatively soft lens in the plane of the iris until it is consumed (Fig. 15.1.5). Small amounts of ultrasound energy can be used when needed. Care should be taken to avoid directing the infusion flow toward the phaco needle tip to prevent dislodging nuclear material from the tip. While infusion is maintained with the irrigating hand piece, the phaco needle is removed and the aspiration hand piece is inserted to remove residual cortex and polish the posterior capsule. If subincisional cortex is difficult to extract, the irrigating/aspirating (I/A) hand pieces can be alternated be-

tween the two incisions to gain easier access to the subincisional capsule fornix (Fig. 15.1.6). In post-RK patients, it is important to try to maintain a radial orientation of the hand pieces as oar-like movements of the hand pieces can stress the adjacent radial incisions, which may lead to focal rupture.

Once all cortex has been removed, the aspiration hand piece is removed and viscoelastic is injected into the capsular bag and anterior chamber while the irrigating hand piece is withdrawn (Fig. 15.1.7). The viscoelastic cannula is removed from the eye and a new 2.2- to 2.5-mm clear corneal incision is placed between the two micro-incisions for IOL insertion. After IOL insertion, stromal hydration of the incision is performed to assist in self-sealing. Bimanual I/A is performed to remove all viscoelastic. The aspiration hand piece is then removed and irrigation of the anterior chamber maintained. Stromal hydration of the empty incision is performed to assist in closure of the micro-incision. The irrigation hand piece is then removed, followed by stromal hydration of that incision. In this manner, the eye is fully formed and pressurized throughout the procedure, avoiding hypotony and shallowing of the anterior chamber. If a rupture of a radial incision occurs with minimal leakage and maintenance of a full anterior chamber, then it may be possible to proceed without suturing the incision, waiting for an opportune time in the procedure to place a suture. However, in most cases it is best to fill the anterior chamber with viscoelastic and suture the rupture right away.

Bimanual micro-incision phacoemulsification offers advantages over traditional phacoemulsification techniques for routine cataract extraction and refractive lens exchange. Although coaxial phacoemulsification is an excellent procedure with low amounts of induced astigmatism [7], bimanual phacoemulsification offers the potential for truly astigmatic-neutral incisions. In addition, these micro-incisions should behave similar to a paracentesis incision with less likelihood for leakage and, theoretically, a lower incidence of endophthalmitis.

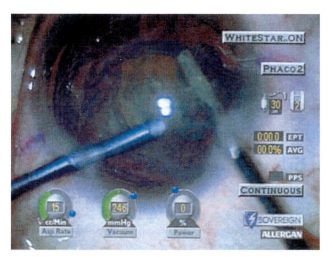

Fig. 15.1.5 The soft lens is carouselled in the iris plane and consumed using high vacuum levels. Forward movement of the lens is prevented with the irrigating hand piece

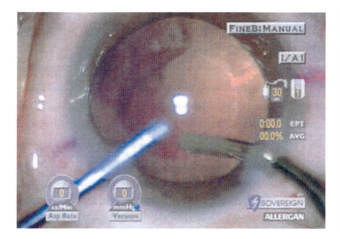

Fig. 15.1.6 Subincisional cortex is easily removed using bimanual I/A hand pieces

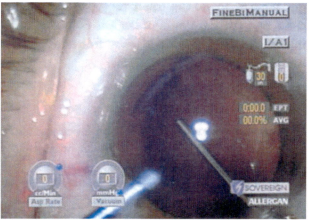

Fig. 15.1.7 Viscoelastic material is injected into the capsular bag while infusion is maintained with the irrigating hand piece.

The major advantage of bimanual micro-incisions that we see is an improvement in control of most endocapsular surgery steps. Because viscoelastics do not leave the eye easily through these small incisions, the anterior chamber is more stable during capsulorhexis construction and there is much less likelihood for an errant capsulorhexis to develop. Hydrodelineation and hydrodissection can be performed more efficiently because of a higher level of pressure building in the anterior chamber before eventual prolapse of viscoelastic through the micro-incisions.

In addition, separation of irrigation from the aspirating phaco needle allows for improved followability by avoiding competing currents at the needle tip. In some instances, the irrigation flow from the second hand piece can be used as an adjunctive surgical device, flushing nuclear pieces from the angle or loosening epinuclear or cortical material from the capsular bag.

Perhaps the greatest advantage of the bimanual technique lies in its ability to easily remove subincisional cortex. As originally described by Brauweiler [8], by switching infusion and aspiration hand pieces between two micro-incisions, 360° of the capsular fornices are easily reached, and cortical clean-up can be performed quickly and safely.

The disadvantages of bimanual phacoemulsification are easy to overcome. Maneuvering through 1.2-mm incisions can be awkward when first learning the technique, and additional equipment is necessary (e.g., small-incision keratomes, capsulorhexis forceps, irrigating choppers [for dense nuclei], and bimanual I/A hand pieces). All major instrument companies are currently working on irrigating choppers and other micro-incision adjunctive devices for micro-incision surgery. For refractive lens exchanges, irrigation can be accomplished with the bimanual irrigation hand piece that can also function as the second side-port instrument, negating the need for an irrigating chopper.

The greatest criticism of bimanual phacoemulsification lies in the fluidics and the limitations in IOL technology that can be used through these micro-incisions. By nature of the incision sizes, less fluid flows into the eye than with coaxial techniques. Most irrigating choppers integrate a 20-ga lumen that limits fluid inflow. This can result in significant chamber instability when high vacuum levels are used, and occlusion from nuclear material at the phaco tip is cleared. Thus, infusion must be maximized by placing the infusion bottle on a separate intravenous pole that is set as high as possible. Also, vacuum levels usually need to be lowered below 350 mmHg to avoid significant surge flow. In post-RK patients it is important to lower the bottle as low as possible without compromising chamber stability in order to avoid rupturing the radial incisions.

Several micro-incision lenses are available outside of the United States, including the AcriSmart IOL (Acri.Tec, AG, Berlin, Germany), and the UltraChoice 1.0 Rollable Thin-Lens IOL (ThinOptX, Abingdon, Va.) .

Several new micro-incision lenses are under development. Medennium (Irvine, Calif.) is developing its SmartI-OL⁻, a thermodynamic accommodating IOL. It is a hydrophobic, acrylic rod that can be inserted through a 2-mm incision and expands to the dimensions of the natural crystalline lens (9.5 × 3.5 mm). A 1-mm version of this lens is also being developed. Finally, injectable polymer lenses are being researched by Calhoun Vision [9, 10]. If viable, the Calhoun Vision injectable polymer would permit a light-adjustable IOL through a 1-mm incision that can then be refined postoperatively to eliminate lower-order and higher-order optical aberrations, and fashion multifocal optics.

The use of bimanual micro-incision phacoemulsification for refractive lens exchange and routine cataract surgery maintains a more stable intraocular environment during lens removal. This may be especially important in patients with high myopia, many of whom have had radial keratotomy, and who are at a greater risk for retinal detachment following lens extraction [11–13]. Maintaining a formed and pressurized anterior chamber throughout the procedure should decrease the tendency for anterior movement of the vitreous body with a theoretical lower incidence of posterior vitreous detachment occurring from intraoperative manipulations. The many advantages of bimanual micro-incision phacoemulsification should be considered by surgeons performing refractive lens exchange.

Suturing of ruptured radial incisions has a minimal effect on altering the corneal curvature and the immediate postoperative refraction. That is because the sutures are peripheral and limbus parallel, so they have little effect on central corneal curvature. However, the pressurization of the eye during phacoemulsification surgery tends to stretch healed radial incisions and flatten the cornea for a period of time that lasts for several weeks to months after surgery, with a resultant hyperopic spherical equivalent during that period.

We have found that patients in whom more than eight radial incisions have been placed have an added risk of a weakened zonular apparatus. One possible reason for this is the surgeon was likely to have been striving for a maximum effect because of a high myopic pre-RK spherical equivalent and the incidents in these patients of micro and macro-perforations leading to shallowing or flattening of the anterior chamber is higher than for less myopic patients requiring fewer radial incisions. With that shallowing of the anterior chamber, a forward movement of the lens may stretch the zonules and make them weaker. Our impression, after having performed multiple post-radial keratotomy phacoemulsifications, is that in these cases capsules frequently wrinkle during capsulorhexis, indicating a loss of zonular integrity. We routinely and uniformly use capsular tension rings, easily implantable through one of the micro-incisions prior to hydroexpression of the crystalline lens, in all patients who have had more than eight incisions at the time of radial keratotomy.

Because of the potential for additional, unwanted retinal images, including halos, starbursts, glare, etc., we tend to prefer the Crystalens (Eyeonics, Aliso Veijo, Calif.) over multifocal IOLs, post-RK, especially where small optical zones have been utilized.

It is our practice not to alter anything until a period of several months has elapsed before we consider enhancing our results [1]. The most frequent way in which we would enhance spherical equivalent after phacoemulsification in post-RK patients would be piggyback IOLs because they are safe, predictable, and very accurate utilizing the Holladay consultant formula [14].

Take-Home Pearls

■ Post-RK patients must be extensively counseled regarding the difficulties of lens power calculation, the increased potential for intraoperative complications, and the high potential for hyperopia in the early postoperative period.

■ K readings taken only from the central portion of the cornea, such as effective refractive power (EffRP, Holladay Diagnostic Summary, EyeSys, Topographer), are better able to accurately predict postoperative refractive results for IOL power calculations than standard K readings.

■ To avoid rupturing incisions, make scleral tunnel incisions and avoid going directly under a radial incision. Our preferred method is to use bimanual micro-incision phacoemulsification and go between the RK incisions.

■ Zonular weakness, leading to movement of the lens, is sometimes a complication of post-RK patients who have had more than eight incisions. The use of bimanual micro-incision phacoemulsification and capsular tension rings help manage this complication.

■ To help prevent unwanted retinal images, our preference is to use the Eyeonics Crystalens, rather than a multifocal IOL.

■ Do not make any alterations or enhancements for at least three months. If enhancements are necessary, we recommend implanting a piggyback IOL.

References

1. Packer M, Brown LK, Hoffman RS, Fine IH (2004) Intraocular lens power calculation after incisional and thermal keratorefractive surgery. J Cataract Refract Surg 30:1430–1434
2. Holladay JT (1995) Understanding corneal topography: the Holladay Diagnostic Summary. User's guide and tutorial. EyeSys Technologies, Houston
3. Celikkol L, Pavlopoulos G, Weinstein, B et al (1995) Calculation of intraocular lens power after radial keratotomy with computerized videokeratography. Am J Ophthalmol 120:739–750
4. Chen L, Mannis MJ, Salz JJ et al (2003) Analysis of intraocular lens power calculation in post-radial keratotomy eyes. J Cataract Refract Surg 29:65–70
5. Fine IH, Hoffman RS, Packer M (2004) Optimizing refractive lens exchange with bimanual micro-incision phacoemulsification. J Cataract Refract Surg 30:550–554
6. Fine IH (1992) Cortical cleaving hydrodissection. J Cataract Refract Surg 18:508–512
7. Masket S, Tennen DG (1996) Astigmatic stabilization of 3.0 mm temporal clear corneal cataract incisions. J Cataract Refract Surg 22:1451–1455
8. Brauweiler P (1996) Bimanual irrigation/aspiration. J Cataract Refract Surg 22:1013–1016
9. Groot JH de, van Beijma JF, Haitjema HJ et al (2001) Injectable intraocular lens material based upon hydrogels. Biomacromolecules 2:628–634
10. Hoffman RS, Fine IH, Packer M (2004) Light adjustable lens. In Agarwal S, Agarwal A, Sachdev MS et al (eds) Phacoemulsification, laser cataract surgery, and foldable IOLs, 3rd edn. SLACK, Thorofare, N.J.
11. Rodriguez A, Gutierrez E, Alvira G (1987) Complications of clear lens extraction in axial myopia. Arch Ophthalmol 105:1522–1523
12. Ripandelli G, Billi B, Fedeli R, Stirpe M (1996) Retinal detachment after clear lens extraction in 41 eyes with axial myopia. Retina 16:3–6
13. Colin J, Robinet A, Cochener B (1999) Retinal detachment after clear lens extraction for high myopia: seven-year follow-up. Ophthalmology 106:2281–2284
14. Packer, Mark (2006) Frequency and risk factor analysis of piggyback IOL enhancement following refractive lens exchange with an accommodative IOL. Refractive surgery: the times they are a-changin'. Sponsored by the International Society of Refractive Surgery of the American Academy of Ophthalmology (ISRS/AAO). American Academy of Ophthalmology 2006 Joint Meeting, Las Vegas, 11 November 2006

Core Messages

- The NearVision CK procedure for presbyopia involves induction of a mild myopia in the non-dominant eye.

- A gain of uncorrected near visual acuity without a marked loss of binocular uncorrected distance acuity has been documented in all CK studies involving the treatment of presbyopic low hyperopes or emmetropes.

- The most common complication following CK is surgically induced astigmatism, and is most frequently caused by errors in intraoperative technique.

- With the NearVision CK with LightTouch nomogram and technique, less cylinder is induced than with the conventional CK nomogram.

- Patient selection is important in avoiding induced astigmatism. Patients with peripheral astigmatism, lenticular astigmatism, or a decentered apex should be avoided.

- Perfect centration of the procedure upon the center of the pupil, accurate corneal marking to delineate the location of spot placement, and symmetrical spot placement in the x-, y-, and z-axes are important to avoiding induced astigmatism.

- Experience with the ring light on the surgical microscope helps in detecting and treating surgically induced astigmatism.

15.2 Complications of Conductive Keratoplasty
Marguerite B. McDonald

15.2.1 Introduction

Conductive Keratoplasty (CK) has improved near vision in well-selected patients, without many of the risks that accompany excimer laser modes of surgical correction [1–9]. The procedure has been especially effective in improving near vision of presbyopic hyperopes or emmetropes through induction of a mild myopia in the non-dominant eye. A large proportion of properly selected patients gain functional near vision, without markedly giving up binocular distance focus. Most achieve a high degree of spectacle independence. Can such effectiveness be achieved without sacrificing safety? In this chapter, I attempt to answer this question, and, in addition, present the most common CK complications and discuss their prevention and management.

15.2.2 Presbyopia Multicenter Clinical Trial

This US Food and Drug Administration (FDA)-approval study was conducted at five centers to determine the safety and efficacy of CK for the treatment of presbyopic symptoms in emmetropic or mildly hyperopic eyes. Eligible patients had to have a preoperative spherical equivalent (SE) of plano (+0.50 to –0.50 D) to +2.00 D, less than or equal to 0.75 D of cycloplegic refractive astigmatism, and a documented history of successful monovision contact lens wear or completion of a contact lens monovision trial. A total of 83 patients were treated unilaterally in the non-dominant eye with an intended correction of up to 2.00 D to attain near vision in that eye. The ViewPoint CK System (study device) and the conventional CK nomogram and technique were used for all patients. Enrolled patients had a mean age of 53 years; the mean target refraction was –1.41 D.

At 12 months postoperatively, 89% of the eyes had binocular uncorrected near visual acuity (UCVA-NEAR) of Jaeger (J)3 or better. A total of 77% had binocular 20/25 or better UCVA-Distance together with J2 or better near, and 89% had 20/32 or better distance together with J3 or better near. According to the patient questionnaire, 86% of eyes treated for near could read newspaper print and had good distance vision, as indicated by the 100% who could see a street sign.

Although two eyes (2%) lost more than two lines of BCVA at 1 month, no eyes lost two lines or more of BCVA beyond 1 month (Table 15.2.1). There were no cases of BCVA worse than 20/40, no increases of 2.00 D or more of cylinder, and no eyes that had 20/20 or better BCVA preoperatively had worse than 20/25 postoperatively. No eye lost two or more lines of BCVA-Near or had BCVA-Near worse than J3 at any follow-up visit through 24 months. No intraoperative complications or adverse events occurred during any of the surgeries. At all follow-up time points, absolute increases in cylinder were 1.75 D or less. No increases in cylinder were seen at months 3, 12, and 24 in 83, 92, and 97%, respectively. There was no loss of two lines or more of BCVA-Near at any follow-up time for any level of induced cylinder. Few eyes were markedly undercorrected or overcorrected in the study.

15.2.3 NearVision CK with LightTouch

The FDA study for the approval of the presbyopia treatment indication, described above, involved treatment of a patient's non-dominant eye with what is known as the conventional or standard technique and nomogram. Recently a modification known as NearVision CK with LightTouch was developed (Fig. 15.2.1), which achieves the same amount of refractive change as does the conventional CK technique, but with fewer spots applied at a larger optical zone. The major difference between the two techniques is that less pressure is applied during energy delivery with the LightTouch technique, and the result is a more robust refractive response.

15

Table 15.2.1 Safety results of CK studies on the treatment of presbyopia

Safety variable	Multicenter Presbyopia Study[a] (%)		LightTouch multicenter study (%)		LightTouch McDonald personal (%)		Multicenter post-LASIK (%)	
	Month 1	Month 3	Month 1	Month 3	Month 1	Month 3	Month 1	Month 3
Loss of >2 lines BCVA-Distance	2	0	0	NA	0	0	0	0
Loss of >2 lines BCVA-Distance	3	1	0	NA	0	NA	0	0
BCVA-Distance worse than 20/40	0	0	0	NA	0	NA	0	0
Increase >2.00 D cylinder	0	0	0	NA	NA	NA	0	0
Patients ≤20/20 distance preop who change to ≥20/25 postop	0	0	0	NA	0	NA	0	0
Quality of depth perception (excellent, very good, good)	100	93	NA	NA	0	NA	89	91
Adverse events or complications	0	0	0	NA	0	NA	0	0

[a]Performed with conventional nomogram
NA data not available

NearVision CK® With LightTouch Nomogram*

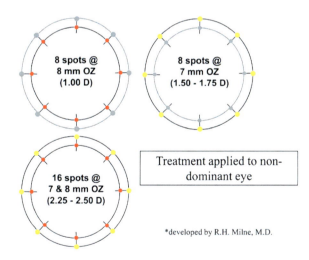

8 spots @ 8 mm OZ (1.00 D)

8 spots @ 7 mm OZ (1.50 - 1.75 D)

16 spots @ 7 & 8 mm OZ (2.25 - 2.50 D)

Treatment applied to non-dominant eye

*developed by R.H. Milne, M.D.

Fig. 15.2.1 NearVision CK with LightTouch Nomogram

With the earlier conventional nomogram, some surgeons were obtaining variable results with CK, as well as induced astigmatism postoperatively. Dr. H.L. Milne, an active CK surgeon, first proposed that a varied degree of corneal compression during treatment spot application could account for some of the undesirable outcomes. His observations led to the development of the NearVision CK with LightTouch technique and nomogram. In the conventional CK treatment, the cornea is compressed with the Keratoplast tip to create a 5- to 7-mm dimple on the cornea. With the NearVision CK with LightTouch technique, however, the cornea is only minimally depressed with the tip to create a 2- to 3-mm dimple. Dr. Milne also observed that induced astigmatism was probably caused by poor Keratoplast tip alignment and asymmetrical placement of spots. (H.L. Milne, "LightTouch technique for Conductive Keratoplasty." Presented at ASCRS, April 2005, Washington, D.C.). Individual surgeons' results may vary when performing CK with LightTouch based on Dr. Milne's nomogram, and it is strongly recommended that a physician develop his or her own CK nomogram based on personal practice results.

15.2.4 NearVision CK after Excimer Laser Surgery

Efficacy and safety of NearVision CK is also being evaluated in a prospective, multicenter, FDA-approval study of patients previously treated with LASIK who are now presbyopic (M. Gordon, "NearVision CK in Post-LASIK Emmetropes: FDA Clinical Trial Update." Presented at the Refractive Subspecialty Day meeting, November 2006, Las Vegas). A notable safety advantage of a NearVision CK procedure in presbyopic eyes in lieu of an excimer laser treatment is that no flap re-cutting or lifting is needed, thereby avoiding any risk of epithelial ingrowth or dry eye [10]. An additional safety advantage is the likelihood that the CK procedure will not jeopardize distance visual acuity.

As with eyes without previous refractive surgery, treatment involves inducing a mild myopia in the non-dominant eye. However, because the NearVision CK procedure has been observed to have a greater effect in post-LASIK eyes than in previously untreated eyes, a conservative approach is recommended. Thus, treatment should be limited to eight spots applied to the 7.5- to 8-mm optical zone with the LightTouch technique. The treatment goal in this study was a +1.25-D add, which can be achieved with eight spots at the 7.5- to 8-mm optical zone.

A total of 55 emmetropic presbyopic patients who have previously had LASIK to correct myopia have undergone the procedure in the multicenter trial. They had a mean age of 52, a mean pre-CK manifest refraction spherical equivalent (MRSE) of +0.50 D, less than 0.75 D of cylinder, residual central pachymetry greater than 400 µm, and peripheral pachymetry greater than 560 µm. At 1 month postoperatively, 88% could read newspaper-sized print, compared with 24% preoperatively. The improvements in near vision came with only slight loss of distance vision. Mean mesopic contrast sensitivity with glare showed mostly better results postoperatively than preoperatively.

Regarding safety, no eyes lost more than two lines of BCVA-Distance. At 1 month, 88% showed no change from preoperative in induced cylinder, 4% showed induction of 1.00 D, and 8% showed induction of >1.00 D. Of the 12% (six eyes) with induced cylinder, all had J1 or J1+ near acuity. There were no adverse events or complication with the corneal flap that had been created during the previous LASIK procedure. At 1 month, 43/50 (86%) of patients were satisfied or very satisfied with their CK procedure.

The evaluation of the safety and effectiveness of treating post–excimer laser patients with CK is ongoing. It is important to note that a greater refractive effect from NearVision CK treatment has been observed in post–excimer laser eyes compared with eyes that have not undergone excimer laser surgery, and the nomogram must be adjusted in view of this. All use of CK following previous excimer laser treatment is empirical and off-label at this time. It is best to treat these patients very conservatively and informed that they may need additional treatments later if they are over- or undercorrected.

15.2.5 Complications and Their Management

In general, complications are rare after a CK procedure for any indication, and most can be avoided by careful patient selection and screening. Patients suitable for the NearVision CK procedure should have good bilateral BCVA, a healthy cornea with average curvature and thickness, no keratoconus, nuclear sclerotic cataract less than +2, and no previous corneal incisional refractive surgery, especially radial keratotomy. Preoperative topography, preferably by Orbscan, is essential. Avoid atypical or unusual corneas, such as those with keratoconus or pellucid marginal degeneration and be aware of potential sources of induced cylinder. These include corneas with a decentered apex or peripheral, asymmetric, or non-orthogonal astigmatism. Although CK does not induce neurotrophic dry eye symptoms commonly seen after LASIK, significant dryness or tear-function compromise may limit improvement in function. Amblyopic patients or those with >1.00 D of cylinder do not make good candidates.

Contact lens wearers should have a stable refraction, regular mires, two central keratometry readings one week apart or more that differ by no more than 0.50 D. Hard lens wearers should discontinue lens use three weeks and soft contact lens wearers two weeks before the procedure. Since the NearVision CK procedure for presbyopia is performed on the non-dominant eye, eye dominance must be determined preoperatively. Several tests can be used including the "hole-in-the-hand," the plus-lens test, alternate occlusion, or the camera-to-the-eye method. A "loose-lens test" is useful to assess monovision tolerance and to determine the amount of surgical correction.

An important part of patient selection is patient education. The surgeon must make sure that patients have reasonable goals and expectations and understand that they will be having surgery to improve vision for daily life, i.e., to be able to see most reading material, food, price tags, games, and computers. They must also understand that they will have limited vision for very small material, i.e., the telephone book, accounting ledgers, and maps. The necessity of binocular vision for the postoperative effect and the difference in distance capability in each of their two eyes should be explained.

15.2.6 Surgical Technique for the Primary Procedure

Carefully align the patient's head to center the cornea in the microscope field, with the iris parallel to the floor and the fixation light equally spaced between oculars in the patient's view. Gently indent a Sinskey hook over the center of the entrance pupil to aid centration of corneal marking. For corneal marking, dampen an eight-intersection CK corneal marker with gentian violet or rose bengal stain, center the marker over the pupil center, and apply to the corneal epithelium with light pressure to make a circular mark. Well-placed corneal marks are essential for accurate spot placement, which, in turn, helps to prevent induced astigmatism. Then set the appropriate treatment parameters on the console, according to the nomogram (LightTouch or conventional).

Following marking, treatment can be applied. Insert the Keratoplast tip (Fig. 15.2.2) into the stroma, perpendicular to surface (perpendicular placement is highly important), at the marked spots around the peripheral cornea. The desired technique is to penetrate the corneal stroma with the Keratoplast tip to full-probe depth (450 µm) while applying only minimal compression on the corneal surface so that a 2- to 3-mm dimple forms on the cornea. This LightTouch technique is in contrast to the conventional NearVision CK technique in which the cornea is compressed more firmly to create a 5- to 7-mm corneal dimple (Fig. 15.2.3). After penetration, pull back to minimize striae around the tip, apply energy by depressing the foot pedal, follow the cornea down with the Keratoplast tip to ensure complete and full depth of treatment, and remove the tip. Attempt to apply a

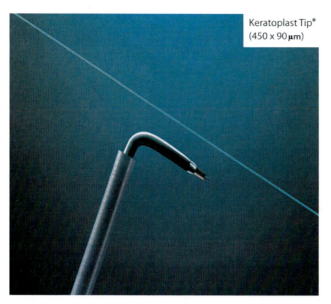

Fig. 15.2.2 Keratoplast Tip. The CK procedure is performed with the ViewPoint CK System. The console weighs about 16 kg (about the size of a VCR) and is portable. It can be easily moved from minor OR suite to examination lane and throughout your office. (1) Briefly explain here the components of the ViewPoint System and how the radio frequency (RF) energy exits the machine, travels through the cable, into the hand piece and through the tip to enter intrastromally. (2) Explain that the cornea's natural conductive properties "resists" the RF energy and creates heat from the bottom of the tip to the top. (3) When the energy reaches the corneal surface, it looks for somewhere to go (a ground) which is why we always use a speculum with this procedure. (4) The RF energy reaches the speculum and travels back through that cable back to the machine. The Keratoplast tip (shown on the right, next to a 7-0 suture) is held in the hand piece and is used to deliver radio frequency energy (350 kHz) into the corneal stroma at 8 to 32 treatment points. Energy release is controlled with a foot pedal

consistent amount of pressure at each spot in the ring during energy application, as variable degrees of compression can produce variable results. Maintaining a steady hand position during the procedure is important. To assist with intraoperative identification and management of surgically induced astigmatism, a microkeratoscope (also called a ring light) attachment may be used with the operating microscope. Look for the ring light reflex pushed to opposite side of pupil, and try to maintain relative roundness of the mire at the time of energy delivery.

15.2.7 Managing Astigmatism

Despite strict adherence to proper technique, induced astigmatism can occur occasionally, and can be observed through an operating microscope that incorporates a ring-light attachment. Typically, cylinder appears as an elongated or pear-shaped distortion to the ring reflection on the cornea and is commonly observed if there are more than 2.00 D of astigmatism. The elongation corresponds to a sector of the cornea that was asymmetrically or incompletely flattened during the primary CK procedure.

If you have not previously treated astigmatism intraoperatively, begin by observing the effect of light corneal touch with the Keratoplast tip on the shape of the ring light and attempt to make the shape round. Record the amount of observed cylinder and the axis based on the appearance of the ring light. One week postoperatively, confirm presence of cylinder and its axis and magnitude using topography/Orbscan, and keratometric readings. This approach helps develop the skills for interpreting ring light shapes, which can lead to incorporation of intraoperative astigmatism management into your primary procedure. It is best to treat CK induced cylinder within one month of the primary NearVision CK procedure.

The elongation of the ring light reflection on the cornea indicates the axis of induced astigmatism. This should correspond to flat axis on the topography map and the axis of minus cylinder in the refraction. Treatment involves applying a "bonus CK spot" to the tip of the narrowed end of the

Conventional-pressure technique

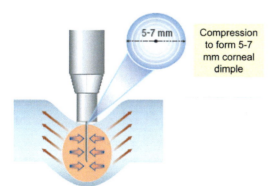

Compression to form 5-7 mm corneal dimple

CK with LightTouch technique

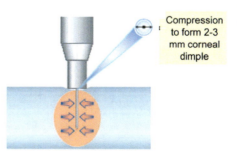

Compression to form 2-3 mm corneal dimple

Fig. 15.2.3 Conventional-pressure and light-pressure CK techniques. Ring light identifies axis of astigmatism where bonus spot is to be placed

ring light refection to balance the vector forces around the ring, as shown in Fig. 15.2.4. To test for ideal placement of the bonus spot, apply light pressure on the flat axis with the Keratoplast tip without puncturing Bowman's membrane. The oval ring-light reflection should become round. Repeat this maneuver several times until you are confident that the correct axis of astigmatism has been identified. If placement is not ideal, then the treated side will not flatten and the ring shape will skew.

Before placing the bonus spot, ensure that all measurements confirm the axis you are about to treat, and be sure you are evaluating a stable ring light image. Lift the speculum to remove all pressure from the globe before treating. Never treat inside the 7-mm optical zone using the Light-Touch technique. Treating within the band of striae on the cornea is recommended. Apply only one bonus spot. Figure 15.2.5 shows a decision flow chart that can be helpful to the surgeon regarding the decision to place a bonus spot.

Typically, the optical zone selected for astigmatic spot placement is determined by the optical zones that were used for the primary treatment rings. If a single ring treatment was executed, place the astigmatic spot in the same optical zone. In other words, if treatment was with one ring at the 7-mm optical zone, place one bonus spot at the 7-mm optical zone, and if treatment was with one ring at the 8-mm optical zone, place one bonus spot at the 8-mm optical zone (Fig. 15.2.6). If two treatment rings were used, then place the astigmatic spot between those two zones (at 7.5 mm). Spots should never overlap; always treat in virgin cornea. After placing the balancing spot, the shape to the ring light will change immediately, although it is not uncommon to see a less than a perfectly rounded ring (only qualitatively rounder). Do not place an additional spots at this time in pursuit of a rounder ring. Instead, retreat if necessary at one week postoperatively. Figure 15.2.7 shows the topography of a post-CK patient (plano –1.00 × 135) treated with a bonus spot.

15.2.8 Undercorrection and Overcorrection

Additional management challenges can arise following CK that will require further surgical attention. Typically, this will be an undercorrection or suboptimal effect resulting in less improvement in near vision than the patient expected, usually J3. Approximately 20% relaxation of effect from 1 to 6 months postoperatively can be expected. Undercorrection is most commonly observed in patients under 45 years of age or when more than 2.25 D of effect were required. Be-

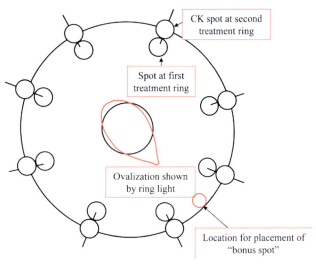

Fig. 15.2.4 Use of ring light and placement of bonus spot

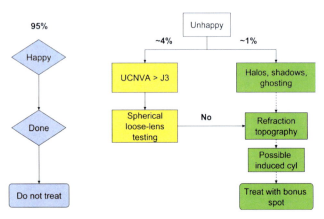

Fig. 15.2.5 Decision tree for further treatment vs. no treatments

Single ring of treatment: one spot *within* the ring   Double ring of treatment: one spot *between* the rings

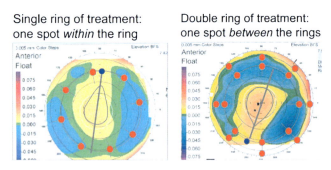

Fig. 15.2.6 Bonus spot placement. Treatment with single spot in the flatter hemi-meridian, as identified by elevation map

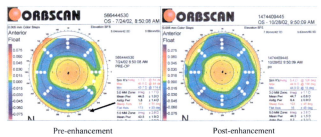

Pre-enhancement   Post-enhancement

Fig. 15.2.7 The pre-enhancement Orbscan map shows the treatment spot added in the flat meridian to treat plano –1.00 × 135. The 3-month post-enhancement Orbscan shows spherical topography with a large optical zone. (Courtesy Jason Stahl, M.D.)

15

fore discussing enhancement surgery with the patient, rule out the possibility of induced astigmatism as the potential cause by checking the patient's topography/Orbscan, refraction, and keratometry.

If induced astigmatism is absent, then the benefit of adding another ring of treatment spots to treat undercorrection can be determined by holding a +0.75-D sphere loose lens in front of the CK-treated eye. If the patient is within two lines of target vision and achieves near visual acuity of J3 or better with the lens, then adding another ring of CK spots is likely to produce an excellent result. Make the decision about enhancement 1 month after the primary procedure. To mark the cornea before adding a new ring of treatment, rotate the axis of the marker approximately 22.5° away from the previous CK treatment spots. Add a single ring of treatment at the 7.5-mm optical zone.

If a +0.75-D sphere loose lens does not produce J3 near vision, then a surface excimer laser procedure can be performed. The appropriate refractive error to be corrected is determined, once again, by loose lens testing. Currently, LASIK is not recommended, as a LASIK flap would cut some of the tension lines induced by the primary CK procedure and potentially reduce the refractive result. Overcorrected CK procedures are very rare and can be usually avoided by proper preoperative discussions and planning. Three to 6 months of observation are recommended to allow for potential regression of effect before taking any action.

Occasionally, patients may present with nonspecific functional complaints after a NearVision CK procedure. First, ask the patient about the location, time of day, lighting conditions, specific activity, etc., when the problem occurs and perform objective measurements. If all objective measurements indicate that the CK procedure was accurately performed and there is minimal or no astigmatism and good near vision in the treated eye, then discuss the outcome with the patient and remind him or her that J3 near vision is the target and that spectacles may be needed for certain activities and lighting conditions. Often patients with functional complaints have unrealistic expectations of the procedure and, in reality, are doing quite well, except for rare occasions of blurred near vision. Often the latter will resolve on its own as a patient becomes more accustomed to the "blended vision" effect of CK.

Rarely, patients may experience temporary glare, photosensitivity, and poor night vision after CK. Photosensitivity can be helped by the administration of topical nonsteroidal anti-inflammatory agents and night vision difficulties by the wearing of spectacles. These problems will usually resolve spontaneously with no further treatment required. Spectacles are the best treatment for night driving complaints.

15.2.9 Conclusion

In clinical trials for the treatment of presbyopia with the conventional nomogram, the LightTouch nomogram, and

in the treatment of presbyopia in patients who have previously had LASIK, CK has shown a remarkable record of safety. Loss of BCVA-Distance is minimal or absent, and contrast sensitivity and stereopsis are essentially maintained postoperatively. These safety findings with CK stand in contrast to findings seen after monovision LASIK procedures. Furthermore, the CK procedure is not susceptible to surgical flap complications or postoperative dry eye seen after LASIK procedures.

Complications management after conductive keratoplasty is a strategy that begins with appropriate patient selection and counseling regarding expectations, and progresses through a properly performed procedure that encompasses attention to centration, spot placement, and detection of surgically induced astigmatism. Postoperatively, if necessary, visual outcomes can be refined by selective spot placement for any induced astigmatism or rings of treatment added to augment the effect. Ultimately, mastery of complications management affords the patient and surgeon a rewarding experience and outcome from the procedure.

Take-Home Pearls

- Intraoperatively induced astigmatism is more commonly observed early in the surgeon's experience and generally decreases with greater experience. Most cases of induced cylinder are the result of inconsistent placement of treatment spots.
- Induced astigmatism can be observed through an operating microscope that incorporates a ring-light attachment. Typically, it appears as an elongated or pear-shaped distortion to the ring reflection.
- Treatment of induced astigmatism involves applying a bonus CK spot to balance the vector forces around the ring light mire.
- To test for ideal placement of the bonus spot, apply light pressure on the flat axis with the Keratoplast tip without puncturing Bowman's membrane. The oval ring-light reflection should become round.
- Undercorrection is most commonly observed in patients under 45 years of age or when more than 2.25 D of effect were required.
- The benefit of adding another ring of treatment spots in undercorrection or less-than-expected postoperative near vision can be determined by holding a +0.75 D sphere loose lens in front of the CK-treated eye.
- If the patient is within two lines of target vision and achieves near visual acuity of J3 or better with the lens, then adding another ring of CK spots is likely to produce an excellent result.

References

1. Asbell PA, Maloney RK, Davidorf J, Hersh P, McDonald M, Manche E (2001) Conductive Keratoplasty Study Group. Conductive keratoplasty for the correction of hyperopia. Trans Am Ophthalmol Soc 99:79–84

2. McDonald MB, Hersh PS, Manche EE, Maloney RK, Davidorf J, Sabry M (2002) Conductive keratoplasty for the correction of low to moderate hyperopia: US clinical trial 1-year results on 355 eyes. Ophthalmology 109:1978–1989

3. Alió JL, Ramzy MI, Galal A, Claramonte PJ (2005) Conductive keratoplasty for the correction of residual hyperopia after LASIK. J Refract Surg 2:698–704

4. Pallikaris IG, Naoumidi TL, Astyrakakis NI (2005) Long-term results of conductive keratoplasty for low to moderate hyperopia. J Cataract Refract Surg 31:1520–1529

5. Haji SA, Ramonas K, Potapova N, Wang G, Asbell PA (2005) Intraoperative correction of induced astigmatism after spherical correction of hyperopia with conductive keratoplasty. Eye Contact Lens 31:76–79

6. Naoumidi TL, Kounis GA, Astyrakakis NI, Tsatsaronis DN, Pallikaris IG (2006) Two-year follow-up of conductive keratoplasty for the treatment of hyperopic astigmatism. J Cataract Refract Surg 32:732–741

7. McDonald, MB, Durrie DS, Asbell PA, Maloney R, Nichamin L (2004) Treatment of presbyopia with conductive keratoplasty: six-month results of the United States FDA clinical trial. Cornea 23:661–668

8. Stahl JE (2006) Conductive keratoplasty for presbyopia: 1-year results. J Refract Surg 22:137–144

9. Durrie DS, McDonald M, Asbell PA, Maloney RK, Nichamin LD (2007) Conductive Keratoplasty* for the treatment of presbyopic emmetropes and hyperopes to improve near vision: 24-month results of the United States FDA clinical trial. J Cataract Refract Surg (in press)

10. De Paiva CS, Chen Z, Koch DD, Hamill MB, Manuel FK, Hassan SS, Wilhelmus KR, Pflugfelder SC (2006) The incidence and risk factors for developing dry eye after myopic LASIK. Am J Ophthalmol 141:438–445

15

Chapter 16

Complications of Intrastromal Corneal Ring Segments

16

Mohamed H. Shabayek and Jorge L. Alió

Contents

Core Messages

- Intrastromal corneal ring segments are gaining popularity with time as a surgical alternative for correcting corneal ectatic disorders. With an increase in frequency of using such a technique, it is important that ophthalmic surgeons become oriented with the complications of this surgical procedure as well as the best way to handle these complications.

- There are two commercially available types of Intrastromal corneal ring segments, Intacs® and KERARING®.

- Intraoperative, during surgical semiautomated manual tunnel creation or the femtosecond laser tunnel creation, and postoperative, clinical, as well as visual, complications are briefed in this chapter.

16.1 Introduction

Intrastromal corneal ring segments were first proposed by Fleming and Reynolds, in the late seventies, for the correction of various degrees of myopia [19]. The initial implant was a complete ring inserted through a peripheral single corneal incision. Due to technical surgical difficulties, it was re-fashioned into an incomplete ring and finally to two C-shape rings, hence the name intrastromal corneal ring segments [11, 22, 28–30]. Intrastromal corneal ring segments (ICRS) act as a spacer element between arching bundles of corneal lamellae, producing a shortening of the central arc length (arc shortening effect) with almost a linear relationship between the thickness of the spacer elements and the degree of the corneal flattening [31].

In 2000, Colin et al. [13] proposed ICRS as an additive surgical procedure for keratoconus correction, which provide an interesting surgical alternative aiming to delay if not to avoid corneal grafting in keratoconus patients [2–4, 6, 7, 10, 13]. The effect of ICRS on soft ectatic corneal tissue (keratoconus or post-LASIK ectasia) is much greater than that on more or less normal corneas of myopic patients [8, 14, 24, 27, 37]. The aim from implanting ICRS is not to treat

Table 16.1 Technical specification of both types of intrastromal corneal ring segments

	Intacs	KERARING
Design (cross section)	Hexagonal	Triangular
Inner diameter	6.77 mm	5.4 mm
Outer diameter	8.1 mm	6.6 mm
Implantation in respect to	Center of the cornea	Center of the pupil
Implantation depth	70% of the corneal thickness	70% of the corneal thickness
Arc length	150°	120 and 160°
Available segment thickness	0.25, 0.3, 0.35, 0.4, and 0.45 mm	0.15, 0.2, 0.25, 0.3, and 0.35 mm
Material	Polymethylmethacrylate (PMMA)	PMMA or acrylic Perspex CQ
Method of implantation	Surgical or with femtosecond laser	Surgical or with femtosecond laser

or eliminate the existing disease, or to consider it as a traditional refractive surgical procedure with high predictability and safety indices, but as a surgical alternative aiming to increase the visual acuity to acceptable limits by correcting the accompanying irregular astigmatism and corneal curvature abnormality. Moreover, ICRS may be used to delay, if not eliminate, the need of corneal grafting, especially in young patients with vision threatening pathology and long life expectancy [2–4, 13, 15, 23].

ICRS have gained popularity, overtime, as a surgical alternative for correcting corneal ectatic disorders. With the increasing frequency of such a technique, it is important that ophthalmic surgeons become oriented with the complications of this surgical procedure as well as the best way to handle these complications.

Complications (whether intraoperative or postoperative) that may result from ICRS vary, and mainly depend on the implantation technique. In addition to ICRS complications and in order to achieve a more systematic understanding, this chapter provides a brief overview of the different implantation techniques as well as different ICRS types.

16.2　Types of ICRS

Two types of ICRS are used by ophthalmic surgeons. The first is known under the trade name Intacs* (Addition Technologies, Fremont, Calif.) and KERARING*, which was originally designed by Pablo Ferrara (Mediphacos, Belo Horizonte, Brazil) [1]. Technical specification and differences between both types are shown in Table 16.1.

16.3　Complications Due to Implantation Techniques

ICRS can be implanted after creating corneal tunnels either with a semi-automated device (manual dissection) technique or with the aid of the femtosecond laser [1].

16.3.1　Manual Tunnel Dissection

The procedure is performed mainly under topical anaesthesia after marking the geometrical center of the cornea for Intacs implantation and center of the pupil for KERARING implantation (Intacs are implanted in respect to the corneal center, while in KERARINGs are implanted in respect to the pupil center). Intraoperative ultrasonic pachymetry is performed at the site of the incision. After seven readings, the highest and lowest measurements are discarded and the average of the remaining five readings is considered as the corneal thickness [1, 4, 6]. A calibrated diamond knife is set at 70–80% (Intacs and KERARING, respectively) of the mean measured corneal thickness and a 1.8-mm radial incision is made. The incision is sited at 5- to 7-mm (KERARING and Intacs, respectively) from the previously marked center.

The stromal pocket is dissected on both sides of the incision using a modified Suarez spatula. For KERARING implantation, widening the tunnels is made manually with a 270° dissecting spatula (Fig. 16.1), followed by segments implantation and wound suturing.

Intacs requires a semiautomated vacuum device (Fig. 16.2a), this device has a suction ring (Fig. 16.2b) that is placed around the limbus guided by the previously marked geometrical center of the cornea. After careful checking of the suction pressure, two semicircular lamellar dissectors are placed sequentially into the lamellar pocket and steadily advanced by a rotational movement into the corneal stroma, resulting in two 180° circular tunnels with an approximate diameter of 7.5 mm. Then the Intacs segment is inserted into the corneal tunnel [4, 6].

16.3.2　Operative Complications with the Manual Tunnel Dissection Technique

Anterior or posterior perforations may occur during manual dissection. Such complications occur mainly due to (1) inaccurate measurements of the corneal thickness, (2) inadequate pressure, or (3) segment implantation in the wrong plane.

16

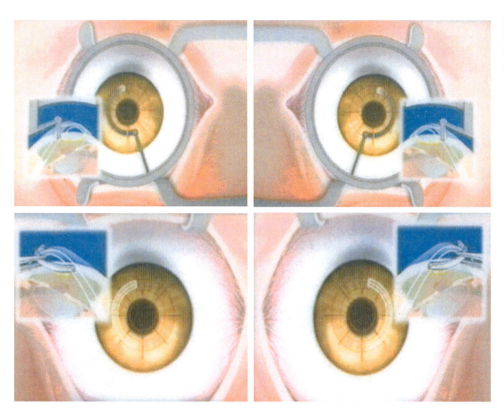

Fig. 16.1 Diagram showing KERARING implantation with the 270° dissecting spatula

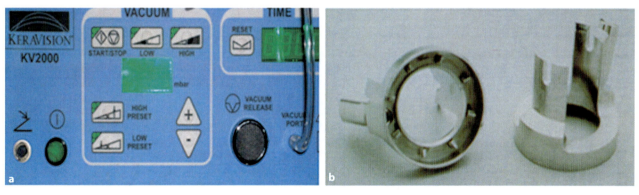

Fig. 16.2 **a** Intacs semi automated vacuum device with the suction ring (**b**)

Proper and accurate measurements of the corneal thickness may avoid perforations. It is advised to measure corneal thickness at the incision site. Commonly used contact ultrasonic pachymeters are not highly accurate in measuring the paracentral or the peripheral cornea (7-mm zone in the case of Intacs implantation); hence, an average of multiple measurements is taken as the corneal thickness. This can aid in having a more precise measurement at the implantation site. Also using new non-contact pachymetry as the very high frequency optical coherence tomography (Visante™ OCT, Carl Zeiss Meditec, Jena, Germany) with the generated pachymetry map (Fig. 16.3) can aid in providing a more accurate measurement of the corneal thickness especially at the paracentral area, usually the thinnest area in keratoconus and other ectatic disorders.

In addition, checking the pressure during manual dissection and performing a steady uniform rotational movement with a dissecting spatula is mandatory, not only to avoid anterior or posterior perforation, but also to achieve a uniform tunnel depth.

Lastly, if the surgeon experiences resistance during segment implantation, then the segment is in the wrong plane. Minimal resistance is observed during segment implantation in a properly dissected plane.

The procedure must be aborted, in the event of such complications, and postponed for at least 3 months and during the next attempt, the previous incision and tunnel site should be avoided.

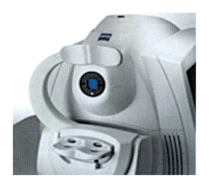
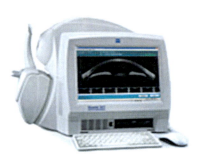
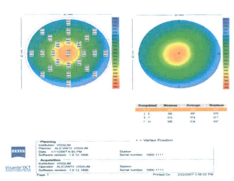

Fig. 16.3 Visante™ OCT with the generated pachymetry map

16.3.3 Femtosecond Laser IntraLase Tunnel Dissection

The femtosecond laser (IntraLase, Irvine, Calif.) is an infrared, neodymium glass, ultrafast (10^{-15} s) laser with a wavelength of 1,053 nm. The laser beam, which is of 3-μm diameter spot size is optically focused to a specific predetermined intrastromal depth by means of a computer scanner, which gives a focus range between 90 and 400 μm from the anterior corneal surface. This laser beam forms plasma photodisruption, resulting in cavitations (microbubbles) of carbon dioxide and water vapor. The interconnection of this series of micro–gas bubbles leads to the formation of a precise planar dissection plane [36].

A disposable low-vacuum suction ring provided by the manufacturer is applied to the surface of the globe, and then a disposable glass lens applanates the cornea to maintain a precise focal distance between the laser emission aperture and the desired focal point, as well as to flatten the anterior corneal surface in order to achieve a planer tunnel (tunnel of equal in depth all through 360°). The procedure takes approximately 10 s with the 60-KHz femtosecond laser. The 60-KHz IntraLase parameters for both ICRS types are shown in Table 16.2. After intracorneal ring segment placement, usually no suture is required [1].

16.3.4 Operative Complications with Femtosecond Laser Tunnel Dissection

With this new technology, which provides a precise planar tunnel and easy segments implantation, operative complications such as anterior or posterior perforation are rare to occur, especially after proper and accurate corneal thickness measurement. However, and due to inaccurate corneal thickness measurement, posterior perforation can occur with femtosecond laser, but contrary to the manual dissection technique, there is no need to postpone the surgery. Another tunnel at the same site, but more superficially, (40 μm) is performed by changing the software parameters followed by ICRS implantation. Table 16.3 summarizes the reported postoperative clinical complications after manual and femtosecond tunnel creation.

Table 16.2 60-KHz IntraLase parameters for intrastromal corneal ring segments implantation.

	Intacs	KERARING
Inner diameter	6.6 mm	4.8 mm
Outer diameter	7.4 mm	5.4 mm
Incision length	1 mm	1mm
Tunnel energy	2.5 mJ	2.5 mJ
Incision energy	2.5 mJ	2.5 mJ

16.4 Postoperative Complications

Various postoperative complications whether clinical or visual have been reported after intrastromal corneal ring segments implantation with the manual dissection as well as after the femtosecond laser technique.

16.4.1 Postoperative Clinical Complications after Manual Dissection Technique

16.4.1.1 Infectious Keratitis

Infectious keratitis [21, 25, 26] (Fig. 16.4) has been reported by sporadic case reports in the literature. Until now, the literature lacks a known incidence due to small published reports. Kwitko and Severo [22] reported an incidence of 1.9% (1 out of 52 eyes) after manually implanting Ferrara rings for keratoconus correction. This devastating complication is either an early postoperative complication (due to intraoperative infection) or late postoperative, mostly occurring in contact lens patients. Dealing with such complications is by properly identifying the causative organism whether by culture and sensitivity or PCR [18]. Sampling may be difficult as the site is usually deep and localized around the segment. The treatment should be started immediately after tissue sampling, with heavy doses of fortified topical antibiotic drops that cover both aerobic and anaerobic organisms, with small doses of topical corticosteroids in case of suspected bacterial infectious keratitis

Table 16.3 Reported complications after manual and femtosecond laser tunnel creation

	Shabayek and Alió [27]	Kwitko and Severo [6]	Boxer Wachler et al. [14]	Alió et al. [10]	Alió et al. [13]	Colin [24]
Tunnel Creation	F	M	M	M	M	M
No. of eyes	21	51	74	20	26	57
Type of segment	Ferrara	Ferrara	Intacs	Intacs	Intacs	Intacs
Operative anterior perforation	0	0	1	0	0	0
Deposits	0	X	2	3	C	C
Extrusion	0	10		7	0	0
Decentration	0	2	1	0	0	0
Keratitis	1	2	0	0	0	0
Vascularization	0	0	0	2	3	0

X did not comment on deposits, C did not comment on the exact number but commented that the complication was common

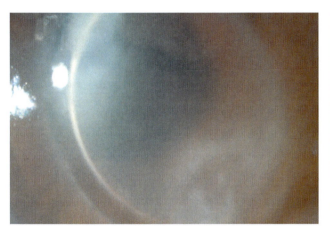

Fig. 16.4 Infectious keratitis after Intacs implantation with the manual tunnel creation

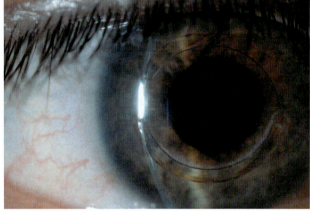

Fig. 16.5 Segment extrusion

[27] and topical antifungal medications in case of suspected fungal infectious keratitis. Unfortunately, segment removal sometimes is the ultimate solution, followed by flushing the tunnel with buffered salt solution, and administering topical antibiotics and corticosteroids until corneal clarity is achieved again [33]. Segment explantation should not be the first choice, and only must be considered when medical treatment fails.

16.4.1.2 Segment Extrusion and Migration

Segment extrusion (Fig. 16.5) has been reported with an incidence of 19.6% (10 out of 51 eyes) after Ferrara ring implantation with the manual dissection technique by Kwitko and Severo [22]. Alió et al. [3], however, reported this complication in 7 eyes after Intacs with the manual dissec-

tion technique. Although segment extrusion seems to be an uncommon early complication, late segment extrusion can occur especially in atopic patients with frequent eye rubbing. Management of segment extrusion is with topical antibiotics to guard against secondary bacterial infection and therapeutic contact lens application.

Segment migration or decentration (superficial or horizontal displacement) (Fig. 16.6) occurs mainly with allergic and atopic patients. High degrees of migration can cause change in the refraction or to segment extrusion. Patient education, especially atopic (allergic) patients, is important to prevent such complications. In addition, topical anti histaminic is helpful in relieving allergy symptoms. However, segment explantation is indicated with severe migration with corneal edema (Fig. 16.7).

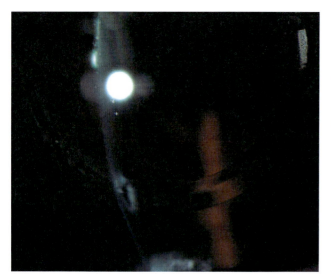

Fig. 16.6 Segment decentration (the *arrow* pointing at the touching lower ends)

16.4.1.3 Tunnel Neovascularization

Tunnel neovascularization (Fig. 16.8) is a complication that was reported [6] in five eyes after Intacs implantation; this complication usually subsides during the first postoperative year. Intacs segments implantation with respect to the geometrical corneal center can avoid such a complication by avoiding the vascularized limbus, apically in contact lens patients.

16.4.1.4 Tunnel Deposits

Tunnel deposits (Fig. 16.9), with no accurate incidence rates, are reported to occur as the most common complication after ICRS implantation. Such complications do not require any management as long as they do not interfere with the central visual axis [3, 6, 10, 16].

16.4.2 Postoperative Clinical Complications after Femtosecond Laser Tunnel Dissection

Recent studies [17, 32, 33], reported few and irrelevant complications after intrastromal ring segments (Intacs and KERARING) implantation after femtosecond tunnel creation. Other studies did not report any clinical complications. In our latest report, we reported clinical complications after KERARING implantation following femtosecond tunnel creation such as; Subconjunctival hemorrhage, superficial corneal "incision" opacification, and infectious keratitis.

16.4.2.1 Subconjunctival Hemorrhage

Subconjunctival hemorrhage (Fig. 16.10) results from the suction ring and subsides after 1 or 2 weeks [33] .

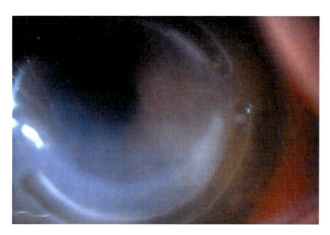

Fig. 16.7 Severe migration with corneal edema

16

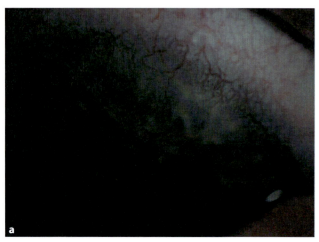

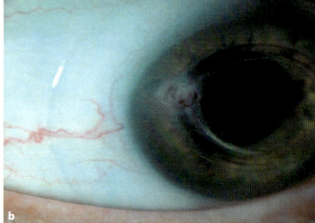

Fig. 16.8 Tunnel neovascularization (**a**) tunnel vascularization with extrusion (**b**)

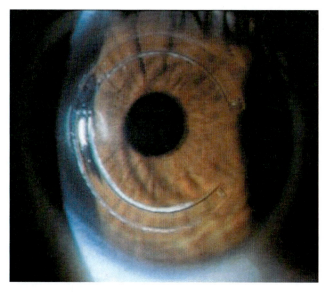

Fig. 16.9 Tunnel deposits

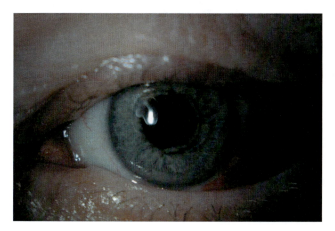

Fig. 16.10 Subconjunctival hemorrhage with KERARING after tunnel creation with the femtosecond laser

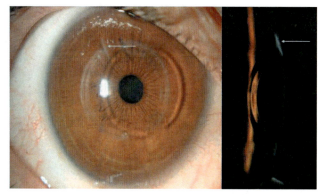

Fig. 16.11 Superficial corneal opacification coinciding with the incision site after femtosecond laser tunnel creation

and the fortified antibiotics were stopped with continuation of antibiotic (Tobramycin 3 mg/ml) and steroid (Dexamethasone 1mg/ml) eye drops five times daily for 2 weeks ,with complete visual recovery, but due to traces of small localized infectious pockets that existed around the lower segment end, (Fig. 16.12b) and also due to tapering the medications, exacerbation of the infection re-occurred (Fig. 16.12c). One month later, (2 months after the surgery) the segment was explanted by dissecting the incision with a 21-ga blade and explanting the segment with Sinskey hook, followed by tunnel irrigation with buffered saline solution and vancomycin. In spite of the negative culture and sensitivity results of the explanted segment, electron microscopy pictures (Fig. 16.13a, b) showed debris and necrotic tissue around the segment. One month after the explantation of the lower segment, corneal clarity was recovered but with minimal scarring "stromal opacification" which coincided with the site of the localized keratitis (Fig. 16.12d) and the best spectacle-corrected visual acuity (BSCVA) was restored to the initial preoperative level but with an increase in the spherical equivalent by 11.25 D when compared to pre-explantation data of the lower segment [33].

16.4.3 Postoperative Visual Complications

16.4.3.1 Decrease in BSCVA

Decrease in BSCVA after intrastromal corneal ring segments is mainly due to poor patient selection, advanced keratoconus [4] (grade IV) with or without corneal opacity, or improper decision-making regarding symmetrical or asymmetrical segment implantation [6]. The distribution of the ectatic area and spherical equivalent should be taken in consideration in the decision-making, as previous reports demonstrated that asymmetrical ectatic cones achieve better visual outcome with asymmetrical implantation, while symmetrical central cones obtain better visual outcome with symmetrical implantation [4, 6, 12, 22]. Previous studies reported a better visual outcome with symmetrical implantation in central cones than with symmetrical implantation with asymmetrical or peripheral cones [22]. Also the

16.4.2.2 Superficial Corneal "Incision" Opacification

Superficial corneal opacification, which was coinciding with the incision site (Fig. 16.11), was reported [33] with an incidence of 38% (8 out of 21 eyes). This complication most probably occurred due to high energy of first generation, the 15-KHz femtosecond laser on the superficial corneal stroma.

16.4.2.3 Infectious Keratitis

Only one case of late localized infectious keratitis was reported after tunnel creation using the femtosecond laser [33] (1 [4.8 %] eye out of 21) 1 month after surgery (Fig. 16.12a) with uncorrectable visual acuity of 0.05. Intensive fortified antibiotic and corticosteroid combination was prescribed every two hours for 3 days with a good response after 48 h. Corneal clarity was achieved one week after treatment (Fig. 16.12b),

16

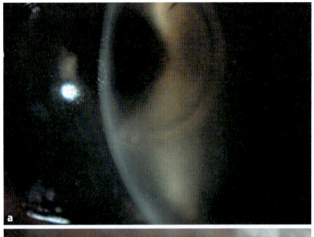

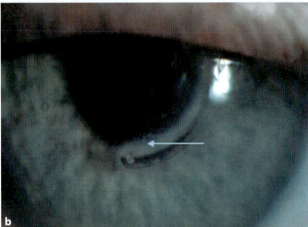

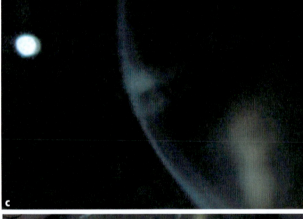

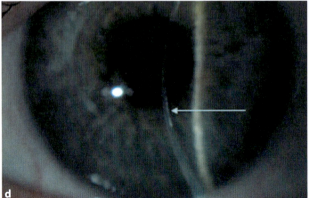

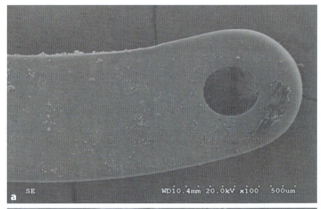

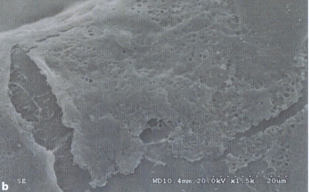

Fig. 16.13 Electron microscopy pictures showing debris and necrotic tissue around the segment (**a**) low magnification and (**b**) high magnification

placement of the relatively thicker segment in asymmetrical implantation in the inferior corneal half (coinciding to the ectatic area) provides better visual outcome [2, 12].

Decrease in the visual acuity after Intacs implantation for keratoconus correction has been previously reported. We reported that this decrease in the BSCVA occurred in advanced or grade IV keratoconus (keratoconus with mean K value > 55 D) and with high spherical equivalent (SE) [4]. Boxer Wachler et al. [10] also reported such decrease in the BSCVA after Intacs implantation in keratoconic eyes with high preoperative SE. This visual complication can be avoided as mentioned by proper patient selection. However, with decrease in the BSCVA the segment explantation and corneal grafting in advanced keratoconus grade IV are the last solution for these patients. Also in our latest report [27], we found similar results after KERARING implantation for keratoconus correction in advanced keratoconus grade IV. In addition, a negative significant correlation was

Fig. 16.12 a Late localized infectious keratitis. **b** Corneal clarity was achieved one week after treatment. Traces of small localized infectious pockets that might have caused exacerbation of the infection. **c** Exacerbation of the localized infectious keratitis. **d** Mild stromal opacification, which coincided with the site of the localized infectious keratitis after lower segment explantation

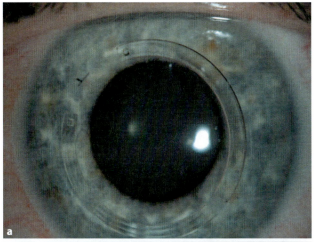

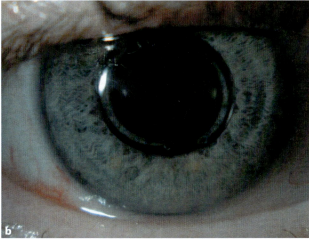

Fig. 16.14 Uncomplicated (normal) clinical outcome after Intacs implantation after manual tunnel creation (**a**) and KERARING after tunnel creation with the femtosecond laser (**b**)

also observed between the keratoconus grade and preoperative mean K value and the final BSCVA obtained after surgery [33].

Another cause of decrease in the BSCVA is the placement of the relatively thicker segment in asymmetrical implantation in the upper corneal half or opposite to the ectatic area. Previous case reports [2, 12] dramatically demonstrated improvement in visual acuity and K values after re-implanting the thicker segment inferiorly or adjacent to the ectatic area.

16.4.3.2 Increase in Corneal Higher-Order Aberrations

A nonsignificant increase in the total corneal higher order aberrations was reported after KERARING implantation with femtosecond laser, this finding was observed only in grade I and II keratoconus [5] or in eyes with initial preoperative coma and coma-like aberration <3.0 μm. To our knowledge, this is the only report detailing the evaluated

changes in corneal higher aberrations after intrastromal corneal ring segments implantation [33].

16.4.4 Conclusion

In conclusion, complications after intrastromal corneal ring segments occur and seem to be of low incidence due to the small cohort of individuals reported as well as the few reports published, so the exact incidence is not yet clear; further larger studies will reveal the real incidence of the more serious complications such as infectious keratitis and segment extrusion. Clinical complications are mainly due to the manual tunnel creation, as femtosecond laser tunnel creation provides better clinical outcomes with no serious complications (Fig. 16.14), while good patient selection and proper decision-making can avoid the postoperative visual complications.

Take-Home Pearls

- Intrastromal corneal ring segments are a new surgical alternative for correcting irregular astigmatism associated with ectatic corneal disorders. The aim of this surgical alternative is not to treat the corneal pathology but to correct the associated irregular astigmatism and increase the visual acuity to acceptable limits as a way to delay the need of corneal grafting.
- Operative complications occur mainly with manual tunnel creation, minimal complications were reported after femtosecond tunnel creation. Accurate pachymetry is essential in achieving a reliable depth of implantation and, hence, decreasing the rate of extrusion.
- Femtosecond laser provides a better modality for ICRS implantation. It decreases the clinical operative and postoperative complications, providing a better visual outcome.
- Proper patient selection and decision making regarding symmetrical or asymmetrical implantation and placement of the thicker segment can prevent postoperative decrease in the BSCVA.

References

1. Alió JL, Shabayek MH (2006) Intracorneal implants. In: Kohen T, Koch D (eds) Essentials in ophthalmology—cataract and refractive surgery II. Springer, Berlin Heidelberg New York, pp 159–169
2. Alió JL, Shabayek MH (2006) Intracorneal asymmetrical rings for keratoconus: Where should the thicker segment be implanted? J Refract Surg 22:307–309
3. Alió JL, Shabayek MH, Artola A (2006) ICRS (INTACS) for Keratoconus correction: Long term follow up. J Cataract Refract Surg 32:978–85
4. Alió JL, Shabayek MH, Belda JI et al (2006) Analysis of results related to good and bad outcome of INTACS implantation for correction of keratoconus. J Cataract Refract Surg 32:756–761

5. Alió JL, Shabayek MH (2006) Corneal higher order aberrations: a method to grade keratoconus. J Refract Surg 22:539–545

6. Alió AJ, Artola A, Hassanein A et al (2005) One or two INTACS segments for the correction of keratoconus. J Cataract Refract Surg 31:943–53

7. Alió JL, Artola A, Ruiz-Moreno JM et al (2004) Changes in keratoconic corneas after intracorneal ring segment explantation and reimplantation. Ophthalmology 111:747–751

8. Alió J, Salem T, Artola A et al (2002) Intracorneal rings to correct corneal ectasia after laser in situ keratomileusis. J Cataract Refract Surg 28:1568–1574

9. Bourcier T, Borderie V, Laroche L (2003) Late bacterial keratitis after implantation of intrastromal corneal ring segments. J Cataract Refract Surg 29:407–409

10. Boxer Wachler BS, Christie JP, Chandra NS et al (2003) Intacs for keratoconus. Ophthalmology 110:1031–1040

11. Burris TE, Baker PC, Ayer et al (1993) Flattening of the curvature with intrastromal corneal rings of increasing thickness-an eye bank eye study. J Refractive Surg. 19:182–187

12. Chan CC, Wachler BS (2007) Reduced best spectacle-corrected visual acuity from inserting a thicker Intacs above and thinner Intacs below in keratoconus. J Refract Surg 23:93–955

13. Colin J, Cochener B, Savary G et al (2000) Correcting keratoconus with intracorneal rings. J Cataract Refract Surg 26:1117–1122

14. Colin J, Malet FJ (2007) Intacs for the correction of keratoconus: two-year follow-up. J Cataract Refract Surg 33:69–74

15. Colin J (2006) European clinical evaluation: use of Intacs for the treatment of keratoconus. J Cataract Refract Surg 32:747–755

16. Ertan A, Kamburoglu G, Bahadir M (2006) Intacs insertion with the femtosecond laser for the management of keratoconus: one-year results. J Cataract Refract Surg 32:2039–2042

17. Ferrer C, Colom F, Frases S et al (2001) Detection and identification of fungal pathogens by PCR and by ITS2 and 5.8s ribosomal DNA typing in ocular infections. J Clin Microbiol 39:2873–2879

18. Fleming JR, Reynolds AI, Kilmer L (1987) The intrastromal corneal ring-two cases in rabbits. J Refractive Surg 3:227–232

19. Hofling-Lima AL, Branco BC, Romano AC et al (2004) Corneal infections after implantation of ICRS. Cornea 23:547–549

20. Katsoulis K, Sarra GM, Schittny JC et al (2006) Bilateral central crystalline corneal deposits four years after Intacs for myopia. J Refract Surg 22:910–3

21. Kwitko S, Severo NS (2004) Ferrara ICRS for keratoconus. J Cataract Refract Surg 30:812–820

22. Kymionis GD, Siganos CS, Tsiklis NS et al (2007) Long-term follow-up of Intacs in keratoconus. Am J Ophthalmol 143:236–244

23. Lovisolo CF, Fleming JF (2002) ICRS for iatrogenic keratectasia after laser in situ keratomileusis or photorefractive keratectomy. J Refract Surg 18:535–441

24. McAlister JC, Ardjomand N, Ilari L et al (2006) Keratitis after intracorneal ring segment insertion for keratoconus. J Cataract Refract Surg 32:676–68

25. Mondino BJ, Rabin BS, Kessler E et al (1977) Corneal rings with gram-negative bacteria. Arch Ophthalmology 95:2222–2225

26. Mularoni A, Torreggiani A, di Biase A et al (2005) Conservative treatment of early and moderate pellucid marginal degeneration: A new refractive approach with intracorneal rings. Ophthalmology 112:660–666

27. Nosé W, Neves RA, Burris TE et al (1996) Intrastromal corneal ring—12 months sighted myopic eyes. J Refract Surg 12:20–28

28. Nosé W, Neves RA, Schanzlin DJ et al (1993) Intrastromal corneal ring-one year results of first implant in humans: a preliminary non-functional eye study. Refract Corneal Surg 9:452–458

29. Patel S, Marshall J, Fitzke FW (1995) Model for deriving the optical performance of the myopic eye corrected with an intracorneal ring. J Refract Surg 11:248–252

30. Pinsky PM, Datye DV, Silvestrini TA (1995) Numerical simulation of topographical alterations in the cornea after intrastromal corneal ring (ICR) placement. Invest Ophthalmol Vis Sci 36(Suppl):308

31. Rabinowitz YS, Li X, Ignacio TS, Maguen E (2006) Intacs inserts using the femtosecond laser compared to the mechanical spreader in the treatment of keratoconus. J Refract Surg 22:764–771

32. Shabayek MH, Alió JL (2007) Intrastromal corneal ring segment implantation by femtosecond laser for keratoconus correction. Ophthalmology (in press)

33. Sharma M, Boxer Wachler BS (2006) Comparison of single-segment and double-segment Intacs for keratoconus and post-LASIK ectasia. Am J Ophthalmol 41:891–895

34. Shehadeh-Masha'our R, Modi N, Barbra A (2004) Keratitis after implantation of intrastromal ring segments. J Cataract Refract Surg 30:1802–1804

35. Tran DB, Schanzlin DJ, Traub IR et al (2002) IntraLase femtosecond laser for INTACS implantation. In Lovisolo CF, Fleming JF, Pesando PM (eds) Intrastromal corneal ring segments. Fabiano, Milan, pp, 365–374

36. Tunc Z, Deveci N, Sener B et al (2003) Corneal ring segments (INTACS) for the treatment of Asymmetrical astigmatism of the keratoconus. Follow up after 2 years. J Fr Ophthalmol 26:824–830

16

Chapter 17

Corneal Inlays (Synthetic Keratophakia)

17

M. Emilia Mulet, Jorge L Alió, and Michael Knorz

Contents

Core Messages

- The inlay implant technique is associated with specific complications; the most frequent are inlay displacements and intracorneal deposits.

- Inlay implants correct low hyperopia with poorer results than the LASIK technique with increased ocular aberrations

- Inlay explantations serve to eliminate complications.

- Posterior retreatment of cases with explanted inlays is safe.

17.1 Introduction

The goal of refractive corneal procedures is to modify the anterior curvature of the cornea to yield appropriate refractive change. In the commonly performed laser assisted in situ keratomileusis (LASIK), the corneal curvature is modified by ablation of corneal tissue after lamellar keratotomy. Hyperopic results following LASIK may vary with respect to irregular astigmatism, where some degree of regression may be observed with complaints of halos and glare [4, 19].

Refractive errors can be corrected by placing pre-formed tissue, biological (epikeratophakia) or synthetic material (synthetic keratophakia), onto or into the cornea. This modifies the optical power of the cornea by changing the shape of the anterior corneal surface or by creating a lens with a higher index of refraction than the corneal stroma. This method is additive refractive keratoplasty.

Tissue addition procedures, such as epikeratoplasty, have fallen out of favor because of the difficulty of obtaining donor tissue as well as poor predictability of refractive and visual results [3, 10, 21, 22].

Epikeratoplasty involves suturing a preformed lenticule of human donor corneal tissue directly onto Bowman's layer of the host cornea. Re-epithelialization over the lenticule is a major complication. Other complications and causes for lenticule removal included graft haze/scar, infection, stromal infiltrates, melt, dehiscence, refractive error, irregular astigmatism, epithelial ingrowth and interface cysts, and severe glare symptoms.

Synthetic inlays offer several potential advantages, such as the ability to be mass-produced in a wide range of sizes and powers that can be measured and verified. Also, synthetic material may have optical properties superior to tissue lenses, which are difficult to accurately lathe. Unlike synthetic material, tissue lenticules can become distorted upon insertion and may undergo remodeling, which can prolong postoperative visual recovery and can lead to refractive instability. This method creates the potential for reversibility. If necessary, the implant may be removed, and other treatments may still be available to the patient [2, 10, 19, 22].

Synthetic stromal inlays or intracorneal inlay implants have been investigated for nearly half a century. Barraquer [5] was the first, in 1949, followed by many researchers who used an implantable inlay to modify the refraction of the cornea [6, 28–30, 41, 43, 44]. They used flint glass and Plexiglass in their studies. Synthetic materials hold greater promise because they can be shaped to greater precision than tissue and can be mass-produced. Because of problems with re-epithelialization, synthetic material generally has to be placed in the corneal stroma. The materials used in the first implants caused anterior stromal necrosis because these substances are impermeable to water and nutrients, followed by extrusion in the eyes implanted with this inlay [27, 38]. The limitations of this impermeable membrane developed in previous studies could be avoided by the use of more permeable materials such as hydrogels. Permeability of hydrogel material is similar to the corneal stroma, allowing the exchange of water and nutrients between the posterior and anterior layers of the cornea, maintaining normal physiological characteristics [27, 38]. The first hydrogel to be evaluated for refractive keratoplasty was hydroxyethyl methacrylate, by Dohlman [15] in 1967 and later on by other researchers in the area of refractive keratoplasty [30, 44, 45]. They reported excellent tolerance of hydrogel lens in corneas of rabbits [20, 28] and humans [6, 17, 41]. No signs of keratocytic activity of intrastromal fibrosis, inflammation, ulceration, or neovascularization were found [17, 39].

17.2 Inlay Characteristics

There are different types of materials, but hydrogels, with their different pore sizes and water and nutrient permeability, have been the most popular until now. There are two models used in clinical trials with small differences between them and with a refractive index of approximately 1.39, which is very close to that of the cornea 1.376.

lidofilcon A (Kougar, Advanced Medical Optics [AMO], Irvine, Calif.) is a non-ionic copolymer of N-vinyl-2-pyrrolidone (NVP) and methylmethacrylate (MMA) having a water content of 67.3 % when fully hydrated at 33°C. Lidofilcom A is soft, flexible, autoclavable, non-toxic and biocompatible [41]. The material is permeable to water, glucose, and oxygen in order to meet corneal nutrition needs when implanted. The Permalens (PermaVision, Anamed, Lake Forest, Calif.) is composed of hydrogel material called Nutrapore. The water content varies from 67.3% (Kougar) to 78% (Permalens). The thickness in the center is from 0.115- to 0.35-μm-D dependent (Kougar) to 48–92μm (Permalens), and the edge of the inlay 0.05–0.09 μm, with a base curve of 7.35 mm. The diameter is from 4.75 for more than of 6.00 D, to 5.25 mm for 2.00–6.00 D. The power of the inlay ranges from +2 to +8 in +0.50-D increments in human clinical trials. In primates, the power range used was +6 to +20 [30, 31, 34].

There is another type of inlay designed to correct presbyopia without intraocular surgery. These lenses are implanted in the non-dominant eye either under a LASIK flap or in a corneal pocket. These implants are made of various materials, hydrogels (Bausch & Lomb's Chiron lens, Biovision's Invue Intracorneal Microlens system, ReVision Opticc's Optics PresbyLens) and ultrathin 10-μm discs made of biocompatible polymer called Kynar (Bausch & Lomb's AcuFocus ACI 7000), and measure 2–4 mm in diameter.

17.3 Surgical Technique

The method by which intracorneal inlays are implanted within the cornea consists of creating a corneal flap with an automated microkeratome [1], and more recently by femtosecond laser [34], followed by inlay implantation onto the corneal stromal bed over the pupillary aperture, and covered by the corneal flap (Fig. 17.1). We created a 180-μm corneal flap with a diameter of 8.5 mm, or an 8.5-mm inferior hinged corneal flap [1]. We must maintain a hinged flap of constant thickness and a desired corneal depth for inlay placement. Previous experimental studies have demonstrated that hydrogel lenses need to be placed at a depth between 36 and 60% of the corneal thickness for success [13, 31]. During the procedure, corneal pachymetry was used to measure the cornea and residual stromal bed by using an ultrasonic pachymeter. Following the manufacturer's indications, a "dry technique" was used for the implantation of the inlay. Hence, the interface was not irrigated after the microkeratome cut or the implantation. Immediately after the microkeratome cut was performed, the stromal bed was carefully dried with a sponge, and the inlay was placed over the pupil by means of a specific manual vacuum device, as recommended by the different manufacturers. The hinged corneal flap was replaced onto the bed without sutures. The gutter around the edge of the flap was dried with a sponge, and the flap was allowed to settle for 2 min.

At the end of the procedure, the eye was occluded for 24 h postoperatively. We administered 0.3 % Ofloxacin four times per day for 1 week and combined tobramycin and 0.1% Dexamethasone four times a day for 1 week.

17.4 Results

The results in this chapter include 32 eyes of 23 patients from J.L. Alió and M. Knorz. All the patients underwent

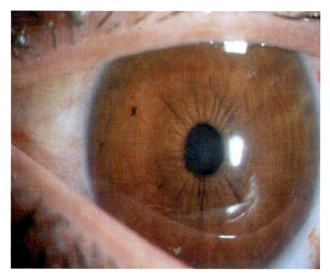

Fig. 17.1 month after inlay implantation

the same implantation technique performed by both surgeons.

Uncorrected visual acuity improved significantly during the first three months and was generally stable from 3 months to 2 years. The recovery of best-corrected visual acuity (BCVA) was similar through 1 year. Other authors [1, 17] report that the BCVA improves up to 12 months postoperatively.

In our study (a clinical trial with selected patients without important ocular diseases corneal, retinal or inflammatory diseases that can compromise the results) the follow-up period was 5 years. We had a predictability ±0.50 D in 67% of eyes and ±1.00 D in 86 % of the eyes that were not explanted in the first month. We had a visual acuity loss of two lines in 32% at 2 years, and the loss was even higher in later years of follow-up because of an increase in the deposits on the inlay surface with visual acuity loss of three or more lines in 40.6 % of the eyes between 3 and 5 years follow-up. Other authors reported a predictability ±0.50 D in 83% at 3 months to 100% at 6 and 12 months. Eighty-three percent maintained the same spectacle-corrected visual acuity at 12 months [17]. However, these good results were in a small group of patients.

Refractive predictability was poor with 88% of the eyes ± 3.00 D of emmetropia. At 2 years, these findings may favorably be compared with results of epikeratophakia, in which 75% of the eyes were within ±3.00 D of emmetropia, with a mean follow-up time of 6 months [22, 34]. Other authors confirmed in primates a slight overcorrection and slight undercorrection in 10.3% [30]. In eyes that had preoperative diseases with prior surgical procedures, stability of mean spherical equivalent remained stable during a 2-year follow-up period. The proportion of patients with residual refractive errors of ±3.00 D was 88%; 75% with refractive errors of ±2.00 D and 50% with ±1.00 D [41].

17.5 Complications

There is a large list of complications described in animal models [7, 34] with different inlay materials due to the technical difficulty of the surgical procedure very severe complications on the surface or in the eye occur, which do not occur in humans. Therefore, in this chapter we describe the complications observed in human studies only.

The intracorneal lens implant was well tolerated in the human cornea [6, 17, 41]. In most eyes, the cornea was clear at 1 day postoperatively. The most common complication were intracorneal deposits, corneal edema, corneal haze, irregular astigmatism, implant migration, undercorrection, epithelial perilenticular opacity and in consequence implant removal.

In some patients, complications were associated with technical difficulties during the microkeratome cut, whereas in other patients the cause was unknown.

Possible causes for the removal of the implant include an irregular microkeratome resection, interface epithelial ingrowth, and implant migration. There are several possible causes for corneal damage related to the inlay. In thin flaps, the mechanical pressure of the lids against the implant may cause flap melting. In thick inlays, the thick material may not allow nutrients of aqueous or tear film to pass. In spite of the porosity of the material, we believe that the inlay used is too thick to allow a good passage of different nutrients [32] or that passage is sufficient initially but decreases with time as those pores become obstructed by the deposits accumulating [1].This hypothesis is also supported by the fact that it is a convex lens with very thin external edges, but much thicker and with less permeability in the center [34].

17.5.1 Inlay Displacement

Inlay displacements or decentrations greater than 1 mm occurred in approximately 30% of the eyes. Different degrees of decentration required repositioning or change of the inlay in 20% of the eyes. Specific manual vacuum devices are recommended by the manufacturer. The excessive irrigation or washing of the stromal bed or flap to eliminate particles can also influence displacements or even loss of the inlay. As a result, the dry technique is recommended.

17.5.2 Small Tears or Holes in the Inlay

The thinness of the inlay does not allow repositioning. Small decentrations over the pupil area are very difficult to manage, and some instruments or forceps used can damage and break the inlay. These breaks or holes in the inlay deposit substances with greater ease in the affected area, changing the optic quality of the inlay (Fig. 17.2).

17.5.3 Loss of Inlay

Sometimes extrusion of the implant occurs through the wound. The loss of the implant, which is the place of the

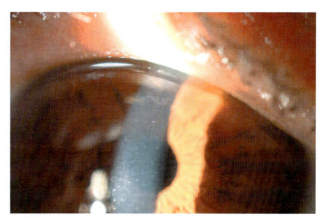

Fig. 17.2 Small holes: epithelization or depositing of substances with greater ease in the affected area

hinge, brings into question whether it is necessary to suture the flap. We used an inferior hinge to avoid the strength of the blinking and the loss of the inlay through the inferior area of the flap without suturing. The percentage inlay loss during the first night was approximately 10%.

17.5.4 Corneal Edema

In most eyes, the cornea was clear in the early postoperative period. In a few cases, a flap edema can occur because of surgical complication; in our case, it varied from 8.5 to 21.8%. It disappeared within 1 week with anti-inflammatory treatment [41]. Many eyes with early postoperative edema eventually formed deposits in the ensuing months. Excessive microkeratome suction during the surgery appeared to be a major contributor to early edema. It has been reported that cholesterol crystals can be deposited because of degenerative changes occurring after corneal edema [35, 40]. These crystals can accumulate as degenerating cells fail to metabolize fats [11, 16].

17.5.5 Deposits

A progressive depositing of amorphous material and numerous highly reflective, irregularly shaped keratocyte nuclei were observed [11]. Deposits started at the edge of the inlay and covered the implant. The incidence of corneal deposits seemed to be related to the inlay design. These deposits did not affect the overall clarity of the cornea. Small deposits along the intracorneal lens-stromal interface developed in 29% [34] and 37% [41] to 86% in our study. Although the deposited material was slightly opaque, the corneas remained clear (Fig. 17.3).

This occurred in almost every patient. In some patients, it produced an encapsulation of the implant, and a progressive visual acuity loss. Contrary to other authors [17], who state that the deposits were non-progressive after 6 months, we observed that the deposits adjacent or in the lens surface were progressive up to three years. Many corneal changes appeared to be reversible upon inlay removal. On the other hand, the deposits remain in the corneal interface more than 6 months post–inlay explantation (Fig. 17.4). In some eyes that had developed corneal deposits, 10 months after the inlay was removed, the deposits were barely detectable under the slit lamp [34].

17.5.6 Haze

Haze was produced by interface deposits of variable degrees. Deposits were usually seen along the anterior or posterior interface of the implant and stroma. Often they appeared in eyes that encountered surgical difficulties or developed complications in the early postoperative period. A thin, fibrous layer encircled the inlay. This may have been collagen material deposited along the inlay–stromal inter-

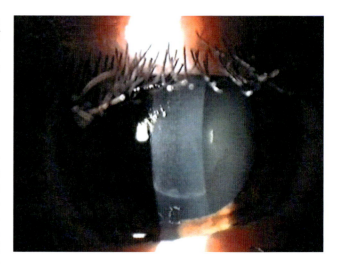

Fig. 17.3 Deposits on edges and surface of the inlay

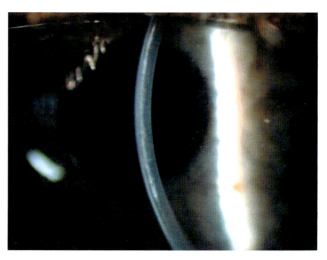

Fig. 17.4 Deposits remain in cornea 6 months after inlay explantation.

face. There was an increase of keratocyte density, and collagen fibrils were somewhat disrupted in the compressed area between stroma and inlay by the rapid change in curvature. They produced progressive visual acuity loss.

The minimum tissue requirements necessary to maintain cell viability in the cornea are not precisely known. Nutritional factors probably do not play a major role, considering that similar epithelial changes have been observed after other keratorefractive procedures that alter the anterior surface curvature using corneal lenses [10, 48]. Percentage of haze was 14% [41] to 46% in our study.

17.5.7 Halos and Glare

Independent of the deposits and corneal opacities or haze degree, there are patients with few deposits who suffer an important glare grade that reduces a good visual acuity. They suffer glare symptoms between a moderate grade in 32% and a severe grade in 43%, with diurnal fluctuation in their visual acuity.

17.5.8 Irregular Astigmatism

Irregular astigmatism can be due to the microkeratome used and could produce irregular tissue resections and an irregular stromal bed, affecting the optical quality and producing visual aberrations. The incidence varied from 25.7% [41] to 15.5%.

17.5.9 Epithelial Perilenticular Opacity

This is the most serious complication in patients with intracorneal inlay implantation. This complication occurred in 45% of the eyes [1]. The opacity was evident after 1 week's follow-up. The inlays developed deposits on and around the surface. The appearance was very similar to the diffuse lamellar keratitis (DLK), leading to the initial diagnosis, but the corneal opacity was limited to the edges of the inlay. Otherwise, the rest of the cornea was not affected by opacity (Fig. 17.5). These cases had previously required flap lifting and inlay repositioning because of inlay decentration shortly after the first repositioning after the first implantation. No case showed evidence of epithelial ingrowth from the edge of the flap. The symptoms were night glare, moderate photophobia, starbursts, and blurry vision. They received antibiotic and anti-inflammatory treatment. A study of the corneal stroma using confocal microscopy showed that the corneal epithelium and the stroma behind the basal membrane were normal. The keratocytes of the anterior stroma were activated and a zone of apoptotic keratocytes was found on the anterior inlay surface. We observed many epithelial cells in the posterior inlay and around the edge and epithelioid cells (Fig. 17.6). The posterior stroma and endothelium were normal. Explantation of the inlay was performed after 1 month of follow-up. During the explantation procedure when the flap was lifted, a thin membrane was observed between the posterior inlay surface and the stromal bed (Fig. 17.7). After explantation, topical steroids and antibiotics were used. Corneal transparency improved in all the eyes, although some eyes still showed mild stromal peripheral opacity around the central cornea. Histopathological studies were also carried out, and microbiological analysis and cultures of corneal specimens from all patients were negative for bacteria, fungi, and mycobacteria (Fig. 17.8). The complications of epithelial perilenticular opacity are distinctly different from DLK. The infiltration was confined to the limits of the inlay, did not respond to steroids, and had a different clinical evolution from DLK. A possibility that could be considered with our cases is a hypersensitivity reaction type 4 [14]. Immunological rejection depends on whether the host recognized the implanted material as foreign and produced specific persistent antibod-

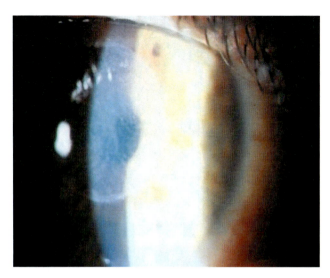

Fig. 17.5 Perilenticular opacity

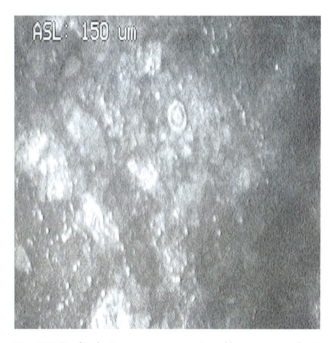

Fig. 17.6 Confocal microscopy image: activated keratocytes and epithelioid cells

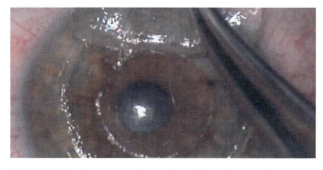

Fig. 17.7 Inflammatory membrane in perilenticular opacity

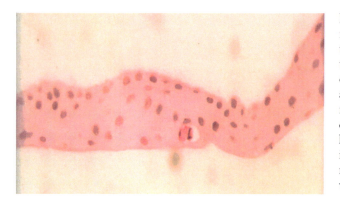

Fig. 17.8 Histopathology of inflammatory membrane in perilenticular opacity

ies, as in the case of intracorneal inlay. According to pathologic and confocal microscopy analysis, the implantation of epithelial cells and their further ingrowth on the inlay surface was the cause of the perilenticular opacity. The implantation of epithelial cells in the interface may occur during the microkeratome cut, through backflow during irrigation, carrying floating epithelial cells, and through migration under the flap [18].

17.5.10 Explant of the Inlay

The explant of the inlay was necessary in 44% [41] to 56% of eyes because of undercorrection, intracorneal deposits in the visual axis, irregular astigmatism, reduced vision, severe haze, implant decentration, or perilenticular opacity .

Many corneal changes appeared to be reversible upon inlay removal. The feasibility of inlay removal and replacement has been documented by other authors [9, 34]. They found that the epithelium was uniform over the corneal surface in eyes from which implants has been removed 8–10 months previously. In eyes that had developed corneal deposits when inlays were in place and 10 months after inlay was removed, the deposits were detectable by slit lamp. Extracellular matrix material accumulated along the inlay–stromal interface. This material appeared to be acellular in nature [47]. This amorphous material is most likely secreted by keratocytes to fill in the space between intrastromal lens and stroma. Fibroblasts could have deposited this material in other places within the stroma. The long-term effects of this material are not known, and studies to identify its composition histologically are underway. Deposition of amorphous material has been used to fill empty space within the stromal layers.

17.6 Conclusion

The long-term tolerance of hydrogel intracorneal inlays has been reported previously in monkey eyes [30, 31, 34], rabbits [20], and humans [1, 6, 17, 41]. The clinical experience

has demonstrated the feasibility of using hydrogel intracorneal lenses to achieve good refractive predictability, stability, and biocompatibility in adult patients. However, limitations to this procedure have also been demonstrated. Postoperative lens migrations, interface deposits, and irregular astigmatism necessitated lens removal, repositioning, or replacement of the inlay. One of the theoretical advantages of the inlay is that the refractive results are potentially reversible and adjustable by removing the lens or replacing it with another of different power. However, if it was removed, then the corneal changes such as deposits and haze were not reversible in many cases.

For this and other reasons, a careful review of the surgical process involved in the inlay implantation, substantial advances of microkeratomes and the use of new material for inlays could potentially lead to improved results using inlays and should be carefully investigated in future research. Nevertheless, inlays offer an alternative to invasive surgery for patients who at the time were considered ineligible for secondary intraocular lenses.

Take-Home Pearls

- The inlay implantation is a simple technique but is associated with a large list of complications, with the most severe complication derived from excess manipulation of the implant.
- Visual acuity may be affected by progressive depositing of amorphous material that started at the edge of the inlay and covered the implant.
- Apart from the deposits and corneal opacities, some patients may suffer a high degree of glare that reduces visual acuity.
- The symptoms of epithelial perilenticular opacity are similar to DLK, but the corneal opacity was limited to the inlay. The opacity appears after 1 week and does not improve with corticosteroids therapy, but requires inlay explantation.

References

1. Alió JL, Mulet ME, Zapata JL, Vidal MT, De Rojas V, Javaloy J (2004) Intracorneal inlay complicated by intrastromal epithelial opacification. Arch Ophthalmol 122:1441–446
2. Alió JL, Shabayek MH (2006) Hyperopic LASIK following intracorneal hydrogel lens explantation. J Refract Surg 22:205–207
3. American Academy of Ophthalmology (1996) Epikeratoplasty: ophthalmic procedure assessment. Ophthalmology 103:983–991
4. Arbealaez MC, Perez-Santonja JJ, Ismail MM et al (1977) Automated lamellar keratoplasty (ALK) and laser in situ keratomileusis (LASIK). In: Serdarevic ON (ed) Refractive surgery: current techniques and management. Igaku-Shoin, New York, pp 131–150
5. Barraquer JL (1966) Modification of refraction by means of intracorneal inclusions. Int Ophthalmol Clin 6:53–78
6. Barraquer JI, Gomez L (1987) Permalens hydrogel ultracorneal lenses for spherical ametropia. J Refract Surg 13:342–348

7. Beekhuis WH, McCarey BE, Rij GV, Waring GO III (1987) Complications of hydrogel intracorneal lenses in monkeys. Arch Ophthalmol 105:116–122

8. Binder PS, Deg JK, Zavala EY, Grossman KR (1982) Hydrogel keratophakia in non human primates. Curr Eye Res 1:535–542

9. Binder PS, Zavala EY, Deg JK (1983) Hydrogel refractive keratoplasty. Lens renoval and exchanges. Cornea 2:119–125

10. Binder PS, Zavala EY, Deg JK (1987) Why do some epikeratoplasties fail? Arch Ophthalmol 105:63–69

11. Bleckmann H, Schnoy H, Keuch R (2004) Removal of epikeratophakia lenticules and implantation of intraocular lenses. Ophthalmologe 101,:285–289

12. Cavanagh H, Sameh M, Petroll M, Jester J (2000) Specular microscopy confocal, and ultrasound biomicroscopy. Cornea 19:712–722

13. Climenhaga H, McCarey BE (1986) Biocompatibility of polysulfone intracorneal lenses in the cat model. Invest Ophthalmol Vis Sci 27(Suppl):14

14. Cotran RS, Kumar V, Collins T (2006) Patologia structural y funcional, 6th edn. McGraw-Hill Interamericana de España, Madrid, Spain, p 208–276

15. Dohlman CH, Refojo MF, Rose J (1967) Synthetic polymers in corneal surgery:glyceryl methacrylate. Arch Ophthalmol 177:52–58

16. Fine BS, Townsed WM, Zimmerman LE, Lashkari MH (1974) Preliminary lipoidal degeneration of the cornea. Am J Ophthalmol 78:12–23

17. Guell JL,Velasco F, Guerrero E, Gris O, Pujol J (2004) Confocal microscopy of cornea with an intracorneal lens for hyperopia. J Refract Surg 20.6:778–782

18. Helena MC, Baeveldt F, Kim WJ, Wilson SE (1997) Epithelial growth within the lamellar interface alter laser in situ keratomileusis (LASIK). Cornea 16:300–305

19. Ismail MM (1999) Management of post-Lasik overcorrections. In: Machat JJ, Slade SG, Probst LE (eds) The art of LASIK, 2nd edn. Slack, Thorofare, NJ, pp 451–457

20. Ismail MM (2002) Correction of hyperopia with intracorneal implants. J Cataract Refract Surg 28:527–530

21. Kaminski SL, Biowski R, Koyuncu D, Lukas JR, Grabner G (2003) Ten year follow-up of epikeratophakia for the correction of high myopia. Ophthalmology 110:2147–2152

22. Kaufman HE (1980) The correction of aphakia. Am J Ophthalmol 89:1–10

23. Keates RH, Martines E, Tennen DG, Reich C (1995) Small-diameter corneal inlay in presbyopic or pseudophakic patients. J Cataract Refract Surg 21:519–521

24. Lee WB, Mannis MJ (2003) Lasik after epikeratophakia. Cornea 22:382–384

25. Martinez I, Mendicute J, AsensioAB, Madarieta I, Alava JI, Garagorri N, Aldazabal P (2005) Two different intracorneal inlay surgical technique in rabbit eyes. Arch Soc Esp Oftalmol 80:581–587

26. Masters B, Böhnke M (2001) Confocal microscopy of the human cornea in vivo. Int Ophthalmol 23:192–206

27. Maurice DM (1969) Nutritional aspects of corneal grafts and prostheses. In: Rycrofts PV (ed) Corneo-plastic conference. Pergamon, Elmsford, N.Y., pp 197–207

28. McCarey BE (1986) Alloplastic refractive keratoplasty. In: Sanders D (ed) Refractive surgery: a text of radial keratotomy. Slack, Thorofare, N.J., p 530–548

29. McCarey BE, Andrews DM (1981) Refractive keratoplasty with intrastromal lenticular implants. Invest Ophthalmol Vis Sci 21:107–115

30. McCarey BE, McDonald MB, Rij GV, Salmeron B, Pettit DK, Knight PM (1989) Refractive results of hyperopic hydrogel intracorneal Lenses in primate eyes. Arch Ophthalmol 107:724–730

31. McCarey BE, Storie BR, Rij GV, Knight PM (1990) Refractive predictability of myopic hydrogel Intracorneal lenses in nonhuman primate eyes. Arch Ophthalmol 108:1310–1315

32. Mccarey BE, Schmidt FH (1990) Modeling glucose distribution in the cornea. Curr Eye Res 9:1025–1039

33. McCarey BE, Waring GO III, Street DA (1987) Refractive keratoplasty in Monkeys using intracorneal lenses of various refractive indexes. Arch Ophthalmol 105:123–126

34. McDonald MB, McCarey BE, Storie B, Beuerman RW, Salmeron B, Rij GV, Knight PM (1993) Assessment of the long –term corneal response to hydrogel intrastromal lenses implanted in monkey eyes four to five years. 19:213–222

35. Miller KH, Green WR, Stark WJ et al (1980) Immunoprotein deposition in the Cornea Ophthalmology 87:944–950

36. Montes R, Rodriguez A, Aliò JL (2006) Femtosecond laser versus mechanical keratome LASIK for myopia. Ophthalmology 114:62–68

37. Peyman GA, Beyer CF, Bezerra Y, Vincent JM, Arosemena A, Friedlander MH, Hoffman L, Kangeler J, Roussau D (2005) Photoablative inlay laser in situ keratomileusis (PAI-LASIK) in the rabbit model. J Cataract Refract Surg 389–397

38. Refojo MF (1968) Artificial membranes of corneal surgery. J Biomed Mater Res. 3:333–337

39. Sendele DD, Abelson MB, Kenyon KR, Haninen CA (1983) Intracorneal lens implantation. Arch Ophthalmol 101:940–944

40. Shapiro LA, Farkas TG (1977) Lipid keratopathy following corneal hydrops. Arch Ophthalmol 95:456–458

41. Steirnet RF, Storie B, Smith P, Mcdonald MB, Rij GV, Bores LD et al (1996) Hydrogel intracorneal lenses in Aphakic eyes. Arch Ophthalmol 114:135–141

42. Stone W, Herbert E (1953) experimental study of plastic material as replacement for the cornea. Am J Ophthalmol 36:168–173

43. Wasty MA, McCarey BE, BeeKhuis WH (1985) Predicting refractive alterations with hydrogel keratophakia. Invest Ophthalmol Vis Sci 26:240–243

44. Werblin TP, Blaydes JE, Fryezkowski A et al (1982) Refractive corneal surgery: The use of implantable alloplastic lens material. Aust J Ophthalmol 11:325–331

45. Werblin TP, Patel AS, Barraquer JL (1992) Initial hydrogel intracorneal lens implants. Refract Corneal Surg 8:23–26

46. Xie RZ, Evans MD, Bojarski B, Hughes TC, Chan GY, Nguyen X, Wilkie JS, Mclean KM, Vannas A Sweeney DF (2006) Two-year preclinical testing of perfluoropolyether as a corneal inlay. Invest Ophthalmol Vis Sci 4:574–581

47. Yamaguchy T, Koening SB, Hamano T et al (1984) Electron microscopic study of intracorneal hydrogel implants in primates. Ophthalmology 91:1170–1175

48. Zavala EY, Krrumeich J, Binder PS (1988) Clinical pathology of non-freeze lamellar refractive keratoplasty. Cornea 7:223–230

The Patient

Contents

Core Messages

- The relationship between patient expectations, the medical outcome, and patient satisfaction is complex.

- It is important to determine patient's motivations and expectations before surgery.

- Patients should be educated on the potential side effects of refractive surgery.

- In case of complications, patients should be informed as soon as possible, whereby the doctor should try to maintain their trust.

18.1 Predicting the Unhappy Patient and Patient Expectations
Nayyirih G. Tahzib and Rudy M.M.A. Nuijts

18.1.1 Introduction

With the increasing amounts of new and improved keratorefractive surgery treatments for the correction of the refractive error, the importance of systematic evaluation of the treatment outcome has grown. Until recently, the evaluation and comparison of refractive surgery techniques were mainly focused on the objective, clinical outcome such as the residual refraction, the visual acuity, and the number of Snellen acuity lines lost or gained after the procedure.

Patient satisfaction after cataract and refractive surgery, however, entails the greater area of quality of life and functional status as perceived by the patient. The area of measuring patient satisfaction is complex and multidimensional, since it is influenced by the combination of subjective quality of vision, personal expectations, and personality type [1–3]. It is important that refractive surgeons understand patient motivations for seeking surgery, since this can influence their postoperative satisfaction. In order to predict the unhappy patient it is important to:

- Identify what the expectations and motivations of patients are before undergoing refractive surgery
- Describe the population of satisfied and dissatisfied patients
- Identify parameters responsible for patient dissatisfaction

Patient satisfaction can be defined by the difference between the patient's expectation before surgery and the outcome after surgery. An example is the "disconfirmation-of-expectations" model, which dictates that if perceived performance is evaluated as worse than the expectation, then negative disconfirmation results in dissatisfaction (Fig. 18.1.1). This model closely adheres to the current theory of "undersell and overdeliver" to achieve satisfied patients in corneal and lenticular refractive surgery.

18.1.2 Patient Questionnaires

One of the most effective and efficient ways to study patient expectations and motivations is by using validated questionnaires, which systematically ask patients about their experiences [3, 5–8]. Self-administered questionnaires, rather than physician-administered questionnaires, enable a more objective view of patient satisfaction and quality of vision. When a test is administered by a physician, results may be biased and patients might feel compelled to answer always in the affirmative.

Several studies have used questionnaires for the assessment of patient expectations and satisfaction. Realistic preoperative patient expectations seem to correlate well with postoperative patient satisfaction, meaning that a good

understanding of patient motivation for seeking refractive surgery is important [9]. Primary reasons for seeking refractive surgery such as laser in situ keratomileusis (LASIK) are a desire for freedom from spectacles or contact lenses (32.1%) and spectacle or contact lens intolerance (30.4%) [10–12].

Many studies in the literature show that the level of patient satisfaction after refractive surgery was generally higher than 90%. However, these studies also show that there are night vision complaints (NVC) which range from about 5 to 30%, depending on the time these complaints were measured [6, 8, 9, 13]. We recently described patient satisfaction and perceived quality of vision after myopic LASIK and ARTISAN lens implantation and tried to define clinical parameters of patient satisfaction after these procedures. We used a validated questionnaire which covered seven quality-of-vision scales, including global satisfaction, quality of uncorrected and corrected vision, quality of night vision, glare, daytime driving, and night driving [5, 6]. In terms of overall satisfaction, we found that more than 90% of patients in both groups were satisfied their visual outcome and would be willing to have the surgery done again if they could do it over. For uncorrected vision, about 65% of patients in both groups said that their uncorrected vision after surgery was better than their best-corrected vision before surgery. About 65% of patients reported that their night vision was the same or better after surgery, however, a group of about 35% reported that their night vision was worse. It is important to add however, that about 35% of patients with NVC reported having them before surgery. Glare complaints increased in about 50% of patients in both groups after surgery.

18.1.3 Clinical Parameters as Predictors of Patient Satisfaction. Two Examples of Refractive Surgery Techniques

18.1.3.1 ARTISAN Phakic Intraocular Lens Implantation Patients

Clinical parameters that can predict patient satisfaction after ARTISAN lens implantation are the refractive outcome (uncorrected and corrected visual acuity, sphere, cylinder, and spherical equivalent), pupil size, lens centration, the pupil–optical zone disparity (meaning, the disparity between the pupil size and the optical zone of the lens) and higher-order aberrations (HOA). Our results showed higher levels of global satisfaction and subjective uncorrected vision when the residual error was small. Glare complaints did not depend on lens decentration, which was probably related to the fact that about 90% of these cases had lens decentrations lower than 0.5 mm. Pupil sizes were measured with a digital infrared pupillometer (P2000 SA pupillometer, Procyon Instruments, London, UK). We found that glare complaints increased with higher amounts of pupil–optical zone disparity in scotopic light conditions (Fig. 18.1.2), but not in mesopic-low conditions. Study of optical aberrations (Zywave aberrometer, software version 3.21, Bausch

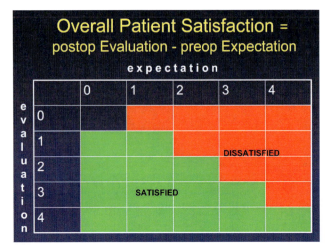

Fig. 18.1.1 The "disconfirmation-of-expectations" model; when perceived performance is evaluated as worse than the expectation, negative disconfirmation results in dissatisfaction

18

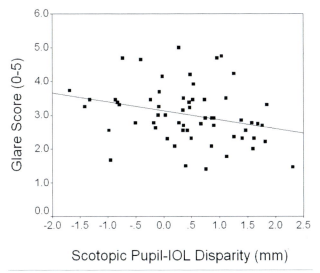

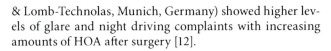

Fig. 18.1.2 Glare score versus the scotopic pupil–optical zone disparity after ARTISAN phakic intraocular lens implantation for the correction of myopia ($r = -0.28$, $p = 0.03$)

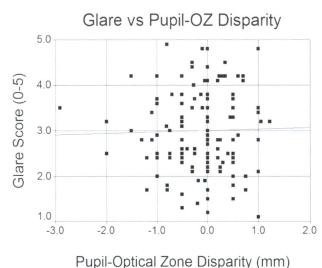

Fig. 18.1.3 Glare score versus the scotopic pupil–optical zone disparity after myopic LASIK ($r = 0.03$, $p = 0.75$)

& Lomb-Technolas, Munich, Germany) showed higher levels of glare and night driving complaints with increasing amounts of HOA after surgery [12].

18.1.3.2 LASIK Patients

Clinical parameters that can predict patient satisfaction after LASIK are also the refractive outcome, the ablation depth, and the pupil–optical zone disparity. Our results showed higher levels of subjective uncorrected vision when the residual error was small. There was no correlation between night vision and the ablation depth or between glare and the scotopic pupil–optical zone disparity (Figs. 18.1.3, 18.1.4) [11].

18.1.4 Discrepancy in Patient Satisfaction and Night Vision Complaints

NVC are the main downsides after refractive surgery and have been reported in the literature, ranging from 12 to 57% in patients; they appear to diminish after the first six postoperative months [6, 8, 13–18]. It seems that there is a discrepancy between patient satisfaction and NVC. Despite the relatively high occurrence rate of NVC, patients are generally very satisfied after surgery. Possible explanations for this discrepancy may be that patients simply adapt to their new condition [6, 13]. In addition, the benefits of surgery such as the reduction in contact lens and spectacle dependence might be greater than the disadvantages of NVC. Also, patients who wore rigid gas-permeable contact lenses and spectacles before surgery might show an easier acceptance and an increased level of tolerance to glare and halos.

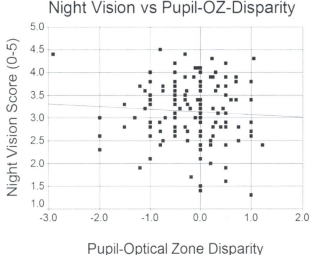

Fig. 18.1.4 Night vision score versus the scotopic pupil-optical zone disparity after myopic LASIK ($r = -0.06$, $p = 0.50$)

18.1.4.1 Risk Factors for Night Vision Complaints

Three reports on patient satisfaction after LASIK treatment [8, 13, 17] showed that predictors for NVC had:

- Preoperative level of myopia (more than 5.00 D)
- Preoperative uncorrected visual acuity
- Preoperative contrast sensitivity levels
- Increasing age
- A flatter preoperative corneal curvature
- Surgical enhancements

- Optical zones smaller than 6 mm
- Postoperative residual error higher than 0.50 D from emmetropia
- The postoperative residual cylinder

The pupil size was not shown to be a significant predictor of NVC in any of these studies.

18.1.4.2 Other Postoperative Reasons for Dissatisfaction

Common subjective complaints after refractive surgery in dissatisfied patients are blurred distance vision (59%), glare and night-vision disturbances (44%) [8, 13, 15, 19, 20]. Common complications are under- and overcorrection (30%), irregular astigmatism (30%), dry eyes (4% to 30%), glare (up to 48%), and difficulty with night driving (17%) [19–24]. Common recommendations for management are non-surgical treatments (68%) consisting primarily of medication and contact lenses [19, 23].

18.1.5 Managing the Unhappy Patient

Clinical diagnoses that may lead to a suboptimal outcome after laser surgery are:

- Myopia higher than 12 D and/or high astigmatism (20.7%)
- Patients with thin corneas or insufficient corneal thickness (8.2%)
- Keratoconus (6.4%)
- Cataract (5.7%)
- Hyperopia and/or hyperopic astigmatism (4.1%) [4]

There are some ways to try to prevent dissatisfying postoperative outcomes and resulting unhappy patients.

1. Carefully consider the pupil size and the choice of optical zone size.
2. There is variable evidence in the literature on excluding patients with large pupils [8, 13, 15, 25]. Higher myopic corrections generally require smaller optical zones, which in turn increased ablation depth and risk of NVC [13]. Our earlier-mentioned study showed increased glare with higher amounts of pupil–optical zone disparity in scotopic light conditions, but not with the "real-life" mesopic-low pupil size [12]. Pupil measurements can be biased and should be standardized and improved [26].
3. Apply wavefront-guided treatments.
4. Wavefront technology was developed to categorize and treat HOA induced by refractive surgery. HOA can cause glare and halos and lead to decreased quality of vision. A few studies have shown increased satisfaction, a reduction in HOA and night vision complaints after wavefront-guided treatments [16, 27, 28]. Current problems with wavefront-guided treatments are the lack of predictability for correcting the amount of HOA by the treatment [28–35]. Several studies have indicated the advantages of wavefront-guided over conventional ablations in terms of decreased HOA and subjective complaints, but more and larger good randomized studies are needed to analyze this further [36–38].
5. Topography-guided ablation for irregular corneas
6. HOA in symptomatic post-LASIK corneas have been shown to be an average of 2.3 times greater in comparison to normal post-LASIK corneas [31]. Recent studies indicate that customized ablation based on corneal topography is safe and effective, can lead to fewer NVC and less increase of HOA compared to conventional ablation [39–41].
7. Patients with visual symptoms should be advised to be patient and wait for healing or "adaptation."
8. Try and treat the residual cylinder if there is a low uncorrected visual acuity with glasses or additional procedures.
9. Use pharmacological pupillary constriction methods to reduce NVC and HOA.

Take-Home Pearls

- Uneventful refractive surgery with a good clinical outcome would be expected to lead to a high level of patient satisfaction, unless the patient's preoperative expectations were unrealistic.
- It is important to determine patient's motivations and expectations before surgery, since the relationship between patient expectations, the medical outcome, and patient satisfaction is complex and the clinical outcome does not always directly correlate with the subjective outcome. We should inform patients of complications as soon as possible, maintain their trust and try to reassure them.

References

1. McGhee CN, Orr D, Kidd B, Stark C, Bryce IG, Anastas CN (1996) Psychological aspects of excimer laser surgery for myopia: reasons for seeking treatment and patient satisfaction. Br J Ophthalmol 80:874–879
2. Houtman DM (2000) Managing patient expectations. Int Ophthalmol Clin 40:29–34
3. Nijkamp MD, Nuijts RM, Borne B, Webers CA, van der Horst F, Hendrikse F (2000) Determinants of patient satisfaction after cataract surgery in 3 settings. J Cataract Refract Surg 26:1379–1388
4. Hori-Komai Y, Toda I, Asano-Kato N, Tsubota K (2002) Reasons for not performing refractive surgery. J Cataract Refract Surg 28:795–797
5. Brunette I, Gresset J, Boivin JF, Boisjoly H, Makni H (2000) Functional outcome and satisfaction after photorefractive keratectomy, part 1: development and validation of a survey questionnaire. Ophthalmology 107:1783–1789

18

6. Brunette I, Gresset J, Boivin JF et al (2000) Functional outcome and satisfaction after photorefractive keratectomy, part 2: survey of 690 patients. Ophthalmology 107:1790–1796

7. McDonnell PJ, Mangione C, Lee P et al (2003) Responsiveness of the National Eye Institute Refractive Error Quality of Life instrument to surgical correction of refractive error. Ophthalmology 110:2302–2309

8. Bailey MD, Mitchell GL, Dhaliwal DK, Boxer Wachler BS, Zadnik K (2003) Patient satisfaction and visual symptoms after laser in situ keratomileusis. Ophthalmology 110:1371–1378

9. McGhee CN, Craig JP, Sachdev N, Weed KH, Brown AD (2000) Functional, psychological, and satisfaction outcomes of laser in situ keratomileusis for high myopia. J Cataract Refract Surg 26:497–509

10. Khan-Lim D, Craig JP, McGhee CN (2002) Defining the content of patient questionnaires: reasons for seeking laser in situ keratomileusis for myopia. J Cataract Refract Surg 28:788–794

11. Tahzib NG, Bootsma SJ, Eggink FA, Nabar VA, Nuijts RM (2005) Functional outcomes and patient satisfaction after laser in situ keratomileusis for correction of myopia. J Cataract Refract Surg 31:1943–1951

12. Tahzib NG, Bootsma SJ, Eggink FA, Nuijts RM (2006) Functional outcome and patient satisfaction after ARTISAN phakic intraocular lens implantation for the correction of myopia. Am J Ophthalmol 142:31–39

13. Pop M, Payette Y (2004) Risk factors for night vision complaints after LASIK for myopia. Ophthalmology 111:3–10

14. Brown SM, Khanani AM (2004) Night vision complaints after LASIK. Ophthalmology 111:1619–1620; author reply 1920

15. Hammond SD Jr, Puri AK, Ambati BK (2004) Quality of vision and patient satisfaction after LASIK. Curr Opin Ophthalmol 15:328–332

16. Nuijts RM, Nabar VA, Hament WJ, Eggink FA (2002) Wavefront-guided versus standard laser in situ keratomileusis to correct low to moderate myopia. J Cataract Refract Surg 28:1907–1913

17. Schallhorn SC, Kaupp SE, Tanzer DJ, Tidwell J, Laurent J, Bourque LB (2003) Pupil size and quality of vision after LASIK. Ophthalmology 110:1606–1614

18. Salz JJ, Boxer Wachler BS, Holladay JT, Trattler W (2004) Night vision complaints after LASIK. Ophthalmology 111:1620–1621; author reply 1621–1622

19. Jabbur NS, Sakatani K, O'Brien TP (2004) Survey of complications and recommendations for management in dissatisfied patients seeking a consultation after refractive surgery. J Cataract Refract Surg 30:1867–1874

20. El Danasoury MA, El Maghraby A, Gamali TO (2002) Comparison of iris-fixed ARTISAN lens implantation with excimer laser in situ keratomileusis in correcting myopia between -9.00 and -19.50 diopters: a randomized study. Ophthalmology 109:955–964

21. McDonald MB, Carr JD, Frantz JM et al (2001) Laser in situ keratomileusis for myopia up to –11 diopters with up to –5 diopters of astigmatism with the summit autonomous LADARVision excimer laser system. Ophthalmology 108:309–316

22. Schallhorn SC, Amesbury EC, Tanzer DJ (2006) Avoidance, recognition, and management of LASIK complications. Am J Ophthalmol 141:733–739

23. Melki SA, Azar DT (2001) LASIK complications: etiology, management, and prevention. Surv Ophthalmol 46:95–116

24. Iskander NG, Peters NT, Penno EA, Gimbel HV (2000) Postoperative complications in laser in situ keratomileusis. Curr Opin Ophthalmol 11:273–279

25. Lee YC, Hu FR, Wang IJ (2003) Quality of vision after laser in situ keratomileusis: influence of dioptric correction and pupil size on visual function. J Cataract Refract Surg 29:769–777

26. Pop M, Payette Y, Santoriello E (2002) Comparison of the pupil card and pupillometer in measuring pupil size. J Cataract Refract Surg 28:283–288

27. Carones F, Vigo L, Scandola E (2003) Wavefront-guided treatment of abnormal eyes using the LADARVision platform. J Refract Surg 19:S703–S708

28. Lawless MA, Hodge C, Rogers CM, Sutton GL (2003) Laser in situ keratomileusis with Alcon CustomCornea. J Refract Surg 19:S691–S696

29. Kohnen T, Mahmoud K, Buhren J (2005) Comparison of corneal higher-order aberrations induced by myopic and hyperopic LASIK. Ophthalmology 112:1692

30. Kohnen T, Buhren J, Kuhne C, Mirshahi A (2004) Wavefront-guided LASIK with the Zyoptix 3.1 system for the correction of myopia and compound myopic astigmatism with 1-year follow-up: clinical outcome and change in higher order aberrations. Ophthalmology 111:2175–2185

31. McCormick GJ, Porter J, Cox IG, MacRae S (2005) Higher-order aberrations in eyes with irregular corneas after laser refractive surgery. Ophthalmology 112:1699–1709

32. Kohnen T, Kuhne C, Buhren J (2007) The future role of wavefront-guided excimer ablation. Graefes Arch Clin Exp Ophthalmol (in press)

33. Buhren J, Kohnen T (2006) Factors affecting the change in lower-order and higher-order aberrations after wavefront-guided laser in situ keratomileusis for myopia with the Zyoptix 3.1 system. J Cataract Refract Surg 32:1166–1174

34. Chalita MR, Chavala S, Xu M, Krueger RR (2004) Wavefront analysis in post-LASIK eyes and its correlation with visual symptoms, refraction, and topography. Ophthalmology 111:447–453

35. Oshika T, Klyce SD, Applegate RA, Howland HC, El Danasoury MA (1999) Comparison of corneal wavefront aberrations after photorefractive keratectomy and laser in situ keratomileusis. Am J Ophthalmol 127:1–7

36. Kim TI, Yang SJ, Tchah H (2004) Bilateral comparison of wavefront-guided versus conventional laser in situ keratomileusis with Bausch and Lomb Zyoptix. J Refract Surg 20:432–438

37. Netto MV, Dupps W, Jr., Wilson SE (2006) Wavefront-guided ablation: evidence for efficacy compared to traditional ablation. Am J Ophthalmol 141:360–368

38. Waheed S, Krueger RR (2003) Update on customized excimer ablations: recent developments reported in 2002. Curr Opin Ophthalmol 14:198–202

39. Farooqui MA, Al-Muammar AR (2006) Topography-guided CATz versus conventional LASIK for myopia with the NIDEK EC-5000: A bilateral eye study. J Refract Surg 22:741–745

40. Kermani O, Schmiedt K, Oberheide U, Gerten G (2006) Topographic- and wavefront-guided customized ablations with the NIDEK-EC5000CXII in LASIK for myopia. J Refract Surg 22:754–763

41. Du CX, Yang YB, Shen Y, Wang Y, Dougherty PJ (2006) Bilateral comparison of conventional versus topographic-guided customized ablation for myopic LASIK with the NIDEK EC-5000. J Refract Surg 22:642–646

Core Messages

■ Informed consent is a process, not just a signed document.

■ The process begins with the first patient encounter.

■ Informed consent should explain the proposed procedure, list alternatives, benefits, and common and serious complications in language the patient can understand.

■ Unusual or abnormal findings that potentially can negatively influence the outcome should be explained and documented in the record.

■ Videos, pamphlets, documents, and interactions with staff members are not a substitute for face-to-face discussion with the surgeon.

■ The surgeon should make a dated note in the record that the risks, benefits, side effects, and alternatives were discussed with the patient.

■ The written informed consent should be provided well before the surgery so the patient can read it without the influence of drugs or dilating drops and have an opportunity to ask questions on the day of surgery or earlier.

18.2 Informed Consent

James J. Salz

18.2.1 Introduction

My interest in refractive surgery began with radial keratotomy around 1980. Ophthalmic surgery at that time was performed primarily to cure pathology, and the majority of ophthalmologists did not consider myopia to truly represent a pathologic condition. Dr. Jerome Bettman, considered by many at that time to be the foremost authority on medical ethics and medical legal matters, was invited to speak in Los Angeles at a symposium about radial keratotomy. Jerry was a delightful, humble man with an infectious sense of humor and an ability to tell it like it is.

Many respected ophthalmologists at that time were highly critical of those of us who would dare to operate on "normal eyes" and articles about greedy, "buccaneer" eye surgeons were not uncommon. Jerry spoke eloquently that day about informed consent, and I believe he covered most of what I wrote in this chapter. I edited a textbook on refractive corneal surgery, and Jerry wrote the chapter [1] on medical legal aspects of refractive keratoplasty, which I read in preparation for writing this chapter.

He was not at all critical of the surgery itself and was in fact quite interested in the technique of performing the incisions, the number and depth of incisions, size of the op-

tical zone, and complications and side effects. As I recall it, the main thrust of his talk was that "performing surgery on an essentially normal 20/20 eye placed a heavy burden on the surgeon" to properly inform the patient of the alternatives, risks, side effects, and most likely outcomes. He later wrote in the book chapter, "The need for fully informed consent is geometrically greater in elective procedures. In cases of refractive keratoplasty, fully informed consent is of the greatest importance from both legal and ethical standpoints" [1].

In other words, refractive surgery, more than other ophthalmic surgery, requires an especially thoughtful informed consent. It is far different from both a surgeon and patient perspective to perform LASIK on a –2.00-D myopic eye than to operate on a patient with a detached retina, dense cataract, or uncontrolled glaucoma.

18.2.2 Informed Consent as a Process

It is a common misconception that as long as the patient signs the written informed consent, he or she was properly informed. From a legal standpoint, nothing could be further from the truth. Consider a –10-D myopic patient who fist learns about LASIK in a newspaper ad sponsored by Dr. X at the 20/20 LASIK Center. The ad touts, "Throw away your glasses after LASIK, a 10-minute painless laser procedure." Neither Dr. X nor his staff explains to the patient that the –10-D correction is not likely to result in 20/20 vision, and that there is some discomfort during the creation of the LASIK flap as well as some discomfort in the postoperative period. Nevertheless, the patient signs a detailed informed consent that does discuss under- and overcorrection, infections, corneal abrasions, etc. If the patient had a complication that led to loss of vision, the patient could claim that the advertisement led him/her to choose Dr. X, with the expectation of 20/20 vision, and the advertisement would most likely be admitted as evidence. A jury could conclude that the advertisement was more important than the written consent, and that the patient was not informed properly.

Figure 18.2.1 is an example of a newspaper ad that mentions in fine print "over 20,000 microsurgical procedures performed." This would certainly imply an experienced surgeon. Although the owner of the center may well have performed 20,000 cataract operations, he/she employed a newly trained LASIK surgeon who had performed less than 100 LASIK procedures. A patient who suffered complications at that center, which normally would have been defensible, claimed he would not have had the procedure if he realized the surgeon was less experienced than the ad implied. The case was settled without a trial since the defense attorney knew the ad was admissible as part of the informed consent process.

Years ago, we formed a group of refractive surgeons so we could cooperatively market refractive surgery. An advertising agency came up with what we all agreed was a clever ad for LASIK (Fig. 18.2.2). We thought by placing a

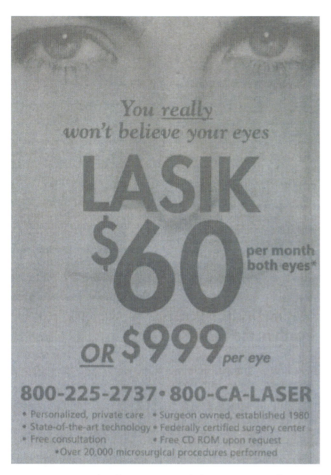

Fig. 18.2.1 Example of a newspaper ad that mentions in fine print "over 20,000 microsurgical procedures performed"

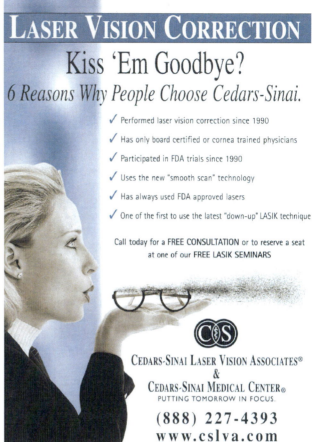

Fig. 18.2.2 "Kiss them goodbye?"

question mark around the text, "Kiss them goodbye?" we were not really guaranteeing the elimination of the glasses. On the advice of an attorney, we quickly withdrew the ad because the implication was that the glasses would be eliminated. The informed consent process begins with the patient's first encounter with your office, whether that be by radio, television or newspaper add, or statements on your webpage. Be careful that none of the statements from any of these sources could be potentially used against you by an unhappy patient or one who sustains a complication. Complications are not usually considered a deviation from the standard of care but misleading advertising could be.

18.2.3 Language of Informed Consent

The proposed procedure, the alternatives to the procedure, the risks, and benefits should all be explained in language the average patient can comprehend. Consider the language of the sample LASIK consent recommended by the Ophthalmic Mutual Insurance Company (OMIC) included at the end of this chapter. Technically, LASIK involves a lamellar dissection of the cornea with a microkeratome to create a flap. The flap is reflected, and an excimer laser corrects the refractive error by ablating the corneal stroma. The OMIC explanation of the procedure is as follows: "In LASIK, the microkeratome is used to shave the cornea to create a flap. The flap then is opened like the page of a book to expose tissue just below the cornea's surface. Next, the excimer laser is used to remove ultra-thin layers from the cornea to reshape it to reduce nearsightedness. Finally, the flap is returned to its original position, without sutures."

The reader can find examples of OMIC-approved informed consents for common refractive surgery procedures such as LASIK, intra-LASIK, photorefractive keratectomy (PRK), phakic implants, and refractive lensectomy by going to www.omic.com. These consents can be downloaded at no charge and modified to meet the needs of an individual practice.

18.2.3.1 Additions to the Generic Informed Consent
Informed consent is designed to help inform the average patient with typical findings on examination and no unusual risk factors. If the patient presents with findings that could *potentially* increase the risk of complications or decrease

the likelihood of a satisfactory outcome, then an additional consent would be wise. Examples would include borderline dry eye, unusual but not clearly abnormal topography, borderline pachymetry for correction required, large scotopic pupils, high myopia, hyperopia, or astigmatism. Opinions about all of these examples are varied and the literature can be confusing. How much inferior steepening on topography is acceptable as a normal variant? Does a large scotopic pupil increase the risk of night vision problems? Is 250 µm the minimum safe value to avoid post-LASIK ectasia? If a surgeon encounters any of these findings, then it would be wise to have an extra detailed discussion with the patient about the potential increased risks. This discussion should simply be documented with a brief dated note in the record. For example, several years ago one of my 30-year-old patients presented with inferior steepening on topography in just one eye. His topography was not as abnormal as the topography in two recent high-profile medical malpractice cases that resulted in large awards. There were no clinical signs of keratoconus, and the family history was negative. I explained to him that I felt that LASIK was contraindicated and that many surgeons would feel that PRK was also contraindicated. In fact, the VISX surgeon's manual lists "abnormal topography" as a contraindication to PRK. I told him that removing corneal stroma to correct his −5.00-D refractive error might accelerate his progression to keratoconus, and the risk of this happening in terms of a percentage was unknown. I also explained that keratoconus was usually a bilateral disease and both of his eyes could eventually develop it, whether he had the PRK or not. I documented this discussion with a brief note in the record. He proceeded to have the PRK in each eye, several months apart. He did well for 5 years, but at 6 years post-PRK he developed ectasia in the eye with the abnormal topography but the other eye is uninvolved at present. He requires a Synergis (hybrid gas perm, soft contact) lens to see well in that eye. He accepted this outcome and felt that he was fully informed about the risk before he consented to have the surgery.

Some myopic patients who have absolutely no abnormalities suggestive of keratoconus at the time of their surgery will develop ectasia, unrelated to their laser surgery. Two such cases have recently come to trial, and the plaintiff's have prevailed with substantial awards. Because of the complexity of this issue and the difficulties that can arise in trying to explain how this can happen to a jury, OMIC has added a separate paragraph pertaining to this possibility to the informed consent documents for LASIK and PRK (see example at the end of this chapter, no. 6 under "Vision-Threatening Complications").

Similarly, patients with borderline dry eyes, thin corneas (where the post-ablation thickness may be close to or less that 250 µm), scotopic pupils larger than 6.5 mm, or high corrections should all have a special discussion about the possible increase risk of complications or the decreased likelihood of obtaining 20/20 vision.

18.2.4 Personal Interaction with the Surgeon

Many practices use videos and pamphlets as part of the informed consent. These visual aids can be helpful in explaining the details of the procedure, but they should never be a substitute for a direct discussion with the surgeon. Dr. Richard Abbott analyzed 100 consecutive OMIC LASIK and PRK claims and lawsuits to try to identify predictors that increase the risk of malpractice liability [2]. The data showed that when the surgeon spent more time with the patient there was a decreased risk of a claim or lawsuit ($p = 0.003$). This was even more significant with higher-volume surgeons ($p = 0.0001$). This finding is of course not surprising. If a patient feels some connection with the surgeon, established during the preoperative examination and discussion, then they will be far less likely to sue in the event of an unexpected outcome or complication. An ideal time to establish this rapport with the patient is to personally go over the examination results, likelihood of success, alternative treatments, and complications and side effects of the surgery. This is the part of the informed consent process that is the most important, far more important than the patient's signature on a form.

After this important discussion with the patient, the surgeon should make a brief note in the record that: "The risks, benefits, and alternatives to the proposed procedure were discussed with the patient and the patient had an opportunity to ask questions." As Dr. Bettman said in his lecture to us, "If the surgeon takes the time to write and date a note in the record that this discussion took place, a jury will likely believe it happened."

18.2.5 Timing of the Informed Consent

What if the patient arrives at the laser center, receives a drug to help them relax, has their pupil dilated, and the staff realizes that the written informed consent has not been signed? If the patient signs this consent under those circumstances, the signed consent has virtually no value for obvious reasons. If the surgeon has not documented in the record that the procedure was discussed with the patient during the pre-operative evaluation, then the surgery should be cancelled. If a previous discussion did take place, if a staff member, or family member of the patient witnessed and remembers this discussion are facts that should be documented in the record if the surgeon and patient decide to proceed with surgery. In the event of a lawsuit, a jury would most likely believe the patient had been properly informed, and the circumstances of the written consent could be neutralized. The best way to avoid this scenario is to set up a system in the practice to allow the patient to discuss the surgery with the surgeon well ahead of the surgical date. The informed consent document should be provided so that the patient can take it home, read it, and bring it back on day of surgery with an opportunity to question the surgeon about any issues. Then before any sedation or eye drops, the patient should sign the consent in front of a witness. Thus, the written, signed informed consent supplements the oral informed consent and the process is completed.

Take-Home Pearls

- Remember your advertising and marketing materials, including your webpage, initiate the informed consent process so be careful of the content.
- If the examination reveals risk factors that may potentially increase the risk of complications and side effects, or decrease the possibility of an excellent outcome, then document in the record that these issues were discussed.
- Do not rely on videos, pamphlets, and signed documents. The surgeon has a duty to personally participate in the informed consent process.
- In your own handwriting, date and sign a note stating that the risk, benefits, and alternatives to the proposed procedure have been discussed with the patient and all questions were answered.

Sample OMIC informed consent for LASIK

NOTE: THIS FORM IS INTENDED AS A SAMPLE ONLY. PLEASE REVIEW IT AND MODIFY TO FIT YOUR ACTUAL PRACTICE. IT DOES NOT CONTAIN INFORMATION ABOUT LIMBAL RELXING INCSIONS (LRI), SO INCLUDE THAT IF YOU PERFORM LRI DURING CATARACT SURGERY.

Version 071906

Informed Consent For Laser In-situ Keratomileusis (Lasik)

Introduction

This information is being provided to you so that you can make an informed decision about the use of a device known as a microkeratome, combined with the use of a device known as an excimer laser, to perform LASIK. LASIK is one of a number of alternatives for correcting nearsightedness, farsightedness, and astigmatism. In LASIK, the microkeratome is used to shave the cornea to create a flap. The flap then is opened like the page of a book to expose tissue just below the cornea's surface. Next, the excimer laser is used to remove ultra-thin layers from the cornea to reshape it to reduce nearsightedness. Finally, the flap is returned to its original position, without sutures.

LASIK is an elective procedure: There is no emergency condition or other reason that requires or demands that you have it performed. You could continue wearing contact lenses or glasses and have adequate visual acuity. This procedure, like all surgery, presents some risks, many of which are listed below. You should also understand that there may be other risks not known to your doctor, which may become known later. Despite the best of care, complications and side effects may occur; should this happen in your case, the result might be affected even to the extent of making your vision worse.

Alternatives To Lasik

If you decide not to have LASIK, there are other methods of correcting your nearsightedness, farsightedness, or astigmatism. These alternatives include, among others, eyeglasses, contact lenses and other refractive surgical procedures.

Patient Consent

In giving my permission for LASIK, I understand the following: The long-term risks and effects of LASIK are unknown. I have received no guarantee as to the success of my particular case. I understand that the following risks are associated with the procedure:

Vision-threatening Complications

1. I understand that the microkeratome or the excimer laser could malfunction, requiring the procedure to be stopped before completion. Depending on the type of malfunction, this may or may not be accompanied by visual loss.
2. I understand that, in using the microkeratome, instead of making a flap, an entire portion of the central cornea could be cut off, and very rarely could be lost. If preserved, I understand that my doctor would put this tissue back on the eye after the laser treatment, using sutures, according to the ALK procedure method. It is also possible that the flap incision could result in an incomplete flap, or a flap that is too thin. If this happens, it is likely that the laser part of the procedure will have to be postponed until the cornea has a chance to heal sufficiently to try to create the flap again.
3. I understand that irregular healing of the flap could result in a distorted cornea. This would mean that glasses or contact lenses may not correct my vision to the level possible before undergoing LASIK. If this distortion in vision is severe, a partial or complete corneal transplant might be necessary to repair the cornea.
4. I understand that it is possible a perforation of the cornea could occur, causing devastating complications, including loss of some or all of my vision. This could also be caused by an internal or external eye infection that could not be controlled with antibiotics or other means.
5. I understand that mild or severe infection is possible. Mild infection can usually be treated with antibiotics and usually does not lead to permanent visual loss. Severe infection, even if successfully treated with antibiotics, could lead to permanent scarring and loss of vision that may require corrective laser surgery or, if very severe, corneal transplantation or even loss of the eye.
6. I understand that I could develop keratoconus. Keratoconus is a degenerative corneal disease affecting vision that occurs in approximately 1/2000 in the general population. While there are several tests that suggest which patients might be at risk, this condition can develop in patients who have normal preoperative topography (a map of the cornea obtained before surgery) and pachymetry (corneal thickness measurement) . Since keratoconus may occur on its own, there is no absolute

test that will ensure a patient will not develop keratoconus following laser vision correction. Severe keratoconus may need to be treated with a corneal transplant while mild keratoconus can be corrected by glasses or contact lenses.

7. I understand that other very rare complications threatening vision include, but are not limited to, corneal swelling, corneal thinning (ectasia), appearance of "floaters" and retinal detachment, hemorrhage, venous and arterial blockage, cataract formation, total blindness, and even loss of my eye.

Non–vision-threatening Side Effects

1. I understand that there may be increased sensitivity to light, glare, and fluctuations in the sharpness of vision. I understand these conditions usually occur during the normal stabilization period of from one to three months, but they may also be permanent.

2. I understand that there is an increased risk of eye irritation related to drying of the corneal surface following the LASIK procedure. These symptoms may be temporary or, on rare occasions, permanent, and may require frequent application of artificial tears and/or closure of the tear duct openings in the eyelid.

3. I understand that an overcorrection or undercorrection could occur, causing me to become farsighted or nearsighted or increase my astigmatism and that this could be either permanent or treatable. I understand an overcorrection or undercorrection is more likely in people over the age of 40 years and may require the use of glasses for reading or for distance vision some or all of the time.

4. After refractive surgery, a certain number of patients experience glare, a "starbursting" or halo effect around lights, or other low-light vision problems that may interfere with the ability to drive at night or see well in dim light. The exact cause of these visual problems is not currently known; some ophthalmologists theorize that the risk may be increased in patients with large pupils or high degrees of correction. For most patients, this is a temporary condition that diminishes with time or is correctable by wearing glasses at night or taking eye drops. For some patients, however, these visual problems are permanent. I understand that my vision may not seem as sharp at night as during the day and that I may need to wear glasses at night or take eye drops. I understand that it is not possible to predict whether I will experience these night vision or low light problems, and that I may permanently lose the ability to drive at night or function in dim light because of them. I understand that I should not drive unless my vision is adequate.

5. I understand that I may not get a full correction from my LASIK procedure and this may require future enhancement procedures, such as more laser treatment or the use of glasses or contact lenses.

6. I understand that there may be a "balance" problem between my two eyes after LASIK has been performed on one eye, but not the other. This phenomenon is called anisometropia. I understand this would cause eyestrain and make judging distance or depth perception more difficult. I understand that my first eye may take longer to heal than is usual, prolonging the time I could experience anisometropia.

7. I understand that, after LASIK, the eye may be more fragile to trauma from impact. Evidence has shown that, as with any scar, the corneal incision will not be as strong as the cornea originally was at that site. I understand that the treated eye, therefore, is somewhat more vulnerable to all varieties of injuries, at least for the first year following LASIK. I understand it would be advisable for me to wear protective eyewear when engaging in sports or other activities in which the possibility of a ball, projectile, elbow, fist, or other traumatizing object contacting the eye may be high.

8. I understand that there is a natural tendency of the eyelids to droop with age and that eye surgery may hasten this process.

9. I understand that there may be pain or a foreign body sensation, particularly during the first 48 hours after surgery.

10. I understand that temporary glasses either for distance or reading may be necessary while healing occurs and that more than one pair of glasses may be needed.

11. I understand that the long-term effects of LASIK are unknown and that unforeseen complications or side effects could possibly occur.

12. I understand that visual acuity I initially gain from LASIK could regress, and that my vision may go partially back to a level that may require glasses or contact lens use to see clearly.

13. I understand that the correction that I can expect to gain from LASIK may not be perfect. I understand that it is not realistic to expect that this procedure will result in perfect vision, at all times, under all circumstances, for the rest of my life. I understand I may need glasses to refine my vision for some purposes requiring fine detailed vision after some point in my life, and that this might occur soon after surgery or years later.

14. I understand that I may be given medication in conjunction with the procedure and that my eye may be patched afterward. I therefore, understand that I must not drive the day of surgery and not until I am certain that my vision is adequate for driving.

15. I understand that if I currently need reading glasses, I will still likely need reading glasses after this treatment. It is possible that dependence on reading glasses may increase or that reading glasses may be required at an earlier age if I have this surgery.

16. Even 90% clarity of vision is still slightly blurry. Enhancement surgeries can be performed when vision is stable UNLESS it is unwise or unsafe. If the enhancement is performed within the first six months following surgery, there generally is no need to make another cut with the microkeratome. The original flap can usually be lifted with specialized techniques. After 6 months of

healing, a new LASIK incision may be required, incurring greater risk. In order to perform an enhancement surgery, there must be adequate tissue remaining. If there is inadequate tissue, it may not be possible to perform an enhancement. An assessment and consultation will be held with the surgeon at which time the benefits and risks of an enhancement surgery will be discussed.

17. I understand that, as with all types of surgery, there is a possibility of complications due to anesthesia, drug reactions, or other factors that may involve other parts of my body. I understand that, since it is impossible to state every complication that may occur as a result of any surgery, the list of complications in this form may not be complete.

For Presbyopic Patients (those requiring a separate prescription for reading): The option of monovision has been discussed with my ophthalmologist.

Patient's Statement Of Acceptance And Understanding
The details of the procedure known as LASIK have been presented to me in detail in this document and explained to me by my ophthalmologist. My ophthalmologist has answered all my questions to my satisfaction. I therefore consent to LASIK surgery on:

Right eye: _____

Left eye: _____

Both eyes: _____

I give permission for my ophthalmologist to record on video or photographic equipment my procedure, for purposes of education, research, or training of other health care professionals. I also give my permission for my ophthalmologist to use data about my procedure and subsequent treatment to further understand LASIK. I understand that my name will remain confidential, unless I give subsequent written permission for it to be disclosed outside my ophthalmologist's office or the center where my LASIK procedure will be performed.

Patient Name: _____   Date: _____

Witness Name: _____   Date: _____

I have been offered a copy of this consent form
(please initial): _____

References

1. Sanders DR, Hofman RF, Salz JJ (1986) Refractive corneal surgery. Slack, Thorofare, N.J.
2. Abbott RL, Ou RJ, Bird M (2003) Medical malpractice predictors and risk factors for ophthalmologists performing LASIK and photorefractive keratectomy surgery. Ophthalmology 110:2137–2146

Core Messages

- Strabismus and binocular vision impairment are uncommon yet significant complications associated with refractive surgery.

- Strabismus and disturbance of binocular vision post–refractive procedures are most commonly secondary to a decompensation of a preexisting ocular misalignment.

- Thorough preoperative evaluation for latent strabismus and phorias is the most effective measure to prevent postoperative strabismus complications.

- Contact lens trial should be performed in patients with preoperative latent strabismus who choose monovision to prevent ocular misalignment post-procedure.

18.3 Effect of Refractive Surgery on Strabismus and Binocular Vision

Bharavi Kharod and Natalie A. Afshari

18.3.1 Background

In 1948, Jose Barraquer pioneered the field of altering corneal shape and curvature to correct refractive errors. He developed surgical techniques to remove portions of cornea, freeze and reshape them, and then resuture them back to the cornea. His work was the driving force behind the development of modern-day refractive procedures. In the 1960s, Svyatoslav Fyodorov introduced radial keratotomy in Russia. However, the introduction of excimer laser technology in the 1970s revolutionized the world of ophthalmology. Patients who had been confined to spectacle or contact lens correction were now able to get "corrected" vision from their waking moments to the time they retired at night. Ophthalmologists and patients alike embraced refractive surgery and all the advances in this field with open arms, as it allowed patients to gain independence from corrective lenses and significantly improved their quality of life. Refractive surgery gained momentum rapidly and soon became a highly demanded ophthalmic procedure. In fact, since its introduction in the 1990s, refractive surgery has had a mass following and has become one of the leading elective ophthalmic procedures.

Though refractive surgery literally transformed the quality of vision and quality of life for millions around the globe, there were some setbacks of this procedure. The most well-known and well-published side effects of refractive procedures include glare, halos, and starbursting. Complications such as infections, dehisced flaps, epithelial ingrowth, and buttonholes are also well studied in the literature. One of the less commonly recognized effects of refractive surgery is decompensation of vision in patients who have latent or manifest strabismus. Many of these patients presented with symptoms of binocular visual impairment or frank diplopia and ocular misalignment following a refractive procedure. This chapter discusses the cause, prevention, and treatment of this post refractive complication.

18.3.2 Causes of Strabismus and Binocular Vision Impairment in Refractive Patients

In many of the early studies, patients who had preoperative strabismus were noted to have orthophoria after undergoing refractive surgery. However, as more time elapsed after their procedure, strabismus-related problems started surfacing in these patients. Another subset of patients had well-controlled strabismus preoperatively with spectacle correction but suffered either from ocular misalignment or diplopia immediately postoperatively. Finally, there was a subset of patients who had "de novo" strabismus or binocular vision impairment after refractive surgery. Initially, these patients presented an enigma to ophthalmologists. What caused this decompensation? We now know that several factors attributed to these symptoms.

18.3.2.1 Patients with Delayed Decompensation of Strabismus after Refractive Surgery

In the early postoperative period, many patients with preoperative strabismus had orthophoric outcomes. However, as more time elapsed after their procedure, decompensation of their strabismus occurred. What causes this delayed decompensation? A major factor in these cases is regression toward the preoperative refractive error. High myopes and hyperopes often have regression after refractive procedures. In most patients without strabismus, this does not pose any significant problems except blurry vision. However, in patients with preexisting strabismus, a regression (even if it would be considered minimal under other circumstances) is adequate to affect their binocular vision. Their decompensation, thus, is a function of the sensorimotor alteration following their refractive procedure.

18.3.2.2 Patients with Spectacle-Corrected Preoperative Strabismus

Another scenario included patients with preoperative strabismus that was adequately controlled with glasses. These patients returned with strabismus after their refractive procedure. If patients wearing glasses had no symptoms of diplopia or signs of strabismus, then how did refractive surgery induce ocular misalignment in these patients? It is important to realize that refractive surgery does not cause ocular misalignment; rather, it only allows the manifestation of the ocular misalignment that was previously present.

Glasses have a prismatic effect on both eyes. Patients who are accustomed to wearing glasses are used to this prismatic effect. Refractive surgery eliminates the prismatic effect in these patients and induces a "reverse prismatic effect" after their procedure. This offsets their retinal correspondence and falsely gives the illusion of an abnormal retinal correspondence (ARC). This causes nonphysiologic diplopia in these patients. This problem is usually associated with patients who are highly myopic or hyperopic or have anisometropia. These patients would have a similar effect with contact lenses as the contact lens removes the prismatic effect of spectacles.

18.3.3 Patients with Preoperative Latent or Manifest Strabismus

Many patients were noted to have strabismus de novo following refractive surgery. This created quite a stir in the ophthalmic community. However, on further research and reflection on previous exams, it was realized these patients had either an *eso* or *exo* phoria before their refractive procedure was performed. The procedure, however, caused a decompensation of their phorias.

In another scenario, patients with preoperative latent or manifest strabismus had strabismus or frank diplopia after their refractive procedure. One of the attributing factors in such cases is inaccuracy in their refractive correction. An undercorrection or overcorrection in these cases, no matter how minimal, is often adequate to cause strabismus-related problems. It is important to realize that patients with latent or manifest strabismus have fragile binocular fusion reserve. Thus, disturbing their refractive balance offsets this reserve and causes decompensation of their preexisting strabismus. Furthermore, over- or undercorrection changes their nodal point, which also impairs their functional binocular vision.

Decentration of the flap and/or treatment is an intraoperative cause of postoperative deviations, especially vertical deviations. When the treatment in one eye is in the visual axis and the treatment in another eye is decentered, the eye with the eccentric treatment will deviate in the direction of the best treatment zone. For example, if the flap or the treatment in the eye is decentered temporally (especially in someone with a preexisting exophoria or exotropia), then the patient will have an exotropia after the refractive procedure. If the flap and/or treatment are decentered superiorly or inferiorly, then the patient will have a vertical deviation. Patients with a preexisting horizontal phoria or tropia often develop a V- or A-pattern deviation if their treatment is decentered vertically. Furthermore, patients with a congenital superior oblique palsy may manifest their deviation and present with diplopia following a decentered flap/treatment.

18.3.3.1 Monovision and Strabismus

Patients with preoperative strabismus who opt for monovision require special evaluation. In these patients, binocular fusion is very fragile. They require both of their eyes aligned and require their vision similar in both eyes to maintain fusion. Therefore, disrupting this fusion by creating partial or complete monovision (especially with the dominant eye corrected for near vision and non-dominant eye corrected for distance) places them at a high risk for binocular vision impairment after surgery. However, some patients who have a mild degree of phoria or tropia might be able to tolerate partial monovision. Therefore, a trial with contact lenses or monovision trial frames is imperative in such circumstances to determine if the patient is a good candidate for monovision.

18.3.4 Prevention of Strabismus and Binocular Vision Impairment in Refractive Patients

The degree of strabismus may be a determining force in whether a patient will develop strabismus-related problems postoperatively. The most important intervention to prevent strabismus and binocular vision impairment in patients undergoing refractive surgery is a thorough preoperative evaluation. Patients should be asked extensively about their ocular history. Have they had previous muscle surgery? Have they suffered from double vision at the end of the day or when tired? Has anyone in the family noticed a "wandering eye," especially when the patient is tired? Have they had difficulties with binocular vision with contact lenses? This is especially important in someone considering monovision.

Equally important is a thorough exam—this includes a cover–uncover test, an alternate cover test, and sometimes even a Maddox rod evaluation. In patients who have established strabismus, it may be wise to try them in contact lenses to evaluate the role of prismatic effect from their glasses. In strabismic patients considering monovision, it is almost essential to try them with monovision contact lenses to simulate the effects of refractive surgery.

Finally, intraoperative care should be taken to ensure that the flaps and the treatment are not decentered. In addition, under- or overcorrection may throw the patient's binocular vision off and cause decompensation of a phoria into a tropia or cause a persistent tropia or vertical deviation.

Ultimately, it is critical to recognize that patients with a preoperative history of latent or manifest strabismus have fragile binocular fusion. They are at risk of disruption of

ocular alignment and fusion with minimal alteration in their refractive balance. This should be discussed extensively with the patients preoperatively.

18.3.5 Treatment of Decompensated Strabismus

The treatment in cases where refractive surgery has induced a decompensation of strabismus depends on the underlying cause. If the decompensation is determined to be secondary to an undercorrection or regression, then an enhancement may be a suitable option. In cases of overcorrection, spectacle correction might be useful. In these cases, the hope would be for the patient to regress eventually to emmetropia. If the decompensation is secondary to a decentered treatment, then the management is more challenging. Some experts recommend determining the postoperative refractive error and treating the refractive error with centration in the central visual axis. Often times, however, these patients require spectacle correction. In cases of vertical deviations, patients often require prisms to maintain fusion.

Take-Home Pearls

- Careful selection of patients for refractive surgery is especially important in avoiding strabismus-related complications after refractive surgery.
- A thorough preoperative evaluation of phorias and latent strabismus can reduce the rates of manifest strabismus post refractive procedures.
- An accurate manifest and cycloplegic refraction are essential in preventing strabismus associated with under- or overcorrection.
- Centration of flaps and treatment is an important intraoperative measure of reducing strabismus following refractive procedures.
- Monovision should be approached with care in patients with latent or manifest strabismus.
- Patients with a preoperative strabismus have fragile binocular fusion and are at risk of disruption of ocular alignment and fusion with minimal alteration in their refractive balance.

Bibliography

Godts D, Tassignon MJ, Gobin L (2004) Binocular vision impairment after refractive surgery. J Cataract Refract Surg 30:101–109

Godts D, Trau R, Tassignon MJ (2006) Effect of refractive surgery on binocular vision and ocular alignment in patients with manifest or intermittent strabismus. Br J Ophthalmol 90:1410–1413

Kowal L, Battu R, Kushner B (2005) Refractive surgery and strabismus. Clin Experiment Ophthalmol 33:90–96

Krasny J, Brunnerova R, Kuchynka P, Novak P, Cyprichova J, Modlingerova E (2003) Indications for refractive procedures in adult patients with strabismus and results of the subsequent therapeutic procedures. Cesk Slov Oftalmol 59:402–414

Mandava N, Donnenfeld ED, Owens PL et al (1996) Ocular deviation following excimer laser photorefractive keratectomy. J Cataract Refract Surg 22:504–505

Marmer RH (1987) Ocular deviation induced by radial keratotomy. Ann Ophthalmol 19:451–452

Nemet P, Levenger S, Nemet A (2002) Refractive surgery for refractive errors which cause strabismus: a report of 8 cases. Binocul Vis Strabismus Q 17:187–190

Sabetti L, Spadea L, D'Alessandri L, Balestrazzi E (2005) Photorefractive keratectomy and laser in situ keratomileusis in refractive accommodative esotropia. J Cataract Refract Surg 31:1899–1903

Snir M, Kremer I, Weinberger D, Sherf I, Axer-Siegel R (2003) Decompensation of exodeviation after corneal refractive surgery for moderate to high myopia. Ophthalmic Surg Lasers Imaging 34:363–370

Stidham DB, Borissova O, Borissov V, Prager TC (2002) Effect of hyperopic laser in situ keratomileusis on ocular alignment and stereopsis in patients with accommodative esotropia. Ophthalmology 109:1148–1153

Sugar A, Rapuano CJ, Culberston WW (2002) Laser in situ keratomileusis for myopia and astigmatism safety and efficacy (ophthalmic technologies assessment), A report by the American Academy of Ophthalmology. Ophthalmology 109:175–187

18

Peer-Reviewed Literature

Contents

Core Messages

- The excimer laser is one of the most widely used tools in ophthalmology for correcting refractive error, with an estimated 1.5 million procedures per year.

- LASIK complications persist even with recent advancements in excimer laser technology.

- Reported complications associated with LASIK include corneal flap abnormalities, epithelial ingrowth, corneal ectasia, diffuse lamellar keratitis, dry eyes, and infectious keratitis.

- Reported complications associated with PRK and LASEK include many of the non flap-related complications seen after LASIK, such as corneal subepithelial haze/glare/halos and optical aberrations.

19.1 10-Year Classified Review of the Peer Review Literature on Excimer Laser Refractive Complications

Takashi Kojima, Tatsuya Ongucci, Joelle Hallak, and Dimitri Azar

19.1.1 Introduction

In this chapter, we summarize the complications of excimer laser surgery, including laser in situ keratomileusis (LASIK), photorefractive keratectomy (PRK), and laser epithelial keratomileusis (LASEK), which were reported between 1996 and 2006. The information is presented in table format for easy reference. We attempted to calculate an approximate incidence using weighted averages when the number of studies was sufficient to draw meaningful conclusions.

Table 19.1.1 Intraoperative flap complications

Author	Total no. of eyes	Cases	Incidence rate (%)	Comment
Incomplete flap				
Gimbel et al. 1998 [2]	1,000	12	1.2	
Lin et al. 1999 [3]	1,019	3	0.29	
Stulting et al. 1997 [4]	1,062	8	0.75	
Al-Swailem et al. 2006 [5]	500	10	2	Cases treated by a clinical fellow
Al-Swailem et al. 2006 [5]	200	3	1.5	Cases treated by an attending
Total	3,781	36	0.95	
Irregular flap				
Lin et al. 1999 [3]	1,019	9	0.88	
Thin flap				
Gimbel et al. 1998 [2]	1,000	3	0.3	
Lin et al. 1999 [3]	1,019	2	0.2	
Stulting et al. 1997 [4]	1,062	1	0.09	
Total	3,081	6	0.19	
Button hole				
Gimbel et al. 1998 [2]	1,000	3	0.3	
Lin et al. 1999 [3]	1,019	2	0.2	
Stulting et al. 1997 [4]	1,062	6	0.56	
Al-Swailem et al. 2006 [5]	500	3	0.6	Cases treated by a clinical fellow
Al-Swailem et al. 2006 [5]	200	1	0.5	Cases treated by an attending
Total	3,781	15	0.4	
Dislodged flap				
Gimbel et al. 1998 [2]	1,000	2	0.2	
Free cap				
Gimbel et al. 1998 [2]	1,000	1	0.1	
Lin et al. 1999 [3]	1,019	10	0.98	
Stulting et al. 1997 [4]	1,062	10	0.94	
Al-Swailem et al. 2006 [5]	500	2	0.4	Cases treated by a clinical fellow
Al-Swailem et al. 2006 [5]	200	0	0	Cases treated by an attending
Total	3,781	23	0.61	

The excimer laser is regarded as the most successful and widely used tool for correcting refractive errors. Through using argon fluoride gases to emit ultraviolet laser pulses, the excimer reshapes the cornea into its normal curvature. Excimer laser techniques have evolved rapidly to meet increasing patients' expectations. Nevertheless, as with any surgical procedure, intraoperative and postoperative complications may occur. Several complications have been identified. These include anatomic complications (corneal flap abnormalities, epithelial ingrowth, and corneal ectasia), diffuse lamellar keratitis, dry eyes, and infectious kera-

Table 19.1.2 Flap folds

Author	Total no. of eyes	Cases	Incidence rate (%)	Comment
Binder 2006 [6]	1,000	4	0.4	IntraLase was used for all cases
Gimbel et al. 1998 [2]	1,000	6	0.6	
Lin et al. 1999 [3]	1,019	11	1.08	
Stulting et al. 1997 [4]	1,062	2	0.19	
Al-Swailem et al. 2006 [5]	500	4	0.8	Cases treated by a clinical fellow
Al-Swailem et al. 2006 [6]	200	2	1	Cases treated by an attending
Total	4,781	29	0.61	

titis. These complications and their management have been described elsewhere in the book.

19.1.2 LASIK Complications

19.1.2.1 Flap Complications

LASIK has rapidly become the most frequently performed refractive surgical procedure, with an estimated 1.5 million annual procedures [1]. It involves the use of a microkeratome to create a thin corneal flap followed by excimer laser ablation of the corneal stroma. LASIK is not a complication-free procedure; it mainly involves flap related complications that can occur intraoperatively or postoperatively.

Intraoperative flap complications mainly involve incomplete, irregular, thin, buttonhole, dislodged, and free cap. The incidence rates from several studies with large case series are presented in Table 19.1.1. Incomplete flap has the highest incidence rate among flap complications, with an estimated 0.95% occurrence. Incomplete flaps are created when the microkeratome blade comes to a halt prior to reaching the intended location of the hinge. Microkeratome jamming due to either electrical failure or mechanical obstacles may be the most common cause of incomplete flaps.

Postoperative flap complications involve dislocated flaps and flap folds. Binder et al. reported an incidence rate of 2% (20 cases out of 1,000) of dislocated flaps using the IntraLase microkeratome [6].

Several studies have reported the occurrence of flap folds following LASIK (Table 19.1.2). Flap folds can induce irregular astigmatism with optical aberrations and loss of best spectacle-corrected visual acuity (BSCVA), especially if they involve the visual axis [7, 8].

Until recently, the lamellar flap could only be made with a microkeratome. The femtosecond laser provides increased accuracy in flap thickness than previous methods, avoiding all of the flap related complications. LASEK is a relatively new laser surgical procedure that has been developed to combine certain elements of both LASIK and PRK to improve the risk/benefit ratio. In this procedure, an epithelial flap is fashioned using either dilute alcohol or microkeratome (epi-LASIK) is used to loosen the epithelial adhesion to the corneal stroma. The loosened epithelium is moved aside from the treatment zone as a hinged sheet. Laser ablation of the subepithelial stroma is performed before the epithelial sheet is returned to its original position [9].

19.1.2.1.1 Diffuse Lamellar Keratitis

Diffuse lamellar keratitis (DLK) was first reported as a complication of LASIK in a published case-series review in 1998 (Table 19.1.3) [10]. It is characterized by proliferation of presumably inflammatory cells at the LASIK interface. It can lead to stromal corneal melting with induced hyperopia or hyperopic astigmatism. Additional symptoms include loss of BSCVA with optical aberrations secondary to irregular astigmatism. In a recent case series, Binder et al. reported 50 cases with DLK out of 1,000 eyes [2].

19.1.2.1.2 Interface Fluid

Fluid collection in the interface is one of the unusual complications after LASIK. It is reported to result from increased intraocular pressure, decreased endothelial cell density, or uveitis [12]. The first case of interface fluid collection following LASIK was reported in 1999 [13]. Steroid-induced intraocular pressure elevation and epithelial ingrowth were notable features in this case. Various case reports on this complication are listed in Table 19.1.4, from the year 1999 to 2006.

19.1.2.1.3 Dry Eye

Dry eye is defined as a disorder of the tear film caused by tear deficiency or excessive tear evaporation, which, in turn, causes damage to the interpalpebral ocular surface and is associated with symptoms of ocular discomfort [28]. Symptoms of ocular dryness are most common after ophthalmic surgical procedures. Cutting a LASIK flap and performing a stromal ablation disrupts the corneal nerve innervation and produces a relative loss of corneal sensation for up to

Table 19.1.3 DLK

Author	Total no. of eyes	Cases	Incidence rate (%)	Comment
Bigham et al. 2005 [11]	72,360	482	0.67	The data was derived from the survey at community-based clinics. 64% of cases occurred in an outbreak
Binder 2006 [2]	1,000	50	5	IntraLase was used for all cases
Lin et al. 1999 [3]	1,019	18	1.77	
Stulting et al. 1997 [4]	1,062	2	0.19	
Al-Swailem et al. 2006 [5]	500	3	0.6	Cases reported by a fellow, grade >2+
Al-Swailem et al. 2006 [5]	200	0	0	Cases reported by an faculty, grade >2+

Table 19.1.4 Interface fluid

Author	Total no. of eyes	No. of eyes (patient)	Incidence rate (%)	Condition before LASIK	Comment
Lyle et al. 1999 [13]	6,000	1	0.02	Ocular hypertension	
Najman-Vainer et al. 2000 [14]	CR	1			
Rehany et al. 2000 [15]	CR	2 (1)		Primary open-angle glaucoma	
Portellinha et al. 2001 [16]	CR	2 (1)			
Fogla et al. 2001 [17]	CR	2 (1)			
Parek et al. 2001 [18]	CR	1		Penetrating keratoplasty	
Shaikh et al. 2002 [19]	CR	4 (2)		Glaucoma suspect, juvenile glaucoma	
Hamilton et al. 2002 [20]	CR	6 (4)			
Dawson et al. 2003 [21]	CR	1		After penetrating keratoplasty	
Lyle et al. 2003 [22]	6,000	1	0.02	After penetrating keratoplasty	
Bushleyet al. 2005 [23]	CR	1		Occurred after traumatic corneal perforation	Occurred after traumatic corneal perforation
Mcleod et al. 2005 [24]	CR	1			
Kang et al. 2006 [25]	CR	1		Chronic angle-closure glaucoma	
Bacsal et al. 2006 [26]	CR	1			
Galal et al. 2006 [27]	CR	13 (8)			All cases were misdiagnosed as DLK or infectious keratitis at first visit

CR case reports

19

Table 19.1.5 Dry eyes

Author	Total no. of eyes	Preoperative	1 week	1 month	3 months	6 months	12 months	Comments
Yu et al. 2000 [31]	96	15 (15.6%)	82 (85.4%)	57 (59.4%)				Based on the symptoms
Hovanesian et al. 2001 [32]	587		Various time points at least 6 month after surgery, 266 (45.3%)					
Albietz et al. 2005 [29]	878	20	NA	32	38	39	29	Based on the symptoms
De Paiva et al. 2006 [33]	35	0	17 (48.6%)		7 (20%)	8 (22.9%)		The criteria for dry eye is the total corneal fluorescent staining score ≥3

NA not applicable

6 months after surgery [29] According to the 2003 Refractive Surgery Survey, dry eye symptoms are the most common problem encountered after LASIK and occur in 15–25% of patients [30]. Table 19.1.5 presents different studies that show the prolonged symptoms of dry eye after LASIK.

19.1.2.1.4 Infectious Keratitis
In 1999, Lin et al. reported the incidence of bacterial keratitis after LASIK to be 0.1% [34]. In November 2001, the American Society of Cataract and Refractive Surgery developed a post-LASIK infectious keratitis survey. One hundred sixteen post-LASIK infections were reported by 56 LASIK surgeons who had performed an estimated 338,550 procedures (an incidence of 1 infection in every 2,919 procedures) [35]. The most common organisms cultured were atypical mycobacteria and staphylococci [35]. Excimer refractive surgery techniques should be approached in a manner similar to other surgical procedure even if low incidence rates of infection are reported. Several investigators have analyzed the incidence and visual outcomes of infectious keratitis after LASIK (Table 19.1.6).

19.1.2.1.5 Epithelial Ingrowth
Implantation of epithelial cells in the interface occurs either due to seeding during surgery or migration under the flap [1]. More concerning is epithelial ingrowth that is contiguous with the flap edge. This can progress to involve the visual axis with irregular astigmatism and possible overlying flap melting [1]. The incidence rate of epithelial in-

growth has been retrospectively determined by several investigators (Table 19.1.7).

19.1.2.1.6 Ectasia
Corneal ectasia remains one of the most serious complications after LASIK. It has mainly been reported in patients with keratoconus, forme fruste keratoconus, and high myopia [38]. The first reports of this complication were by Seiler and colleagues in 1998 [39]. Fewer than 150 cases have been reported in ophthalmic literature [39]. Initially patients may be managed with hard contact lens wear, but many progress to require penetrating keratoplasty. Several investigators have retrospectively analyzed the incidence of ectasia at different follow-up durations (Table 19.1.8). However, the true incidence of this complication might not emerge until longer term follow-up studies are conducted.

19.1.2.1.7 Night Vision
LASIK candidates typically have healthy eyes; hence, high levels of satisfaction levels and quality of vision are essential. Estimates of patient satisfaction with LASIK range from 82 to 98% [42]. Patients may be highly satisfied with the overall outcomes of refractive surgery, but not necessarily with individual facets such as night vision. The potential for excimer laser refractive surgery to induce clinically important night vision complaints (NVCs) was recognized soon after its introduction in 1992, when investigators theorized that small optical zones would diverge marginal rays and, thereby, might produce visual aberrations in low light

Table 19.1.6 Infectious keratitis

Author	Total no. of eyes	Cases	Incidence rate (%)	Comment
Lin et al. 1999 [34]	1,019	1	0.1	
Pirzada et al. 1997 [36]	85	1	1.17	
Perez-Santonja et al. 1997 [37]	801	1	0.12	
Stulting et al. 1999 [4]	1,062	2	0.18	Bilateral case
Solomon et al. 2003 [35]	338,550	116	0.03	Questionnaire from ASCRS member
Al-Swailem et al. 2006 [5]	500	0	0	Cases reported by a clinical fellow
Al-Swailem et al. 2006 [5]	200	0	0	Cases reported by a faculty attending

ASCRS American Society of Cataract and Refractive Surgery

Table 19.1.7 Epithelial ingrowth

Author	Total no. of eyes	Cases	Incidence rate (%)	Comment
Binder 2006 [2]	1,000	0	0.00	IntraLase was used for all cases. Three eyes developed epithelial ingrowth after enhancement
Lin et al. 1999 [3]	1,019	22[a]	2.16[a]	
Stulting et al. 1997 [4]	1,062	123 (23)[a]	11.5 (2.16)[a]	
Al-Swailem et al. 2006 [5]	500	1	0.20	Cases in fellow
Al-Swailem et al. 2006 [5]	200	0	0.00	Cases in faculty

[a]Requiring surgical intervention

Table 19.1.8 Corneal ectasia

Author	Total no. of patients	Cases	Incidence rate (%)	Mean follow-up (months)	Comment
Pallikaris et al. 2001 [40]	2,873	19	0.66	16.32	
Rad et al. 2004 [41]	6,941	14	0.2		
Al-Swailem et al. 200 [65]	500	2	0.4	4.9	Cases reported by clinical fellows
Al-Swailem et al. 2006 [5]	200	0	0	4.3	Cases reported by faculty attendings
Total	10,514	35	0.33		

illumination [43]. Clinically important NVCs are mainly as the ones having an impact on important daily activities, such as driving. In 1996, concerns were brought forward about potential adverse consequences of excimer laser surgery in eyes with a pupil size larger than 8 mm [43]. Various studies have evaluated and assessed the visual experiences, quality of life, and patient satisfaction following excimer refractive surgery (Table 19.1.9).

Table 19.1.9 Night vision complaints

Author	Total no. of patients	Cases	Incidence rate (%)	Comment
Schein et al. 2001 [44] Patients who reported difficulty driving after surgery	176		41.5	Data from 2 to 6 months after surgery
Bailey et al. 2003 [45]	604		Glare, 27.2; halo, 30; starburst, 27.2	Questionnaire from the patient who completed at least 6 months' follow-up
Pop et al. 2004 [43]				
1 month postoperatively	655	172	26.3	
3 months postoperatively	460	58	12.6	
6 months postoperatively	427	31	7.3	
12 months postoperatively	325	16	4.9	
Hammond et al. 2005 [42]	8,528	2	0.02	Study for army service member
O'Doherty et al. 2007 [46]	49	12	24	5 years' follow-up

Table 19.1.10 Retinal detachment

Author	Total no.	Cases	Incidence rate (%)
Ruiz-Moreno et al. 1999 [47]	1,554	4	0.26
Arevalo et al. 2000 [48]	29,916	20	0.07
Arevalo et al. 2002 [49]	38,823	33	0.09
Faghihi et al. 2006 [50]	59,424	49	0.08
Total	129,717	106	0.08

19.1.2.1.8 Retinal Detachment

The first case of retinal detachment after LASIK was reported in 1998 and was associated with a giant retinal tear [47]. Ruiz Moreno et al. in 1999 retrospectively studied the retinal detachments observed in 1,544 consecutive eyes (878) patients undergoing LASIK for myopia. Retinal detachment occurred in four eyes [47]. The incidence of retinal detachment is higher in myopic patients than in patients with emmetropia [47]. In eyes in which the myopia has been corrected by LASIK, the risk of development of retinal detachment is initially a result of the myopia itself. Table 19.1.10 shows the number of cases reported by several investigators with retinal detachment after LASIK for high myopia.

19.1.3 PRK and LASEK Complications

19.1.3.1 PRK Haze

The major limitations of PRK are subepithelial haze, postoperative pain, and prolonged visual rehabilitation brought by epithelial removal. Corneal subepithelial haze is commonly seen as part of the normal corneal healing response following PRK. This subepithelial scarring of the cornea peaks 3–6 months after PRK, with a steady decrease in severity until 18 months postoperatively (Table 19.1.11). Haze is associated with loss of BSCVA, regression of treatment effect, decreased contrast sensitivity, and light scatter around bright light sources, especially at night [51]. The use of prophylactic mitomycin C may reduce the corneal haze after PRK or LASEK [51].

Table 19.1.11 Haze after PRK (grade 1 or more)

Author	1 month Total no. of eyes	1 month Cases (incidence %)	3 months Total no.	3 months Cases (incidence %)	6 months Total no.	6 months Cases (incidence %)	12 months Total no.	12 months Cases (incidence %)	Comment
Hammond 2005 [52]			21,428	30 (0.14)					
Lee 2004 [53]					168	41 (24.4)			
Claringbold 2002 [54]				29 (13)			84	0	
El Danasoury 1999 [55]					24	6 (25.0)			
Pop 2000 [56]	686	0	578	0	647	1 (0.16)	646	1 (0.15)	
Lee 2001 [57]	27	20 (74.07)	27	7 (25.93)					
Carones 2002 [58]		8 (26.7)		24 (82.%)		12 (40%)			Without MMC
Carones 2002 [58]		16 (53.3)		23 (76.7)		24 (80%)			With MMC

MMC mitomycin C

Table 19.1.12 Haze following LASEK (grade 1 or more)

Haze (grade 1 or more) Author	1 month No. of eyes	1 month Cases (incidence %)	3 months No. of eyes	3 months Cases (incidence %)	6 months No. of eyes	6 months Cases (incidence %)	12 months No. of eyes	12 months Cases (incidence %)	Comments
Kim 2004 [59]	146	21 (14.4%)			146	88 (60.27%)	146	83 (56.8%)	
Wu 2006 [60]			NA	NA	NA	NA			Low–moderate
Wu (2006) [60]			NA	(16.67%)	NA	NA (22.23%)			High
Anderson 2002 [61]			313	5 (1.6%)					Clinically significant haze
Shahinian 2002 [62]	85	3 (3.53%)	71	1 (1.41%)	55	0	23	0	<6
Shahinian 2002 [62]	60	2 (3.33%)	46	2 (4.35%)	40	0	32	2 (6.25%)	>6
Feit 2003 [63]			163	29 (17.79%)					

NA not applicable

19.1.3.2 LASEK Haze

As with PRK, corneal subepithelial haze may occur following LASEK, but some studies have shown that LASEK reduced the incidence of significant postoperative pain and corneal haze (Table 19.1.12) [57].

19.1.4 Conclusion

The advancements in excimer laser refractive technology (such as laser design and eye tracking) have yielded improved visual and refractive outcomes. Patient expectation and demand for high standards in quality of vision will rise further, which may bring new unanticipated complications. Refractive surgeons' effort to minimize and control these complications and to share their experiences and continuously report unexpected results, will allow continued smooth transitions to more successful correction techniques in the future.

Take-Home Pearls

- The femtosecond laser used in LASIK may provide increased accuracy in flap thickness and reduced incidence of flap related complications.
- Longer-term follow-up studies are needed to determine the true incidence of ectasia following LASIK.
- In eyes in which the myopia has been corrected by LASIK, the risk of development of retinal detachment is initially a result of the myopia itself.
- The use of prophylactic mitomycin C may reduce the corneal haze after PRK or LASEK.
- Refractive surgeons are advised to continuously share their experiences and report unexpected complications.

References

1. Melki SA, Azar DT (2001) LASIK complications: etiology, management, and prevention. Surv Ophthalmol 46:95–116
2. Gimbel HV, Penno EE, van Westenbrugge JA, Ferensowicz M, Furlong MT (1998) Incidence and management of intraoperative and early postoperative complications in 1000 consecutive laser in situ keratomileusis cases. Ophthalmology 105:1839–1847
3. Lin RT, Maloney RK (1999) Flap complications associated with lamellar refractive surgery. Am J Ophthalmol 127:129–316
4. Stulting RD, Carr JD, Thompson KP, Waring GO III, Wiley WM, Walker JG (1999) Complications of laser in situ keratomileusis for the correction of myopia. Ophthalmology 106:13–20
5. Al-Swailem SA, Wagoner MD (2006) Complications and visual outcome of LASIK performed by anterior segment fellows vs.experienced faculty supervisors. Am J Ophthalmol 141:13–23
6. Binder PS (2006) One thousand consecutive IntraLase laser in situ keratomileusis flaps. J Cataract Refract Surg 32:962–969
7. Lyle WA, Jin GJ (2000) Results of flap repositioning after laser in situ keratomileusis. J Cataract Refract Surg 26:1451–1457
8. Steinemann TL, Denton NC, Brown MF (1998) Corneal lenticular wrinkling after automated lamellar keratoplasty. Am J Ophthalmol 126:588–590
9. Taneri S, Zieske JD, Azar DT (2004) Evolution, techniques, clinical outcomes, and pathophysiology of LASEK: review of the literature. Surv Ophthalmol 49:576–602
10. Smith RJ, Maloney RK. Diffuse lamellar keratitis (1998) A new syndrome in lamellar refractive surgery. Ophthalmology 105:1721–1726
11. Bigham M, Enns CL, Holland SP, Buxton J, Patrick D, Marion S, Morck DW, Kurucz M, Yuen V, Lafaille V, Shaw J, Mathias R, Van Andel M, Peck S (2005) Diffuse lamellar keratitis complicating laser in situ keratomileusis: post-marketing surveillance of an emerging disease in British Columbia, Canada, 2000–2002. J Cataract Refract Surg 31:2340–2344
12. Kang SJ, Dawson DG, Hopp LM, Schmack I, Grossniklaus HE, Edelhauser HF (2006) Interface fluid syndrome in laser in situ keratomileusis after complicated trabeculectomy. J Cataract Refract Surg 32:1560–1562
13. Lyle WA, Jin GJ (1999) Interface fluid associated with diffuse lamellar keratitis and epithelial ingrowth after laser in situ keratomileusis. J Cataract Refract Surg 25:1009–1012
14. Najman-Vainer J, Smith RJ, Maloney RK (2000) Interface fluid after LASIK: misleading tonometry can lead to end-stage glaucoma. J Cataract Refract Surg 26:471–472
15. Rehany U, Bersudsky V, Rumelt S (2000) Paradoxical hypotony after laser in situ keratomileusis. J Cataract Refract Surg 26:1823–186
16. Portellinha W, Kuchenbuk M, Nakano K, Oliveira M (2001) Interface fluid and diffuse corneal edema after laser in situ keratomileusis. J Refract Surg 17(2 Suppl):S192–S195
17. Fogla R, Rao SK, Padmanabhan P (2001) Interface fluid after laser in situ keratomileusis. J Cataract Refract Surg 27:1526–1528
18. Parek JG, Raviv T, Speaker MG (2001) Grossly false applanation tonometry associated with interface fluid in susceptible LASIK patients. J Cataract Refract Surg 27:1143–1144
19. Shaikh NM, Shaikh S, Singh K, Manche E (2002) Progression to end-stage glaucoma after laser in situ keratomileusis. J Cataract Refract Surg 28:356–359
20. Hamilton DR, Manche EE, Rich LF, Maloney RK (2002) Steroid-induced glaucoma after laser in situ keratomileusis associated with interface fluid. Ophthalmology 109:659–665
21. Dawson DG, Hardten DR, Albert DM (2003) Pocket of fluid in the lamellar interface after penetrating keratoplasty and laser in situ keratomileusis. Arch Ophthalmol 121:894–896
22. Lyle WA, Jin GJ, Jin Y (2003) Interface fluid after laser in situ keratomileusis. J Refract Surg 19:455–459
23. Bushley DM, Holzinger KA, Winkle RK, Le LH, Olkowski JD (2005) Lamellar interface fluid accumulation following traumatic corneal perforation and laser in situ keratomileusis. J Cataract Refract Surg 31:1249–1251
24. McLeod SD, Mather R, Hwang DG, Margolis TP (2005) Uveitis-associated flap edema and lamellar interface fluid collection after LASIK. Am J Ophthalmol 139:1137–1139
25. Kang SJ, Dawson DG, Hopp LM, Schmack I, Grossniklaus HE, Edelhauser HF (2006) Interface fluid syndrome in laser in situ keratomileusis after complicated trabeculectomy. J Cataract Refract Surg 32:1560–1562
26. Bacsal K, Chee SP (2006) Uveitis-associated flap edema and lamellar interface fluid collection after LASIK. Am J Ophthalmol 141:232
27. Galal A, Artola A, Belda J, Rodriguez-Prats J, Claramonte P, Sanchez A, Ruiz-Moreno O, Merayo J, Alió J (2006) Interface corneal edema secondary to steroid-induced elevation of intraocular pressure simulating diffuse lamellar keratitis. J Refract Surg 22:441–447

28. Ang RT, Dartt DA, Tsubota K (2001) Dry eye after refractive surgery. Curr Opin Ophthalmol 12:318–322

29. Albietz JM, Lenton LM, McLennan SG (2005) Dry eye after LASIK: comparison of outcomes for Asian and Caucasian eyes. Clin Exp Optom. 88:89–96

30. Vroman DT, Sandoval HP, Fernandez de Castro LE, Kasper TJ, Holzer MP, Solomon KD (2005) Effect of hinge location on corneal sensation and dry eye after laser in situ keratomileusis for myopia. J Cataract Refract Surg 31:1881–1887

31. Yu EY, Leung A, Rao S, Lam DS (2000) Effect of laser in situ keratomileusis on tear stability. Ophthalmology. 107:2131–2135

32. Hovanesian JA, Shah SS, Maloney RK (2001) Symptoms of dry eye and recurrent erosion syndrome after refractive surgery. J Cataract Refract Surg 27:577–584

33. De Paiva CS, Chen Z, Koch DD, Hamill MB, Manuel FK, Hassan SS, Wilhelmus KR, Pflugfelder SC (2006) The incidence and risk factors for developing dry eye after myopic LASIK. Am J Ophthalmol 141:438–445

34. Lin RT, Maloney RK (1999) Flap complications associated with lamellar refractive surgery. Am J Ophthalmol 127:129–136

35. Solomon R, Donnenfeld ED, Azar DT, Holland EJ, Palmon FR, Pflugfelder SC, Rubenstein JB (2003) Infectious keratitis after laser in situ keratomileusis: results of an ASCRS survey. J Cataract Refract Surg 29:2001–2006

36. Pirzada WA, Kalaawry H (1997) Laser in situ keratomileusis for myopia of –1 to –3.50 diopters. J Refract Surg 13(5 Suppl): S425–S426

37. Perez-Santonja JJ, Sakla HF, Abad JL, Zorraquino A, Esteban J, Alió JL (1997) Nocardial keratitis after laser in situ keratomileusis. J Refract Surg 13:314–317

38. Randleman JB, Russell B, Ward MA, Thompson KP, Stulting RD (2003) Risk factors and prognosis for corneal ectasia after LASIK. Ophthalmology 110:267–275

39. Randleman JB (2006) Post-laser in-situ keratomileusis ectasia: current understanding and future directions. Curr Opin Ophthalmol 17:406–412

40. Pallikaris IG, Kymionis GD, Astyrakakis NI (2001) Corneal ectasia induced by laser in situ keratomileusis. J Cataract Refract Surg 27:1796–1802

41. Rad AS, Jabbarvand M, Saifi N (2004) Progressive keratectasia after laser in situ keratomileusis. J Refract Surg 20(5 Suppl): S718–S722

42. Hammond SD Jr, Puri AK, Ambati BK (2004) Quality of vision and patient satisfaction after LASIK. Curr Opin Ophthalmol 15:328–332

43. Pop M, Payette Y (2004) Risk factors for night vision complaints after LASIK for myopia. Ophthalmology 111:3–10

44. Schein OD, Vitale S, Cassard SD, Steinberg EP. Patient outcomes of refractive surgery (2001) The refractive status and vision profile. J Cataract Refract Surg 27:665–673

45. Bailey MD, Mitchell GL, Dhaliwal DK, Boxer Wachler BS, Zadnik K (2003) Patient satisfaction and visual symptoms after laser in situ keratomileusis. Ophthalmology 110:1371–1378

46. O'Doherty M, O'Keeffe M, Kelleher C (2006) Five year follow-up of laser in situ keratomileusis for all levels of myopia. Br J Ophthalmol 90:20–23

47. Ruiz-Moreno JM, Perez-Santonja JJ, Alió JL (1999) Retinal detachment in myopic eyes after laser in situ keratomileusis. Am J Ophthalmol 128:588–594

48. Arevalo JF, Ramirez E, Suarez E, Morales-Stopello J, Cortez R, Ramirez G, Antzoulatos G, Tugues J, Rodriguez J, Fuenmayor-Rivera D (2000) Incidence of vitreoretinal pathologic conditions within 24 months after laser in situ keratomileusis. Ophthalmology 107:258–262

49. Arevalo JF, Ramirez E, Suarez E, Cortez R, Ramirez G, Yepez JB (2002) Retinal detachment in myopic eyes after laser in situ keratomileusis. J Refract Surg 18:708–714

50. Faghihi H, Jalali KH, Amini A, Hashemi H, Fotouhi A, Esfahani MR (2006) Rhegmatogenous retinal detachment after LASIK for myopia. J Refract Surg 22:448–452

51. Melki SA, Azar DA (2006) Four photorefractive keratotomy, LASEK, and, Epi-LASIK pearls: handling haze and decentration in surface ablation. In: 101 Pearls in refractive, cataract, and corneal surgery, 2nd edn. Slack, Thorofare, N.J., pp 47–49

52. Hammond MD, Madigran WP Jr, Bower KS (2005) Refractive surgery in the United States Army, 2000–2003. Ophthalmology 112:184–190

53. Lee HK, Lee KS, Kim JK, Kim HC, Seo KR, Kim EK (2005) Epithelial healing and clinical outcomes in excimer laser photorefractive surgery following three epithelial removal techniques: mechanical, alcohol, and excimer laser. Am J Ophthalmol 139:56–63

54. Claringbold TV II (2002) Laser-assisted subepithelial keratectomy for the correction of myopia. J Cataract Refract Surg 28:18–22

55. el Danasoury MA, el Maghraby A, Klyce SD, Mehrez K (1999) Comparison of photorefractive keratectomy with excimer laser in situ keratomileusis in correcting low myopia (from –2.00 to –5.50 diopters). A randomized study. Ophthalmology 106:411–420

56. Pop M, Payette Y (2000) Photorefractive keratectomy versus laser in situ keratomileusis: a control-matched study. Ophthalmology 107:251–257

57. Lee JB, Seong GJ, Lee JH, Seo KY, Lee YG, Kim EK (2001) Comparison of laser epithelial keratomileusis and photorefractive keratectomy for low to moderate myopia. J Cataract Refract Surg 27:565–570

58. Carones F, Vigo L, Scandola E, Vacchini L (2002) Evaluation of the prophylactic use of mitomycin-C to inhibit haze formation after photorefractive keratectomy. J Cataract Refract Surg 28:2088–2095

59. Kim JK, Kim SS, Lee HK, Lee IS, Seong GJ, Kim EK, Han SH (2004) Laser in situ keratomileusis versus laser-assisted subepithelial keratectomy for the correction of high myopia. J Cataract Refract Surg 30:1405–1411

60. Wu Y, Chu RY, Zhou XT, Dai JH, Qu XM, Rao S, Lam D (2006) Recovery of corneal sensitivity after laser-assisted subepithelial keratectomy. J Cataract Refract Surg 32:785–788

61. Anderson NJ, Beran RF, Schneider TL (2002) Epi-LASEK for the correction of myopia and myopic astigmatism. J Cataract Refract Surg 28:1343- 7

62. Shahinian L Jr (2002) Laser-assisted subepithelial keratectomy for low to high myopia and astigmatism. J Cataract Refract Surg 28:1334–1342

63. Feit R, Taneri S, Azar DT, Chen CC, Ang RT (2003) LASEK results. Ophthalmol Clin North Am. 16:127–135

19

19.2 10-Year Review of the Literature on Complications of Incisional, Thermal, and Lenticular Refractive Procedures

Tatsuya Ongucci, Takashi Kojima, and Dimitri Azar

19.2.1 Introduction

Excimer laser refractive surgery has enjoyed great popularity and suffers from relatively few serious complications (described in detail elsewhere in this book). In this chapter, we summarize the complications of non–excimer-based refractive surgery such as incisional keratotomy, conductive keratoplasty, and refractive lens exchange, which provide a viable alternative to laser vision correction.

As compared with LASIK, in which the main complications are flap-related (such as thin, incomplete, and buttonhole flaps), complications of many non–excimer-based refractive surgery may be more serious and range from glare and halos to cataracts and retinal detachment.

19.2.2 Complications of Incisional, Thermal, and Inlay Keratorefractive Procedures

19.2.2.1 Complications of Radial Keratotomy and Astigmatic Keratotomy

Keratotomy and Astigmatic Keratotomy Infectious keratitis is the most commonly reported complication after incisional refractive surgery (in the early or late postoperative period). *Staphylococcus* is the most frequently isolated organism in early-onset infections, whereas *Pseudomonas* causes most late-onset infections [1]. *Acanthamoeba* and *Pseudomonas aeruginosa* have also been isolated (Table 19.2.1). In a review, Jain et al. reported 47 cases of infectious keratitis between years 1975 and 1994 [2]. Iatrogenic keratoconus and subepithelial fibrosis have also been reported as complications of incisional refractive surgery (Table 19.2.1). The complications of radial keratotomy (RK) related to dehiscence during cataract surgery are summarized in Table 19.2.1.

19.2.2.2 Complications of Conductive Keratoplasty

Conductive keratoplasty (CK) is a method used mainly to correct low-to-moderate hyperopia. Radio frequencies delivered directly to the peripheral cornea steep the surface of the cornea by contraction of collagen fiber. This method is US Food and Drug Administration (FDA)-approved. Early haze formation (within 6 months postoperatively) and anterior chamber inflammation seem to be the major complications. The incidence of haze formation peaks at 6 months and varies up to 20%, and eventually improves (less than 2%) within a year [13]. Temporary inflammation is very common 1 month postoperatively (50%). Loss of two or more lines of BCVA is less than 2% (Table 19.2.2).

19.2.2.3 Complications of Intacs and Inlay Procedures

19.2.2.3.1 Intra Corneal Ring Segment (Intacs)

Intrastromal corneal ring segments (ICRSs), or Intacs, are placed in the peripheral stroma at approximately two-thirds' depth, outside the central optical zone, to reshape the anterior corneal surface while maintaining the positive asphericity of the cornea. Results of Intacs may be encouraging; however, complications by several refractive surgeons were reported (Table 19.2.3). Schanzlin et al. and Asbell et al. reported the incidence rate of haze to be 96.2 and 75.1% respectively. Other high reported complications include neovascularization, halos, glare, epithelial cyst, and difficulty with night vision (Table 19.2.3).

19.2.2.3.2 Inlay Complications

One of the complications reported with inlay procedures is diffuse perilenticular opacity. Alió et al reported a 45% (5 out of 11 eyes) incidence rate after inlay [31].

19.2.3 Complications of Phakic Intraocular Lenses

Patients who are poor candidates for refractive surgery due to high myopia or hyperopia are considered candidates for visual rehabilitation with phakic intraocular lenses (PIOLs). In 2003, a survey of members of the American Society of Cataract and Refractive Surgery reported 17.4% of respondents inserted PIOLs [32]. The refractive and visual outcomes of PIOLs have been encouraging to date, yet the potential for significant complications exist in angle, iris, and post-supported PIOLs. Evidence from the literature in the past 10 years shows that cataract is a common complication that results following phakic IOLs. The risk of retinal detachment in high myopes is high. Additional complications include elevated intraocular pressure, papillary block, endothelial cell loss, and pupil ovalization.

Table 19.2.1 Infectious keratitis and other complications

Author	Total no. of eyes	Cases	Incidence rate (%)	Comment(s)
Heidemann 1999 [1]	NA	14	NA	10 early, 9 late RK
Utine 2006 [3]	170	1	0.6	
Adrean 2005 [4]	NA	3	NA	Case reports after PK
Friedmann 1997 [5]	NA	1	NA	A case report of *Acanthamoeba*
Erkin 1998 [6]	NA	1	NA	A case report of *P. aeruginosa*
Procope 1997 [7]	NA	1	NA	A case report of *P. aeruginosa*
Jain 1996 [2]	NA	47	NA	1975–1994
Iatrogenic keratoconus				
Shaikh 2002 [8]	NA	1	NA	Case report
Subepithelial fibrosis				
Majmudar 2000 [9]	6	3	50	
Dehiscence of RK incision during cataract operation				
Budak 1998 [10]	1	NA	NA	11 years
Behl 2001 [11]	1	NA	NA	9 months
Freeman 2004 [12]	1	NA	NA	14 years

NA not applicable

19.2.3.1 Cataract

The estimated incidence rate of cataract formation was highest in post supported PIOLs (10.3%) compared to angle and iris supported PIOLs, 3.8 and 1.7% respectively (Table 19.2.4). Cataract after PIOL insertion is not age-related but is due to trauma after surgery.

19.2.3.2 Retinal Detachment

High myopes have a high risk of retinal detachment after insertion of PIOL, with an incidence rate of 1.3% (Table 19.2.5).

19.2.3.3 Intraocular Pressure

A high incidence rate of elevated intraocular pressure (IOP) was estimated from reported cases in the literature with angle-supported phakic IOLs (10.1%), compared with iris (2.7%) and post (3.1%) (Table 19.2.6)

19.2.3.4 Pupillary Block

Pupillary block, a sight-threatening complication, is not rare in spite the routine preoperative YAG iridotomy. The incidence is the highest in posterior chamber phakic IOL. On the other hand, it is very rare in iris-supported phakic IOL (Table 19.2.7).

19.2.3.5 Endothelial Cell Loss

Endothelial cell loss after phakic IOL implantation is caused by many factors. Surgical trauma must be the major factor and explanation of the various rate of cell loss. Long-term studies also reveal the continuous decrease, suggesting the influence of chronic inflammation and intermittent contact between the IOL and endothelium (Table 19.2.8).

19.2.3.6 Pupil Ovalization

Pupil ovalization is one of the most common complications after angle-supported PIOLs. Incidence rates are reported from 6 to 46% (Table 19.2.9). This complication may also occur years later because of angular fibrosis.

19.2.4 Retinal Detachment after Refractive Lens Exchange

Estimates of retinal detachment risk in the un-operated-on highly myopic population vary from 0.4 to 0.68% per person year [71, 72]. The average incidence of retinal detachment is 4.2%. It is possible to say that clear lens extraction can increase the risk of retinal detachment. Despite the technological improvement in cataract surgery, no improvement seems to be confirmed in the literature for the past 10 years (Table 19.2.10).

Table 19.2.2 Complications of CK

Incidence rate of haze (cases/total no [%eyes])						
Author	**1 month**	**3 months**	**6 months**	**9 months**	**12 months**	**24 months**
McDonald 2005 [13]	6/390 (1.5%)	15/392 (3.8%)	12/389 (3.1%)	0/386	0/391	
Lin 2003 [14]	0/25	0/25	0/25	0/25	0/25	0/25
McDonald (2002) 15	6/51(11.76%)		10/51 (19.60%)		1/51 (2%)	
Intraocular pressure >25 mmHg						
McDonald 2005 [13]			2/389 (0.5%)	1/386 (0.3%)	1/391 (0.3%)	
McDonald 2002 [15]			2 /51 (3.9%)			
Iritis						
McDonald 2005 [13]					1/391 (0.3%)	
FDA report 2002 [16]		1/401 (0.3%)				
Lin 2003 [14]		1/25 (4%)				
Moshirfar 2005 [17]	7/14 (50%)					
Loss of two or more lines of BCVA						
McDonald 2005 [13]	33/390 (8.5%)	24/392 (6.1%)	18/389 (4.6%)	15/386 (4%)	9/391 (2.3%)	6/322 (2%)
Fernandez-Suntay 2004 [18]					7/355 (2%)	
Pallikaris 2005 [19]					0/38	
Lin 2003 [14]	0/25	1/25 (4%)	0/24	1/21 (5%)	0/25	0/24
Naoumidi 2006 [20]						0/47
Endothelial cell loss						
McDonald 2005 [13]		0/392	0/389		0/391	
Fernandez-Suntay 2004 [18]		0/162	0/162		0/162	

19.2.5 Conclusion

The advancements in non–excimer laser refractive technology have yielded satisfactory visual and refractive outcomes. The possible main indications of non-excimer procedures are high myopia, presbyopia, and thin cornea. These procedures may have complications that are different from excimer laser complications, and patients should be aware that although complications are infrequent they might result in reduced vision.

Take-Home Pearls

- Phakic IOLs
  - Indications: high myopia or hyperopia
  - Complications: cataract, elevated IOP, papillary block, endothelial cell loss, and pupil ovalization
- CK
  - Indications: presbyopia
  - Complications: early haze formation and surgically induced astigmatism
- Intacs
  - Indications: thin cornea, early keratoconus
  - Complications: haze, neovascularization, halos, glare, epithelial cyst, and difficulty with night vision
- Prospective studies are recommended to evaluate the risk factors and severity of complications in non-excimer refractive surgery.

Table 19.2.3 Intacs complications

Segment move				
Author	**Total no. of eyes**	**Cases**	**Incidence rate (%)**	**Comment**
Kanellopoulos 2006 [21	20	2	10	2 Exposed
Colin 2007 [22]	100	0	0	
Boxer Wachler 2001 [23]	74	1	1.4	
Asbell 2001 [24]	106	0	0	
Total	300	3	1	
Corneal infiltrate/melt				
Kanellopoulos 2006 [21]	20	1	5	Melt
Boxer Wachler 2001 [23]	74	0	0	
McAlister 2006 [25]	NA	1	NA	Case report
Total	94	1	1.1	
Neovascularization				
Colin 2007 [22]	100	0	0	
Kymionis 2007 [26]	17	12	70.6	5 years
Alió 2006 [27]	13	2	15.4	6 months
Siganos 2003 [28]	33	1	3	2 months
Total	163	15	9.2	
Haze surrounding Intacs				
Asbell 2001 [24]	106	102	96.2	Within the stromal channel
Schanzlin 2001 [29]	358	269	75.1	
Total	464	371	80	
Epithelial cyst				
Colin 2007 [22]	100	21	21	
Asbell 2001 [24]	106	3	2.8	
Schanzlin 2001 [29]	358	25	7	24 months
Total	564	49	8.7	
Deposit				
Colin 2007 [22]	100	22	22	2 years
Kymionis 2007 [26]	17	12	70.6	5 years
Asbell 2001 [24]	106	61	57.5	
Alió 2006 [27]	13	4	30.8	
Siganos 2003 [28]	33	Majority	NA	6 months
Total	236	99	41.9	
Iron line				
Asbell 2001 [24]	106	36	34	
Glare				
Asbell 2001 [24]	106	16	15.1	2 Rings removed
Colin 2006 [30]	28	5	17.9	Peak 3 months
Total	134	21	15.7	

19

Table 19.2.3 *continued*

Segment move				
Author	**Total no. of eyes**	**Cases**	**Incidence rate (%)**	**Comment**
Halo				
Asbell 2001 [24]	106	24	22.4	2 Rings removed
Colin 2006 [30]	28	3	10.7	Peak 3 months
Total	134	27	20.1	
Pain/foreign body sensation				
Asbell 2001 [24]	106	1	0.9	Ring removed
Colin 2006 [30]	28	1	3.6	Peak 3 months
Total	134	2	1.5	
Difficulty with night vision				
Asbell 2001 [24]	106	19	17.7	
Colin 2006 [30]	28	3	10.7	Peak 3 months
Total	134	22	16.4	
Infection				
Schanzlin 2001 [29]	449	1	0.2	

NA not available

Table 19.2.4 Phakic IOL complication: Cataract

Cataract					
Author	**Total no. of eyes**	**Cases**	**Incidence rate (%)**	**Lens**	**Comments**	**Age in years (±SD)**
Perez-Santonja 2000 [33]	23	0	0	Angle		31.52±4.77
Alió 2000 [34]	263	9	3.4	Angle		NA
de Souza 2001 [35]	26	3	11.5	Angle		35.9±6.7
Total	312	12	3.8	Angle		
Maloney 1999 [36]	155	4	2.6	Iris		39
Menezo 2004 [37]	137	2	1.46	Iris		36.2±9.6
Menezo 2004 [38]	232	7	3	Iris	Nuclear cataract	
Dick 2003 [39]	70	0	0	Iris		35
Tehrani 2006 [40]	40	0	0	Iris		36
Lifshitz 2005 [41]	31	0	0	Iris		25.7± 5.9
Budo 2000 [42]	249	6	2.4	Iris	–5.00 to ca. –20	36.4± 9.7
Total	914	19	2.1	Iris		
Lackner 2004 [43]	76	11	14.5	Post, STAAR		48.3±7.4
Sarikkola 2005 [44]	38	18	47.4	Post, STAAR		34 (including >45)
Sarikkola 2005 [44]	45	2	7.7	Post, STAAR		34 (all <45)

Table 19.2.4 *continued*

Cataract						
Author	**Total no. of eyes**	**Cases**	**Incidence rate (%)**	**Lens**	**Comments**	**Age in years (±SD)**
Lackner 2003 [45]	75	25	33.5	Post, STAAR		38.3±11.5
Sanchez-Galeana [46]	170	14	8.2	Post, STAAR		37.1± 8.4
Dejaco-Ruhswurm 2002 [47]	34	4	11.8	Post, STAAR		39.8±9.6
Brauweiler 1999 [48]	17	9	52.9	Post, Adatomed		28-53
Pineda-Fernandez 2004 [49]	18	2	11.1	Post, STAAR		34.5±5.7
Pallikaris 2004 [50]	34	1	2.9	Post, Chiba		29±7.9
Uusitalo 2002 [51]	38	2	5.2	Post, STAAR	One is slight	39
Arne 2000 [52]	48	2	4.2	Post, STAAR		NA
Menezo 2004 [37]	59	26	44.1	Post, Adatomed		39.1± 4.5
Menezo 2004 [37]	21	2	9.5	Post, STAAR		31.3± 9.6
Menezo 2004 [38]	89	38	42.7	Post, Adatomed	Anterior subcapsular cataract	
Menezo 2004 [38]	23	3	13	Post, STAAR	Anterior subcapsular cataract	
ITM study group 2004 [53]	526	7	1.4	Post, STAAR	Clinically significant	36.5±5.8
Total	1209	125	10.3	Post		

Table 19.2.5 Phakic IOL complication: retinal detachment

Author	**Total no. of eyes**	**Cases**	**Incidence rate (%)**	**Lens**	**Refraction (±SD)**	**Age years (±SD)**	**Comment**
Gierek-Ciaciura 2007 [54]	20	0	0	Angle	−15.76±3.13	30±8.02	
Ruiz–Moreno 1999 [55]	166	8	4.8	Angle	−18.62±5.00		
Alió 1999 [56]	263	8	3	Angle	NA		
Perez-Santonja 2000 [33]	23	0	0	Angle	−19.56±1.76	31.52±4.77	
Budo 2000 [42]	249	2	0.8	Iris	−5.00 to ca. −20	36.4±9.7	
Dick 2003 [39]	70	0	0	Iris	−6.50 to ca. −21.25	35	
Lifshitz 2004 [41]	31	0	0	Iris	−5.29 to ca. −19		
Tehrani 2006 [57]	40	0	0	Iris	−9.84±4,98	36	
Tahzib 2006 [58]	36	0	0	Iris	−3.19±4.31	63.8±17	Toric
Gierek-Ciaciura 2007 [54]	20	0	0	Iris	−15.73±3.06	32.25±9.5	
Zaldivar 1998 [59]	124	1	0.8	Post, STAAR	−8 to ca. −19		
Arne 2000 [52]	48	0	0	Post, STAAR	−13.85±3.1	NA	
ITM study group 2004 [54]	526	3	0.6	Post, STAAR	−10.06±3.74	age 36.5±5.8	

19

Table 19.2.5 *continued*

Author	Total no. of eyes	Cases	Incidence rate (%)	Lens	Refraction (±SD)	Age years (±SD)	Comment
Pannozo 2001 [60]	NA	4	NA	Post, STAAR	NA		Case report
Uusitalo 2002 [51]	38	0	0	Post, STAAR	−15.10		1 Macular degeneration
Total	1654	22	1.33	Angle, Iris, Post			

NA not available

Table 19.2.6 Phakic IOL complication: IOP

Author	Total no. of eyes	Cases	Incidence rate (%)	Lens	Comment
Baikoff 1998 [61]	133	23	17.3	Angle(ZB5M)	
Alió 1999 [56]	263	19	7.2	Angle	IOP > 21 mmHg
Perez-Santonja 2000 [33]	23	3	13	Angle	
Leccisotti 2005 [62]	43	2	4.7	Angle	
Total	462	47	10.1	Angle	
Maloney 1999 [36]	155	4	2.6	Iris	IOP > 21 mmHg next day
El Danasoury 2002 [63]	90	2	4.4	Iris	
Asano-Kato 2005 [64]	44	2	4.5	Iris	IOP > 21 mmHg
Lifshitz 2004 [41]	31	0	0	Iris	
Tehrani 2006 [40]	40	2	5	Iris	−9.84±4.98
Total	360	10	2.7	Iris	
Arne 2000 [52]	48	2	4.2	Post, STAAR	
Lackner 2002 [43]	75	6	8	Post, STAAR	
Pineda-Fernandez 2004 [49]	18	5	27.8	Post, STAAR	
Pallikaris 2004 [50]	34	8	23.5	post, Chiba	IOP > 20 mmHg
ITM study group 2004 [54]	526	3	0.6	Post, STAAR	IOP > 25 mmHg, or increase >10 mmHg
Total	701	24	3.1	Post, STAAR	

Table 19.2.7 Phakic IOL complication: pupillary block

Author	Total no. of eyes	Cases	Incidence rate (%)	Lens
Perez-Santonja 2000 [33]	23	0	0	Angle
Allemann 2000 [65]	21	0	0	Angle
de Souza 2001 [35]	26	3	11.5	Angle
Leccisotti 2005 [62]	43	1	2.3	Angle
Total	113	4	3.5	Angle
Budo 2000 [42]	249	2	0.8	Iris
Dick 2003 [39]	70	0	0	Iris
Lifshitz 2004 [41]	31	0	0	Iris
Tehrani 2006 [40]	40	0	0	Iris
Total	390	2	0.5	Iris
Brauweiler 1999 [48]	17	3	17.6	Post, Adatomed
Uusitalo 2002 [51]	38	3	7.9	Post, STAAR
Pineda-Fernandez 2004 [49]	18	2	11.1	Post, STAAR
Sarikkola 2005 [44]	45	3	7.7	Post, STAAR
Total	118	11	9.3	Post

Table 19.2.8 Phakic IOL complication: endothelial cell loss

Author	Lens	Total no. of eyes	3 months (%)	6 months (%)	1 year (%)	2 years (%)	3 years (%)	4 years (%)	5 years (%)	6 years (%)	7 years (%)
Baikoff 1998 [61]	Angle ZB5M	133		3.3							
Alió 1999 [56]	Angle	263	3.8	3.4	5.5	6.8	7.5	7.8	8.3	8.7	9.3
Perez-Santonja 2000 [33]	Angle	18	1.4	1.73	4.2						
de Souza 2001 [35]	Angle	26							1.53		
Coullet 2006 [66]	Angle ARTIFLEX	31			9						
Gierek-Ciaciura 2007 [54]	Angle	20			6.8						
Perez-Santonja 1996 [67]	Iris	NA		10.6	13	17.6					
Menezo 1998 [68]	Iris	111		3.9	6.6	9.2	11.7	13.4			
Landesz 2000 [69]	Iris	67		5.5	7.21	9.1	10.9				
Budo 2000 [42]	Iris	129		4.8	7.2	8.9	9.6				
Saxen 2003 [70]	Iris	26				8.5	11.7				
Dick 2003 [39]	Iris	70	4.9	4.5							
Menezo 2004 [37, 38]	Iris	217		3.3	5.5	7.6			10.5		
Lifshitz 2005 [41]	Iris	21	4								
Coullet 2006 [66]	Iris	31			9.4						
Gierek-Ciaciura 2007 [54]	Iris	20			6.1						
Dejaco-Ruhswurm 2002 [47]	Post, STAAR	34	1.8	4.2	5.5	7.9	12.9	12.3			
Pineda-Fernandez 2004 [49]	Post, STAAR	18		4.9	5	5.3	6.1				
ITM study group 2004 [53]	Post, STAAR	526					8.4–9.7				

NA not applicable

19

Table 19.2.9 Ovalization in angle-supported PIOL

Author	Total no. of eyes	Cases	Incidence rate (%)	Comment
Perez-Santonja 2000 [33]	23	4	17.4	12 and 24 months
Alió 1999 [56]	263	16	6.1	7 years
de Souza 2001[35]	26	12	46.1	5 years
Leccisotti 2005 [62]	43	6	13.9	
Total	355	38	10.7	

Table 19.2.10 Retinal detachment after refractive lens exchange

Author	Total no. of eyes	Cases	Incidence rate (%)	Diopter (±SD)	Duration (months)	Comment
Colin 1999 [73]	49	4	8.1	>12	7 years	
Racalico 2003 [74]	388	1	0.3	−15.95±5.86	46.16±32.83	
Chastang 1998 [75]	33	2	6.1	>12	84	
Lee 1996 [76]	24	0	0	>12	NA	
Jimenez-Alfaro 1998 [77]	26	0	0	NA	12	
Gris 1996 [78]	46	1	2.2	−16.05	6 to ca.15	
Ceschi 1998 [79]	40	0	0	−14.50±3.6	45.9	1 Macular edema
Wang 1998 [80]	120	0	0	AX > 28mm	14.5	No macular edema
Lyle 1997 [81]	20	0	0	NA	23.2	
Alldredge 1998 [82]	80	0	0	≤7	43	No intraoperative complication
Guell JL 2003 [83]	44	0	0	−15.77	48	1 retinal tear without detachment
Vicary 1999 [84]	138	1	0.7	−0.25 to −23.75 +0.25 to +11.62 +0.25 to +11.62		No edema
Gabric 2002 [85]	72	1	1.4	NA.	48	1 RD with cystoid macula edema
Jacobi 1997 [86]	386	3	0.8	29.2±1.71 mm	3.8±2 years	1 Expulsive
Tosi 2003 [87]	73	1	1.3	30.22 mm	62.3	All are aphakia
Ku 2002 [88]	125	2	1.6	>26 mm	NA	After YAG
Fan 1999 [89]	118	2	1.7	30.13±2.08 mm	NA	13 patients with retinal tear
Fernandez-Vega 2003 [90]	190	4	2.1		4.78-year range, 3.10-8.03 years	Subfoveal CNV developed in 4 eyes
Horgan 2005 [91]	62	2	3.2	−7.00 to −22.75 −13.7±4.3 D	NA	12 Macular degeneration
Pucci 2001 [92]	25	1	4	>12	42.92±3.76	
Ripandelli 2003 [93]	930	74	8	−15 and −30	36	
Arne 2004 [94]	36	2	5	−16.7±3.8	47.65	
Total	2,215	94	4.2			

NA not available

References

1. Heidemann DG, Dunn SP, Chow CY (1999) Early- versus late-onset infectious keratitis after radial and astigmatic keratotomy: clinical spectrum in a referral practice. J Cataract Refract Surg 25:1615–1619
2. Jain S, Azar DT (1996) Eye infections after refractive keratotomy. J Refract Surg 12:148–155
3. Utine CA, Bayraktar S, Kaya V, Kucuksumer Y, Eren H, Perente I, Yilmaz OF (2006) Radial keratotomy for the optical rehabilitation of mild to moderate keratoconus: more than 5 years' experience. Eur J Ophthalmol 16:376–384
4. Adrean SD, Cochrane R, Reilly CD, Mannis MJ (2005) Infectious keratitis after astigmatic keratotomy in penetrating keratoplasty: review of three cases. Cornea 24:626–628
5. Friedman RF, Wolf TC, Chodosh J (1997) Acanthamoeba infection after radial keratotomy. Am J Ophthalmol 123:409–410
6. Erkin EF, Durak I, Ferliel S, Maden A (1998) Keratitis complicated by endophthalmitis 3 years after astigmatic keratotomy. J Cataract Refract Surg 24:1280–1282
7. Procope JA (1997) Delayed-onset Pseudomonas keratitis after radial keratotomy. J Cataract Refract Surg 23:1271–1272

8. Shaikh S, Shaikh NM, Manche E (2002) Iatrogenic keratoconus as a complication of radial keratotomy. J Cataract Refract Surg 28:553–555

9. Majmudar PA, Raviv T, Dennis RF, Epstein RJ (2000) Subepithelial fibrosis after RK. J Cataract Refract Surg 26:1433–1434

10. Budak K, Friedman NJ, Koch DD (1998) Dehiscence of a radial keratotomy incision during clear corneal cataract surgery. J Cataract Refract Surg 24:278–280

11. Behl S, Kothari K (2001) Rupture of a radial keratotomy incision after 11 years during clear corneal phacoemulsification. J Cataract Refract Surg 27:1132–1134

12. Freeman M, Kumar V, Ramanathan US, O'Neill E (2004) Dehiscence of radial keratotomy incision during phacoemulsification. Eye 18:101–103

13. McDonald MB (2005) Conductive keratoplasty: a radiofrequency-based technique for the correction of hyperopia. Trans Am Ophthalmol Soc 103:512–536

14. Lin DY, Manche EE (2003) Two-year results of conductive keratoplasty for the correction of low to moderate hyperopia. J Cataract Refract Surg 29:2339–2350

15. McDonald MB, Davidorf J, Maloney RK, Manche EE, Hersh P (2002) Conductive keratoplasty for the correction of low to moderate hyperopia: 1-year results on the first 54 eyes. Ophthalmology 109:637–649

16. U.S. Food and Drug Administration, Center for Devices and Radiological Health (200) Ophthalmic Devices Panel meeting summary, 11 April 2002. Available at: http://www.fda.gov/cdrh/pdf/p010018.html

17. Moshirfar M, Feilmeier M, Kumar R (2005) Anterior chamber inflammation induced by conductive keratoplasty. J Cataract Refract Surg 31:1676–1677

18. Fernandez-Suntay JP, Pineda R II, Azar DT (2004) Conductive keratoplasty. Int Ophthalmol Clin 44:161–1618

19. Pallikaris IG, Naoumidi TL, Astyrakakis NI (2005) Long-term results of conductive keratoplasty for low to moderate hyperopia. J Cataract Refract Surg 31:1520–1529

20. Naoumidi TL, Kounis GA, Astyrakakis NI, Tsatsaronis DN, Pallikaris IG (2006) Two-year follow-up of conductive keratoplasty for the treatment of hyperopic astigmatism. J Cataract Refract Surg 32:732–741

21. Kanellopoulos AJ, Pe LH, Perry HD, Donnenfeld ED (2006) Modified intracorneal ring segment implantations (INTACS) for the management of moderate to advanced keratoconus: efficacy and complications. Cornea 25:29–33

22. Colin J, Malet FJ (2007) Intacs for the correction of keratoconus: Two-year follow-up. J Cataract Refract Surg 33:69–74

23. Boxer Wachler BS, Christie JP, Chandra NS, Chou B, Korn T, Nepomuceno R (2003) Intacs for keratoconus. Ophthalmology 110:1031–1040

24. Asbell PA, Ucakhan OO (2001) Long-term follow-up of Intacs from a single center. J Cataract Refract Surg 27:1456–1468

25. McAlister JC, Ardjomand N, Ilari L, Mengher LS, Gartry DS (2006) Keratitis after intracorneal ring segment insertion for keratoconus. J Cataract Refract Surg 32:676–678

26. Kymionis GD, Siganos CS, Tsiklis NS, Anastasakis A, Yoo SH, Pallikaris AI, Astyrakakis N, Pallikaris IG (2007) Long-term follow-up of Intacs in keratoconus. Am J Ophthalmol 143:236–44

27. Alió JL, Shabayek MH, Artola A (2006) Intracorneal ring segments for keratoconus correction: long-term follow-up. J Cataract Refract Surg 32:978–985

28. Siganos CS, Kymionis GD, Kartakis N, Theodorakis MA, Astyrakakis N, Pallikaris IG (2003) Management of keratoconus with Intacs. Am J Ophthalmol 135:64–70

29. Schanzlin DJ, Abbott RL, Asbell PA, Assil KK, Burris TE, Durrie DS, Fouraker BD, Lindstrom RL, McDonald JE II, Verity SM, Waring GO III (2001) Two-year outcomes of intrastromal corneal ring segments for the correction of myopia. Ophthalmology 108:1688–1694

30. Colin J (2006) European clinical evaluation: use of Intacs for the treatment of keratoconus. J Cataract Refract Surg 32:747–55

31. Alió JL, Mulet ME, Zapata LF, Vidal MT, De Rojas V, Javaloy J (2004) Intracorneal inlay complicated by intrastromal epithelial opacification. Arch Ophthalmol 122:1441–1446

32. Solomon R, Donnenfeld ED (2006) Refractive intraocular lenses: multifocal and phakic IOLs. Int Ophthalmol Clin 46:123–143

33. Perez-Santonja JJ, Alió JL, Jimenez-Alfaro I, Zato MA (2000) Surgical correction of severe myopia with an angle-supported phakic intraocular lens. J Cataract Refract Surg 26:1288–1302

34. Alió JL, de la Hoz F, Ruiz-Moreno JM, Salem TF (2000) Cataract surgery in highly myopic eyes corrected by phakic anterior chamber angle-supported lenses(1). J Cataract Refract Surg 26:1303–1311

35. de Souza RF, Forseto A, Nose R, Belfort R Jr, Nose W (2001) Anterior chamber intraocular lens for high myopia: five year results. J Cataract Refract Surg 27:1248–1253

36. Maloney RK, Nguyen LH, John ME (2002) Artisan phakic intraocular lens for myopia:short-term results of a prospective, multicenter study. Ophthalmology 109:1631–1641

37. Menezo JL, Peris-Martinez C, Cisneros AL, Martinez-Costa R (2004) Phakic intraocular lenses to correct high myopia: Adatomed, STAAR, and ARTISAN. J Cataract Refract Surg 30:33–44

38. Menezo JL, Peris-Martinez C, Cisneros-Lanuza AL, Martinez-Costa R (2004) Rate of cataract formation in 343 highly myopic eyes after implantation of three types of phakic intraocular lenses. J Refract Surg 20:317–234

39. Dick HB, Alió J, Bianchetti M, Budo C, Christiaans BJ, El-Danasoury MA, Guell JL, Krumeich J, Landesz M, Loureiro F, Luyten GP, Marinho A, Rahhal MS, Schwenn O, Spirig R, Thomann U, Venter J (2003) Toric phakic intraocular lens: European multicenter study. Ophthalmology 110:150–162

40. Tehrani M, Dick HB (2006) Iris-fixated toric phakic intraocular lens: Three-year follow-up. J Cataract Refract Surg 32:1301–1306

41. Lifshitz T, Levy J, Aizenman I, Klemperer I, Levinger S (2004) Artisan phakic intraocular lens for correcting high myopia. Int Ophthalmol25:233–238

42. Budo C, Hessloehl JC, Izak M, Luyten GP, Menezo JL, Sener BA, Tassignon MJ, Termote H, Worst JG (2000) Multicenter study of the Artisan phakic intraocular lens. J Cataract Refract Surg 26:1163–1171

43. Lackner B, Pieh S, Schmidinger G, Simader C, Franz C, Dejaco-Ruhswurm I, Skorpik C (2004) Long-term results of implantation of phakic posterior chamber intraocular lenses. J Cataract Refract Surg 30:2269–7226

44. Sarikkola AU, Sen HN, Uusitalo RJ, Laatikainen L. Traumatic cataract and other adverse events with the implantable contact lens. J Cataract Refract Surg 2005 31:511–524

45. Lackner B, Pieh S, Schmidinger G, Hanselmayer G, Dejaco-Ruhswurm I, Funovics MA, Skorpik C (2003) Outcome after treatment of ametropia with implantable contact lenses. Ophthalmology 110:2153–2161

46. Sanchez-Galeana CA, Smith RJ, Sanders DR, Rodriguez FX, Litwak S, Montes M, Chayet AS (2003) Lens opacities after posterior chamber phakic intraocular lens implantation. Ophthalmology 110:781–785

47. Dejaco-Ruhswurm I, Scholz U, Pieh S, Hanselmayer G, Lackner B, Italon C, Ploner M, Skorpik C (2002) Long-term endothelial changes in phakic eyes with posterior chamber intraocular lenses. J Cataract Refract Surg 28:1589–1593

19

48. Brauweiler PH, Wehler T, Busin M (1999) High incidence of cataract formation after implantation of a silicone posterior chamber lens in phakic, highly myopic eyes. Ophthalmology 106:1651–1655

49. Pineda-Fernandez A, Jaramillo J, Vargas J, Jaramillo M, Jaramillo J, Galindez A (2004) Phakic posterior chamber intraocular lens for high myopia. J Cataract Refract Surg 30:2277–2283

50. Pallikaris IG, Kalyvianaki MI, Kymionis GD, Panagopoulou SI (2004) Phakic refractive lens implantation in high myopic patients: one-year results. J Cataract Refract Surg 30:1190–1197

51. Uusitalo RJ, Aine E, Sen NH, Laatikainen L (2002) Implantable contact lens for high myopia. J Cataract Refract Surg 28:29–36

52. Arne JL, Lesueur LC (2000) Phakic posterior chamber lenses for high myopia: functional and anatomical outcomes. J Cataract Refract Surg 26:369–374

53. Sanders DR, Doney K, Poco M; ICL in Treatment of Myopia Study Group (2004) United States Food and Drug Administration clinical trial of the Implantable Collamer Lens (ICL) for moderate to high myopia: three-year follow-up. Ophthalmology 111:1683–1692

54. Gierek-Ciaciura S, Gierek-Lapinska A, Ochalik K, Mrukwa-Kominek E (2007) Correction of high myopia with different phakic anterior chamber intraocular lenses: ICARE angle-supported lens and Verisyse iris-claw lens. Graefes Arch Clin Exp Ophthalmol 245:1–7

55. Ruiz-Moreno JM, Alió JL, Perez-Santonja JJ, de la Hoz F (1999) Retinal detachment in phakic eyes with anterior chamber intraocular lenses to correct severe myopia. Am J Ophthalmol 127:270–275

56. Alió JL, de la Hoz F, Perez-Santonja JJ, Ruiz-Moreno JM, Quesada JA (1999) Phakic anterior chamber lenses for the correction of myopia: a 7-year cumulative analysis of complications in 263 cases. Ophthalmology 106:458–466

57. Tehrani M, Dick HB (2006) Iris-fixated toric phakic intraocular lens: Three-year follow-up. J Cataract Refract Surg 32:1301–6

58. Tahzib NG, Cheng YY, Nuijts RM (2006) Three-year follow-up analysis of Artisan toric lens implantation for correction of postkeratoplasty ametropia in phakic and pseudophakic eyes. Ophthalmology 113:976–984

59. Zaldivar R, Davidorf JM, Oscherow S (1998) Posterior chamber phakic intraocular lens for myopia of -8 to -19 diopters. J Refract Surg 14:294–305

60. Panozzo G, Parolini B (2001) Relationships between vitreoretinal and refractive surgery. Ophthalmology 108:1663–1668

61. Baikoff G, Arne JL, Bokobza Y, Colin J, George JL, Lagoutte F, Lesure P, Montard M, Saragoussi JJ, Secheyron P (1998) Angle-fixated anterior chamber phakic intraocular lens for myopia of −7 to −19 diopters. J Refract Surg 14:282–293

62. Leccisotti A (2005) Bioptics by angle-supported phakic lenses and photorefractive keratectomy. Eur J Ophthalmol 15:1–7

63. El Danasoury MA, El Maghraby A, Gamali TO (2002) Comparison of iris-fixed Artisan lens implantation with excimer laser in situ keratomileusis in correcting myopia between −9.00 and -19.50 diopters: a randomized study. Ophthalmology 109:955–964

64. Asano-Kato N, Toda I, Hori-Komai Y, Sakai C, Fukumoto T, Arai H, Dogru M, Takano Y, Tsubota K (2005) Experience with the Artisan phakic intraocular lens in Asian eyes. J Cataract Refract Surg 31:910–915

65. Allemann N, Schneider A (2000) ATP production in isolated mitochondria of procyclic Trypanosoma brucei. Mol Biochem Parasitol 111:87–94

66. Coullet J, Guell JL, Fournie P, Grandjean H, Gaytan J, Arne JL, Malecaze F (2006) Iris-supported phakic lenses (rigid vs foldable version) for treating moderately high myopia: randomized paired eye comparison. Am J Ophthalmol 142:909–916

67. Perez-Santonja JJ, Iradier MT, Sanz-Iglesias L, Serrano JM, Zato MA (1996) Endothelial changes in phakic eyes with anterior chamber intraocular lenses to correct high myopia. J Cataract Refract Surg 22:1017–1022

68. Menezo JL, Cisneros AL, Rodriguez-Salvador V (1998) Endothelial study of iris-claw phakic lens: four year follow-up. J Cataract Refract Surg 24:1039–1049

69. Landesz M, Worst JG, van Rij G (2000) Long-term results of correction of high myopia with an iris claw phakic intraocular lens. J Refract Surg 16:310–316

70. Saxena R, Landesz M, Noordzij B, Luyten GP (2003) Three-year follow-up of the Artisan phakic intraocular lens for hypermetropia. Ophthalmology 110:1391–1395

71. Burton TC (1989) The influence of refractive error and lattice degeneration on the incidence of retinal detachment. Trans Am Ophthalmol Soc 87:143–515

72. Perkins ES (1979) Morbidity from myopia. Sight Sav Rev 49:11–19

73. Colin J, Robinet A, Cochener B (1999) Retinal detachment after clear lens extraction for high myopia: seven-year follow-up. Ophthalmology 106:2281–2284

74. Ravalico G, Michieli C, Vattovani O, Tognetto D (2003) Retinal detachment after cataract extraction and refractive lens exchange in highly myopic patients. J Cataract Refract Surg 29:39–44

75. Chastang P, Ruellan YM, Rozenbaum JP, Besson D, Hamard H. Phacoemulsification for visual refraction on the clear lens (1998) Apropos of 33 severely myopic eyes. J Fr Ophtalmol 21:560–566

76. Lee KH, Lee JH (1996) Long-term results of clear lens extraction for severe myopia. J Cataract Refract Surg 22:1411–1415

77. Jimenez-Alfaro I, Miguelez S, Bueno JL, Puy P (1998) Clear lens extraction and implantation of negative-power posterior chamber intraocular lenses to correct extreme myopia. J Cataract Refract Surg 24:1310–6

78. Gris O, Guell JL, Manero F, Muller A (1996) Clear lens extraction to correct high myopia. J Cataract Refract Surg 22:686–689

79. Ceschi GP, Artaria LG (1998) Clear lens extraction (CLE) for correction of high grade myopia. Klin Monatsbl Augenheilkd 212:280–282

80. Wang W, Yang G, Nin W, Fang J (1998) Phacoemulsification in myopia and negative or low powered posterior chamber intraocular lens implantation. Zhonghua Yan Ke Za Zhi 34:294–297

81. Lyle WA, Jin GJ (1997) Clear lens extraction to correct hyperopia. J Cataract Refract Surg 23:1051–1056

82. Alldredge CD, Elkins B, Alldredge OC Jr (1998) Retinal detachment following phacoemulsification in highly myopic cataract patients. J Cataract Refract Surg 24:777–780

83. Guell JL, Rodriguez-Arenas AF, Gris O, Malecaze F, Velasco F (2003) Phacoemulsification of the crystalline lens and implantation of an intraocular lens for the correction of moderate and high myopia: four-year follow-up. J Cataract Refract Surg 29:34–38

84. Vicary D, Sun XY, Montgomery P (1999) Refractive lensectomy to correct ametropia. J Cataract Refract Surg 25:943–948

85. Gabric N, Dekaris I, Karaman Z (2002) Refractive lens exchange for correction of high myopia. Eur J Ophthalmol 12:384–387

86. Jacobi FK, Hessemer V (1997) Pseudophakic retinal detachment in high axial myopia. J Cataract Refract Surg 23:1095–1102

87. Tosi GM, Casprini F, Malandrini A, Balestrazzi A, Quercioli PP, Caporossi A (2003) Phacoemulsification without intraocular lens implantation in patients with high myopia: long-term results. J Cataract Refract Surg 29:1127–1131

88. Ku WC, Chuang LH, Lai CC (2002) Cataract extraction in high myopic eyes. Chang Gung Med J 25:315–320

89. Fan DS, Lam DS, Li KK (1999) Retinal complications after cataract extraction in patients with high myopia. Ophthalmology 106:688–691
90. Fernandez-Vega L, Alfonso JF, Villacampa T (2003) Clear lens extraction for the correction of high myopia. Ophthalmology 110:2349–2354
91. Horgan N, Condon PI, Beatty S (2005) Refractive lens exchange in high myopia: long term follow up. Br J Ophthalmol 89:670–672
92. Pucci V, Morselli S, Romanelli F, Pignatto S, Scandellari F, Bellucci R (2001) Clear lens phacoemulsification for correction of high myopia. J Cataract Refract Surg 27:896–900
93. Ripandelli G, Scassa C, Parisi V, Gazzaniga D, D'Amico DJ, Stirpe M (2003) Cataract surgery as a risk factor for retinal detachment in very highly myopic eyes. Ophthalmology 110:2355–2361
94. Arne JL (2004) Phakic intraocular lens implantation versus clear lens extraction in highly myopic eyes of 30- to 50-year-old patients. J Cataract Refract Surg 30:2092–2096

19

Epilog: Preventing Complications in Refractive Surgery – Present and Future

George O. Waring III

There are two approaches to dealing with complications in refractive surgery, avoid them and manage them. This textbook by Alió and colleagues presents a breadth and depth of information in managing complications. I emphasize here the general principles of avoiding complications.

Read

The foundation, the cornerstone, the bedrock, the root, and the underpinning of complication avoidance is education, which is still centered around reading, whether print or electronic text.

- "I just don't have time to read."
- "I subscribe to all the journals–they are in an organized pile in my office."
- "Reading the peer-reviewed journals is difficult and boring."
- (You make up the next excuse.)

No one debates that the peer-reviewed literature is the gold standard for accurate information. We frequently hear the question, "What is the most important technique in refractive surgery?" The surprise answer is, "The prospective randomized clinical trial as reported in the peer-reviewed literature." Indeed, the randomized clinical trial technique has had as big an influence on medicine as did the invention of the microscope; both allow us to see things that were previously not seen or known. Even a well-structured prospective trial without randomization or specific controls can contribute valuable information. For example, postoperative hyperopic shift over time was identified in a clinical series about 10 years after Fyodorov introduced anterior radial keratotomy in humans, and the continued progression of a hyperopic shift up to 10 years after radial keratotomy was documented by the Prospective Evaluation of Radial Keratotomy (PERK) study.

Yes, yes, it is easier, more fun, and more relaxing to read the ophthalmology newspapers and colloquial magazines. Everyone gets their say, it is the latest news, and there are no boring "patients and methods." But consider what we get when we read the peer-reviewed literature: (1) the careful and thoughtful work of the authors through multiple revisions often with high scientific principles, (2) the fruits of peer review–the critical assessment of experts in the field that has led to improvements in the paper, and, (3) prov-

en information that is more clinically and scientifically valid and can lead to better patient treatment, with the more likely avoidance of complications. As in most of life, "you get what you pay for," and in this case we pay with our time and energy to read the peer-reviewed literature, and we get much more for it.

For example, those whose reading was limited to the ophthalmology news magazines were much more likely to enthusiastically treat their patients with hexagonal keratotomy for hyperopia, automated lamellar keratoplasty for myopia, and thermokeratoplasty flattening of keratoconus–procedures that generated complications and quickly feel by the wayside.

You get my point.

Textbooks represent an interesting median between newspapers and tabloids and the peer-reviewed periodical literature; books can contain a wealth of information, especially for surgical techniques that are seldom subjected to prospective randomized trials, but suffer from the lack of peer review, having only the self-critique of the author and the keen eye of the editor for quality control.

No, there is no time. Yes, we must make time–to read.

Listen

This is easier. We have all been listening to lectures since high school, and we will continue to do so throughout our practice lifetimes. Individual lectures and symposia at meetings, courses on a particular topic, and debates as part of a scientific program; all can provide information that can help us avoid complications. There is one prerequisite: We have to show up!

- "I am so busy in the office; I can't get away for meetings."
- "The meetings are so big and complicated. I just get frustrated."
- "The technical exhibits are so fascinating. I just never get to the lectures and courses."
- (Add your own excuse here.)

Many of us will spend enormous amounts of time planning in detail a splendid vacation, with the right location, the right hotel, the right suite, the right transportation, the right golf course, the right tee time, the right restaurant, etc. Similar planning is necessary in advance for our modern complex ophthalmology meetings. Most organizations publish the program far in advance, and the prescient refractive surgeon will plan and fill out a weekly schedule to access the information desired.

Moreover, with a little more effort, one can ask questions in a course or corral a speaker after their talk to listen to their response to specific questions.

Talk

Talk is usually cheap, but not always. The most valuable type of talk is to become the presenter–allowing others to listen.

■ (Insert three objections here.)

Reporting a complication on an individual case or a series of complications on a particular technique has great value. Not only does it inform your colleagues who are listening, but also it requires the speaker to analyze in more detail the complication at hand, to seek insight into why it occurred, to devise techniques of intraoperative prevention and management, and to work out the details of postoperative care.

The aphorism, "You don't know it 'til you teach it," is true enough.

There is another type of talk: conversation. Talking with colleagues about complications is a fundamental mode of self-education: a discussion with practice partners, a call to a trusted surgical colleague or teacher, hall-side consultations on a case at meetings, an informal presentation in local rounds or study groups all can generate helpful information on handling complications.

Watch

All surgeons–including refractive surgeons–learn first by watching a procedure. Initially, this is often by DVD, video tape, or live surgical broadcast, but always leads to watching surgery in the operating room at the hands of a more experienced colleague. Invariably in the OR, the surgeon–teacher will be discussing steps and techniques to avoid complications and–even on a bad day–will be able to demonstrate in real life the intraoperative management of a complication.

Watching is easy in training–residencies automatically provide for it. What about us practitioners? We still have to make time–just like reading–to watch DVDs, online simulcasts, and other recorded modes. However, there is no substitute for buying a cheap plane ticket and showing up in the practice of a willing expert who fulfills his or her Hippocratic Oath by freely allowing us to observe his or her surgery and absorb their skills in preventing or handling complications.

Practice

Yes, we are in the "practice of medicine"; our seeing refractive surgical patients and doing refractive surgery each week allows us to remain "in practice." However, when addressing new surgical techniques, with the goal of avoiding complications, hands-on practice should precede actual surgical cases. Here, the secret weapon is the wet lab–most of them supported by industry.

■ (Insert three objections here.)

There are formal skills transfer labs that are set up at major ophthalmology meetings. There are wet labs given as part of industry-sponsored courses that introduce new technology. There are wet labs on the technical exhibit floor of meetings, in which one can make an appointment for some direct teaching by technical staff or other surgeons.

Such labs are expensive to setup and run and, of course, time-consuming for both instructors and us participants; they fill up, so seek them out, and register early. My encouragement: Take your time in the lab, stay for the duration of the lab, practice with the instruments and maneuvers as many times as possible to develop rhythm, and be the last person out of the room. This approach will create the difference between true skills transfer as opposed to mere familiarization, and will decrease complications in the operating room.

Teach

Do you really want to learn how to deal with complications of refractive surgery? Well then, participate in a teaching program, the most accessible being resident teaching programs. All residency programs are in dire need of talented, dedicated surgeon–teachers.

■ It takes way too much time to go to the hospital and the OR, especially since they are always running late."
■ "It is so repetitious; it's the same thing with every new resident."
■ "Some of the residents are so cocky; they just won't listen."
■ (Add your own excuse here.)

Almost all residents have complications when learning surgical procedures. As their teachers, we have the opportunity to minimize those complications, to instruct in the management when they occur, and to forestall the sadness and discouragement that inevitably accompany such problems by positive support. As we deal with the residents' complications, we increase our own skill in avoiding and managing them.

Mentoring budding ophthalmologists is not only emotionally satisfying, but also helps to fulfill our Hippocratic obligation to give back to our profession–a profession that provides a deep personal satisfaction as well as our livelihood.

Teaching in the practice labs mentioned above is another excellent place to refine pedagogical skills and to gain new insights about refractive surgery complications.

Write

I emphasized reading as a cornerstone of the lifelong education that diminishes one's complications in refractive surgery. Try the other side: Write. It is surprising how much we can learn by writing a simple case report of a complication.

- "I have never written anything. I don't know how."
- "I tried and submitted a paper, but it was trashed by the reviewers."
- "Researching those references…it's just impossible."
- (Add your own excuse here.)

It was not until I started writing about pseudo–diffuse lamellar keratitis (DLK)–that is, interface stromal edema after LASIK associated with elevated intraocular pressure–that I became aware of the very clear distinction between that entity and inflammatory, exotoxin-induced DLK. Had I not taken the time to write up the case report, I would not have delved deeply into that complication and would not have collaborated with colleagues in laboratory experiments that led to a full description of the three stages of the fluid interface syndrome (FIS).

To lighten the burden of manuscript preparation, approach an academic type who seems to turn out a paper a week, and propose a joint paper based upon your observations. In addition, there are professional writing services that can help organize the information that you have assembled and get it into good draft format for you to refine. Online reference services, such as PubMed (www.pubmed.gov) can assist with literature review, as can many medical libraries. Or take advantage of "free labor" and bring a medical student, resident, or fellow into your practice with the specific goal of writing a paper on a topic drawn from your experience, often describing complications.

OK, OK…all reviewers are ignorant slobs who have no understanding of what you are saying, and all journal editors are obstructionists whose one goal in life is preventing you from publishing your work. Nevertheless, relax for 48 h after you receive their comments, realize that they have some great insights, incorporate their critiques into your paper, and re-submit the revision. It is fun (!) and amazing how much we can learn in that process.

Participate

To stay on the front edge of ophthalmic development, participate in clinical trials. It is complex, bureaucratic, and expensive in terms of time and personnel, but terribly gratifying. It will also introduce new sets of complications that are unfamiliar, because the technology is new, and will make us as investigators much wiser in terms of complication prevention and management.

- "It's all political. I couldn't possibly break into the system."
- "My practice is so busy now. How could I add anything new?"
- "Let them figure it out. I'll use it when it's FDA approved."
- (Add your own excuse.)

The best way to start is to speak personally to those ophthalmologists who are active in clinical trials, and who are presenting at meetings. In addition, the local industry representative can be a good source of information and can open doors at companies that are seeking clinical investigators. Above all, we must be sure that our clinical staff is up to the job, because clinical trials are very demanding on them.

Serve

One of the best circumstances for learning about and managing complications is working in the developing world.

- "Where do you find such places?"
- "They want too much time, sometimes a whole week!"
- "I'm afraid. What if I screw up?"
- (Make up your own excuse.)

Serve as a volunteer in eye camps, mission hospitals, established centers, and planes and boats that go to different countries for teaching and service–there are myriad venues. Not only do we get a chance to see other surgeons working–and dealing with their own types of complications–but we are often called on to operate ourselves in unfamiliar circumstances, which will increase our complication rate and make us even more knowledgeable in complication management.

The Still Small Voice

At any level of education and experience, we refractive surgeons may find a sense of caution, an inkling that something is not right, a gentle nudge to change direction, a surge of anxiety, a still small voice that says, "Stop here and reassess." Surgeons in a hurry may suppress such a gentle inner urge and barrel forward into trouble. Some of us simply are not attuned to these internal reminders. Inexperienced surgeons may confuse their own trepidation during a procedure with this important sense of caution.

This sense may be as important in avoiding complications as any specific technical skill.

In the preoperative clinic, we all confront patients who give us a feeling that we should not operate on this person. They may have unrealistic expectations, be too much of a perfectionist, or have a work environment not conducive to refractive surgery. Recently, I was confronted by a hard-charging senior manager at the Center for Disease Control (CDC) who informed me of the exact date and time when she wanted her LASIK for near-sightedness and let me know of her terribly heavy travel schedule immediately thereafter. She was taken aback when I told her I would not operate on her, but seemed to acquiesce when I explained she was simply too much of a perfectionist and would not be satisfied with any outcome. Maybe that was not a still small voice, but a large shout. Nevertheless, I followed my intuition wisely.

Intraoperatively, a subtle hint that all is not right–a funny shift of the nucleus toward an unseen tear in the capsule, a strange movement of an intraocular lens forward in front of an unanticipated choroidal hemorrhage, the strange behavior of a floppy iris, or the wrestling match to get a microkeratome seated into the deep orbit of someone with "Cro-Magnon" facies–all are subtle warning to stop, reassess and proceed slowly, forestalling a complication.

Conclusion

In the face of the marvelous information presented by experts in this textbook, the educational principles I have enunciated may seem pedantic, unexciting, unnecessary, and certainly unsophisticated. Nevertheless, I think they are fundamental in helping us all avoid complications, by staying truly proficient in our practice of refractive surgery.

Subject Index

Erratum

© Springer-Verlag Berlin Heidelberg 2008
ISBN 978-3-540-37583-8
ISBN 978-3-540-37584-5 (eBook)

Management of Complications in Refractive Surgery
Jorge L. Alió · Dimitri T. Azar (Eds.)

Chapter 7.3 Decentration
Jonathan H. Talamo

Unfortunately the legend of Figure 7.3.4 on page 139 contained a typo, and the corrected version is given below.

Fig. 7.3.4 Corneal topography after ablation decentration and wavefront-guided retreatment. This patient complained of significant glare disability and monocular/ghosting due to temporal ablation decentration with respect to the pupil center seen on Orbscan testing after LASIK for approximately –5.00 D (a). UCVA was 20/40, and BCVA 20/25, with a manifest refraction of –.25 –.75 × 94. Wavefront analysis showed a profound degree of horizontal coma (b). Eight months after wavefront-guided custom retreatment, UCVA improved to 20/25 and 20/20, with manifest refraction using plano –0.50 × 80 and complete resolution of glare/ghosting symptoms. As expected, ablation centration as assessed by corneal topography also improved dramatically (c, upper right) when compared with preoperative topography (c, upper left). The preferential flattening achieved nasally by custom retreatment is depicted in the difference map (c, below center). Wavefront sensing showed reduction in horizontal coma of almost 50% (d)

The Figure 7.3.5 on page 139 is wrong. The correct figure is given below.

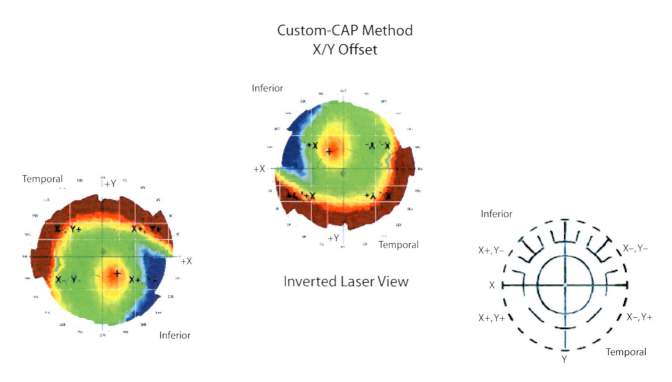

Fig. 7.3.5 Custom contoured ablation for irregular corneas. This picture depicts the ability of the VISX excimer laser system to program and precisely decenter topography-derived custom programmed photoablation (using C-CAP software) with respect to the pupil center after capture by an active eye tracking system. Intentional decentration allows application of a asymmetric ablations to improved corneal topographic symmetry

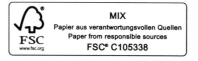

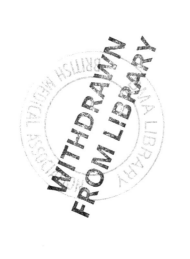